Surgery of the Cranio-Vertebral Junction

Enrico Tessitore • Amir R. Dehdashti
Claudio Schonauer • Claudius Thomé
Editors

Surgery of the Cranio-Vertebral Junction

Springer

Editors
Enrico Tessitore
Neurosurgical Unit
Geneva University Hospitals
Geneva
Switzerland

Amir R. Dehdashti
Department of Neurosurgery
North Shore University Hospitals
Manhasset, NY
USA

Claudio Schonauer
Neurosurgical Unit
ASL Napoli 2 Nord
Naples
Italy

Claudius Thomé
Department of Neurosurgery
Innsbruck University Hospitals
Innsbruck
Austria

ISBN 978-3-030-18699-9 ISBN 978-3-030-18700-2 (eBook)
https://doi.org/10.1007/978-3-030-18700-2

This Springer imprint is published by the registered company Springer Nature Switzerland AG
The registered company address is: Gewerbestrasse 11, 6330 Cham, Switzerland

Preface

This excellent and insightful book details abnormalities and treatments of the craniovertebral junction. It provides an overview of the human anatomy, with an emphasis on biomechanics, including the sagittal balance concept of surgical techniques. Even more so, it describes important perioperative considerations, such as the planning of surgical incisions, anesthesiological considerations, and types of preoperative and intraoperative image guidance.

In particular, the authors thoroughly explain surgery techniques per se. These include the traditional anterior, posterior, and posterolateral approaches, as well as innovative minimally invasive and endovascular approaches.

The last part of the book describes in detail how best to treat many of the wide variety of abnormalities that can afflict the craniovertebral junction. It examines both trauma and tumors, not only extra-axial tumors but also inflammatory tumors and foramen magnum tumors.

The authors close with a review of the vascular abnormalities that can afflict the craniovertebral junction and how best to treat them. Lastly, they discuss infectious metabolic diseases that can affect the craniovertebral junction.

This text is a comprehensive review of craniovertebral surgical techniques, anatomy, and abnormalities. The only aspect not covered is the embryological development of this area of the spine, but the authors do not purport to do so. Other authors have written tomes addressing the treatment of craniovertebral junction abnormalities. In this book, however, the authors describe techniques and provide added information gleaned from the surgical literature published during the past several years. These include the sagittal balance concept applied to the craniovertebral junction; innovative approaches, such as the far-lateral transventricular, the extreme lateral, and the anterolateral approaches; innovative techniques applied to neurosurgery techniques; and recent minimally invasive and endovascular approaches. Subsequently, it provides much information to the reader that can aid diagnosis and treatment considerations to address abnormalities of the craniovertebral junction in the modern arena.

This comprehensive textbook on the management of abnormalities that can present at the craniovertebral junction should be in the library of every surgeon who diagnoses and treats problems in this very complex area of the spine.

Phoenix, AZ, USA Volker K. H. Sonntag

Contents

Part I

Introduction

Relevant Anatomy of the Craniovertebral Junction

1

Elena d'Avella, Luigi Maria Cavallo, Matteo De Notaris, Jose Pineda, Alberto Di Somma, Paolo Cappabianca, and Alberto Prats-Galino

1.1 Introduction

Craniovertebral junction (CVJ) refers to the complex transition from the skull to the spine. Its bony structure consists of the occipital bone, atlas (C1), and axis (C2) (Fig 1.1) [1–3]. The occipital bone surrounds the foramen magnum and has three parts: a squamosal part located behind the foramen magnum, a clival portion located anterior to the foramen magnum, and a condylar part that connects the squamosal and clival parts. The atlas, the first cervical vertebra, is ring shaped and consists of two thick lateral masses situated at the anterolateral parts of the ring connected with short anterior and longer posterior arches. The upper facet of each lateral mass articulates with the occipital condyle that protrudes from the condylar part of the occipital bone (atlanto-occipital joints). The inferior facet of each lateral mass articulates with the superior articular facet of the axis. The axis, the second cervical vertebra, is distinguished by the odontoid process (dens), which projects upward from the body. On the front of the dens is an articular facet that forms a joint with the facet on the back of the anterior arch of the atlas. The body is connected to the lateral mass by short and strong pedicles. Articular facets of the axis extend lateral

E. d'Avella (✉) · L. M. Cavallo · P. Cappabianca
Division of Neurosurgery, Department of Neurosciences and Reproductive and Odontostomatological Sciences, Università di Napoli "Federico II", Naples, Italy

M. De Notaris
Neurosurgery Operative Unit, Department of Neurosciences, "G.Rummo" Hospital, Benevento, Italy

J. Pineda · A. Prats-Galino
Laboratory of Surgical NeuroAnatomy (LSNA), Human Anatomy and Embriology Unit, Faculty of Medicine, Universidad de Barcelona, Barcelona, Spain

A. Di Somma
Institut Clínic de Neurociències (ICN), Department of Neurological Surgery Hospital Clínic de Barcelona, Universidad de Barcelona, Barcelona, Spain

E. Tessitore et al. (eds.), *Surgery of the Cranio-Vertebral Junction*,
https://doi.org/10.1007/978-3-030-18700-2_1

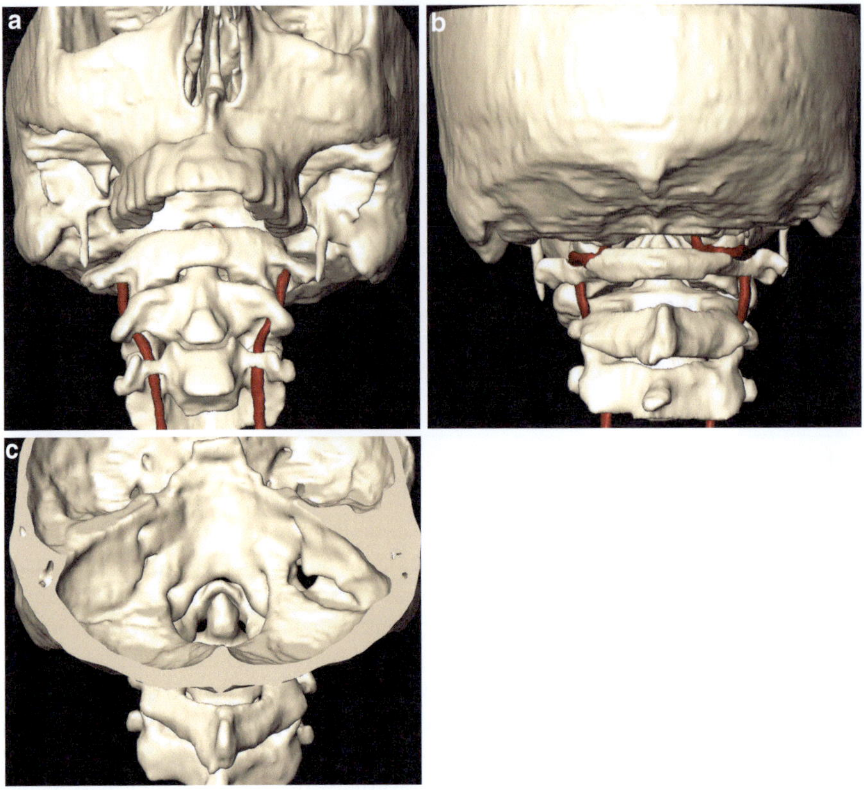

Fig. 1.1 3D anatomical model of the craniovertebral junction (CVJ). Its bony structure consisting in the occipital bone, atlas and axis is shown as seen from an anterior (**a**), posterior (**b**), and superior-posterior intracranial perspective (**c**). The extracranial course of the vertebral artery, which is the major vessel related to the CVJ, is represented

from the body and articulate superiorly with the inferior facets of the atlas [1–5]. Muscles, ligaments, and membranes that provide stability and mobility to the craniovertebral junction support the bony structure of this critical region [2, 5].

Major neurovascular structures are intimately related to the CVJ where they transverse membranous and bony orifices. These include the lower cranial and upper spinal nerves, the caudal brainstem and rostral spinal cord, the vertebral artery and its branches, and the venous drainages through the jugular vein and the vertebral plexus [1, 3, 6, 7]. Anatomy of the vertebral artery will be further detailed in a dedicated chapter.

A thorough understanding of three-dimensional (3D) CVJ anatomy and relations with surrounding neurovascular structures is paramount for the surgical management of pathologies in this region. The aim of this chapter is to describe the relevant anatomy of the CVJ as seen from a posteromedial, posterolateral, anterolateral and anteromedial perspectives. Anatomical dissection through the anteromedial corridor was carried out by an endoscopic endonasal access whereas posterior and lateral corridors were studied by microscopic vision.

Merging together anatomical information coming from endoscopic and microsurgical investigations with the reconstruction of 3D computed models might provide a 360° full and clear understanding of this complex area, more readily applicable to the operative setting.

1.2 Posteromedial Perspective of the CVJ (Fig. 1.2)

1.2.1 Bony Structures

The posteromedial perspective of the CVJ is focused on the squamosal part of the occipital bone bordering the foramen magnum and on the posterior arch of C1 and C2 (Fig. 1.3).

The posterior surface of the squamosal part of the occipital bone in its medial portion has some relevant protuberances on which muscles of the neck attach: the external occipital protuberance (EOP), situated at the central part of the external surface; the superior nuchal line (SNL) and the inferior nuchal lines (INL) that radiate laterally from the protuberance; the posterior border of foramen magnum (FM); and the midline occipital crest, a vertical ridge that descends from the EOP to the midpoint of the posterior margin of the foramen magnum. The area below and between the superior and inferior nuchal lines is rough and irregular and serves as the site of attachment of numerous muscles. There is great variability in the position of the superior nuchal line, and therefore, it does not reflect the internal position of

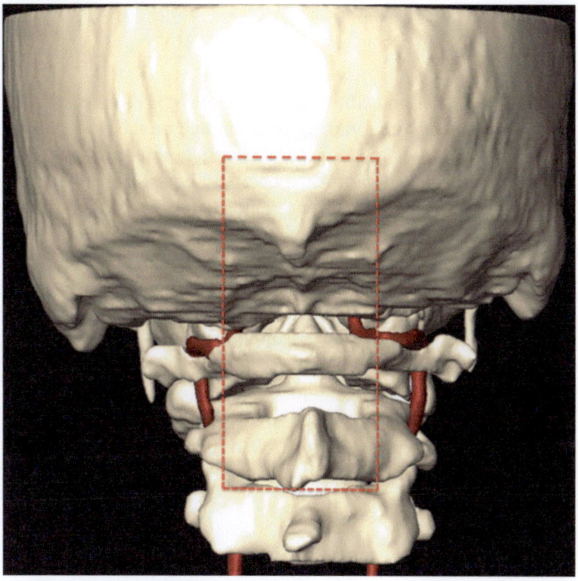

Fig. 1.2 3D anatomical model of the CVJ as seen from a posterior view. The area corresponding to the posteromedial perspective is highlighted with red dotted lines

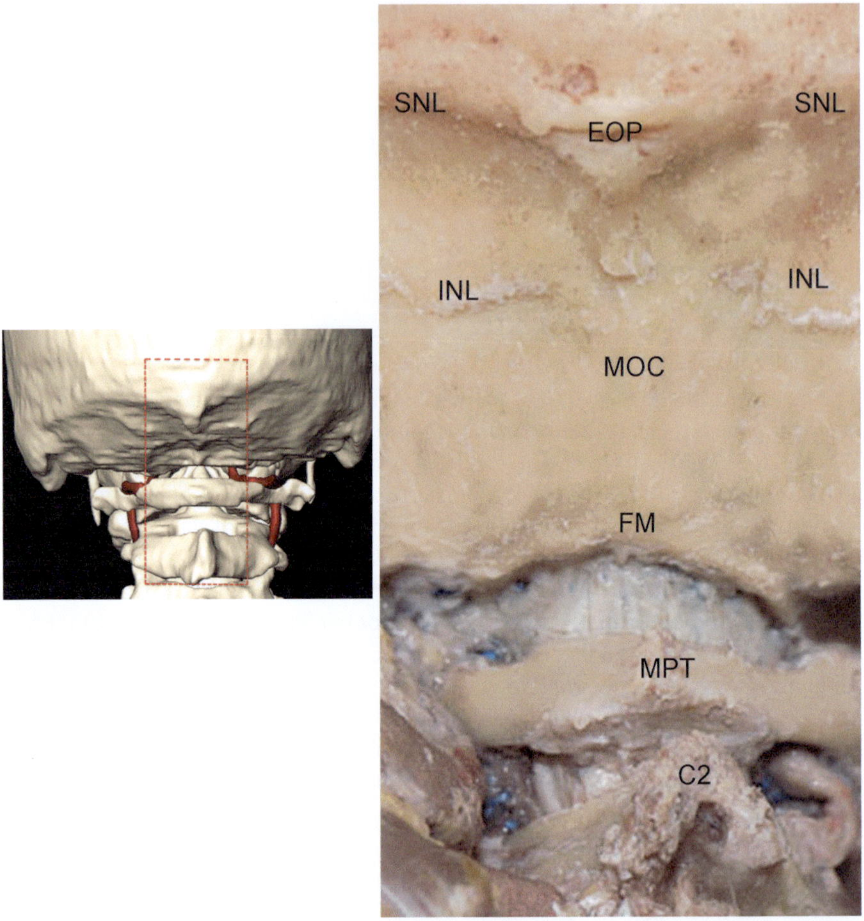

Fig. 1.3 The posteromedial perspective of the CVJ is focused on the squamosal part of the occipital bone bordering the foramen magnum and on the posterior arch of C1 and C2. On the left side of the image, the 3D model is for anatomical reference for the area of interest. The posterior surface of the squamosal part of the occipital bone in its medial portion has some relevant protuberances on which muscles of the neck attach: the external occipital protuberance; the superior nuchal line and the inferior nuchal lines; the posterior border of foramen magnum; the midline occipital crest. The area below and between the superior and inferior nuchal lines is rough and irregular and serves as the site of attachment of numerous muscles. On the posterior arch of the atlas is the median posterior tubercle, which substitutes the spinous process of any other vertebra. The posterior arch of the axis distinguishes by harboring the thickest lamina than on any other cervical vertebrae and a large spinous process serving as an attachment point of important suboccipital triangle muscles and the nuchal ligament. *C2* spinous process of the axis; *EOP* external occipital protuberance; *FM* posterior border of foramen magnum; *INL* inferior nuchal line; *MOC* midline occipital crest; *MPT* median posterior tubercle of the atlas; *SNL* superior nuchal line

transverse sinus accurately. The relation of confluence of the sagittal sinus with the transverse sinus (torcular Herophili) to EOP is more consistent [2, 4, 8].

On the posterior arch of the atlas is the median posterior tubercle, which substitutes the spinous process of any other vertebra. The posterior arch of the axis distinguishes by harboring the thickest lamina than on any other cervical vertebrae and a large spinous process serving as an attachment point of important suboccipital triangle muscles and the nuchal ligament [1, 5].

1.2.2 **Muscular Relationships** (Fig. 1.4)

The trapezius is the most superficial muscle that is encountered when exploring the CVJ through a posteromedial corridor. It extends from the medial half of the SNL, the EOP, and the spinous processes of the cervical and thoracic vertebrae and converges on the shoulder to attach to the scapula and the lateral third of the clavicle. In a deeper layer, the splenius capitis is exposed in its medial half running to the spinous processes of the lower cervical and upper thoracic vertebrae. Deep to the splenius capitis, the semispinalis capitis begins medially at the midline occipital crest in the area between the superior and inferior nuchal lines and attaches below to the upper thoracic and lower cervical vertebrae (Fig. 1.5) [4, 8, 9]. In the next layer, along the posteromedial corridor, the rectus capitis posterior minor can be seen extending from the medial part and below the inferior nuchal line to the tubercle of the posterior arch of the atlas (Fig. 1.6) [6, 10].

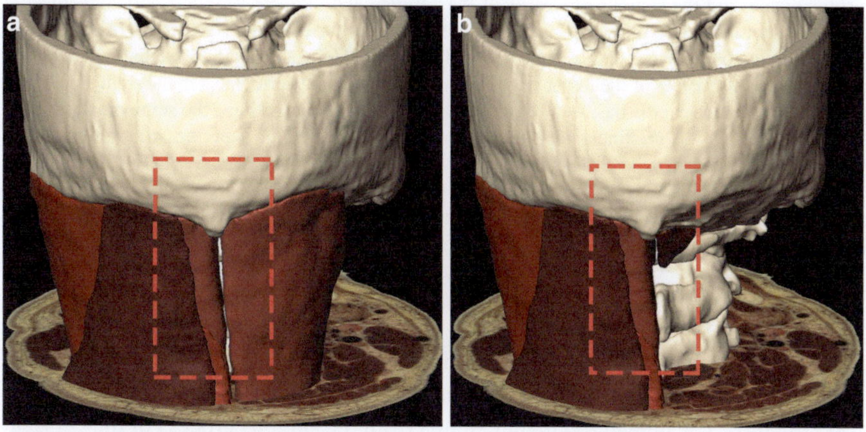

Fig. 1.4 3D model of the muscular layers visible through a posteromedial perspective to the CVJ. The anatomical area of interest is limited by the red dotted lines. The superficial layer (**a**) is represented by the trapezius muscle (dark brown), splenius capitis muscle (dark orange), and semispinalis capitis (light brown). On the right half of the picture, trapezius and splenius capitis muscles have been removed, revealing the semispinalis capitis muscle. The deep muscular layer (**b**) is represented by rectus capitis posterior minor muscles (dark brown), exposed after the removal of the superficial layer muscles on the left side of the picture

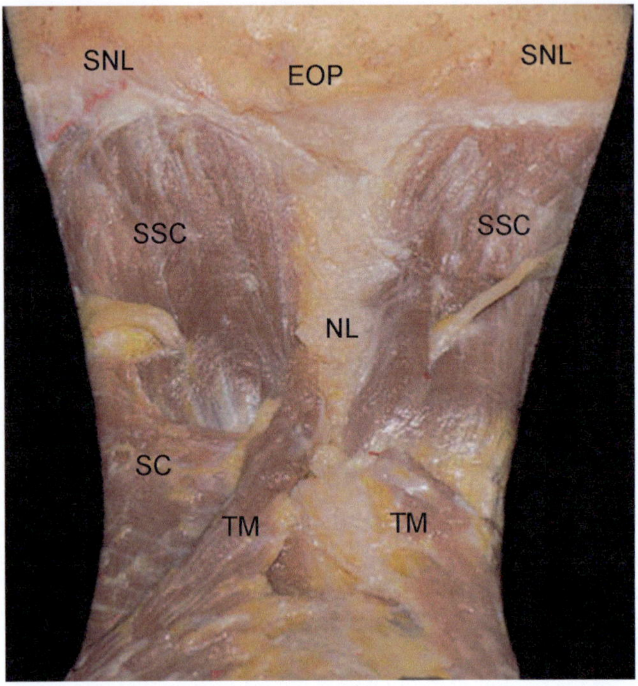

Fig. 1.5 Posteromedial perspective of the CVJ: muscular relationships. Trapezius is the most superficial muscle. It extends from the medial half of the superior nuchal line, the external occipital protuberance, and the spinous processes of the cervical and thoracic vertebrae and converges on the shoulder to attach to the scapula and the lateral third of the clavicle. Here, it has been partially resected in its rostral part to expose in a deeper layer the splenius capitis in its medial half, running to the spinous processes of the lower cervical and upper thoracic vertebrae. On the right side of the picture the splenius capitis has been resected. Deep to the splenius capitis, the semispinalis capitis begins medially at the midline occipital crest in the area between the superior and inferior nuchal lines and attaches below to the upper thoracic and lower cervical vertebrae. In the midline, the nuchal ligament forms a septation dividing the posterior neck muscles on the left and right sides. Moreover, some of these muscles attach medially to this structure. The nuchal ligament extends from the spinous process of the cervical vertebrae to the external occipital protuberance. *EOP* external occipital protuberance; *NL* nuchal ligament; *SC* splenius capitis; *SNL* superior nuchal line; *SSC* semispinalis capitis; *TM* trapezius muscle

In the midline, the nuchal ligament forms a septation dividing the posterior neck muscles on left and right sides. Moreover, some of these muscles attach medially to this structure. The nuchal ligament extends from the spinous process of the cervical vertebrae to the EOP [11].

1.2.3 Extradural Structures

The posterior border of the foramen magnum and the upper border of the posterior arch of the atlas are connected by the posterior atlanto-occipital membrane (PAOM)

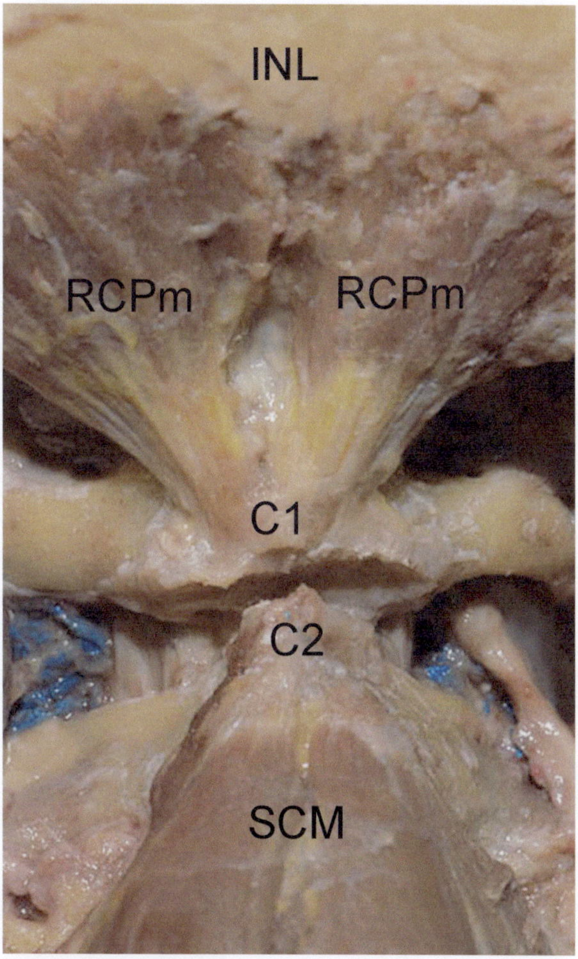

Fig. 1.6 Posteromedial perspective of the CVJ: muscular relationships. The deepest layer of muscle consists of the rectus capitis posterior minor muscles. The muscles extend from the medial part and below the inferior nuchal line to the tubercle on the posterior arch of the atlas. *C1* median posterior tubercle of the atlas; *C2* spinous process of the axis; *INL* inferior nuchal line; *RCPm* rectus capitis posterior minor muscle; *SCM* semispinalis cervicis muscle

that runs adjacent to the rectus capitis posterior minor posteriorly and the dura mater anteriorly. Connection or interdigitation of the PAOM with both the rectus capitis posterior minor muscles and the spinal dura mater can be observed. The PAOM is continuous inferiorly with a thin membrane named the posterior atlanto-axial membrane, which is attached above to the lower border of the posterior arch of the atlas and below to the upper edges of the laminae of the axis, in series with the ligamentum flavum [4, 12]. The posterior opening of the FM is wider posteriorly than anteriorly and transmits the medulla (Fig. 1.7).

The venous channels in the dura mater surrounding the foramen magnum in its posteromedial aspect are the marginal sinus and the occipital sinus. The marginal sinus is located between the layers of the dura in the rim of the foramen magnum. It communicates posteriorly with the occipital sinus. The occipital sinus courses in the cerebellar falx [9, 13].

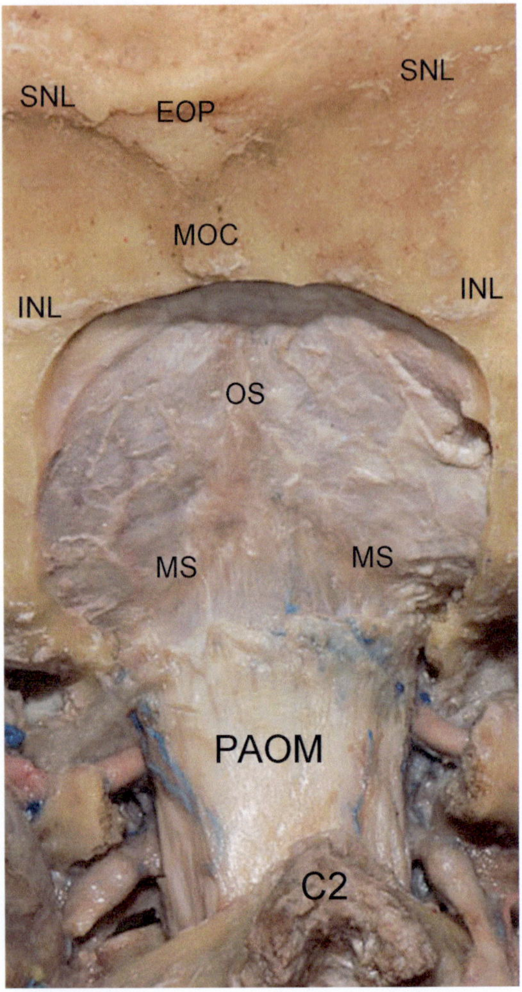

Fig. 1.7 Posteromedial perspective of the CVJ. The middle portion of the squamosal part of the occipital bone and the posterior arch of the atlas have been removed. The posterior border of the foramen magnum has been opened. The posterior border of the foramen magnum and the upper border of the posterior arch of the atlas are connected by the posterior atlanto-occipital membrane that runs adjacent to the rectus capitis posterior minor posteriorly and the dura mater anteriorly. The venous channels in the dura mater surrounding the foramen magnum in its posteromedial aspect are the marginal sinus and the occipital sinus. The marginal sinus is located between the layers of the dura in the rim of the foramen magnum. It communicates posteriorly with the occipital sinus. The occipital sinus courses in the cerebellar falx. *C2* spinous process of the axis; *EOP* external occipital protuberance; *INL* inferior nuchal line; *MOC* middle occipital crest; *MS* marginal sinus; *OS* occipital sinus; *PAOM* posterior atlanto-occipital membrane; *SNL* superior nuchal line

1.2.4 **Intradural Anatomy** (Fig. 1.8)

Through a posteromedial perspective, the medulla can be exposed, occupying the foramen magnum. The medulla blends indistinguishably into the spinal cord at a level arbitrarily set to be at the upper limit of the dorsal and ventral rootlets forming the first cervical nerve. Posteromedially, the spinal cord is divided by the posteromedian sulcus into symmetrical halves. Each half is occupied by the posterior funiculus. At the upper cervical level, the surface of the posterior funiculus is divided by another shallow longitudinal furrow, the posterior intermediate sulcus, into the fasciculus gracilis medially and the fasciculus cuneatus laterally. Superiorly, the posterior surface of the medulla is composed in the midline of the inferior half of the fourth ventricle and laterally by the inferior cerebellar peduncles. Inferiorly the posterior surface is composed of the gracile fasciculus and tubercle medially, and the cuneate fasciculus and tubercle laterally [2, 8, 14].

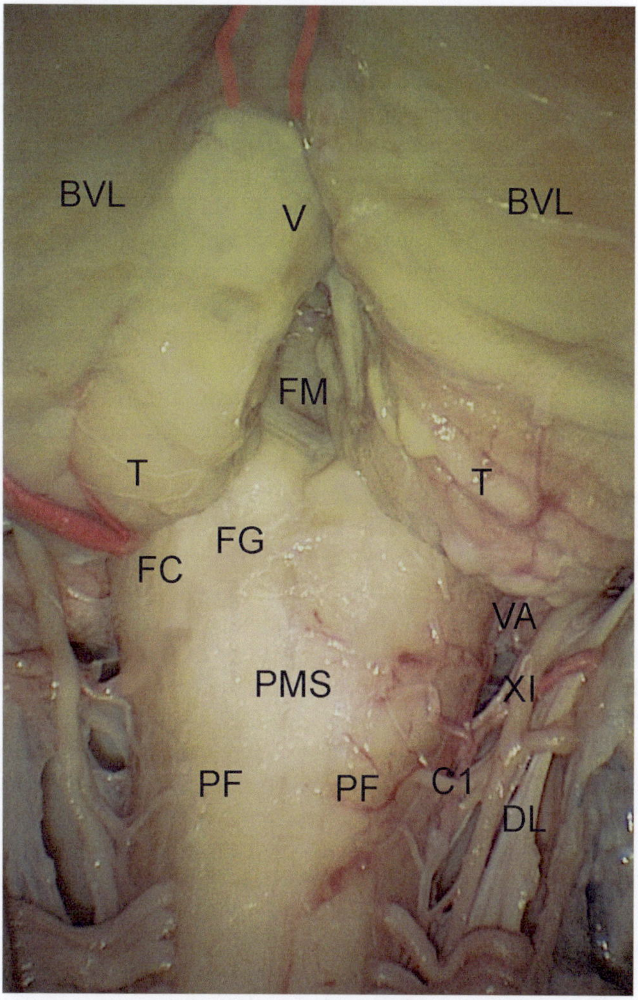

Fig. 1.8 Posteromedial intradural perspective of the CVJ. The medulla is exposed where it blends indistinguishably into the spinal cord at a level arbitrarily set to be at the upper limit of the dorsal and ventral rootlets forming the first cervical nerve. The spinal cord is divided by the posteromedian sulcus into symmetrical halves. Each half is occupied by the posterior funiculus. At the upper cervical level, the surface of the posterior funiculus is divided by another shallow longitudinal furrow, the posterior intermediate sulcus, into the fasciculus gracilis medially and the fasciculus cuneatus laterally. The posteromedial aspect of the cerebellum related to the foramen magnum consists in the lower part of the hemispheres (formed by the tonsils and the biventral lobules) and the lower part of the vermis (formed by the nodule, uvula, and pyramid). Between the tonsils, the foramen of Magendie communicates with the fourth ventricle. The vertebral artery in its third segment (V3) pierces the posterior atlanto-occipital membrane, then dura mater, to enter the posterior fossa. As the artery pierces the dura, it is encased in a fibrous tunnel that binds the posterior spinal artery, dentate ligament, first cervical nerve, and the spinal accessory nerve to the vertebral artery. The C1 nerve root passes through the dura mater on the lower surface of the vertebral artery. The accessory nerve is the only cranial nerve that passes through the foramen magnum, between the dentate ligament and the dorsal spinal roots. *BVL* biventral lobule of the cerebellar hemisphere; *C1* dorsal root of the first cervical nerve; *DL* dentate ligament; *FC* fasciculus cuneatus; *FG* fasciculus gracilis; *FM* foramen of Magendie; *PF* posterior funiculus; *PMS* posteromedial sulcus; *T* tonsil; *V* vermis; *VA* vertebral artery; *XI* accessory nerve

The posteromedial aspect of the cerebellum related to the foramen magnum consists in the lower part of the hemispheres (formed by the tonsils and the biventral lobules) and the lower part of the vermis (formed by the nodule, uvula, and pyramid). The cerebellar surface above the posterior part of the foramen magnum has a deep vertical depression, the posterior cerebellar incisura, which contains the falx cerebelli and extends inferiorly toward the foramen magnum. The vermis is folded into and forms the cortical surface within this incisura. The vermian surface within the incisura is composed of the pyramid in its upper half and of the uvula that projects downward between the tonsils. Inferiorly, the posterior cerebellar incisura is continuous with the vallecula cerebelli, an opening between the tonsils that extends upward through the foramen of Magendie into the fourth ventricle. Each tonsil is an ovoid structure that is attached along its superolateral border to the remainder of the cerebellum. The superior pole faces the inferior half of the roof of the fourth ventricle. The anterior surface of each tonsil faces and is separated from the posterior surface of the medulla by the cerebello-medullary fissure. This fissure extends superiorly to the level of the roof of the fourth ventricle and the lateral recesses of the fourth ventricle. The dorsal wall of the fissure is formed by the uvula in the midline and the tonsils and biventral lobules laterally. The ventral wall is formed by the inferior medullary velum and tela choroidea. The inferior medullary velum is a thin sheet of neural tissue that blends into the ventricular surface of the nodule medially and stretches laterally across the superior pole of the tonsil. The tela choroidea, from which the choroid plexus projects, forms the lowest part of the roof of the fourth ventricle [4, 5, 14, 15].

The vertebral artery in its third segment (V3) pierces the PAOM, then dura mater, to enter the posterior fossa. As the artery pierces the dura, it is encased in a fibrous tunnel that binds the posterior spinal artery, dentate ligament, first cervical nerve, and the spinal accessory nerve to it. The C1 nerve root passes through the dura mater on the lower surface of the vertebral artery. The posterior spinal artery arises from the posteromedial surface of V3 initial just outside or inside the dura mater. In the subarachnoid space, it courses medially between the accessory nerve and the dentate ligament. At the lower medulla, it divides into an ascending branch that supplies the gracile and cuneate tubercles, the rootlets of the accessory nerve, and the choroid plexus near the foramen of Magendie, and a descending branch that supplies the superficial part of the dorsal half of the cervical spinal cord. It anastomoses with the posterior branches of the radicular arteries that enter the vertebral foramen at lower levels. The descending branch gives rise to collateral branches, which course medially across the posterior surface of the spinal cord and join to form an artery that course in the posterior midline [2, 16, 17].

The posterior meningeal artery arises from the posterosuperior surface of the vertebral artery. Its origin may be intra- or extradural and supplies the dura mater of the posterior and posterolateral part of the posterior cranial fossa [4, 17].

The median posterior spinal vein, which courses along the posteromedian spinal sulcus, is continuous above with the main vein on the posterior surface of the medulla and the median posterior medullary vein, which courses along the posteromedian medullary sulcus. The transverse medullary and transverse spinal veins cross the medulla and spinal cord at various levels, interconnecting the major longitudinal channels [3, 5, 14].

The accessory nerve is the only cranial nerve that passes through the foramen magnum between the dentate ligament and the dorsal spinal roots. The main caudal trunk from the spinal cord is exposed through a posteromedial perspective. There are frequently communications between the C1 nerve root and the spinal accessory nerve [18, 19].

The dentate ligament is a white fibrous sheet that is attached to the spinal cord medially and to the dura mater laterally. Its rostral attachment is at the level of the foramen magnum where the vertebral artery pierces the dura. The ligament courses behind the accessory nerve at that level [4, 14].

1.3 Posterolateral Perspective of the CVJ (Fig. 1.9)

1.3.1 Bony Structures

The posterolateral perspective of the CVJ is directed at the condylar part of the occipital bone and lateral masses of atlas and axis (Fig. 1.10).

On the posterolateral external surface of the squamosal part of the occipital bone that extends from the EOP to the mastoid process of the temporal bone, an important bony landmark is the asterion. The asterion is located at the junction of the lambdoid, occipito-mastoid, and parieto-mastoid sutures and is commonly related to the lower half of the junction of the transverse and sigmoid sinuses. The superior and inferior nucal lines cross the posterolateral external surface of the occipital bone radiating laterally from the EOP and serves as the site of attachment of numerous muscles [2, 6].

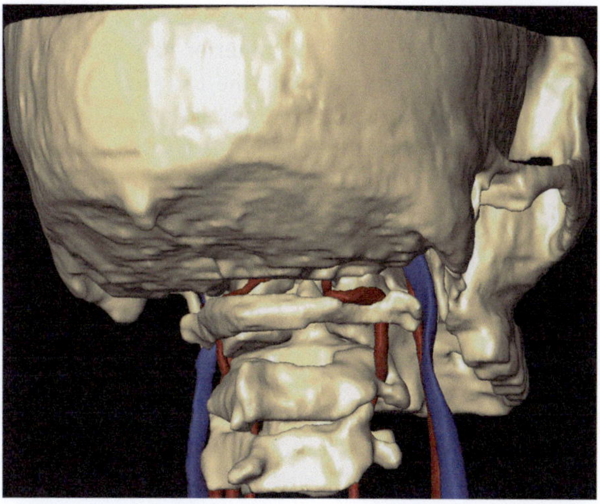

Fig. 1.9 3D anatomical model of the CVJ as seen from a posterolateral perspective. Bony relationships with the main arterovenous structures are shown, i.e., with the vertebral artery, internal jugular vein, and internal carotid artery

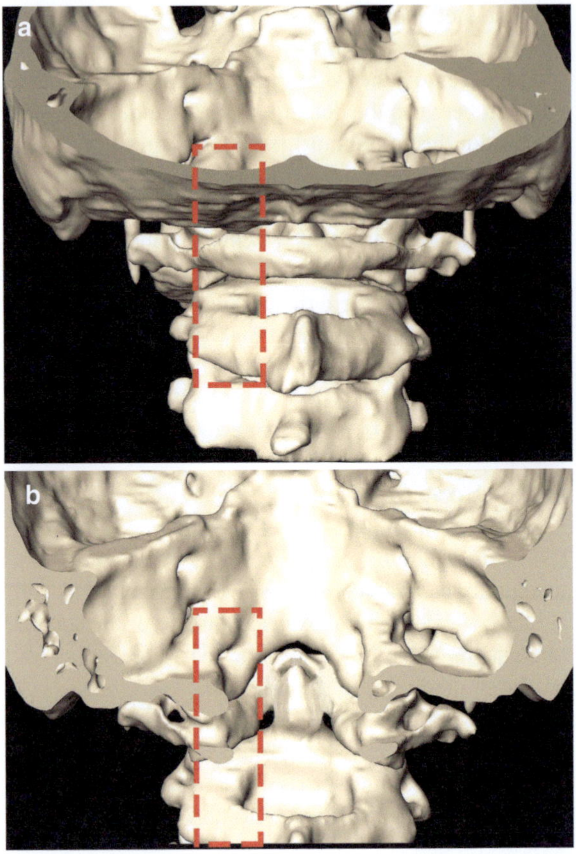

Fig. 1.10 3D anatomical model showing the CVJ bony structures focused by a posterolateral perspective on the extracranial surface (**a**) and on the intracranial surface after removal of the squamous part of the occipital bone and posterior arch of C1. (**b**) The condylar part of the occipital bone and lateral masses of atlas and axis are enclosed in a red dotted rectangular area

The condylar part of the occipital bone includes the occipital condyles and the condylar fossa, and it is situated at the sides of the foramen magnum. The occipital condyles protrude from the external surface of this part. They project downward along the lateral edges of the anterior half of the foramen magnum. The articular surfaces, which are ovoid with the long axis in the anteroposterior direction, are located on the lower-lateral margin of the condyles. They face downward and laterally to articulate with the superior facets of the atlas, which face upward and medially. The condylar fossa is a depression on the external surface of the occipital bone behind the condyle [20, 21].

Lateral masses are the most voluminous bony parts of atlas forming four facet joints. The upper surface of each lateral mass has an oval concave facet that faces upward and medially and articulates with the occipital condyle that faces downward and laterally. The inferior surface of each lateral mass has a circular, flat, or slightly concave facet that faces downward, medially, and slightly backward, and it articulates with the superior articular facet of the axis. The lateral mass of the atlas on its upper-outer surface has a groove in which the V3 segment of the vertebral artery courses. The groove may be partly or fully converted into a foramen by a bridge of bone that arches backward from the posterior edge of the superior articular facet of the atlas to its posterior arch. The medial aspect of each lateral mass has a small tubercle for the attachment of the transverse ligament of the atlas [1, 5, 22, 23].

Each lateral mass of the axis consists of a pair of large oval facets that extend laterally from the vertebral body onto the adjoining parts of the pedicles and articulate with the inferior facets of the atlas superiorly and the superior facet of the third cervical vertebra inferiorly. The superior facets do not form an articular pillar with the inferior facets but are anterior to the latter [5, 20, 23].

1.3.2 Muscular Relationships

The most superficial layer of muscles of the CVJ that is encountered through a posterolateral perspective is formed by the sternocleidomastoid that passes obliquely downward across the side of the neck from the lateral half of the superior nuchal line and mastoid process to the upper part of the sternum and the adjacent part of the clavicle. The splenius capitis in its lateral half is partially covered by the sternocleidomastoid. It extends from the lateral third of the superior nuchal line medially to the spinous processes of the lower cervical and upper thoracic vertebrae. Deep to the splenius capitis and sternocleidomastoid are the semispinalis capitis beginning medially at the midline occipital crest and extending laterally to the occipitomastoid junction in the area between the superior and inferior nuchal lines and the longissimus capitis muscle, which attaches above to the posterior margin of the mastoid process. Both of these muscles attach below to the upper thoracic and lower cervical vertebrae (Fig. 1.11) [4, 22, 24].

The occipital artery is also exposed together with the superficial and deep muscles in this region. It courses medially related to the longissimus capitis and semispinalis capitis just below the superior nuchal line to ascend in the superficial fascia of the posterior scalp. The great occipital nerve ascends with the occipital artery and supplies the scalp as far forward as the vertex and occasionally the back of the ear. It ascends obliquely between the inferior oblique and the semispinalis capitis muscles and pierces the latter and the trapezius muscle near their attachments to the occipital bone [17, 25].

In the next layer, the muscles bounding the suboccipital triangle are covered by the semispinalis capitis medially and by the splenius capitis laterally (Figs. 1.12 and 1.13). The superior oblique muscle extends from the area lateral to the semispinalis capitis between the superior and inferior nuchal lines to the transverse process of the atlas. The inferior oblique muscle extends from the spinous process of the axis to the transverse process of the atlas. The rectus capitis posterior major extends from and below the lateral part of the inferior nuchal line to the spine of the axis. The triangle deep to these muscles is covered by a layer of dense fibro-fatty tissue. The structures in the triangle are the V3 segment of the vertebral artery on the posterior arch of the atlas and the first cervical nerve [10, 17, 22, 25].

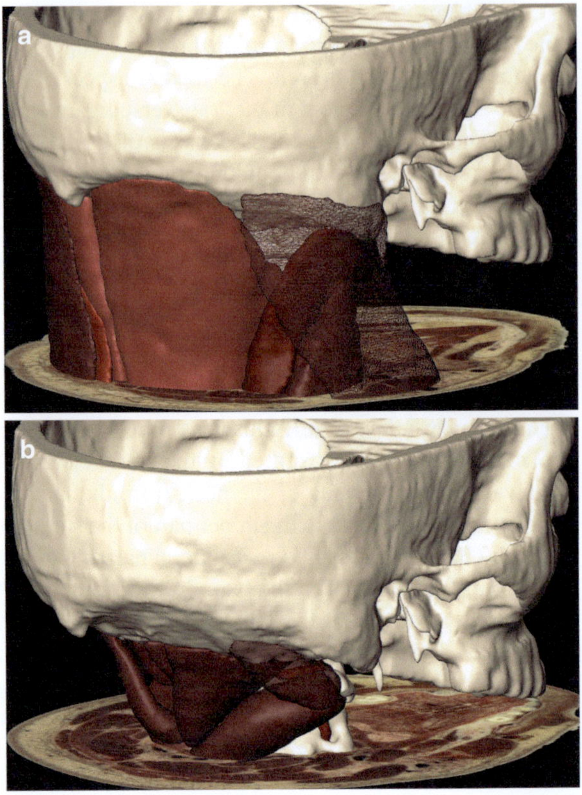

Fig. 1.11 Muscular structures visualized through a posterolateral perspective of the CVJ are represented in a 3D anatomical model. The superficial layer (**a**) with the transparent sternocleidomastoid and the muscles bounding the suboccipital triangle (**b**) are reconstructed

1.3.3 Extradural Structures

Through a posterolateral perspective, the segment of the vertebral artery extending from the transverse foramen of C2 to its entrance to the dura is exposed (V3). The artery, after ascending through the transverse process of the atlas, is located on the medial side of the rectus capitis lateralis muscle. From here it turns medially behind the lateral mass of the atlas and the atlanto-occipital joint and is pressed into the groove on the upper surface of the posterior arch of the atlas, where it courses in the floor of the suboccipital triangle. The triangle is not always easy to identify because of the thick fascia, which covers the deepest layer of the posterior neck muscles. This fascia and the underlying fat and the rich paravertebral venous plexus obscure the anatomical relationship of these muscles (Figs. 1.14 and 1.15) [17, 23].

At the level of the intervertebral foramen dorsal and ventral cervical nerves, roots unite to form the spinal nerve. At the same level, the neurons of the dorsal roots collect to form ganglia. The ganglion associated at the first cervical dorsal root may be absent. The C1, C2, and C3 nerves, distal to the ganglion, divide into dorsal and ventral rami. The dorsal rami divide into medial and lateral branches that supply the skin and muscles of the posterior region of the neck. The C1 nerve, termed the suboccipital nerve, leaves the vertebral canal between the occipital

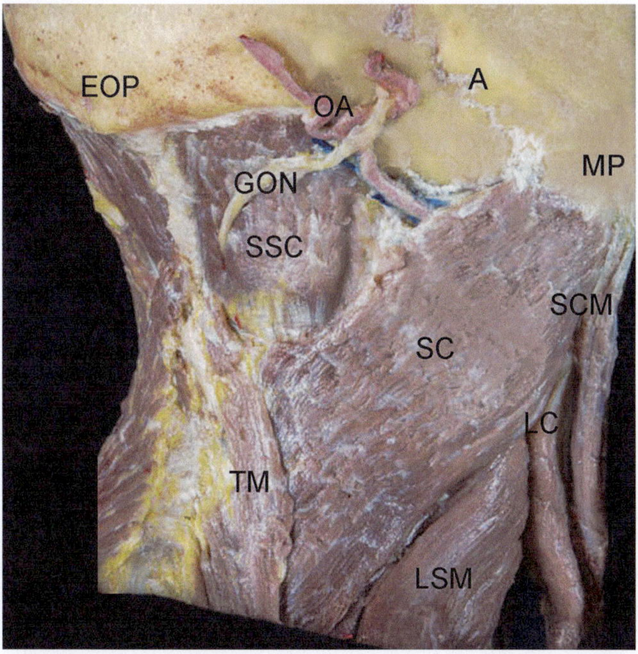

Fig. 1.12 The posterolateral perspective of the CVJ: muscular relationships. The most superficial layer of muscles is formed by the sternocleidomastoid that passes obliquely downward across the side of the neck from the lateral half of the superior nuchal line and mastoid process to the upper part of the sternum and the adjacent part of the clavicle. The splenius capitis in its lateral half is partially covered by the sternocleidomastoid. It extends from the lateral third of the superior nuchal line medially to the spinous processes of the lower cervical and upper thoracic vertebrae. Deep to the splenius capitis and sternocleidomastoid are the semispinalis capitis beginning medially at the midline occipital crest and extending laterally to the occipito-mastoid junction in the area between the superior and inferior nuchal lines, and the longissimus capitis muscle, which attaches above to the posterior margin of the mastoid process. Both of these muscles attach below to the upper thoracic and lower cervical vertebrae. The occipital artery is also exposed together with the superficial and deep muscles in this region. It courses medially related to the longissimus capitis and semispinalis capitis just below the superior nuchal line to ascend in the superficial fascia of the posterior scalp. The great occipital nerve ascends with the occipital artery and supplies the scalp as far forward as the vertex and occasionally the back of the ear. It ascends obliquely between the inferior oblique and the semisplenius capitis muscles and pierces the latter and the trapezius muscle near their attachments to the occipital bone. *A* asterion; *EOP* external occipital protuberance; *GON* great occipital nerve; *LC* longissimus capitis muscle; *LSM* levator scapulae muscle; *MP* mastoid process; *OA* occipital artery; *SC* splenius capitis; *SCM* sternocleidomastoid muscle, partially removed; *SSC* semispinalis capitis; *TM* trapezius muscle

bone and atlas and has a dorsal ramus that is larger than the ventral ramus. The dorsal ramus courses between the posterior arch of the atlas and the vertebral artery to reach the suboccipital triangle, where it sends branches to the rectus capitis posterior major and minor, superior and inferior oblique, and the semispinalis capitis, and occasionally has a cutaneous branch that accompanies the occipital artery to the scalp. The C1 ventral ramus courses between the posterior arch of the

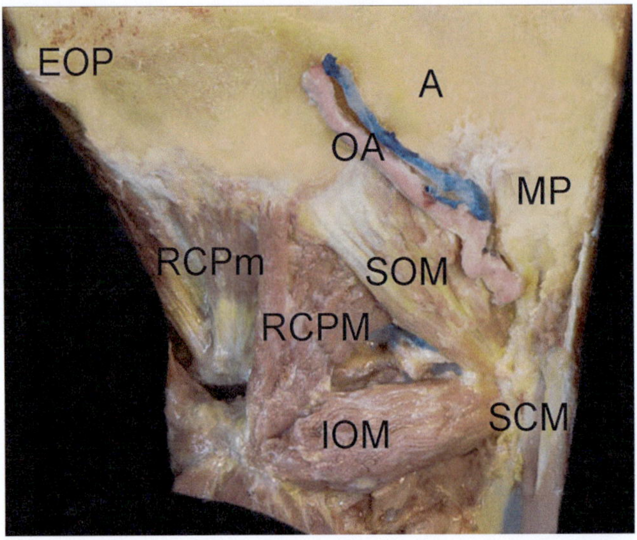

Fig. 1.13 The posterolateral perspective of the CVJ: muscular relationships. The muscles bounding the suboccipital triangle are exposed. The superior oblique muscle extends between the superior and inferior nuchal lines to the transverse process of the atlas. The inferior oblique muscle extends from the spinous process of the axis to the transverse process of the atlas. The rectus capitis posterior major extends from and below the lateral part of the inferior nuchal line to the spine of the axis. The triangle deep to these muscles is covered by a layer of dense fibrofatty tissue. The structures in the triangle are the V3 segment of the vertebral artery on the posterior arch of the atlas and the first cervical nerve. *A* asterion; *EOP* external occipital protuberance; *IOM* inferior oblique muscle; *MP* mastoid process; *OA* occipital artery; *RCPM* rectus capitis posterior major muscle; *RCPm* rectus capitis posterior minor muscle; *SCM* sternocleidomastoid muscle; *SOM* superior oblique muscle

atlas and the vertebral artery and passes forward, lateral to the lateral mass of the atlas and medial to the vertebral artery, and supplies the rectus capitis lateralis. The C2 nerve emerges between the posterior arch of the atlas and the lamina of the axis where the spinal ganglion is located extradurally, medial to the inferior facet of C1 and the vertebral artery. Distal to the ganglion, the nerve divides into a larger dorsal and a smaller ventral ramus. After passing below and supplying the inferior oblique muscle, the dorsal ramus divides into a large medial and a small lateral branch. The medial branch forms the greater occipital nerve. The lateral branch sends filaments that innervate the splenius, longissimus, and semisplenius capitis and is often joined by the corresponding branch from the C3 nerve. The C2 ventral ramus courses between the vertebral arches and transverse processes of the atlas and axis and behind the vertebral artery. Two branches of the C2 and C3 ventral rami, the lesser occipital and greater auricular nerves, curve around the posterior border and ascend on the sternocleidomastoid muscle to supply the skin behind the ear [1, 2, 6, 24].

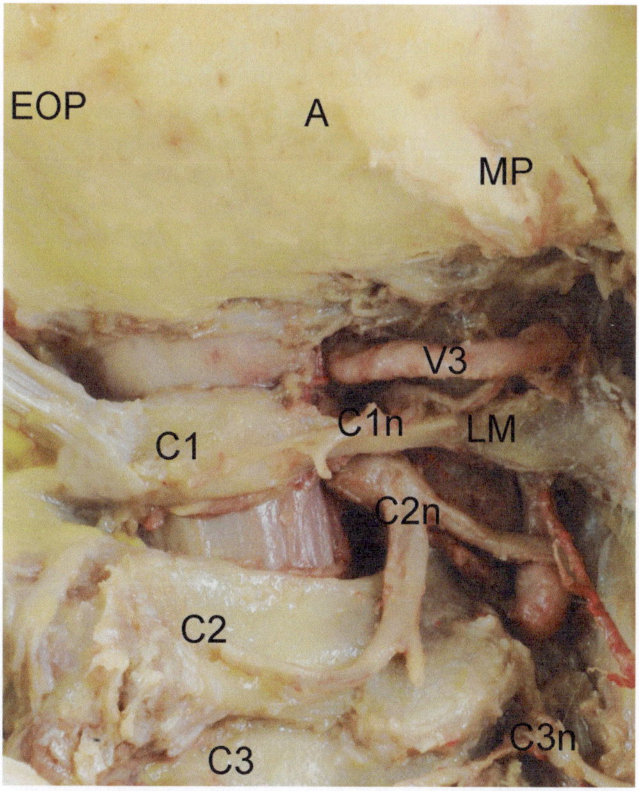

Fig. 1.14 The posterolateral perspective of the CVJ is directed at the external surface of the squamosal part of the occipital bone that extends from the EOP to the mastoid process of the temporal bone. On this surface, an important bony landmark is the asterion, located at the junction of the lambdoid, occipito-mastoid, and parieto-mastoid sutures. The asterion is commonly related to the lower half of the junction of the transverse and sigmoid sinuses. The lateral mass of the atlas on its upper-outer surface has a groove in which the V3 segment of the vertebral artery courses. The groove may be partly or fully converted into a foramen by a bridge of bone that arches backward from the posterior edge of the superior articular facet of the atlas to its posterior arch. *A* asterion; *C1* atlas; *C1n* suboccipital nerve; *C2* axis; *C2n* second cervical nerve; *C3* third cervical vertebra; *C3n* third cervical nerve; *EOP* external occipital protuberance; *LM* lateral mass of the atlas; *MP* mastoid process; *V3* third segment of the vertebral artery

The condylar foramen is present in the condylar fossa posterior to the occipital condyle. It transmits the posterior condylar vein, which is an important emissary vein of the cranium. This vein connects the vertebral venous plexus with the sigmoid-jugular complex. The condylar foramen is one of the largest emissary foramina of the skull and the posterior condylar vein, which traverses it, forms an important alternative source of venous drainage when the venous flow into the sigmoid sinus-jugular complex is impeded [22, 23, 25].

The hypoglossal canal (HC), which transmits the hypoglossal nerve, is situated above the condyle and is directed forward and laterally from the posterior cranial fossa. The canal is surrounded superiorly by the jugular tubercle, supero-laterally by the jugular foramen, laterally by the sigmoid sinus, and inferiorly by the occipital condyle. The intracranial end of the HC is located approximately 5 mm above the junction of the posterior and middle third of the occipital condyle and appropriately 5 mm below the jugular tubercle. The extracranial end is located immediately above the junction of the anterior and middle third of the occipital condyle and medial to the jugular foramen. The HC is surrounded by cortical bone. It consists of the hypoglossal nerve, a meningeal branch of the ascending pharyngeal artery, and the venous plexus of the hypoglossal canal, which communicates the basilar venous plexus with the marginal sinus that encircles the foramen magnum. The hypoglossal nerve enters the canal as two groups of roots that merge just before exiting the canal (Fig. 1.16) [6, 26, 27].

The sigmoid sinus borders the posterior cranial fossa laterally and descends along the sigmoid groove. It exits the cranium through the sigmoid part of the jugular foramen and descends anterolateral to the occipital condyle and anterior to the transverse process of the atlas [8, 13, 23].

Fig. 1.15 Posterolateral perspective of the CVJ. The squamosal part of occipital bone in its posterolateral aspect, from the external occipital protuberance to the asterion and mastoid process, has been removed. The posterior border of the foramen magnum has been opened and the posterior arch of C1 removed. The dura mater covering the cerebellar hemisphere in the posterior cranial fossa is exposed. The sigmoid sinus borders the posterior cranial fossa laterally and descends along the sigmoid groove. It exits the cranium through the sigmoid part of the jugular foramen and descends anterolateral to the occipital condyle and anterior to the transverse process of the atlas. The condylar part of the occipital bone is situated at the sides of the foramen magnum and includes the occipital condyles and the condylar fossa. The condylar fossa is a depression on the external surface of the occipital bone behind the condyle. The occipital condyles, which articulate with the atlas, protrude from the external surface of this part. The articular surfaces are located on the lower-lateral margin of the condyles. They face downward and laterally to articulate with the superior facets of the atlas, which face upward and medially. Lateral masses are the most voluminous bony parts of atlas forming four facet joints. The upper surface of each lateral mass articulates with the occipital condyle. The inferior surface articulates with the superior articular facet of the axis. At the level of the intervertebral foramen dorsal and ventral cervical nerves roots unite to form the spinal nerve. At the same level, the neurons of the dorsal roots collect to form ganglia. The ganglion associated at the first cervical dorsal root may be absent. The C1 nerve, termed the suboccipital nerve, leaves the vertebral canal between the occipital bone and atlas and has a dorsal ramus that is larger than the ventral ramus. The C2 nerve emerges between the posterior arch of the atlas and the lamina of the axis where the spinal ganglion is located extradurally, medial to the inferior facet of C1 and the vertebral artery. Distal to the ganglion, the nerve divides into a larger dorsal and a smaller ventral ramus. *A* asterion; *C1n* suboccipital nerve; *C2* spinous process of the axis; *C2n* second cervical nerve; *CF* condylar fossa; *CHd* dura mater covering the cerebellar hemisphere; *EOP* external occipital protuberance; *IJV* internal jugular vein; *JP* jugular process; *OC* occipital condyle; *PAOM* posterior atlanto-occipital membrane; *SS* sigmoid sinus; *V2* second segment of the vertebral artery; *V3* third segment of the vertebral artery

1.3.4 Intradural Structures

The posterolateral perspective at the CVJ allows for intradural exposure of the cerebello-medullary cistern and posterior spinal cistern. The cerebello-medullary cistern extends from the dorsal margin of the inferior olive around the dorsolateral medulla to the biventral lobule of the cerebellum. The glossopharyngeal (IX) and vagal nerves (X) and the medullary portion of the accessory nerve (XI) arise within and course through this cistern to reach the jugular foramen (Fig. 1.17). The intradural segment of the vertebral artery (V4) can be divided into a lateral medullary

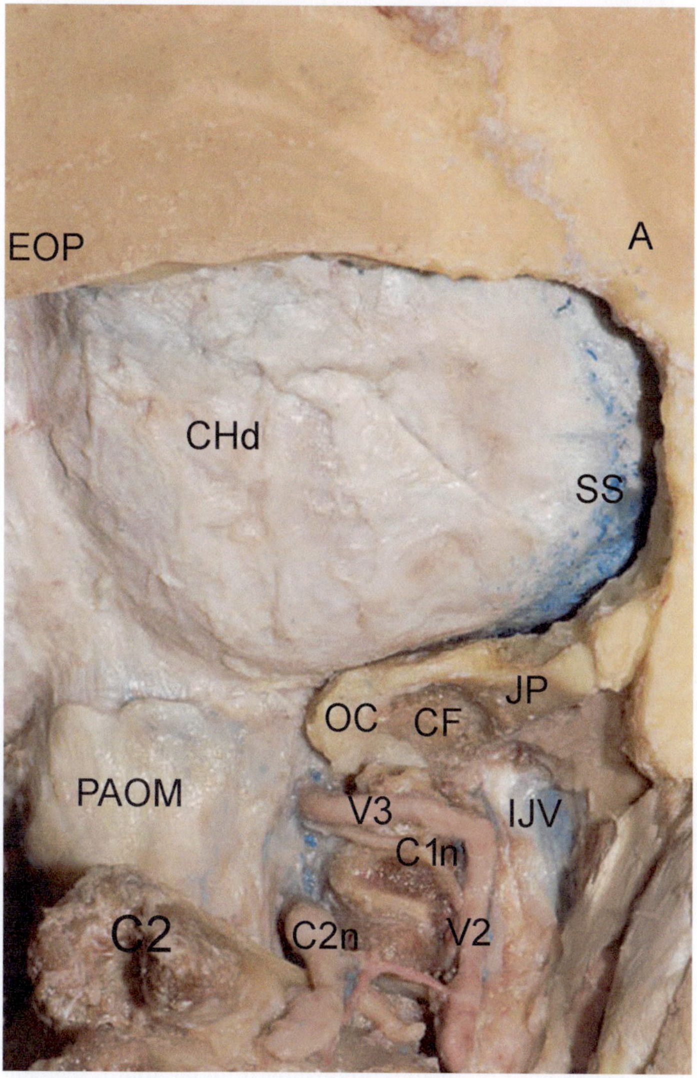

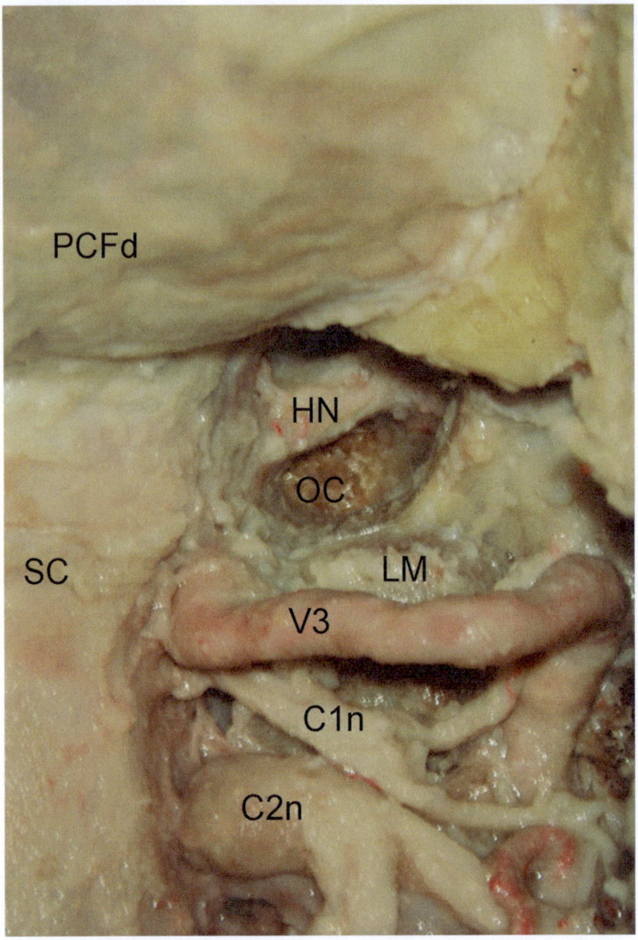

Fig. 1.16 Posterolateral perspective of the CVJ. The hypoglossal nerve is exposed after the opening of the hypoglossal canal. The hypoglossal canal is situated above the condyle and is directed forward and laterally from the posterior cranial fossa. The canal is surrounded superiorly by the jugular tubercle, supero-laterally by the jugular foramen, laterally by the sigmoid sinus, and inferiorly by the occipital condyle. The intracranial end of the hypoglossal canal is located approximately 5 mm above the junction of the posterior and middle third of the occipital condyle and appropriately 5 mm below the jugular tubercle. The extracranial end of the hypoglossal canal is located immediately above the junction of the anterior and middle third of the occipital condyle and medial to the jugular foramen. The hypoglossal canal is surrounded by the cortical bone. *C1n* first cervical nerve; *C2n* second cervical nerve; *HN* hypoglossal nerve; *LM* lateral mass of the atlas; *OC* occipital condyle; *PCFd* dura of the posterior cranial fossa; *SC* spinal cord; *V3* third segment of the vertebral artery

segment and an anterior medullary segment. The V4 lateral medullary segment begins at the dural foramen and passes anterior and superior along the lateral medullary surface to terminate at the pre-olivary sulcus. The posterior inferior cerebellar artery (PICA) enters this cistern after originating from the fourth segment (V4) of

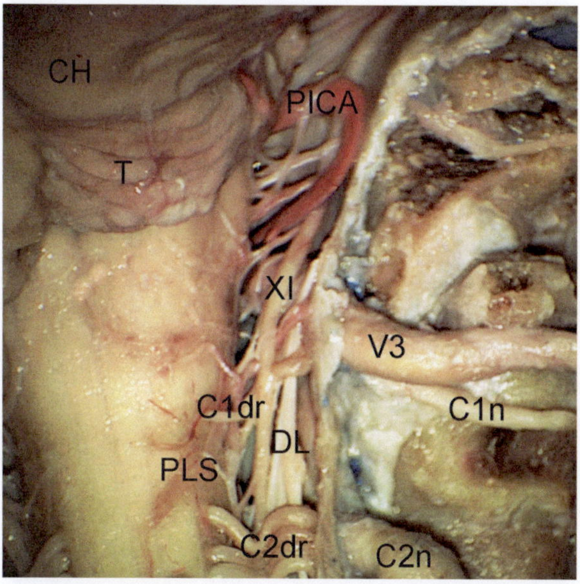

Fig. 1.17 Posterolateral intradural perspective of the CVJ. At the level of the spinal cord, the posterior lateral sulcus is situated along the line where the dorsal roots enter the spinal cord. Each dorsal root is composed of a series of six to eight rootlets. The dorsal roots of the first two cervical nerves pass posterior to the dentate ligament and accessory nerve. *CH* cerebellar hemisphere; *C1dr* dorsal root of the first cervical nerve; *C1n* first cervical nerve; *C2dr* dorsal roots of the second cervical nerve; *C2n* second cervical nerve; *DL* dentate ligament; *PICA* posterior inferior cerebellar artery; *PLS* posterior lateral sulcus; *T* tonsil; *V3* third segment of the vertebral artery; *XI* accessory nerve

the vertebral artery intradurally. In the cerebello-medullary cistern, the PICA passes dorsally between the rootlets of the IX, X, and XI cranial nerves and pursues a posterior course around the medulla (Fig. 1.18) [19, 20, 28, 29].

The lateral surface of the medulla is formed predominantly by the inferior olives. The glossopharyngeal, vagus, and accessory nerves arise from the medulla as a line of rootlets situated along the posterior edge of the inferior olive in the post-olivary sulcus. The only location where the glossopharyngeal nerve may consistently be distinguished from the vagal nerve is just proximal to a dural septum, which separates these nerves as they penetrate the dura to enter the jugular foramen. The hypoglossal nerve arises as a line of rootlets that exit the brainstem along the anterior margin of the lower olive in the pre-olivary sulcus, a groove between the olive and medullary pyramid. The rootlets of the XII pass behind the vertebral artery to reach the hypoglossal canal. The vertebral artery may stretch the hypoglossal rootlets posteriorly over its dorsal surface. The accessory nerve in the cranial fossa is composed of one main trunk from the spinal cord and three to six small rootlets that emerge from the medulla. The nerve joins the vagus nerve entering the jugular foramen (Fig. 1.19) [6, 14].

At the level of the spinal cord, the posterior lateral sulcus is situated along the line where the dorsal roots enter the spinal cord. Each dorsal root is composed of a

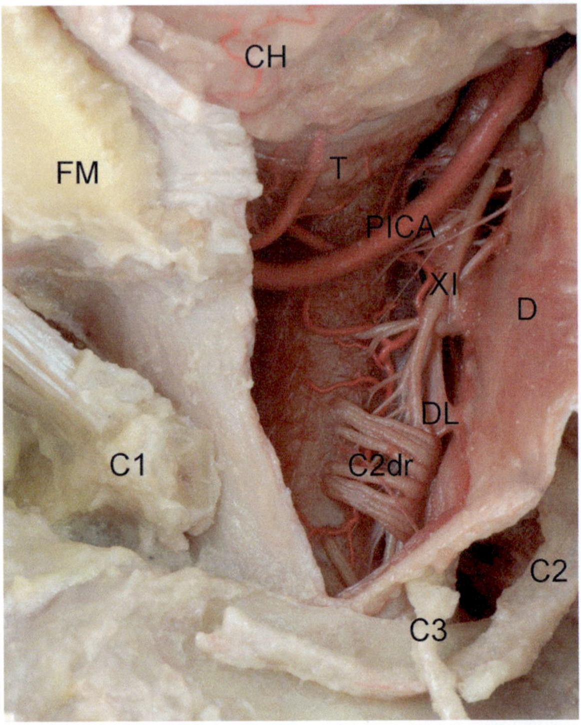

Fig. 1.18 Posterolateral intradural perspective of the CVJ. The posterior inferior cerebellar artery enters the cerebello-medullary cistern after originating from the fourth segment of the vertebral artery. In the cerebello-medullary cistern, the posterior inferior cerebellar artery passes dorsally between the rootlets of the IX, X, and XI cranial nerves and pursues a posterior course around the medulla. *CH* cerebellar hemisphere; *C1* atlas partially removed; *C2* second cervical nerve; *C2dr* dorsal roots of the second cervical nerve; *C3* third cervical nerve; *D* dura mater opened; *DL* dentate ligament; *FM* posterior border of foramen magnum partially opened; *PICA* posterior inferior cerebellar artery; *T* tonsil; *XI* accessory nerve

series of six to eight rootlets that fan out to enter the posterolateral surfaces of the spinal cord. The dorsal roots of the first two cervical nerves pass posterior to the dentate ligament and accessory nerve [2, 9].

The lateral posterior spinal vein, which courses along the line of origin of the dorsal roots in the posterior lateral spinal sulcus, is continuous above with the lateral medullary vein that courses along the retro-olivary sulcus, dorsal to the olive [4, 14].

1.4 Anterolateral Perspective of the CVJ

1.4.1 Bony Structures

The anterolateral perspective of the CVJ is directed to the jugular foramen and transverse process of C1 and C2 (Fig. 1.20).

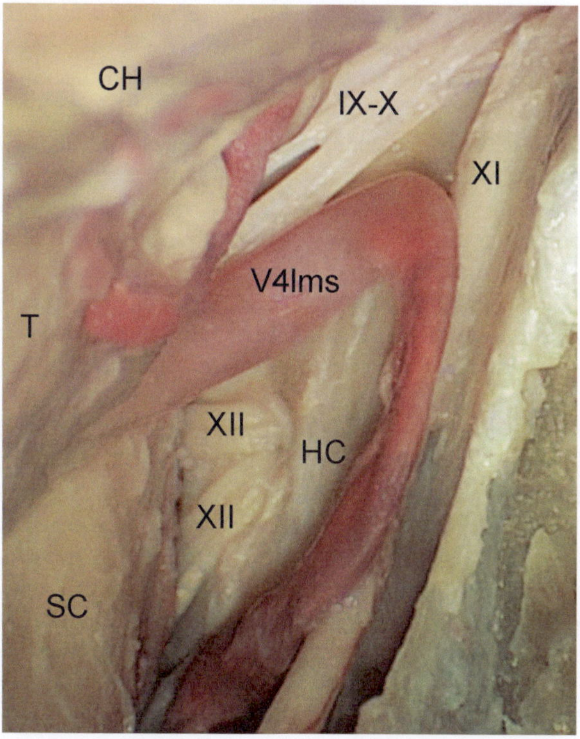

Fig. 1.19 Posterolateral intradural perspective of the CVJ. The lateral medullary segment of the vertebral artery begins at the dural foramen and passes anterior and superior along the lateral medullary surface to terminate at the pre-olivary sulcus in the cerebello-medullary fissure. The hypoglossal nerve arises as a line of rootlets that exit the brainstem along the anterior margin of the lower olive in the pre-olivary sulcus. The medullary trunk of the accessory nerve running toward the jugular foramen together with the glossopharyngeal and vagal nerves is exposed. *CH* cerebellar hemisphere; *HC* hypoglossal canal; *SC* spinal cord; *T* cerebellar tonsil; *V4lms* lateral medullary segment of the fourth segment of the vertebral artery; *IX-X* glossopharyngeal and vagal nerves; *XI* accessory nerve; *XII* hypoglossal nerve

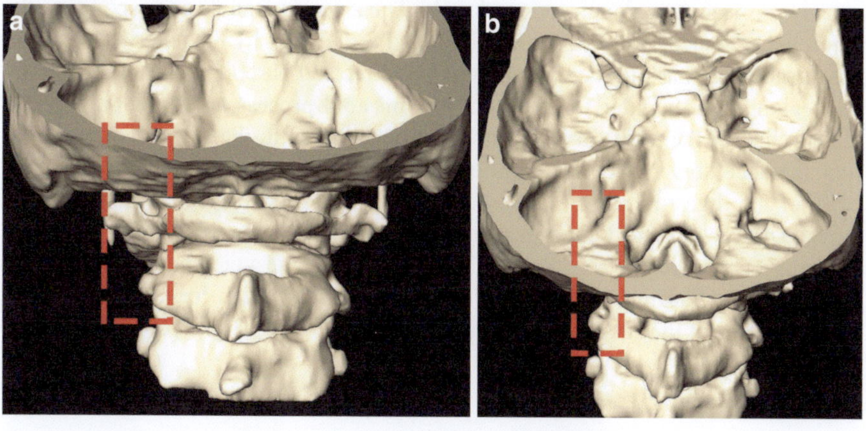

Fig. 1.20 3D reconstruction of the anterolateral perspective to the CVJ limited by a red dotted rectangular area on the extracranial (**a**) and intracranial (**b**) surfaces from a posterior view

The jugular foramen (JF) is a canal-like aperture, which is formed by the combination of the most indented parts of the occipital and temporal bones. The jugular process consists of a quadrilateral plate of bone that extends laterally from the posterior half of the condyle to form the posterior border of the jugular foramen. It serves as a bridge between the condylar and squamosal portions of the occipital bone and forms the posteromedial wall of the foramen. The jugular process is penetrated by the hypoglossal canal. It articulates laterally with the jugular surface of the temporal bone. The jugular process also serves as the site of attachment of the rectus capitis lateralis muscle behind the jugular foramen. The upper surface of the jugular process at the junction of the basilar and condylar parts of the occipital bone presents an oval prominence, the jugular tubercle. It is situated above the hypoglossal canal and medial to the lower half of the intracranial end of the jugular foramen [28, 30–32].

The transverse foramen of the atlas, which transmits the vertebral artery, is situated between the lateral mass and the transverse process. The transverse process of the atlas projects in the area between the mastoid process and the angle of the mandible, further lateral than the transverse processes on the adjacent cervical vertebrae. It has an apex that gives attachment to several muscles: the rectus capitis lateralis arises from the anterior portion; the superior oblique arises from the posterior portion of the upper surface of the transverse process; the inferior oblique muscle inserts on the lateral tip of the transverse process; the levator scapulae, splenius cervicis, and the scalenus medius attach to the inferior and lateral surface of the transverse process [2, 9, 22].

The transverse processes of the axis are small. Each transverse foramen faces supero-laterally, thus permitting the lateral deviation of the vertebral artery as it passes up to the more widely separated transverse foramina in the atlas [5, 9].

1.4.2 Muscular Relationships

The sternocleidomastoid muscle that passes obliquely downward from the lateral half of the superior nuchal line and mastoid process divides the side of the neck into an anterior triangle and a posterior triangle. The anterior triangle corresponds to the anterolateral aspect of the CVJ. It is bounded posteriorly by the anterior border of the sternocleidomastoid, laterally by the mandible and parotid gland, superiorly by the region of the jugular foramen and the mastoid process and anteriorly by the median line of the neck. In the fatty pad situated deep to the sternocleidomastoid runs the accessory nerve that supplies the muscle. In a deeper layer the posterior belly of the digastric muscle arises in the digastric groove located medial to the mastoid process and the longissimus capitis. Reflecting the digastric muscle exposes the transverse process of the atlas, which is covered by the attachments of numerous muscles, including the superior and inferior obliques, which form the upper and lower margins of the suboccipital triangle (Figs. 1.21 and 1.22) [3, 6–8]. The rectus

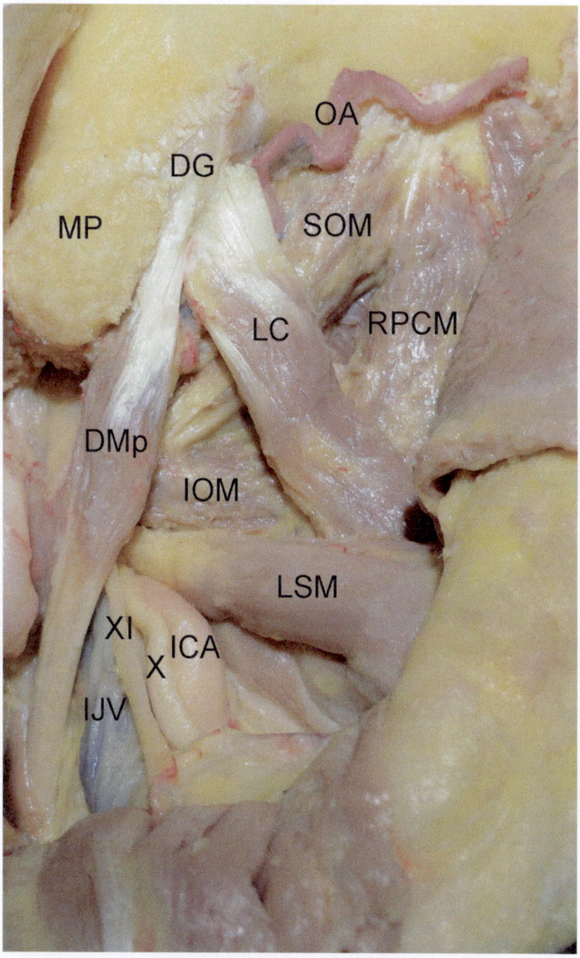

Fig. 1.21 Anterolateral perspective of the CVJ: muscular relationships. The sternocleidomastoid muscle has been reflected inferiorly and the semispinalis capitis laterally. Deeper to the sternocleidomastoid muscle, the posterior belly of the digastric muscle arises in the digastric groove located medial to the mastoid process and the longissimus capitis. Reflecting the digastric muscle exposes the transverse process of the atlas, which is covered by the attachments of numerous muscles, including the superior and inferior obliques, which form the upper and lower margin of the suboccipital triangle. *DG* digastric groove; *DMp* posterior belly of digastric muscle; *ICA* internal carotid artery; *IJV* internal jugular vein; *IOM* inferior oblique muscle; *LC* longissimus capitis muscle; *LSM* levator scapulae muscle; *MP* mastoid process; *OA* occipital artery; *RCPM* rectus capitis posterior major muscle; *SOM* superior oblique muscle; *X* vagal nerve; *XI* accessory nerve

capitis lateralis muscle is the muscle most intimately related to the jugular foramen. It is considered together with the anterior vertebral muscles. It extends vertically behind the internal jugular vein from the transverse process of the atlas to the jugular process of the occipital bone (Fig. 1.23) [34].

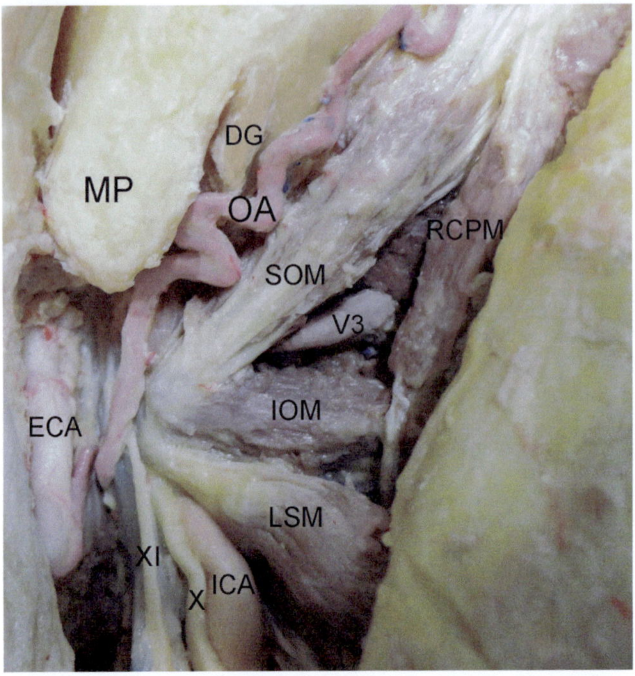

Fig. 1.22 Anterolateral perspective of the CVJ. The relationship between the occipital artery and the muscles on the anterolateral aspect of the CVJ is exposed. It arises from the posterior surface of the external carotid artery at the level of the angle of the mandible and courses obliquely upward between the posterior belly of the digastric muscle and the internal jugular vein, to reach the area posteromedial to the styloid process. At that point, it changes its course to posterior and lateral, passing posterior to the rectus capitis lateralis and then between the superior oblique and the posterior belly of the digastric where it courses in the occipital groove medial to the mastoid notch, in which the posterior belly of the digastric muscle arises. After exiting the area between the superior oblique muscle and the posterior belly of the digastric, it courses medially, being related to the longissimus capitis and semispinalis capitis. It courses medially behind the semispinalis capitis just below the superior nuchal line in the upper part of the posterior triangle to pass between the upper attachment of trapezius and the semispinalis capitis, where it pierces the attachment of the trapezius muscle to the superior nuchal line and ascends in the superficial fascia of the posterior scalp. *DG* digastric groove; *ECA* external carotid artery; *ICA* internal carotid artery; *IOM* inferior oblique muscle; *LSM* levator scapulae muscle; *MP* mastoid process; *OA* occipital artery; *RCPM* rectus capitis posterior major muscle; *SOM* superior oblique muscle; *V3* third segment of the vertebral artery; *XI* accessory nerve; *X* vagal nerve

1.4.3 Extradural Structures

The endocranial surface of the jugular foramen is generally divided into three intrajugular compartments: two venous and a neural compartment (Fig. 1.24). The neural and vascular compartments are generally separated by a bone projection called the intrajugular process. The larger posterolateral venous compartment, the sigmoid compartment, receives the flow of the sigmoid sinus. The sigmoid sinus drains into the internal jugular vein at the jugular bulb. The smaller anteromedial venous

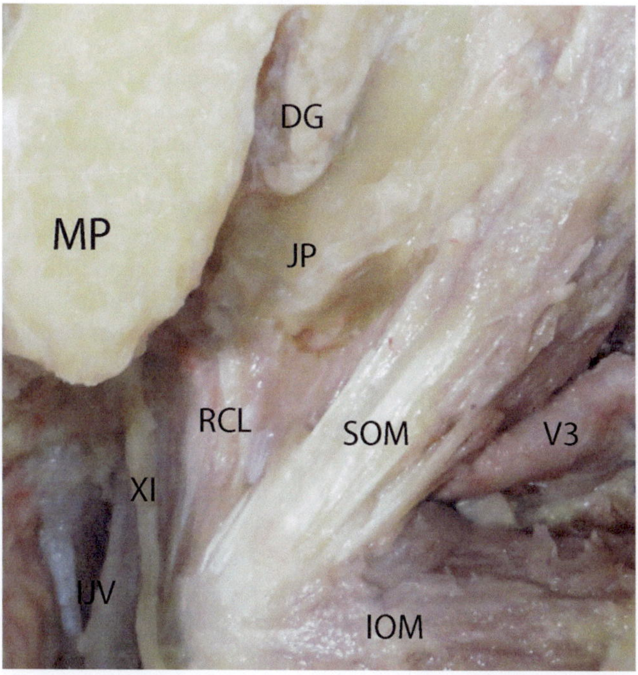

Fig. 1.23 Anterolateral perspective of the CVJ. The rectus capitis lateralis muscle is the muscle most intimately related to the jugular foramen. It is considered together with the anterior vertebral muscles. It extends vertically behind the internal jugular vein from the transverse process of the atlas to the jugular process of the occipital bone. *DG* digastric groove; *IJV* internal jugular vein; *IOM* inferior oblique muscle; *JP* jugular process; *MP* mastoid process; *RCL* rectus capitis lateralis muscle; *SOM* superior oblique muscle; *V3* third segment of the vertebral artery; *XI* accessory nerve

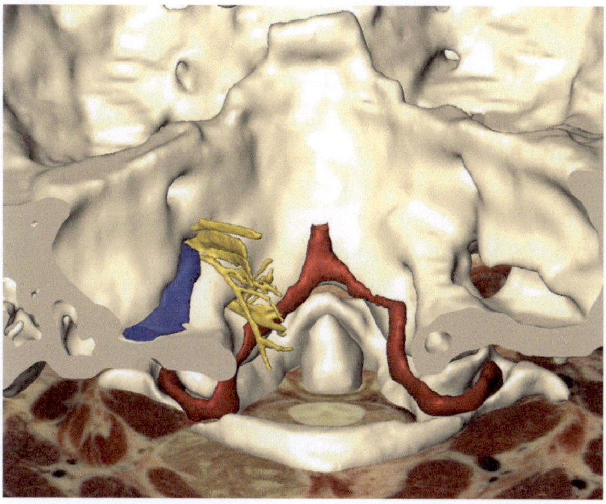

Fig. 1.24 The intracranial surface of the jugular foramen is shown by means of a 3D reconstruction. The neural part is represented in yellow, the venous compartment in blue, and the vertebral arteries joining to form the basilar artery in red

channel, the petrosal part, receives the drainage of the inferior petrosal sinus, besides receiving tributaries from the hypoglossal canal, petroclival fissure, and vertebral venous plexus. The neural part, through which the glossopharyngeal, vagus, and accessory nerves course, is located between the sigmoid and petrosal parts at the site of the intrajugular processes of the temporal and occipital bones, which are joined by a fibrous or osseous bridge. The dura over the neural part of the foramen has two characteristic perforations, a glossopharyngeal meatus, through which the glossopharyngeal nerve passes, and a vagal meatus, through which the vagus and accessory nerves pass. Along their exit from the jugular foramen, the glossopharyngeal, vagus, and accessory nerves penetrate the dura on the medial margin of the intrajugular process of the temporal bone to reach the medial wall of the internal jugular vein [28, 30, 33].

The glossopharyngeal nerve exits the jugular foramen and then turns forward, crossing the lateral surface of the internal carotid artery deep to the styloid process. At the external orifice of the jugular foramen, it gives rise to the tympanic branch (Jacobson's nerve) that provides innervation to the parotid gland. At the level of the vagal meatus, the vagal nerve is joined by the accessory nerve and gives rise to the Arnold's nerve, an auricular branch that join the facial nerve in the temporal bone. The vagal nerve exits the jugular foramen vertically, retaining an intimate relationship to the accessory nerve. At the level the two nerves exit the jugular foramen, they are located behind the glossopharyngeal nerve on the posteromedial wall of the internal jugular vein. As the vagal nerve passes lateral to the outer orifice of the hypoglossal canal, it is joined by the hypoglossal nerve medially. The accessory nerve exiting the jugular foramen descends obliquely laterally between the internal carotid artery and internal jugular vein and then backward across the lateral surface of the vein to reach its muscles. The hypoglossal nerve does not traverse the jugular foramen. However, it joins the nerves exiting the jugular foramen just below the skull and runs with them in the carotid sheath. The nerve exits the inferolateral part of the hypoglossal canal and passes adjacent to the vagal nerve, descends between the internal carotid artery and the internal jugular vein to the level of the transverse process of the atlas, where it turns abruptly forward along the lateral surface of the internal carotid artery toward the tongue (Figs. 1.25 and 1.26) [18, 19, 29, 35].

The internal jugular vein is the most volumetric structure in the JF. The proximal dilated part is called the jugular bulb. Anteriorly the inferior petrosal sinus and posteriorly the sigmoid sinus are the venous structures that drain into the jugular bulb. The top of the jugular bulb may reach out the porus acusticus internus in the temporal bone. The internal jugular vein and its tributaries form the most important drainage system in the craniocervical area [36, 37].

The internal carotid artery passes, almost straightly upward, posterior to the external carotid artery and anteromedial to the internal jugular vein, to reach the carotid canal. At the level of the skull base, the internal jugular vein courses just posterior to the internal carotid artery, being separated from it by the carotid ridge. Between them, the glossopharyngeal nerve is located laterally and the vagus, accessory, and hypoglossal nerves medially [7, 28].

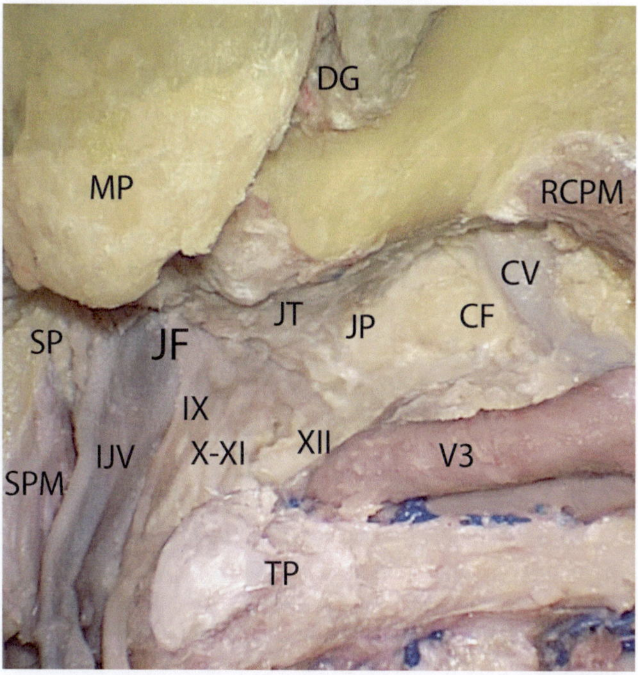

Fig. 1.25 Anterolateral perspective of the CVJ. The extracranial opening of the jugular foramen is exposed. The glossopharyngeal nerve exits the jugular foramen and then turns forward, crossing the lateral surface of the internal carotid artery deep to the styloid process. The vagal nerve exits the jugular foramen vertically, retaining an intimate relationship to the accessory nerve. At the level the two nerves exit the jugular foramen, they are located behind the glossopharyngeal nerve on the posteromedial wall of the internal jugular vein. As the vagal nerve passes lateral to the outer orifice of the hypoglossal canal, it is joined by the hypoglossal nerve medially. The accessory nerve exiting the jugular foramen descends obliquely laterally between the internal carotid artery and internal jugular vein and then backward across the lateral surface of the vein to reach its muscles. The hypoglossal nerve does not traverse the jugular foramen. However, it joins the nerves exiting the jugular foramen just below the skull and runs with them in the carotid sheath. The nerve exits the inferolateral part of the hypoglossal canal and passes adjacent to the vagal nerve, descends between the internal carotid artery and the internal jugular vein to the level of the transverse process of the atlas, where it turns abruptly forward along the lateral surface of the internal carotid artery toward the tongue. *CF* condylar fossa; *CV* condylar vein; *DG* digastric groove; *IJV* internal jugular vein; *JF* jugular foramen; *JP* jugular process; *JT* jugular tubercle; *MP* mastoid process; *RCPM* rectus capitis posterior major muscle; *SP* styloid process; *SPM* stylopharyngeus muscle; *TP* transverse process of the atlas; *V3* third segment of the vertebral artery; *IX* glossopharyngeal nerve; *X* vagal nerve; *XI* accessory nerve; *XII* hypoglossal nerve

The external carotid artery ascends anterior to the internal carotid artery. Proximal to its terminal bifurcation into the maxillary and the superficial temporal arteries, it gives rise to the posterior branches that are related to the jugular foramen: the ascending pharyngeal artery, the occipital artery and the posterior auricular artery [1, 7].

The occipital artery is the largest branch of the posterior group. It arises from the posterior surface of the external carotid artery at the level of the angle of the

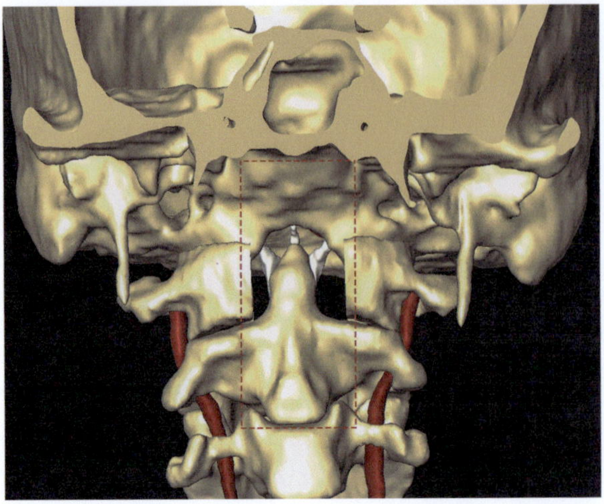

Fig. 1.26 The anteromedial perspective of the CVJ with removal of the anterior arch of C1 is limited by a red dotted rectangular area on a 3D model

mandible and courses obliquely upward between the posterior belly of the digastric muscle and the internal jugular vein, to reach the area posteromedial to the styloid process. At that point, it changes its course to posterior and lateral, passing posterior to the rectus capitis lateralis and then between the superior oblique and the posterior belly of the digastric where it courses in the occipital groove medial to the mastoid notch, in which the posterior belly of the digastric muscle arises. After exiting the area between the superior oblique muscle and the posterior belly of the digastric, it courses medially, being related to the longissimus capitis and semispinalis capitis. It courses medially behind the semispinalis capitis just below the superior nuchal line in the upper part of the posterior triangle to pass between the upper attachment of trapezius and the semispinalis capitis, where it pierces the attachment of the trapezius muscle to the superior nuchal line and ascends in the superficial fascia of the posterior scalp [2, 25].

The vertebral artery, above the transverse foramen of the axis, veers laterally to reach the transverse foramen of the atlas, which is situated further lateral than the transverse foramen of the axis (second segment of the vertebral artery, V2). The artery, after ascending through the transverse process of the atlas, is located on the medial side of the rectus capitis lateralis muscle. From here it turns medially behind the lateral mass of the atlas and the atlanto-occipital joint and is pressed into the groove on the upper surface of the posterior arch of the atlas (V3) [5, 9, 17].

1.5 Anteromedial Perspective of the CVJ

The anteromedial perspective of the CVJ provides exposure of the clival portion of occipital bone, anterior border of foramen magnum, anterior arch of C1, and the odontoid process (Fig. 1.26).

1.5.1 Bony Structures

The clivus, or basilar part of the occipital bone, is a thick quadrangular plate of bone that extends forward and upward, at an angle of about 45° from the foramen magnum. It joins the sphenoid bone at the spheno-occipital synchondrosis just below the dorsum sellae. The clivus is separated on each side from the petrous part of the temporal bone by the petroclival fissure. This fissure has the inferior petrosal sinus on its upper surface and ends posteriorly at the jugular foramen. Clivus is divided into three parts: superior, middle, and inferior. The superior portion is located above the level of the sellar floor; the middle portion extends from the sellar level to the level of sphenoid floor; and the inferior portion from the sphenoid floor to the foramen magnum. On the inferior surface of the basilar part, in front of the foramen magnum, a small elevation, the pharyngeal tubercle, gives attachment to the fibrous raphe of the pharynx (Fig. 1.27) [4, 38, 39].

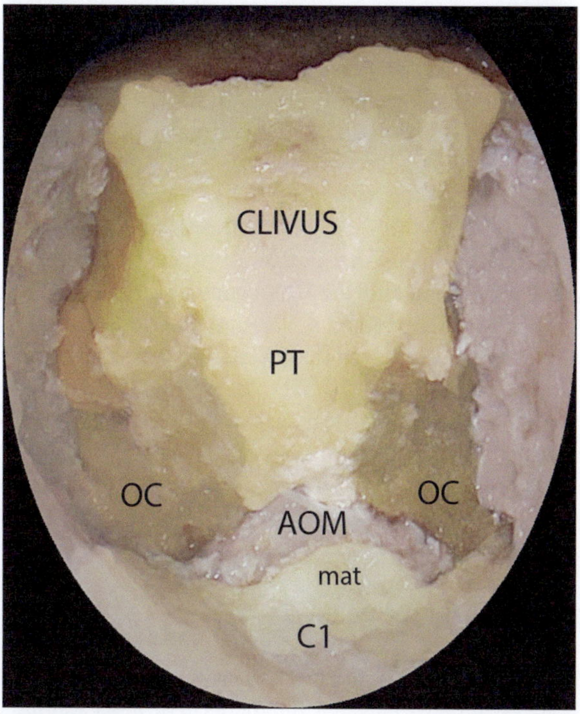

Fig. 1.27 Endoscopic endonasal exposure of the anteromedial aspect of the CVJ. The clivus, or basilar part of the occipital bone, is a thick quadrangular plate of bone that extends forward and upward, at an angle of about 45° from the foramen magnum. On the inferior surface of the basilar part, in front of the foramen magnum, a small elevation, the pharyngeal tubercle, gives attachment to the fibrous raphe of the pharynx. The anterior arch of the atlas is short and convexed forward and has a median anterior tubercle. The anterior atlanto-occipital membrane is a thin structure that attaches the anterior aspect of the atlas to the anterior rim of the foramen magnum. It is located just posterior to the pre-vertebral muscles of the neck. *AOM* anterior occipital membrane; *C1* atlas; *mat* middle anterior tubercle; *OC* occipital condyle; *PT* pharyngeal tubercle

The atlas lacks a vertebral body, whose usual position is occupied by the odontoid process of the axis. The anterior arch is short and convexed forward and has a median anterior tubercle. The internal wall of the anterior arch is in contact with odontoid process forming a facet (fovea dentis). It is the widest cervical vertebra, with its anterior arch approximately half as long as its posterior arch [1, 39, 40].

The dens of the axis, or odontoid process (dens), projects upward from the body of vertebra. The dens has a pointed apex, has a flattened side where the alar ligaments are attached, and is grooved at the base of its posterior surface where the transverse ligament of the atlas passes [1–3].

1.5.2 Muscular Relationships

The anterior vertebral muscles insert on the clival part of the occipital bone anterior to the foramen magnum. The longus colli is located on the anterior aspect of the cervical spine and consists of three portions. The superior oblique portion originates from the anterior tubercle of the transverse processes of the third through fifth cervical vertebrae and inserts on the tubercle of the anterior arch of the atlas; the inferior oblique and vertical portions extend from the fifth cervical vertebra downward to the third thoracic vertebra. The longus capitis originates from tendinous slips from the anterior tubercles of the transverse processes of the third through sixth cervical vertebrae, rising to insert on the basilar portion of the occipital bone. It is supplied by the anterior ramus of first through the third cervical spinal nerves. The rectus capitis anterior, located just deep to the superior aspect of the longus capitis, originates from the anterior surface of the lateral mass and the root of the transverse process of C1. It inserts on the foramen magnum anteriorly and on the basilar portion of the occipital bone. The rectus capitis lateralis has already been described as related to the jugular foramen (Fig. 1.28) [4, 8, 38, 40]. The anterior vertebral muscles are covered by the basipharyngeal fascia and on the midline by the median raphe. Median raphe is a thick band of connective tissue, which is attached to pharyngeal tubercle in the midline at clivus and continues below as anterior longitudinal ligament [12, 39].

1.5.3 Extradural Structures

The two atlanto-occipital joints are true synovial joints. They contain synovial membrane and are covered by capsular ligaments. The atlas and the occipital bone are united anteriorly by the anterior atlanto-occipital membrane. The anterior atlanto-occipital membrane (AAO) is a thin structure that attaches the anterior aspect of the atlas to the anterior rim of the foramen magnum. It is located just posterior to the pre-vertebral muscles of the neck and serves as the anterior wall of the supra-odontoid space, which houses the alar and apical ligaments, as well as fat and veins (Fig. 1.29). The alar ligament attaches the lateral aspects of the odontoid process to the base of the skull on the medial aspect of the occipital condyles. The

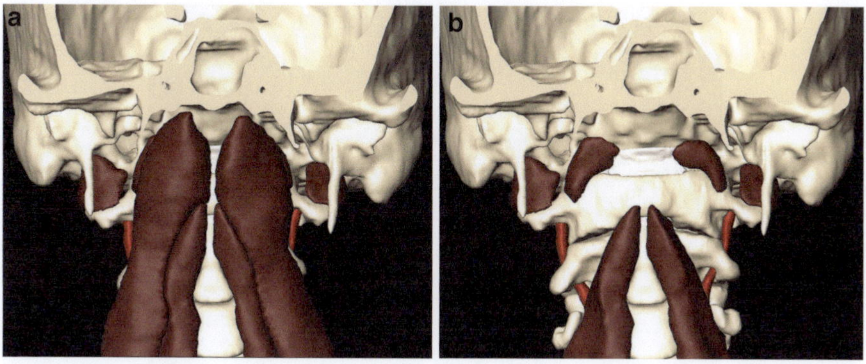

Fig. 1.28 Muscles related to the anteromedial perspective of the CVJ are represented through a 3D model. The superficial layer of the anterior vertebral muscles is exposed. The longus capitis originates from tendinous slips from the anterior tubercles of the transverse processes of the third through sixth cervical vertebrae and inserts on the basilar portion of the occipital bone. Below, the superior oblique portion of the longus colli originates from the anterior tubercle of the transverse processes of the third through fifth cervical vertebrae and inserts on the tubercle of the anterior arch of the atlas (**a**). The rectus capitis anterior, located just deep to the superior aspect of the longus capitis, originates from the anterior surface of the lateral mass and the root of the transverse process of C1. The rectus capitis lateralis extends vertically behind the internal jugular vein from the transverse process of the atlas to the jugular process of the occipital bone (**b**). The anterior vertebral muscles are covered by the basipharyngeal fascia and on the midline by the median raphe. Median raphe is a thick band of connective tissue, which is attached to pharyngeal tubercle in the midline at clivus and continues below as anterior longitudinal ligament

apical ligament, also known as the middle odontoid ligament or suspensory ligament, attaches the tip of the odontoid process to the middle point of the anterior border of the foramen magnum (basion). The ligament runs in the supra-odontoid space between the left and right alar ligaments and travels just posterior to the alar ligaments and just anterior to the superior portion of the cruciform ligament. The cruciform ligament has transverse and vertical parts that form a cross behind the dens. The transverse ligament is the key component of the cruciform ligament and is one of the most important ligaments in the body. It is the largest, strongest, and thickest craniocervical ligament. The superior and inferior limbs of the vertical part of the cruciform ligament are extremely thin. The transverse ligament runs posterior to the odontoid process of the axis and attaches to the lateral tubercles on the lateral mass of the atlas bilaterally. The transverse ligament maintains stability at the CVJ by locking the odontoid process anteriorly against the posterior aspect of the anterior arch of the atlas, and it divides the ring of the atlas into two compartments: the anterior compartment houses the odontoid process and the posterior compartment contains primarily the spinal cord and spinal accessory nerves. A synovial capsule is located between the odontoid process and the transverse ligament. The tectorial membrane, epidural fat, and dura mater are located dorsal to the transverse ligament. The tectorial membrane is a thin structure at the CVJ that serves as the posterior border to the supra-odontoid space. It runs posterior to the cruciform ligament

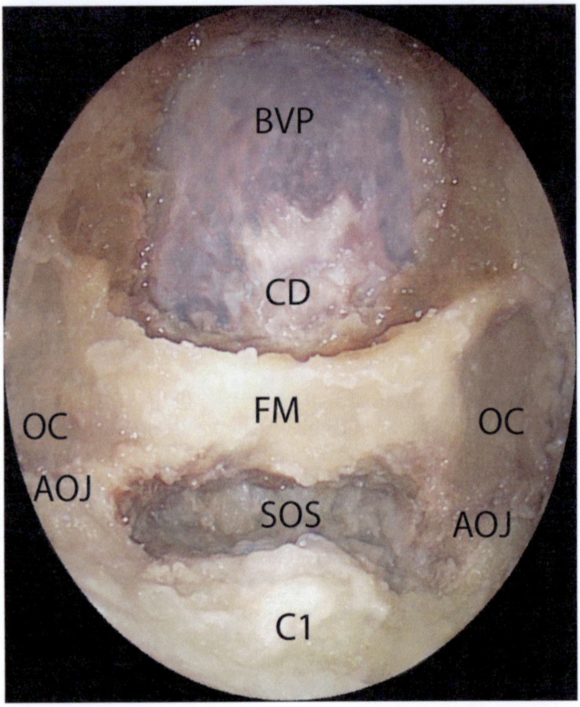

Fig. 1.29 Endoscopic endonasal exposure of the anteromedial aspect of the CVJ. The atlanto-occipital joints consist of the articulation between the upper facet of each lateral mass of the atlas and the occipital condyle that protrudes from the condylar part of the occipital bone. The two atlanto-occipital joints are true synovial joints. They contain synovial membrane and are covered by capsular ligaments. The supra-odontoid space between the anterior arch of the atlas and the anterior border of foramen magnum is exposed. The basilar venous plexus is located between the layers of the dura mater on the clivus. It is formed by interconnecting venous channels that anastomose with the inferior petrosal sinuses laterally, the cavernous sinuses superiorly, and the marginal sinus and epidural venous plexus inferiorly. *AOJ* atlanto-occipital joint; *BPV* basilar venous plexus; *CD* clival dura; *C1* atlas; *FM* foramen magnum; *OC* occipital condyle; *SOS* supra-odontoid space

in intimate contact with the dura mater of the clivus posteriorly. The tectorial membrane firmly adhered to the cranial base and body of the axis, where it is continuous with the posterior longitudinal ligament, but not to the posterior odontoid process. The posterior longitudinal ligament is attached below to the posterior surface of the body of the axis, and above to the transverse part of the cruciform ligament and the clivus. In front, the atlas and axis are connected by the anterior longitudinal ligament, which is a wide band fixed above to the lower border of the anterior arch of the atlas and below to the front of the body of the axis (Fig. 1.30, 3D model with reconstruction of the dens and ligaments) [4, 12, 38].

The basilar venous plexus is located between the layers of the dura mater on the upper clivus. It is formed by interconnecting venous channels that anastomose with

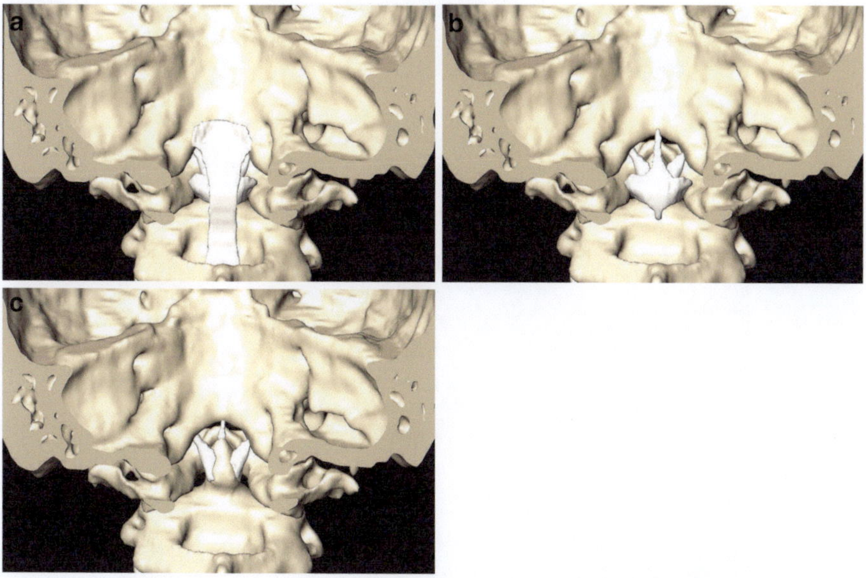

Fig. 1.30 3D model of the odontoid process and ligaments as seen through a posterior view after removal of the posterior arch of C1. The tectorial membrane is a thin structure at the CVJ that runs posterior to the cruciform ligament in intimate contact with the dura mater of the clivus posteriorly. The tectorial membrane firmly adhered to the cranial base and body of the axis, where it is continuous with the posterior longitudinal ligament, but not to the posterior odontoid process. The posterior longitudinal ligament is attached below to the posterior surface of the body of the axis and above to the transverse part of the cruciform ligament and the clivus (**a**). The cruciform ligament has transverse and vertical parts that form a cross behind the dens. The transverse ligament is the key component of the cruciform ligament and is one of the most important ligaments in the body. It is the largest, strongest, and thickest craniocervical ligament. The superior and inferior limbs of the vertical part of the cruciform ligament are extremely thin (**b**). The alar ligament attaches the lateral aspects of the odontoid process to the base of the skull on the medial aspect of the occipital condyles. The apical ligament attaches the tip of the odontoid process to the middle point of the anterior border of the foramen magnum (**c**)

the inferior petrosal sinuses laterally, the cavernous sinuses superiorly, and the marginal sinus and epidural venous plexus inferiorly [4, 38, 39].

On the anteromedial aspect of the CVJ, at the level of the superior surface of the occipital condyle, the supracondylar groove corresponds to an area formed by the insertion of the rectus capitus anterior muscle, anterior atlanto-occipital membrane, and atlanto-occipital capsule joint. The hypoglossal canals are situated posterior and lateral to the supracondylar groove (Fig. 1.31) [41–43].

1.5.4 Intradural Structures

The intradural anteromedial aspect of the CVJ corresponds to the medullary pyramids, which face the clivus, the anterior edge of the foramen magnum, and the

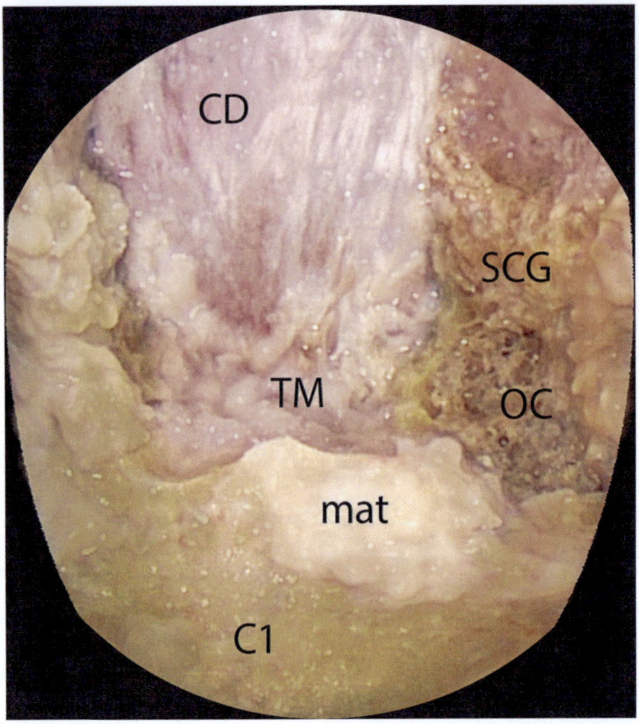

Fig. 1.31 Endoscopic endonasal exposure of the anteromedial aspect of the CVJ. The supracondylar groove corresponds to an area at the level of the superior surface of the occipital condyle formed by the insertion of the rectus capitis anterior muscle, anterior atlanto-occipital membrane, and atlanto-occipital capsule joint, which have been removed. The tectorial membrane is a thin membranous structure at the anteromedial CVJ that serves as the posterior border to the supra-odontoid space. It runs posterior to the cruciform ligament in intimate contact with the dura mater of the clivus posteriorly. The tectorial membrane firmly adhered to the cranial base and body of the axis, where it is continuous with the posterior longitudinal ligament. *CD* clival dura; *C1* atlas; *mat* median anterior tubercle; *OC* occipital condyle; *SCG* supracondylar groove; *TM* tectorial membrane

rostral part of the odontoid process. The anterior median sulcus divides the medulla between the pyramids and is continuous caudally with the anterior median fissure of the spinal cord. The rootlets forming the hypoglossal nerve, the glossopharyngeal, vagus, and accessory nerves run laterally from the lateral surface of the brainstem in the cerebello-medullary cistern (Figs. 1.32 and 1.33) [38–45].

The anterior medullary segment of the vertebral artery (V4) begins at the pre-olivary sulcus, courses in front of, or between, the hypoglossal rootlets, and crosses the pyramid to join with the other vertebral artery at or near the ponto-medullary sulcus to form the basilar artery. Branch of the anterior medullary segment is the anterior spinal artery. The anterior spinal artery is formed by the union of the paired anterior ventral spinal arteries near the origin of the basilar artery. The artery descends through the foramen magnum on the anterior surface of the

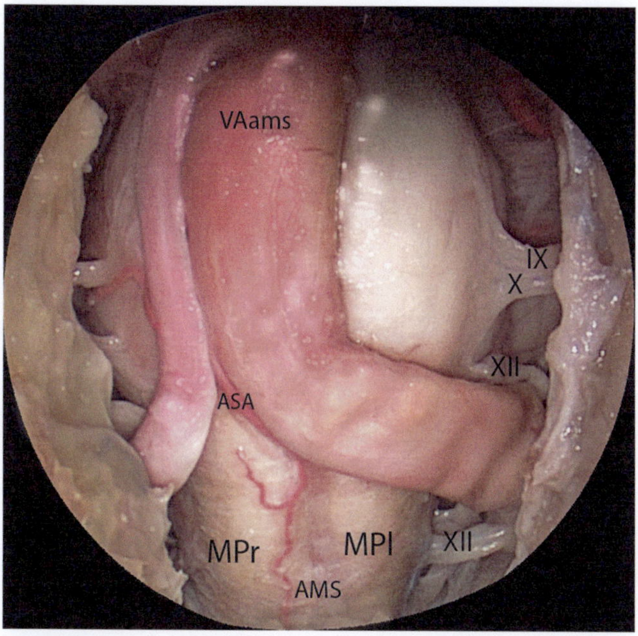

Fig. 1.32 Endoscopic endonasal exposure of the intradural anteromedial aspect of the CVJ. The intradural anteromedial aspect of the CVJ corresponds to the medullary pyramids, which face the clivus, the anterior edge of the foramen magnum, and the rostral part of the odontoid process. The anterior median sulcus divides the medulla between the pyramids and is continuous caudally with the anterior median fissure of the spinal cord. The fourth segment of the vertebral artery (V4) in its anterior medullary segment is visible. This segment begins at the pre-olivary sulcus, courses in front of, or between, the hypoglossal rootlets, and crosses the pyramid to join with the other vertebral artery at or near the ponto-medullary sulcus to form the basilar artery. The anterior spinal artery is formed by the union of the paired anterior ventral spinal arteries near the origin of the basilar artery. The artery descends through the foramen magnum on the anterior surface of the medulla and the spinal cord in or near the anteromedian fissure. The rootlets forming the hypoglossal nerve, the glossopharyngeal, and vagal nerve run laterally from the lateral surface of the brainstem in the cerebello-medullary cistern. The only location where the glossopharyngeal nerve may consistently be distinguished from the vagal nerve is just proximal to its entrance at the jugular foramen. *AMS* anterior median sulcus; *ASA* anterior spinal artery; *MPl* left medullary pyramid; *MPr* right medullary pyramid; *VAams* vertebral artery anterior medullary segment; *IX* glossopharyngeal nerve; *X* vagal nerve; *XII* hypoglossal nerve

medulla and the spinal cord in or near the anteromedian fissure. On the medulla, it supplies the pyramids and their decussation, the medial lemniscus, the interolivary bundles, the hypoglossal nuclei and nerves, and the posterior longitudinal fasciculus. It anastomoses with the anterior branches of the radicular arteries entering the cervical foramina [1, 2, 43]. The median anterior spinal vein, that courses in the anteromedian spinal fissure deep to the anterior spinal artery, is continuous with the median anterior medullary vein that courses on the anteromedian sulcus of the medulla [38–40].

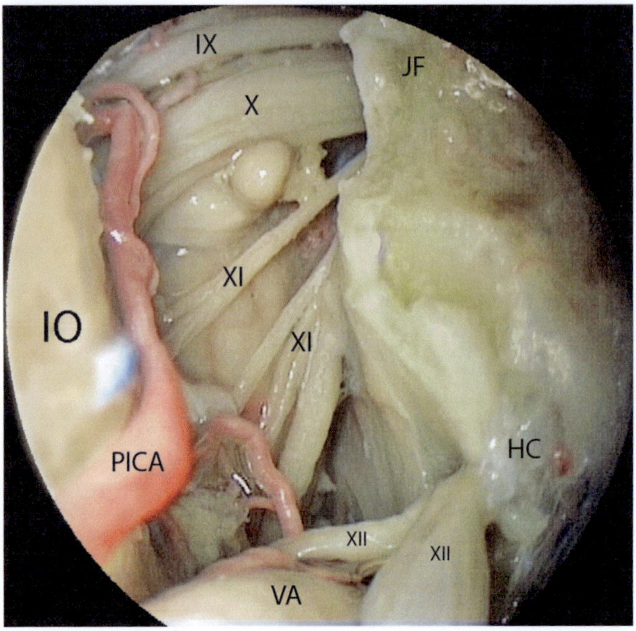

Fig. 1.33 Endoscopic endonasal exposure of the cerebello-medullary fissure through an antero-medial perspective. The glossopharyngeal, vagal, and medullary portions of the accessory nerve origin from the posterior edge of the inferior olive in the post-olivary sulcus. In the cerebello-medullary cistern, the medullary and spinal portions of the accessory nerve unite and run together with the glossopharyngeal and vagal nerves to the jugular foramen. The hypoglossal nerve arises as a line of rootlets that exit the brainstem along the anterior margin of the lower olive in the pre-olivary sulcus, a groove between the olive and medullary pyramid. The rootlets of the hyploglossal nerve pass behind the vertebral artery to reach the hypoglossal canal. The posterior inferior cerebellar artery enters the cerebello-medullary cistern after originating from the fourth segment (V4) of the vertebral artery intradurally. In the cerebello-medullary cistern the artery passes around the rootlets of the glossopharyngeal, vagal, and accessory nerves and pursues a posterior course around the medulla. *HC* hypoglossal canal; *IO* inferior olive; *PICA* posterior inferior cerebellar artery; *IX* glossopharyngeal nerve; *X* vagal nerve; *XI* accessory nerve; *XII* hypoglossal nerve

1.6 Conclusions

The complex anatomy of the CVJ deserves to be unlocked through a chamaleontic perspective based on microsurgical posterior and lateral and anterior endoscopic investigation. The integration of the anatomic knowledge coming from different and complementary perspectives with three-dimensional computer-based information is mandatory to create a safe and effective surgical decision-making process.

References

1. Suchomel P, Choutka O. Reconstruction of upper cervical spine and craniovertebral junction. Berlin: Springer-Verlag; 2011.
2. Rhoton AL Jr, De Oliveira E. Anatomical basis of surgical approaches to the region of the foramen magnum. In: Bambakidis C, Dickman A, Spetzler F, et al., editors. Surgery of the craniovertebral junction. 2nd ed. New York: Thieme; 2013. p. 13–51.
3. Lang J. The cranio-cervical junction—anatomy. In: Voth D, Glees P, editors. Diseases in the cranio-cervical junction. Anatomical and pathological aspects and detailed clinical accounts. Berlin, New York: Gruyter; 1987. p. 27–61.
4. Rhoton AL Jr. The foramen magnum. Neurosurgery. 2000;47(3 Suppl):S155–93.
5. Heller JG, Pedlow FX Jr, Gill SS. Anatomy of the cervical spine. In: Clark CR, editor. The cervical spine. 4th ed. Philadelphia: Lippincott Williams & Wilkins; 2005. p. 3–36.
6. Rhoton AL Jr. The far-lateral approach and its transcondylar, supracondylar, and paracondylar extensions. Neurosurgery. 2000;47(3 Suppl):S195–209.
7. Rhoton AL Jr. Jugular foramen. Neurosurgery. 2000;47(3 Suppl):S267–85.
8. Jhawar SS, Nunez M, Pacca P, et al. Craniovertebral junction 360°: a combined microscopic and endoscopic anatomical study. J Craniovertebr Junct Spine. 2016;7(4):204–16.
9. Pimenta NJ, Gusmão SS, Kehrli P. Posterior atlanto-occipital and atlanto-axial area and its surgical interest. Arq Neuropsiquiatr. 2014;72(10):788–92.
10. Youssef AS, Uribe JS, Ramos E, et al. Interfascial technique for vertebral artery exposure in the suboccipital triangle: the road map. Neurosurgery. 2010;67(2 Suppl Operative):355–61.
11. Dean NA, Mitchell BS. Anatomic relation between the nuchal ligament (ligamentum nuchae) and the spinal dura mater in the craniocervical region. Clin Anat. 2002;15(3):182–5.
12. Tubbs RS, Hallock JD, Radcliff V, et al. Ligaments of the craniocervical junction. J Neurosurg Spine. 2011;14:697–709.
13. Reis CV, Yagmurlu K, Elhadi AM, et al. The anterolateral limit of the occipital lobe: an anatomical and imaging study. J Neurol Surg B Skull Base. 2016;77(6):491–8.
14. Mussi AC, Matushita H, Andrade FG, et al. Surgical approaches to IV ventricle—anatomical study. Childs Nerv Syst. 2015;31(10):1807–14.
15. Matsushima K, Yagmurlu K, Kohno M, et al. Anatomy and approaches along the cerebellar-brainstem fissures. J Neurosurg. 2016;124(1):248–63.
16. Wanibuchi M, Fukushima T, Zenga F, et al. Simple identification of the third segment of the extracranial vertebral artery by extreme lateral inferior transcondylar-transtubercular exposure (ELITE). Acta Neurochir. 2009;151(11):1499–503.
17. Cacciola F, Phalke U, Goel A. Vertebral artery in relationship to C1-C2 vertebrae: an anatomical study. Neurol India. 2004;52(2):178–84.
18. Overland J, Hodge JC, Breik O, et al. Surgical anatomy of the spinal accessory nerve: review of the literature and case report of a rare anatomical variant. J Laryngol Otol. 2016;130(10):969–72.
19. Lloyd S. Accessory nerve: anatomy and surgical identification. J Laryngol Otol. 2007;121(12):1118–25.
20. Verma R, Kumar S, Rai AM, et al. The anatomical perspective of human occipital condyle in relation to the hypoglossal canal, condylar canal, and jugular foramen and its surgical significance. J Craniovertebr Junct Spine. 2016;7(4):243–9.
21. Kalthur SG, Padmashali S, Gupta C, et al. Anatomic study of the occipital condyle and its surgical implications in transcondylar approach. J Craniovertebr Junct Spine. 2014;5(2):71–7.
22. Barut N, Kale A, Turan Suslu H, et al. Evaluation of the bony landmarks in transcondylar approach. Br J Neurosurg. 2009;23(3):276–81.
23. Muthukumar N, Swaminathan R, Venkatesh G, et al. A morphometric analysis of the foramen magnum region as it relates to the transcondylar approach. Acta Neurochir. 2005;147(8):889–95.
24. Cavalcanti DD, Garcia-Gonzalez U, Agrawal A, et al. A clear map of the lower cranial nerves at the superior carotid triangle. World Neurosurg. 2010;74(1):188–94.

25. Alvernia JE, Fraser K, Lanzino G. The occipital artery: a microanatomical study. Neurosurgery. 2006;58(1 Suppl):ONS114–22.
26. Karasu A, Cansever T, Batay F, et al. The microsurgical anatomy of the hypoglossal canal. Surg Radiol Anat. 2009;31(5):363–7.
27. Sreenath SB, Recinos PF, McClurg SW, et al. The endoscopic endonasal approach to the hypoglossal canal: the role of the eustachian tube as a landmark for dissection. Otolaryngol Head Neck Surg. 2015;141(10):927–33.
28. Roche PH, Mercier P, Sameshima T, et al. Surgical anatomy of the jugular foramen. Adv Tech Stand Neurosurg. 2008;33:233–63.
29. Ozveren MF, Türe U, Ozek MM, et al. Anatomic landmarks of the glossopharyngeal nerve: a microsurgical anatomic study. Neurosurgery. 2003;52(6):1400–10.
30. Tekdemir I, Tuccar E, Aslan A, et al. Comprehensive microsurgical anatomy of the jugular foramen and review of terminology. J Clin Neurosci. 2001;8(4):351–6.
31. Suslu HT, Gayretli O, Coskun O, et al. Anatomical and morphometrical evaluation of the jugular tubercle. Br J Neurosurg. 2014;28(4):503–6.
32. Gupta C, Kurian P, Seva KN, et al. A morphological and morphometric study of jugular foramen in dry skulls with its clinical implications. J Craniovertebr Junct Spine. 2014;5(3):118–21.
33. Mei-Hua L, Geng-Sheng X, Zhi-Qun J, et al. Supracondylar transjugular tubercle approach to intradural lesions anterior or anterolateral to the craniocervical junction without resection of the occipital condyle. Turk Neurosurg. 2013;23(2):202–7.
34. Cohen MA, Evins AI, Lapadula G, et al. The rectus capitis lateralis and the condylar triangle: important landmarks in posterior and lateral approaches to the jugular foramen. J Neurosurg. 2017;27:1–9.
35. Keles B, Semaan MT, Fayad JN. The medial wall of the jugular foramen: a temporal bone anatomic study. Otolaryngol Head Neck Surg. 2009;141(3):401–7.
36. Kawashima M, Tanriover N, Rhoton AL Jr, et al. Comparison of the far lateral and extreme lateral variants of the atlanto occipital transarticular approach to anterior extradural lesions of the craniovertebral junction. Neurosurgery. 2003;53:662–74.
37. George B, Dematons C, Cophignon J. Lateral approach to the anterior portion of the foramen magnum: application to surgical removal of 14 benign tumors—technical note. Surg Neurol. 1988;29:484–90.
38. Cavallo LM, Cappabianca P, Messina A, et al. The extended endoscopic endonasal approach to the clivus and cranio vertebral junction: anatomical study. Childs Nerv Syst. 2007;23:665–71.
39. Alfieri A, Jho HD, Tschabitscher M. Endoscopic endonasal approach to the ventral cranio cervical junction: anatomical study. Acta Neurochir. 2002;144:219–25.
40. Kassam AB, Snyderman C, Gardner P. The expanded endonasal approach: a fully endoscopic transnasal approach and resection of the odontoid process: technical case report. Neurosurgery. 2005;57(1 Suppl):E213.
41. Morera VA, Fernandez Miranda JC, Prevedello DM, et al. "Far medial" expanded endonasal approach to the inferior third of the clivus: the transcondylar and transjugular tubercle approaches. Neurosurgery. 2010;66(6 Suppl):211–9.
42. Sekhar LN, Tariq F, Osbun J. Far lateral and far medial approaches to the foramen magnum: microsurgery or endoscopy? World Neurosurg. 2014;81(2):283–4.
43. Solari D, Cappabianca P. Far medial versus far lateral approach: the need of a chamaleontic perspective to unlock a skull base region. World Neurosurg. 2014;81(2):279–80.
44. Benet A, Prevedello DM, Carrau RL, et al. Comparative analysis of the transcranial "far lateral" and endoscopic endonasal "far medial" approaches: surgical anatomy and clinical illustration. World Neurosurg. 2014;81(2):385–96.
45. Morera VA, Fernandez-Miranda JC, Prevedello DM, et al. "Far-medial" expanded endonasal approach to the inferior third of the clivus: the transcondylar and transjugular tubercle approaches. Neurosurgery. 2010;66(6 Suppl Operative):211–9.

Surgical Anatomy of the Vertebral Artery at Craniovertebral Junction Level

2

Michael Bruneau and Bernard George

2.1 Anatomy of the Vertebral Artery V3 Segment

The vertebral artery (VA) course is subdivided into four segments.

The V1 segment, or ostial segment, takes its origin from the subclavian artery and usually ends at the transverse foramen of C6.

The V2 segment, or transversary segment, courses in and between the transverse foramina up to the C2 level. While the VA course is vertical between C6 and C3, its trajectory changes between C3 and C2 because the C2 transverse process is longer than the other ones and then located more laterally, with an orientation obliquely and inferiorly [1]. After exiting the C3 transverse foramen, the VA still runs vertically for 5–6 mm, before sharply bending along the base of the C2 vertebral body and running horizontally a few millimeters below the base of the C2 transverse process toward the C2 transverse foramen [1].

The V3 segment, or suboccipital segment, is located at the level of the craniovertebral junction, between the C2 transverse foramen and the dura mater of the foramen magnum (FM) (Fig. 2.1) [2–6].

The V4 segment, or intradural segment, fuses normally with the contralateral one to form the basilar artery.

M. Bruneau (✉)
Erasme Hospital, Department of Neurosurgery, Free University of Brussels, Brussels, Belgium
e-mail: mbruneau@ulb.ac.be

B. George
Lariboisiere Hospital Department of Neurosurgery, University Paris Descartes, Paris, France

E. Tessitore et al. (eds.), *Surgery of the Cranio-Vertebral Junction*,
https://doi.org/10.1007/978-3-030-18700-2_2

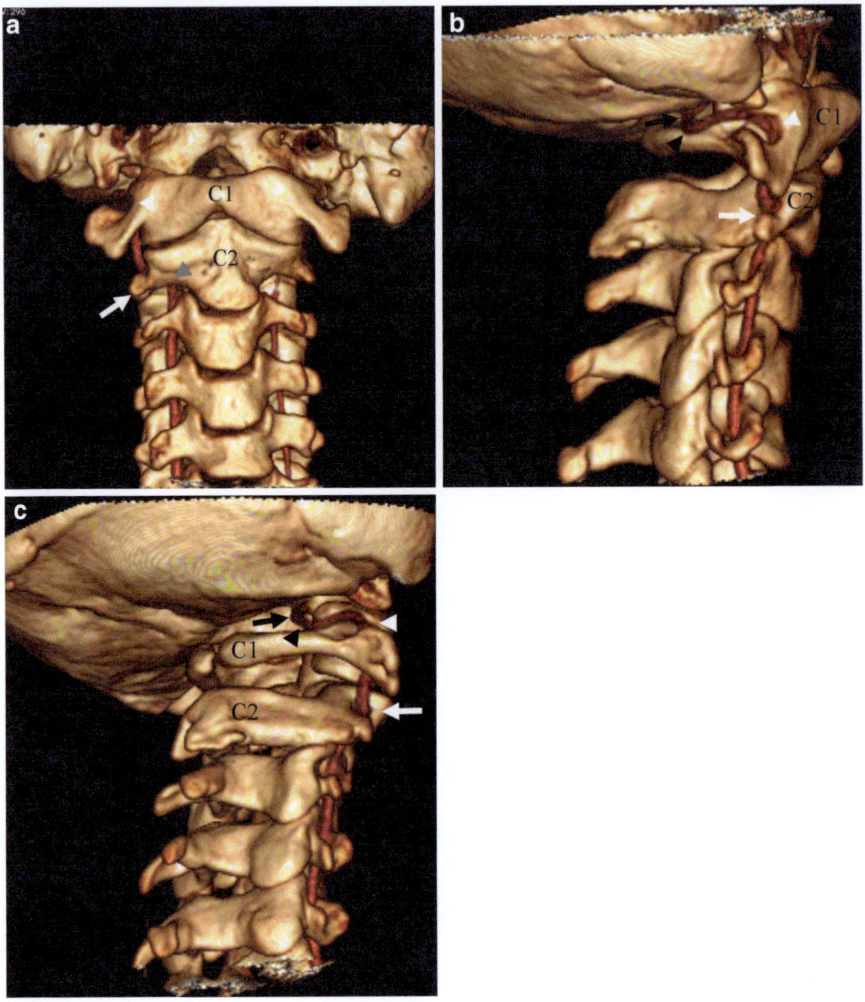

Fig. 2.1 Essential anatomy of the vertebral artery V3 segment on 3D angio-CT, illustrating bone relations. (**a**) Anterior view. (**b**) Lateral view. (**c**) Posterolateral view. The vertebral artery V3 segment extends from the C2 transverse foramen (*white arrow*) to the dura mater of the foramen magnum (*black arrow*). Its course is subdivided into three portions. The vertical portion, its first portion, runs between the C2 (*white arrow*) and C1 (*white arrowhead*) transverse foramina. Then, the artery courses posteriorly around the C1 lateral mass. The horizontal portion, its second portion, runs lateromedially above the C1 posterior arch up to the level of a medial step (*black arrowhead*). At this moment, starts the oblique portion (the third portion) that follows an ascending course up to the dura mater of the foramen magnum (*black arrow*). At each level, the vertebral artery gives off muscular branches. *Note*: The vertical portion of the vertebral artery V3 segment has a course lateral to that of the V2 segment. Under the C2 vertebral body (*gray arrowhead*), a horizontal loop exists in between, which is masked by the bone. The left vertebral artery is hypoplasic. *Pictures created with Osirix software.* (*From George B, Bruneau M, Spetzler RF (eds). Pathology and surgery around the vertebral artery. Springer; 2011*)

2.1.1 V3 Segment Portions

Along its course, the V3 segment is subdivided into three portions (Figs. 2.1 and 2.2). The vertical portion courses between the C2 and C1 transverse foramina. Its name comes from its course orientation when the head is considered in a neutral position. The *horizontal portion* follows the groove situated on the superior aspect of the posterior arch of the atlas. The junction between the vertical and horizontal portions forms a 90° angle in neutral position. The oblique portion prolongs the medial aspect of the horizontal portion toward the dura mater of the foramen magnum. Its course is oblique following the shape of the bone of the posterior arch of the atlas that forms a step at this level.

Bone structures represent crucial landmarks during the exposure of the V3 segment. During a posterolateral approach (Fig. 2.3a), the VA is safely exposed at C1 by a lateromedial subperiosteal dissection along the C1 posterior arch. This technique allows to localize safely the step formed by the bone and then the VA that runs just above it. During an anterolateral approach (Fig. 2.3b), the C1 transverse process represents a crucial landmark that can be palpated 15 mm below the mastoid tip. Dividing the muscles that insert on it (the superior oblique, the rectus capitis lateralis, the inferior oblique, the levator scapulae, the splenius cervicis, and the scalenius medius muscles) will bring the VA into view.

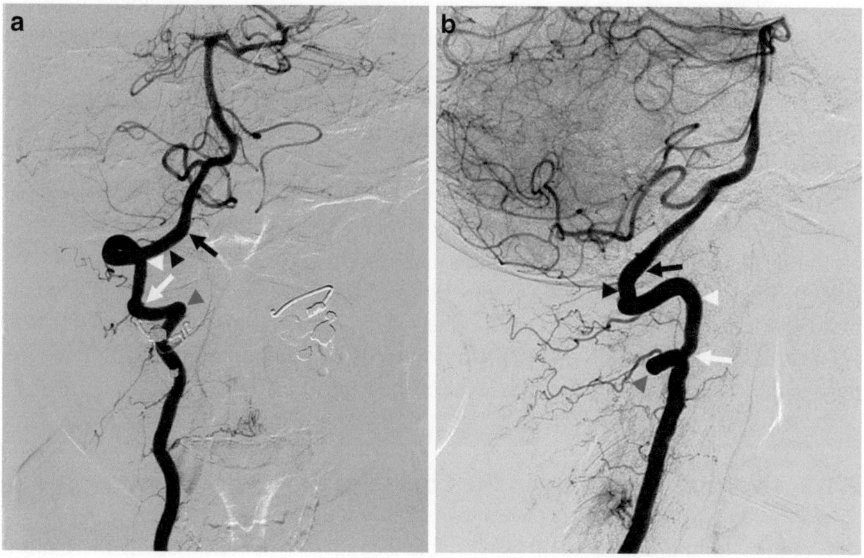

Fig. 2.2 Essential anatomy of the vertebral artery V3 segment on angiography. (**a**) Anterior view. (**b**) Lateral view. The same arrow indications as that on Fig. 2.1 are used. Note the origin of muscular branches at the C1 and C2 levels. (*From George B, Bruneau M, Spetzler RF (eds). Pathology and surgery around the vertebral artery. Springer; 2011*)

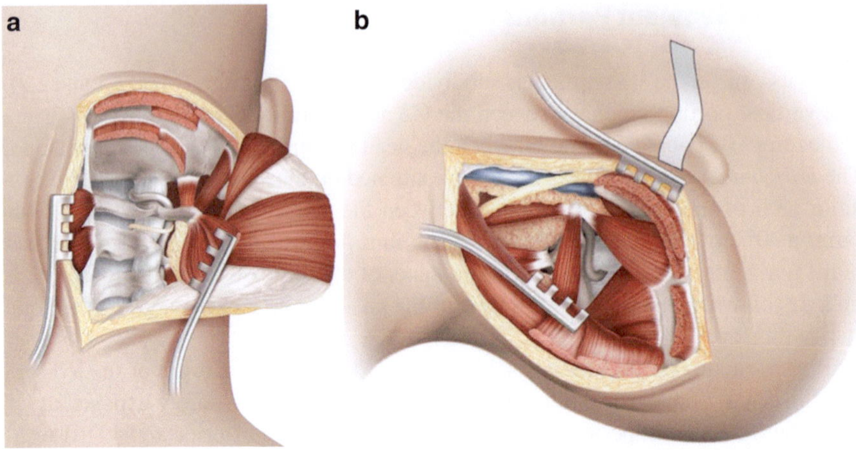

Fig. 2.3 Approaches to the vertebral artery V3 segment. (**a**) The posterolateral approach. (**b**) The anterolateral approach. (*From George B, Bruneau M, Spetzler RF (eds). Pathology and surgery around the vertebral artery. Springer; 2011*)

2.1.2 Periosteal Sheath, Venous Plexus, and Distal Dural Ring

Like the V2 segment, the V3 segment and its venous plexus are enclosed within a periosteal sheath (Fig. 2.4). The periosteal sheath is in fact an extension of the periosteal sheath of the transverse processes [6, 7]. Performing a subperiosteal dissection is a key step in the surgical technique for exposing the VA in safe conditions. This technique avoids to enter inside the periosteal sheath with the subsequent venous bleedings of the venous plexus.

At the FM level, the periosteal sheath fuses tightly with the dura mater forming a ring called the distal dural ring. The ring is located about 10 mm from the midline. At the level of the dural crossing that is 1–2 mm long, the VA cannot be separated from the dura mater due to collagenous fibers of the dura that penetrate the adventitia to reach the media and perforating fibers that really anchor into the arterial wall [8]. For this reason, mobilizing the VA at the V3-V4 junction requires to divide the dura mater circumferentially at the level of the ring.

2.1.3 Normal Variability in the Course of the V3 Segment

The course of the V3 segment is variable because it depends on head rotation (Fig. 2.5). Indeed, since the C1 transverse process moves anteriorly with head rotation as the atlas turns around the axis, the vertical segment becomes more and more oblique anteriorly and the angle between the VA segments above and below C1 becomes acute with increasing angle of rotation. At the maximum of rotation, the horizontal and vertical segments are stretched, so that they run parallel, separated

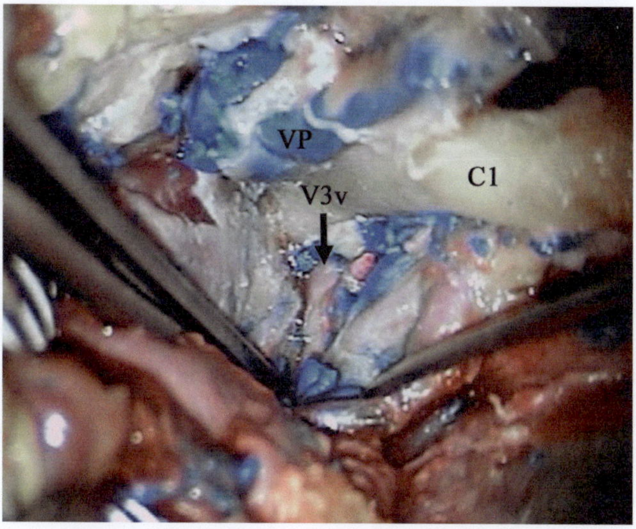

Fig. 2.4 Left-sided cadaver posterolateral approach to the vertebral artery V3 segment. The vertical portion of the V3 segment that runs between the C2 and C1 transverse processes is exposed. The vertebral artery is enclosed within a periosteal sheath surrounded by a huge venous plexus. The plexus has been opened to show the vertical portion of the vertebral artery V3 segment. Above the C1 posterior arch, the horizontal and oblique portions are within the venous plexus. *V3v* vertical portion of the vertebral artery V3 segment, *VP* venous plexus. (*From George B, Bruneau M, Spetzler RF (eds). Pathology and surgery around the vertebral artery. Springer; 2011*)

only by the bone of the posterior arch of the atlas [6, 7]. This anatomical displacement of V3 segment depending on head rotation should be perfectly understood for surgical positioning and for anticipating anatomical relations at surgery.

The displacement of C1 relative to C2 during head rotation explains some motion-related vascular pathologies with VA occlusion during rotation and subsequent strokes, named Bow hunter strokes, or extradural PICA origin occlusion [9, 10].

2.1.4 Branches

Several branches take their origin along the course of the V3 segment (Fig. 2.2):

- A C2 radicular artery. This artery starts in the middle of the posterolateral aspect of the C1-C2 portion. This branch accompanies the C2 nerve laterally and provides the blood supply to the C2 ganglion and nerve.
- A muscular branch that arises posteriorly at the upper exit of the transverse foramen of the atlas.
- A posteromedial branch, located at the junction of the horizontal and oblique portions.

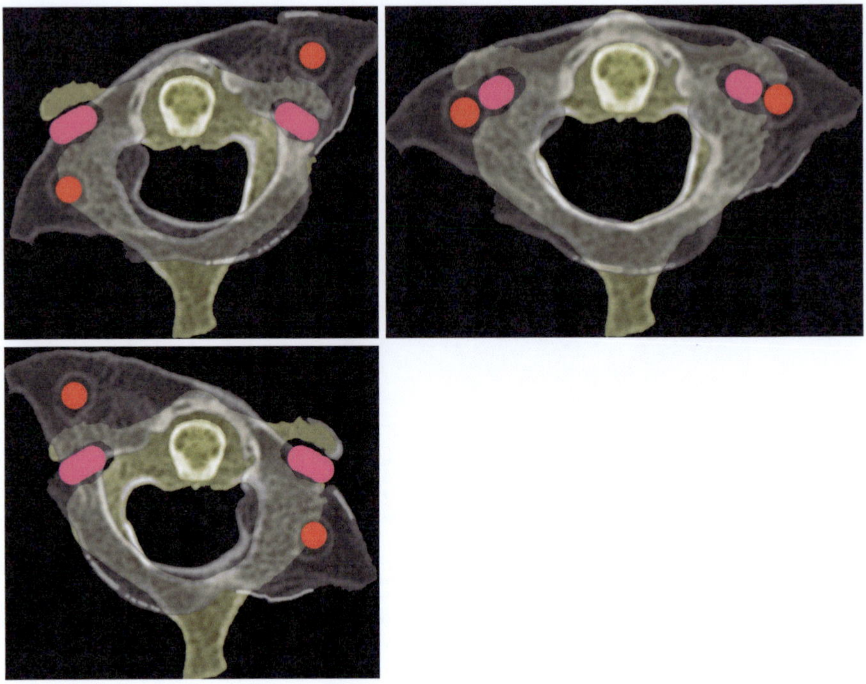

Fig. 2.5 Relative position of the C1 and C2 vertebrae during head rotation. The relations of the vertebral artery move accordingly. Superior views: *left:* head turned to the left; *center:* neutral position; *right:* head turned to the right. When the head is turned to one side, the homolateral C1 transverse process moves posteriorly and the contralateral one anteriorly. (*From George B, Bruneau M, Spetzler RF (eds). Pathology and surgery around the vertebral artery. Springer; 2011*)

2.2 Anatomical Variations

Anatomical variations expose the VA at risk of inadvertent intraoperative traumatism. Their detection is most of the time possible on preoperative workup as soon as the attention is focused on the VA trajectory or subtle bone modifications. The optimal visualization of the VA course is provided by angio-CT or angio-MR (MRA) with 3D reconstructions. Due to its invasive character, angiography is never necessary for this purpose.

2.2.1 Size

In 20–40% of the cases, both VAs may be of different sizes with the left VA usually larger than the right one (Fig. 2.6) [5, 7, 11–13]. The mean size of the left VA at its origin is 5.0 mm (3.3–6.2 mm) compared to 4.1 mm (2.2–5.5 mm) on the right side. The VA and its V3 segment can even be smaller in case of hypoplasia or atresia. This variation is predominantly observed on the right side [14–16]. The size cut-off to

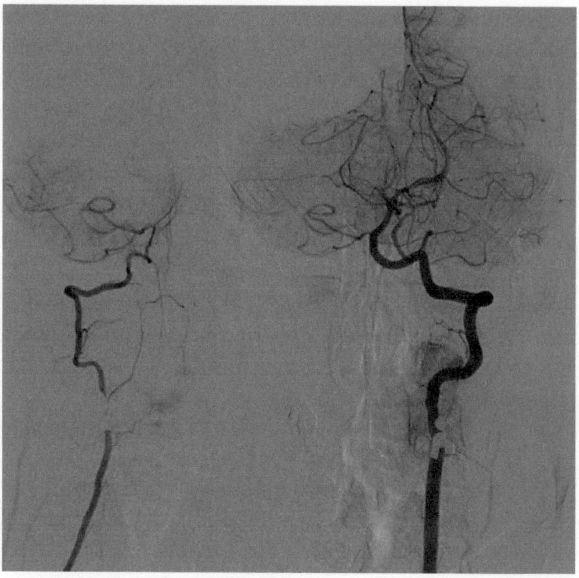

Fig. 2.6 The right VA is smaller than the left one. The artery is considered hypoplasic because it fuses with the contralateral vertebral artery to form the basilar trunk. (*With permission of Erasme Hospital, ULB*)

consider hypoplasia is highly variable in the literature, between 2 and 3.5 mm [14, 15, 17, 18]. Depending on the cut-off considered, the incidence of the variation is reported between 2.34 and 26.5% [14, 15, 17–20]. The difference between hypoplasia and atresia is that in the former condition both VAs fuse to form the basilar trunk, while it is not the case in the latter condition, the VA ending by the PICA (Fig. 2.6) or another vessel such as the occipital artery or a spinal artery [7, 21, 22]. Hypoplasia is relatively common in the general population. Despite being generally an incidental discovery, a high association of VA territory ischemic stroke with ipsilateral hypoplasia has been observed [17, 19]. On the contrary, VA atresia has been reported in a very limited number of cases [22]. At surgery, a hypoplasic VA could be sacrificed (the anterior spinal artery must never be interrupted to avoid a spinal cord infarction, but this branch is never coming from the V3 segment) while an atretic VA ending by the PICA cannot be sacrificed to avoid a posterior fossa stroke.

Anatomical variations are due to the absence of the development of segmental arteries during the embryonic stage; the blood flow is subsequently provided by other vessels that compensate the unformed segment with increased velocity in the contralateral vessel [23]. Bilateral agenesis of the vertebrobasilar junction is exceptional with blood supply to the basilar artery by carotid-vertebral anastomoses [24].

2.2.2 Abnormal Course of the Vessels at the Craniovertebral Junction

Several types of vessels variations can be observed at the craniovertebral junction (CVJ) with an incidence of 5% on MRA [25].

The most common vascular anatomical variation at the CVJ is the extracranial–extradural origin of the PICA. Several other anomalies can be less frequently encountered such as an abnormal course, duplications, fenestrations, and anastomoses. In case of duplication or persisting first intersegmental artery, the abnormal vessel course below C1 in the C1-C2 interspace. Such conditions have direct implications during approaches to the CVJ, and they need to be ruled out by means of a CT angiogram. Many bone variations can also be present and are important to know due to the consequences for the VA exposure and fixation procedures.

2.2.2.1 Extracranial–Extradural Origin of the PICA

The PICA may have an extradural origin in up to 20.8% of the cases (Fig. 2.7) [26–29]. This anomaly is most of the time unilateral but can be encountered bilaterally in few cases [26–28].

A PICA with an extradural origin may arise from the horizontal portion just outside the dura mater, further laterally above the transverse foramen of the atlas, or from the vertical portion of the V3 segment [26].

When arising from the horizontal VA portion, the extradural PICA courses parallel to the VA and the C1 nerve, and these three structures will enter the dura together [26]. Intradurally, the PICA will remain lateral and posterior to the brainstem, providing the blood supply to the lateral and posterior medulla [26]. This situation is different from the one observed with the classical intradural PICA origin in which the first segment of the PICA courses anterior to the medulla and provides blood supply to the anterior aspect of the brainstem [26].

When originating from the vertical portion, the vessel penetrates the dura mater between C2 and C1 [26].

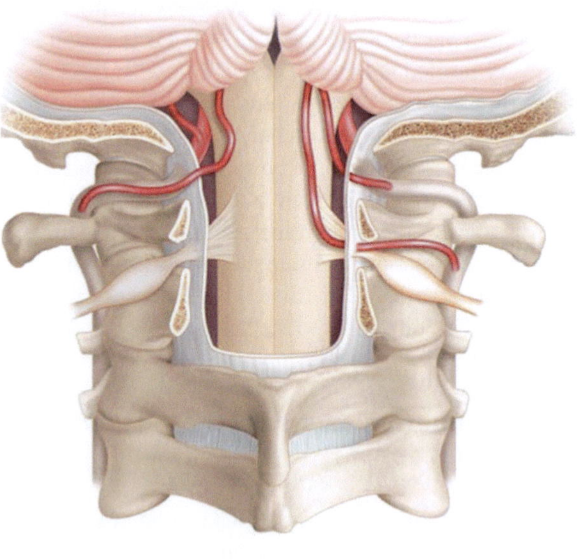

Fig. 2.7 PICA variations: extracranial-extradural origins. (*From George B, Bruneau M, Spetzler RF (eds). Pathology and surgery around the vertebral artery. Springer; 2011*)

An extradural PICA origin is associated with a highest risk of dissection, as is the V3 segment. The risk of inadvertent injury is also higher during posterior approaches to the CVJ, and the PICA may be mistaken for a muscular branch, the posterior meningeal artery, and posterior spinal branches [26]. Extradural PICA origin can be detected on CTA [29]. This anomaly can be missed on a three-vessel angiogram if the contrast medium cannot reflux toward the PICA origin [26]. Extradural origin of the PICA can only be suspected on angiography if the PICA arises below the FM level, but this criterion is not absolute since the PICA may originate intradurally between the atlas and the FM [26].

2.2.2.2 Anastomoses

Proatlantal arteries are developmental anomalies located at the CVJ due to the absence of regression of anastomosing vessels during embryogenesis.

Despite rare, detecting this kind of congenital anomalies is important for explaining some posterior circulation pathologies, before any surgery on the carotid artery that could result in devastating consequence due to flow interruption in the absence of collateral flow [30] and when exposing the VA at the CVJ level.

Two types of proatlantal arteries have been described by Lasjaunias et al. [31] according to their origin from the ICA (type I) (Fig. 2.8) or ECA (type II). They result, respectively, from the persistence of the first and second embryonic intersegmental arteries [32]. These intersegmental arteries arise at the second or third cervical vertebral body level [32].

The type I proatlantal artery takes its origin from the posterior aspect of the cervical ICA; the artery then ascends posteriorly and medially toward the

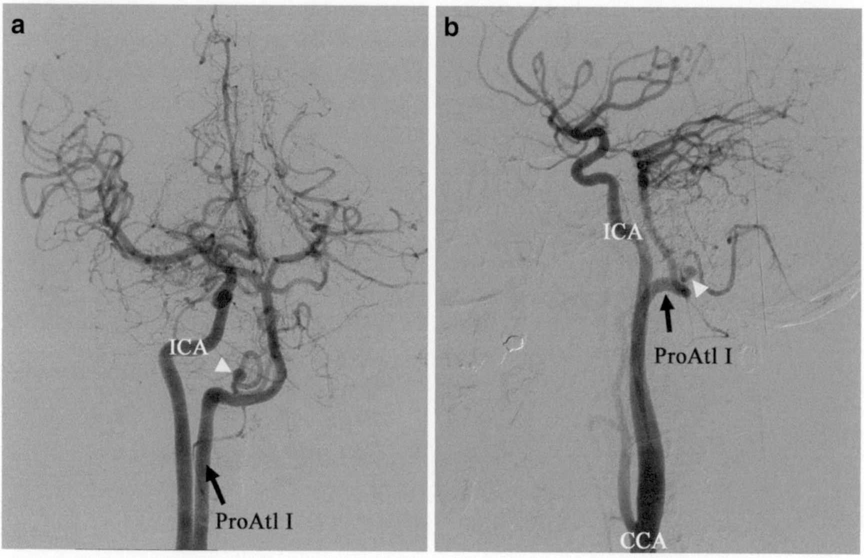

Fig. 2.8 Proatlantal artery type I. Anterior view (**a**), lateral view (**b**). (*From George B, Bruneau M, Spetzler RF (eds). Pathology and surgery around the vertebral artery. Springer; 2011*)

occipitocervical space where it joins the V3 segment before penetrating the foramen magnum [33–35].

The type II proatlantal artery starts shortly after the ECA origin and joins the V3 segment horizontal or vertical portion [33].

More than 40 cases have been reported in the literature [32, 33]. Persistence of bilateral proatlantal arteries is extremely rare [32, 36–38]. The proatlantal artery is commonly associated with other anomalies such as VA agenesis [36, 39, 40], VA hypoplasia, increased incidence of intracranial aneurysms [38], and Galen's vein malformation [32].

At the CVJ level, a hypoglossal artery can be misinterpreted for a proatlantal artery. The distinction between them is based on the vessel trajectory on angiography and on the point of entrance in the skull base on 3D CTA. On lateral digital subtraction angiography, the hypoglossal artery has indeed a less posterior course than the proatlantal artery because the hypoglossal artery passes through the hypoglossal canal which is anterior to the foramen magnum in which passes the proatlantal artery [33].

2.2.2.3 Duplications–Fenestrations

Duplications and fenestrations (Fig. 2.9) are classically incidental findings discovered during MRA, digital subtraction angiography, and autopsies [41–47]. Duplications and fenestrations represent different entities that are often used erroneously as synonyms in the literature [31, 41, 48, 49].

According to Lasjaunias et al. definition [31, 49], in the presence of a duplication, one of the vessels leaves the transverse foramen, enters the spinal canal, and

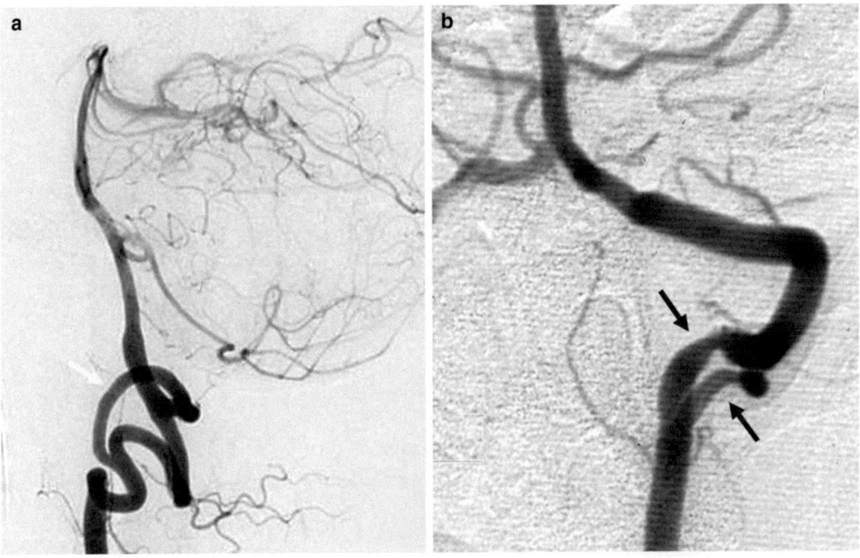

Fig. 2.9 Vertebral artery duplication (**a**) and fenestration (**b**). (*From George B, Bruneau M, Spetzler RF (eds). Pathology and surgery around the vertebral artery. Springer; 2011*)

runs into the subarachnoid space with the nerve root. In the presence of a VA fenestration, a double vessel runs in the transverse foramen as well as in between [31, 49]. Fenestrations result at the V3 level from the persistence of both proatlantal intersegmental artery and first cervical intersegmental artery that normally disappear during the VA development [49, 50].

The incidence of duplications is around 0.7% while the true incidence of cervical VA fenestrations is very low. In fact, several cases reported as fenestrations should in fact be considered as duplications with Lasjaunias's definition [42, 43, 45, 51–53]. Several cases of fenestrations have been reported in the literature, only at high cervical levels [48–50].

2.2.2.4 Intradural Course of the C1–C2 VA

In 0.6% of the cases, the VA may turn medially directly after leaving the C2 transverse foramen. Instead of passing through the C1 transverse foramen, the VA thus enters the spinal canal between C1 and C2 [54–56]. If a congenital osseous anomaly (such as os odontoideum, ossiculum terminale, hypoplastic odontoid, bifid C1 posterior arch, or occipitoatlantal assimilation in case of Chiari malformation [52, 57]) is noted at the CVJ level, the incidence increases up to 19–36.4% [52, 54]. This abnormal VA course is embryologically linked to the persistence of the first intersegmental artery [52]. Despite most anomalies remain asymptomatic, some cases of medulla or cervical cord myelopathy due to a compression and accessory nerve palsy have been described [58–64]. One case of associated PICA aneurysm has been reported [65].

2.2.2.5 High-Riding VA

In case of high-riding vertebral artery (HRVA), the acute lateral bend that makes classically the VA V2 segment at the lower aspect of the axis, just under its superior articular facet is more medial, posterior, or superior resulting in the narrowing of the height and/or the width of the isthmus and pedicle of the axis (Fig. 2.10) [11, 13, 66]. This anatomical situation can be encountered unilaterally in 10–24% of the cases and bilaterally in 3–6% [13, 67–72]. Therefore, the height of the isthmus and pedicle must be evaluated routinely preoperatively on high-resolution CT scans before C1-C2 instrumentation. Screw placement will be contraindicated in the presence of a HRVA due to the risk of inadvertent VA injury. The left side is commonly more affected than the right one [13]. Female sex and age over 70 years are risk factors for HRVA [13] as well as rheumatoid arthritis due to bone osteoporosis.

2.2.3 Bone Anomalies

The groove of the arch of the atlas can be turned into a tunnel due to calcification or ossification of the occipitoatlantal membrane that lies above the groove (Fig. 2.11) [73, 74]. In this situation, it becomes more difficult for exposing the horizontal portion of the V3 segment [11].

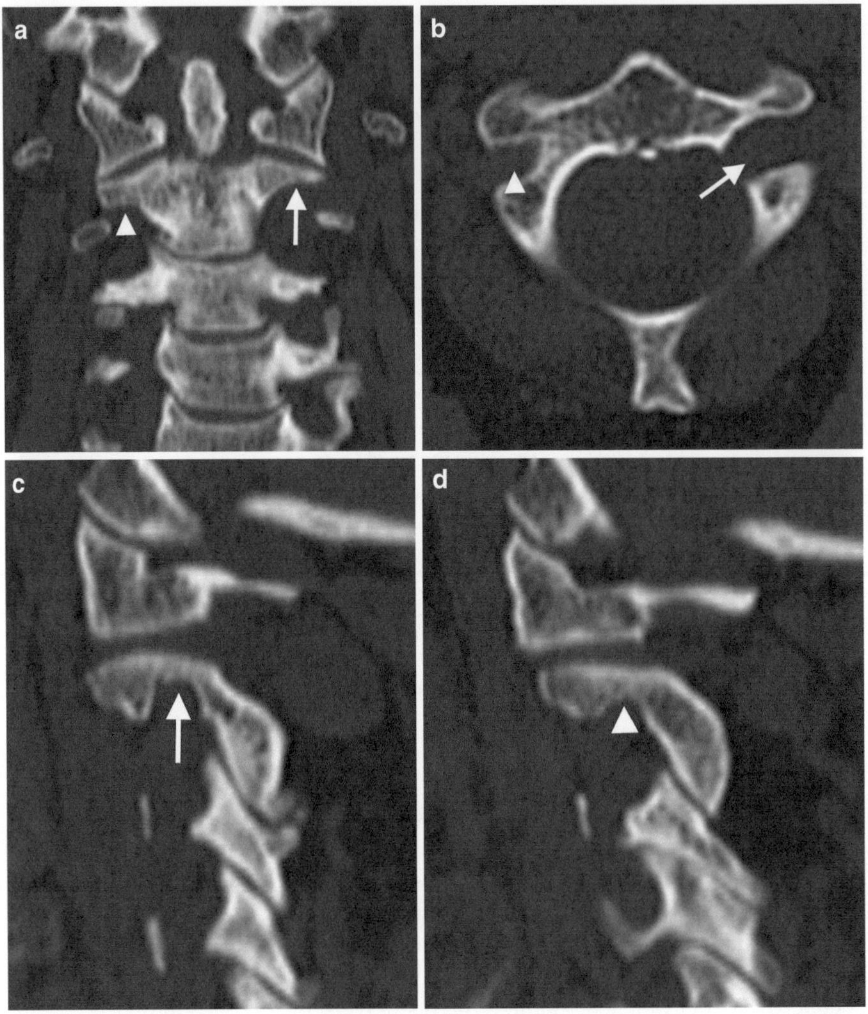

Fig. 2.10 High-riding left vertebral artery. The vertebral artery on the left side (arrow) makes an acute lateral bend at the base of C2 more cranially (**a**) and medially (**b**) than on the right side (arrowhead) narrowing the width (**b**) and height (**c**, abnormal left side; **d**, normal right side) of the isthmus and pedicle of the axis. (*With permission of Erasme Hospital, ULB*)

Posterior bridges are bony spicules that extend from the superior articular facet overhanging the dorsal arch. Partial and complete posterior bridges can be noted in 3.1% and 3.4% of the cases, respectively [74]. Lateral bridges correspond to bone extension from the C1 lateral masses to the transverse process. They have an incidence of 2% [74]. Posterolateral tunnels represent a combination of both posterior and lateral bridges noted in 1.1% of the cases [74]. Several factors influence the incidence of bridges such as age, sex, ethnicity, and type of work with laborers having a higher incidence of bony canal than non-laborers [75, 76].

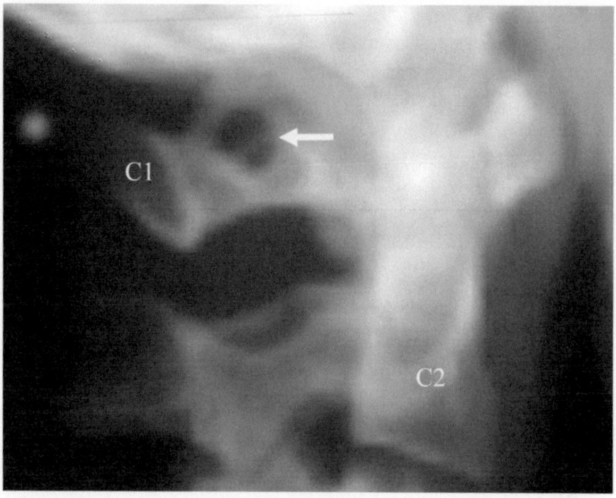

Fig. 2.11 C1 posterior arch turned into a tunnel. (*From George B, Bruneau M, Spetzler RF (eds). Pathology and surgery around the vertebral artery. Springer; 2011*)

Incomplete closure of the C1 posterior arch is another variation that is frequently encountered [11]. In this condition, the classical subperiosteal dissection must be done cautiously and is associated with increased risks.

The presence of an osseous anomaly at the CVJ is associated with a higher incidence of persistent first intersegmental artery, extracranial–extradural origin of the PICA, and high-riding VA [77]. Therefore, the risk for VA injury at surgery is increased. For this reason, in case of CVJ osseous anomaly, it is advised to perform preoperatively a CTA with 3D reconstruction to look for VA anomalies [11].

2.3 Conclusions

The normal anatomy of the suboccipital segment of the VA, as well as all variations, must be perfectly known before any procedure at the level of the craniovertebral junction. It must be remembered that the different portions of this segment are modified by head position. The VA at this level is located inside a periosteal sheath surrounded by a venous plexus.

References

1. George B, Blanquet A, Alves O. Surgical exposure of the vertebral artery. In: Spetzler RF, editor. Operative techniques in neurosurgery. Philadelphia: W.B. Saunders; 2001. p. 182–94.
2. Argenson C, Francke JP, Sylla S, et al. The vertebral arteries (segment V1 and V2). Anat Clin. 1980;2:29–41.
3. George B. Exposure of the upper cervical vertebral artery. In: Dickman CA, Spetzler RF, Sonntag VKH, editors. Surgery of the craniovertebral junction. New York: Thieme; 1998. p. 545–67.
4. Bruneau M, Cornelius JF, George B. Antero-lateral approach to the V3 segment of the vertebral artery. Oper Neurosurg. 2006;58:ONS–29–35. https://doi.org/10.1227/01.NEU.0000193930.74183.42.

5. George B, Cornelius J. Vertebral artery: surgical anatomy. In: Spetzler RF, editor. Operative techniques in neurosurgery. Philadelphia: W.B. Saunders; 2001. p. 168–81.
6. Bruneau M, George B. Surgical approaches to the V3 segment of the vertebral artery. In: George B, Bruneau M, Spetzler RF, editors. Pathology and surgery around the vertebral artery. Berlin: Springer; 2011. p. 329–60.
7. Bruneau M, George B. Surgical technique for the resection of tumors in relation with the V3 and V4 segments of the vertebral artery. In: George B, Bruneau M, Spetzler RF, editors. Pathology and surgery around the vertebral artery. Berlin: Springer; 2011. p. 361–404.
8. Peltier J, Toussaint P, Deramond H, et al. The dural crossing of the vertebral artery. Surg Radiol Anat. 2003;25:305–10. https://doi.org/10.1007/s00276-003-0139-5.
9. Ravindra VM, Neil JA, Mazur MD, et al. Motion-related vascular abnormalities at the craniocervical junction: illustrative case series and literature review. Neurosurg Focus. 2015;38:E6. https://doi.org/10.3171/2015.1.FOCUS14826.
10. Morimoto T, Nakase H, Sakaki T, Matsuyama T. Extrinsic compression Bow Hunter's stroke. In: George B, Bruneau M, Spetzler RF, editors. Pathology and surgery around the vertebral artery. Paris: Springer; 2011. p. 473–87.
11. Bruneau M, De Witte O, Regli L, George B. Anatomical variations. In: George B, Bruneau M, Spetzler RF, editors. Pathology and surgery around the vertebral artery. Paris: Springer; 2011. p. 53–74.
12. Krayenbühl H, Yasargil MG. Cerebral angiography. Stuttgart, NY: Georg Thieme Verlag; 1982.
13. Vaněk P, Bradáč O, Lacy P, et al. Vertebral artery and osseous anomalies characteristic at the craniocervical junction diagnosed by CT and 3D CT angiography in normal Czech population: analysis of 511 consecutive patients. Neurosurg Rev. 2017;40(3):369–76. https://doi.org/10.1007/s10143-016-0784-x.
14. Jeng JS, Yip PK. Evaluation of vertebral artery hypoplasia and asymmetry by color-coded duplex ultrasonography. Ultrasound Med Biol. 2004;30:605–9. https://doi.org/10.1016/j.ultrasmedbio.2004.03.004.
15. Touboul PJ, Bousser MG, LaPlane D, Castaigne P. Duplex scanning of normal vertebral arteries. Stroke. 1986;17:921–3.
16. Francke JP, Di Marino V, Pannier M, et al. Les artères vertébrales, segments atlanto-axo V3 et intracrânien V4. In French. Anat Clin. 1980;2:229–42.
17. Park JH, Kim JM, Roh JK. Hypoplastic vertebral artery: frequency and associations with ischaemic stroke territory. J Neurol Neurosurg Psychiatry. 2007;78:954–8. https://doi.org/10.1136/jnnp.2006.105767.
18. Matula C, Trattnig S, Tschabitscher M, et al. The course of the prevertebral segment of the vertebral artery: anatomy and clinical significance. Surg Neurol. 1997;48:125–31.
19. Chuang YM, Huang YC, Hu HH, Yang CY. Toward a further elucidation: role of vertebral artery hypoplasia in acute ischemic stroke. Eur Neurol. 2006;55:193–7. https://doi.org/10.1159/000093868.
20. Lovrencic-Huzjan A, Demarin V, Bosnar M, et al. Color Doppler flow imaging (CDFI) of the vertebral arteries—the normal appearance, normal values and the proposal for the standards. Coll Antropol. 1999;23:175–81.
21. Cagnie B, Barbaix E, Vinck E, et al. A vertebral artery without Atlantic and intradural sections: a case report and a review of the literature. Ann Anat. 2005;187:271–5. https://doi.org/10.1016/j.aanat.2004.10.003.
22. Cagnie B, Barbaix E, Vinck E, et al. Extrinsic risk factors for compromised blood flow in the vertebral artery: anatomical observations of the transverse foramina from C3 to C7. Surg Radiol Anat. 2005;27:312–6. https://doi.org/10.1007/s00276-005-0006-7.
23. Min JH, Lee YS. Transcranial Doppler ultrasonographic evaluation of vertebral artery hypoplasia and aplasia. J Neurol Sci. 2007;260:183–7. https://doi.org/10.1016/j.jns.2007.05.001.
24. Burger IM, Siclari F, Gregg L, Gailloud P. Bilateral segmental agenesis of the vertebrobasilar junction: developmental and angiographic anatomy. Am J Neuroradiol. 2007;28:2017–22. https://doi.org/10.3174/ajnr.A0719.

25. Uchino A, Saito N, Watadani T, et al. Vertebral artery variations at the C1-2 level diagnosed by magnetic resonance angiography. Neuroradiology. 2012;54:19–23. https://doi.org/10.1007/s00234-011-0849-z.
26. Fine AD, Cardoso A, Rhoton AL. Microsurgical anatomy of the extracranial-extradural origin of the posterior inferior cerebellar artery. J Neurosurg. 1999;91:645–52. https://doi.org/10.3171/jns.1999.91.4.0645.
27. Lasjaunias P, Vallee B, Person H, et al. The lateral spinal artery of the upper cervical spinal cord. Anatomy, normal variations, and angiographic aspects. J Neurosurg. 1985;63:235–41. https://doi.org/10.3171/jns.1985.63.2.0235.
28. Salas E, Ziyal IM, Bank WO, et al. Extradural origin of the posteroinferior cerebellar artery: an anatomic study with histological and radiographic correlation. Neurosurgery. 1998;42:1326–31.
29. Pekcevik Y, Pekcevik R. Variations of the cerebellar arteries at CT angiography. Surg Radiol Anat. 2013;36:455–61. https://doi.org/10.1007/s00276-013-1208-z.
30. Thayer WP, Gaughen JR, Harthun NL. Surgical revascularization in the presence of a preserved primitive carotid-basilar communication. J Vasc Surg. 2005;41:1066–9. https://doi.org/10.1016/j.jvs.2005.03.004.
31. Lasjaunias P, Berenstein A, Ter Brugge KG. Surgical neuroangiography. 2nd ed. Berlin: Springer-Verlag; 2001.
32. Purkayastha S, Gupta AK, Varma R, Kapilamoorthy TR. Proatlantal intersegmental arteries of external carotid artery origin associated with Galen's vein malformation. Am J Neuroradiol. 2005;26:2378–83.
33. Pasco A, Papon X, Bracard S, et al. Persistent carotid-vertebrobasilar anastomoses: how and why differentiating them? J Neuroradiol. 2004;31:391–6.
34. Bahsi YZ, Uysal H, Peker S, Yurdakul M. Persistent primitive proatlantal intersegmental artery (proatlantal artery I) results in "top of the basilar" syndrome. Stroke. 1993;24:2114–7.
35. Hutchinson NA, Miller JD. Persistent proatlantal artery. J Neurol Neurosurg Psychiatry. 1970;33:524–7.
36. Woodcock RJ, Cloft HJ, Dion JE. Bilateral type 1 proatlantal arteries with absence of vertebral arteries. Am J Neuroradiol. 2001;22:418–20.
37. Gumus T, Onal B, Ilgit ET. Bilateral persistence of type 1 proatlantal arteries: report of a case and review of the literature. Am J Neuroradiol. 2004;25:1622–4.
38. Kurose K, Kishi H, Nishijima Y. Type 2 proatlantal artery associated with a ruptured aneurysm—case report. Neurolo Med Chir (Tokyo). 1990;30:191–3.
39. Lui CC, Liu YH, Wai YY, Tsai CC. Persistence of both proatlantal arteries with absence of vertebral arteries. Neuroradiology. 1987;29:304–5.
40. Tsai FY, Mahon J, Woodruff JV, Roach JF. Congenital absence of bilateral vertebral arteries with occipital-basilar anastomosis. Am J Roentgenol Radium Ther Nucl Med. 1975;124:281–6.
41. Ionete C, Omojola MF. MR angiographic demonstration of bilateral duplication of the extracranial vertebral artery: unusual course and review of the literature. Am J Neuroradiol. 2006;27:1304–6.
42. Kowada M, Kikuchi K. Symmetrical extracranial fenestrations of the vertebral artery. Two cases revealed by angiography. Radiology. 1979;131:408. https://doi.org/10.1148/131.2.408.
43. Kowada M, Takahashi M, Tamakawa Y, et al. Fenestration of the basilar and vertebral arteries. In: Kitamura HNT, editor. Recent advances in diagnostic neuroradiology. Tokyo: Igakushoin; 1975. p. 144–9.
44. Kowada M, Takahashi M, Gito Y, Kishikawa T. Fenestration of the vertebral artery: report of 2 cases demonstrated by angiography. Neuroradiology. 1973;6:110–2.
45. Kowada M, Yamaguchi K, Takahashi H. Fenestration of the vertebral artery with a review of 23 cases in Japan. Radiology. 1972;103:343–6. https://doi.org/10.1148/103.2.343.
46. Kowada M, Yamaguchi K, Takahashi H, et al. A case of two fenestrations of the vertebral artery. Brain Nerve. 1970;22:469–72.
47. Carella A, Lamberti P, Federico F, Andreula CF. Double fenestration of the extracranial vertebral artery. Neuroradiology. 1978;15(3):193–4.

48. Sim E, Vaccaro AR, Berzlanovich A, et al. Fenestration of the extracranial vertebral artery: review of the literature. Spine. 2001;26:E139–42.
49. Lasjaunias PL, Berenstein A. Craniofacial and upper cervical arteries: collateral circulations and angiographic protocols. Baltimore/London: Williams and Wilkins; 1983.
50. Lasjaunias P, Braun JP, Hasso AN, et al. True and false fenestration of the vertebral artery. J Neuroradiol. 1980;7:157–66.
51. Hong JT, Lee SW, Son BC, et al. Analysis of anatomical variations of bone and vascular structures around the posterior atlantal arch using three-dimensional computed tomography angiography. J Neurosurg Spine. 2008;8:230–6. https://doi.org/10.3171/SPI/2008/8/3/230.
52. Yamazaki M, Okawa A, Furuya T, et al. Anomalous vertebral arteries in the extra- and intraosseous regions of the craniovertebral junction visualized by 3-dimensional computed tomographic angiography. Spine. 2012;37:E1389–97. https://doi.org/10.1097/BRS.0b013e31826a0c9f.
53. Takahashi M, Kawanami H, Watanabe N, Matsuoka S. Fenestration of the extra-cranial vertebral artery. Radiology. 1970;96:359–60. https://doi.org/10.1148/96.2.359.
54. Tokuda K, Miyasaka K, Abe H, et al. Anomalous atlantoaxial portions of vertebral and posterior inferior cerebellar arteries. Neuroradiology. 1985;27:410–3.
55. Sato K, Watanabe T, Yoshimoto T, Kameyama M. Magnetic resonance imaging of C2 segmental type of vertebral artery. Surg Neurol. 1994;41:45–51.
56. Jian FZ, Santoro A, Wang XW, et al. A vertebral artery tortuous course below the posterior arch of the atlas (without passing through the transverse foramen). Anatomical report and clinical significance. J Neurosurg Sci. 2003;47:183–7.
57. Hotta S, Morita A, Seichi A, Kirino T. Aberrant vertebral artery course in a case of Chiari malformation and occipitoatlantal assimilation. Case report. J Neurosurg Spine. 2005;3:246–8. https://doi.org/10.3171/spi.2005.3.3.0246.
58. Sharma RR, Parekh HC, Prabhu S, et al. Compression of the C-2 root by a rare anomalous ectatic vertebral artery. Case report. J Neurosurg. 1993;78:669–72. https://doi.org/10.3171/jns.1993.78.4.0669.
59. Yano K, Murase S, Kuroda T, et al. Cervical cord compression by the vertebral artery causing a severe cervical pain: case report. Surg Neurol. 1993;40:43–6.
60. Satoh S, Yamamoto N, Kitagawa Y, et al. Cervical cord compression by the anomalous vertebral artery presenting with neuralgic pain. Case report. J Neurosurg. 1993;79:283–5. https://doi.org/10.3171/jns.1993.79.2.0283.
61. Morikawa K, Ohkawa N, Yamashita S. Surgical decompression for the C-1 and C-2 sensory roots and upper cervical cord in a case with cervical myelopathy and occipital neuralgia due to bilateral fenestration of vertebral artery: a case report. No Shinkei Geka. 1993;21:1035–8.
62. Kitagawa M, Nakagawa Y, Kitaoka K, et al. Accessory nerve paralysis due to compression of the fenestrated vertebral artery. No Shinkei Geka. 1988;16:1173–7.
63. Hasegawa T, Kubota T, Ito H, Yamamoto S. Symptomatic duplication of the vertebral artery. Surg Neurol. 1983;20:244–8.
64. Furumoto T, Nagase J, Takahashi K, et al. Cervical myelopathy caused by the anomalous vertebral artery. A case report. Spine. 1996;21:2280–3.
65. Ashley WW, Chicoine MR. Subarachnoid hemorrhage caused by posterior inferior cerebellar artery aneurysm with an anomalous course of the atlantoaxial segment of the vertebral artery. Case report and review of literature. J Neurosurg. 2005;103:356–60. https://doi.org/10.3171/jns.2005.103.2.0356.
66. Neo M, Matsushita M, Iwashita Y, et al. Atlantoaxial transarticular screw fixation for a high-riding vertebral artery. Spine. 2003;28:666–70. https://doi.org/10.1097/01.BRS.0000051919.14927.57.
67. Wakao N, Takeuchi M, Nishimura M, et al. Vertebral artery variations and osseous anomaly at the C1-2 level diagnosed by 3D CT angiography in normal subjects. Neuroradiology. 2014;56:843–9. https://doi.org/10.1007/s00234-014-1399-y.
68. Paramore CG, Dickman CA, Sonntag VK. The anatomical suitability of the C1-2 complex for transarticular screw fixation. J Neurosurg. 1996;85:221–4. https://doi.org/10.3171/jns.1996.85.2.0221.

69. Mandel IM, Kambach BJ, Petersilge CA, et al. Morphologic considerations of C2 isthmus dimensions for the placement of transarticular screws. Spine. 2000;25:1542–7.
70. Song GS, Theodore N, Dickman CA, Sonntag VK. Unilateral posterior atlantoaxial transarticular screw fixation. J Neurosurg. 1997;87:851–5. https://doi.org/10.3171/jns.1997.87.6.0851.
71. Kazan S, Yildirim F, Sindel M, Tuncer R. Anatomical evaluation of the groove for the vertebral artery in the axis vertebrae for atlanto-axial transarticular screw fixation technique. Clin Anat. 2000;13:237–43. https://doi.org/10.1002/1098-2353(2000)13:4<237::AID-CA2>3.0.CO;2-K.
72. Madawi AA, Casey AT, Solanki GA, et al. Radiological and anatomical evaluation of the atlantoaxial transarticular screw fixation technique. J Neurosurg. 1997;86:961–8. https://doi.org/10.3171/jns.1997.86.6.0961.
73. Gupta T. Quantitative anatomy of vertebral artery groove on the posterior arch of atlas in relation to spinal surgical procedures. Surg Radiol Anat. 2008;30:239–42. https://doi.org/10.1007/s00276-008-0313-x.
74. Hasan M, Shukla S, Siddiqui MS, Singh D. Posterolateral tunnels and ponticuli in human atlas vertebrae. J Anat. 2001;199:339–43.
75. Paraskevas G, Papaziogas B, Tsonidis C, Kapetanos G. Gross morphology of the bridges over the vertebral artery groove on the atlas. Surg Radiol Anat. 2005;27:129–36. https://doi.org/10.1007/s00276-004-0300-9.
76. Mitchell J. The incidence of the lateral bridge of the atlas vertebra. J Anat. 1998;193(Pt 2):283–5.
77. Yamazaki M, Koda M, Aramomi M-A, et al. Anomalous vertebral artery at the extraosseous and intraosseous regions of the craniovertebral junction: analysis by three-dimensional computed tomography angiography. Spine. 2005;30:2452–7.

Radiological Assessment of the Craniovertebral Junction

3

Mario Muto, Francesco Giurazza, Carlo Augusto Mallio, Gianluigi Guarnieri, and Roberto Izzo

3.1 Introduction

The craniocervical junction (CCJ) is the transition from the head to the spine, and it carries peculiar anatomical and biomechanical properties in order to dispatch its primary function: ensure a wide mobility of the head for space exploration both visual and auditory in all the three axes.

It is designed to reconcile seemingly opposed necessities being at same time loose enough to allow a great variety of movements and strong enough to preserve the spinal cord and vertebral arteries and to resist the head weight and muscular action.

Occiput, atlas, and *axis* are the three bony elements that form the CCJ, with atlas representing the connecting pivot between the occipital-atlas joint and the atlas-axial joint.

From a radiological point of view, it is crucial to understand the unique atlas anatomy in order to quickly assess a first-look evaluation. Atlas has two peculiar aspects: it presents neither an intervertebral disc nor an anterior vertebral body; therefore, it is "simply" a ring-shaped bone made by two arches, anterior and posterior, connecting two lateral masses. These paired lateral masses articulate superiorly with the condyles of the occiput and inferiorly with the superior articular processes of the axis. Furthermore, the joint composed by the posterior articular facet of the anterior atlas arch and the anterior profile of the odontoid process of the axis should always be evaluated. Finally each lateral mass of atlas presents a groove where the V3 segment of the vertebral artery runs just before entering the foramen magnum.

M. Muto (✉) · G. Guarnieri · R. Izzo
AORN Cardarelli, Naples, Italy

F. Giurazza · C. A. Mallio
Università Campus Bio-Medico di Roma, Rome, Italy
e-mail: c.mallio@unicampus.it

E. Tessitore et al. (eds.), *Surgery of the Cranio-Vertebral Junction*,
https://doi.org/10.1007/978-3-030-18700-2_3

So an initial radiological assessment of the CCJ should be based on a threefold look of atlas: lateral mass articulations both superior and inferior, anterior arch joint with odontoid process, and vertebral artery grooves. All these elements need to be evaluated by computed tomography (CT) with thin layer reconstructions (Fig. 3.1).

The three abovementioned bony structures are linked by multiple ligaments, intrinsic and extrinsic.

Certainly the three intrinsic ligaments of the CCJ represent the most important stabilizers: odontoid ligament, cruciate ligament, and tectorial membrane.

- The *odontoid ligament* is composed of three structures: the alar ligaments, paired lateral elements from the posterolateral surface of the odontoid process to the medial margin of the occipital condyles (Fig. 3.2), the apical ligament, and single anterior element from the tip of the odontoid process to the anterior margin of the foramen magnum (Figs. 3.3 and 3.4).
- The *cruciate ligaments* is composed of three structures: the transverse ligament, the strongest one, connecting just behind the odontoid process, the opposite posterior segments of the anterior atlas arch each other, thus dividing the atlas ring in an anterior compartment including the odontoid process, and a posterior compartment including the thecal sac (Figs. 3.1 and 3.2); the crus superioris, a median

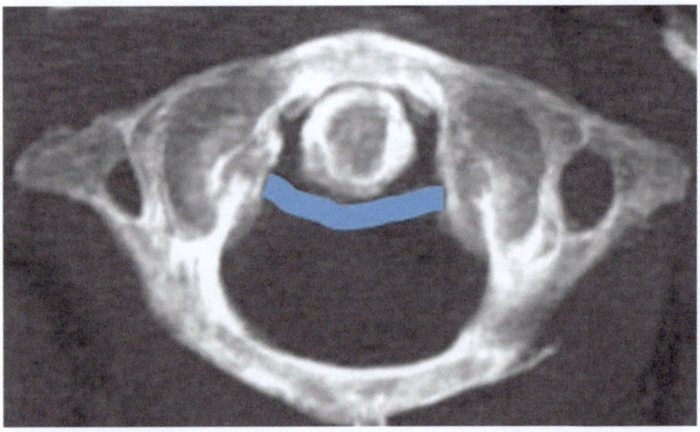

Fig. 3.1 CT scan with 1 mm slice thickness, axial MIP reconstruction: the blue line represents the transverse ligament. Atlas transverse foramina, articular facets for the occipital condyles, and the odontoid process are clearly appreciable

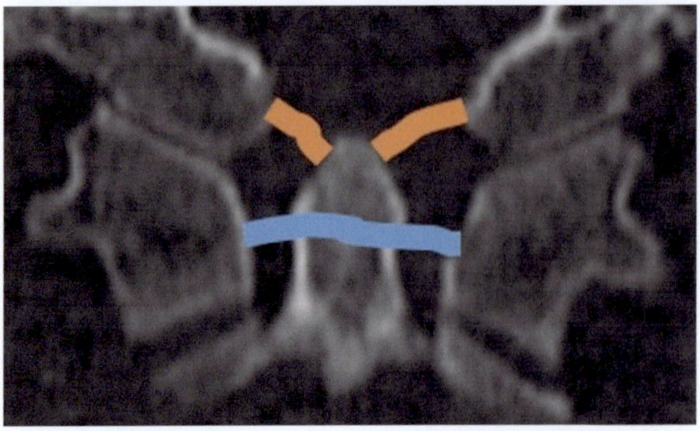

Fig. 3.2 CT scan with 1 mm slice thickness, coronal MPR reconstruction: the orange lines represent the alar ligaments and the blue line the transverse ligament. The odontoid process is visualized in its long axis

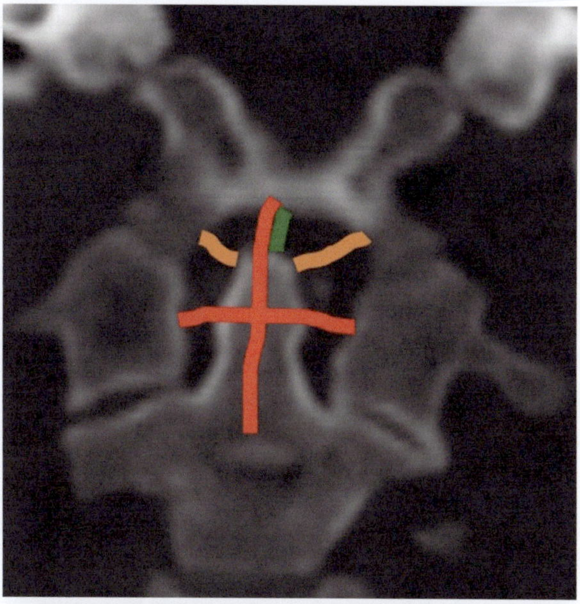

Fig. 3.3 CT scan with 1 mm slice thickness, coronal oblique MPR reconstruction: the orange lines represent the alar ligaments, the green line the apical ligament, and the red line the cruciate ligament. The odontoid process is visualized in its long axis

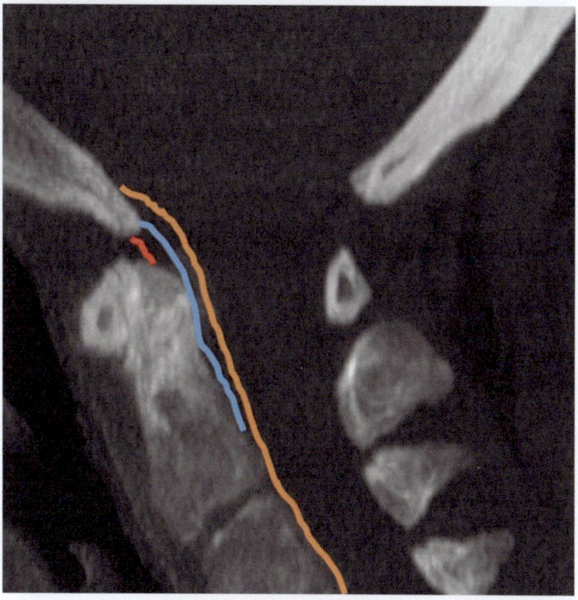

Fig. 3.4 CT scan with 1 mm slice thickness, sagittal MIP reconstruction: the orange line represents the tectorial membrane, the blue line the superior and inferior crus of the cruciate ligament, and the red line the apical ligament

cranial extension of the transverse ligament attaching to the lower margin of the occipital bone; the crus inferioris, a median caudal extension of the transverse ligament attaching to the posterior surface of the axis body (Figs. 3.3 and 3.4).

– The *tectorial membrane* is the cranial continuation of the posterior vertebral longitudinal ligament running from the posterior surface of the body of axis, passing behind the cruciate ligament and attaching on the anterior margin of the foramen magnum (Fig. 3.4).

The occipital-atlas joint is mainly responsible of the flexion-extension movements: the flexion is restricted by the odontoid process, blocking the anterior margin of the foramen magnum while the extension is limited by traction of the tectorial membrane.

The atlas-axis joint is mainly responsible for the rotational movements: the transverse portion of the cruciate ligaments stabilize the rotation while the alar portions of the odontoid ligaments limit the rotation.

So, in terms of radiological assessment of the stability of the CCJ, the evaluation should focus on tectorial membrane, odontoid process, and anterior margin of foramen magnum about the flexion-extension movements related to the occipital-atlas joint; and transverse and alar ligaments about the rotational movements related to the atlas-axial joint.

All these elements need to be evaluated by high-field magnetic resonance imaging (MRI) with thin slice acquisitions (Figs. 3.5, 3.6 and 3.7).

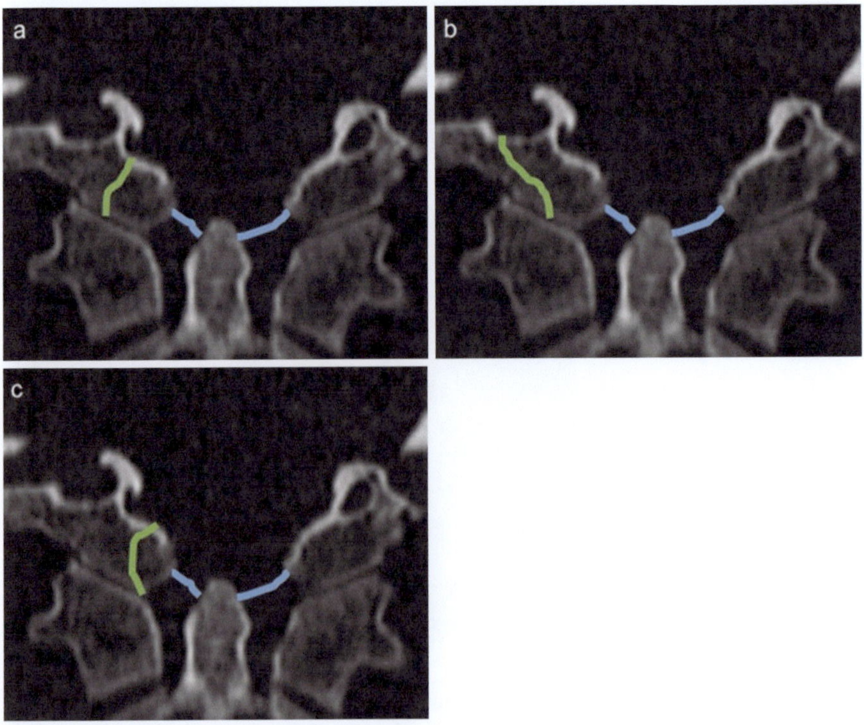

Fig. 3.5 CT scan with 1 mm slice thickness, coronal MPR reconstruction: occipital condylar fractures according to the classification described by Anderson and Montesano (**a** = type 1, **b** = type 2, **c** = type 3); the blue lines represent the alar ligaments, the green line the course of fracture

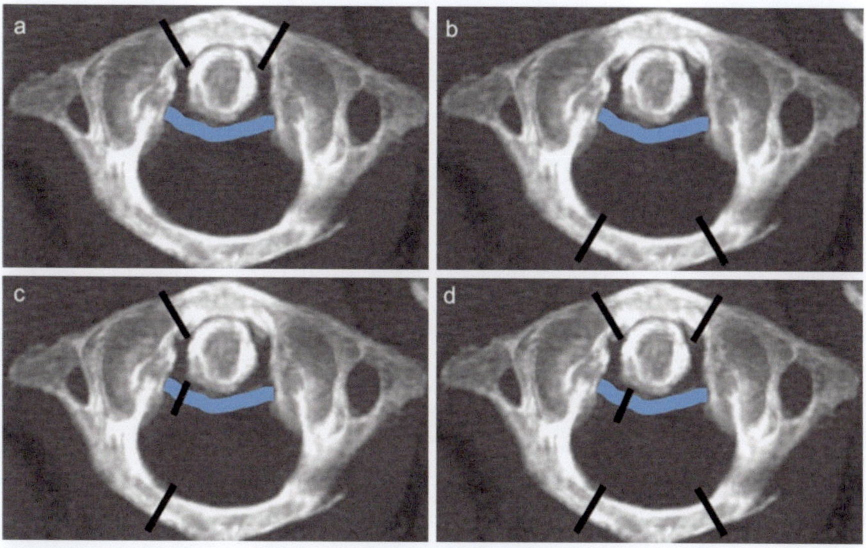

Fig. 3.6 CT scan with 1 mm slice thickness, axial MIP reconstruction: atlas fractures according to the classification described by Jefferson (**a** = anterior arch fracture, **b** = posterior arch fracture, **c** = lateral mass fracture, **d** = burst fracture); the black lines represent the course of fracture, and the blue line the transverse ligament

Thirty percent of all cervical spine injuries occurs at the CCJ, mainly related to motor vehicle accidents [1]; in the past these lesions frequently led patients to death on place. Nowadays the management of this kind of injuries has improved, and this is why lesions affecting the CCJ are more and more encountered in the daily practice in emergency departments.

Furthermore anatomical variants of this district can frequently be observed because of different embryologic developments [2].

The surgical approach to the CCJ, especially with the developing of modern less invasive techniques, requires a clear and accurate preoperative assessment of the anatomy of this area, including bones, ligaments, and also vascular structures [3].

In this scenario, role of imaging is not only to recognize the lesion or the anatomical variants but also to support the surgeon in the choice of the correct treatment planning.

3.2 Imaging in Trauma

Thanks to the spread of CT systems in almost all the emergency departments in Western countries, conventional radiography should not be applied anymore in case of cervical injuries. Furthermore, the continuous technological progress allows to obtain fast acquisitions with thin layer and reformatted multiplanar imaging [4, 5].

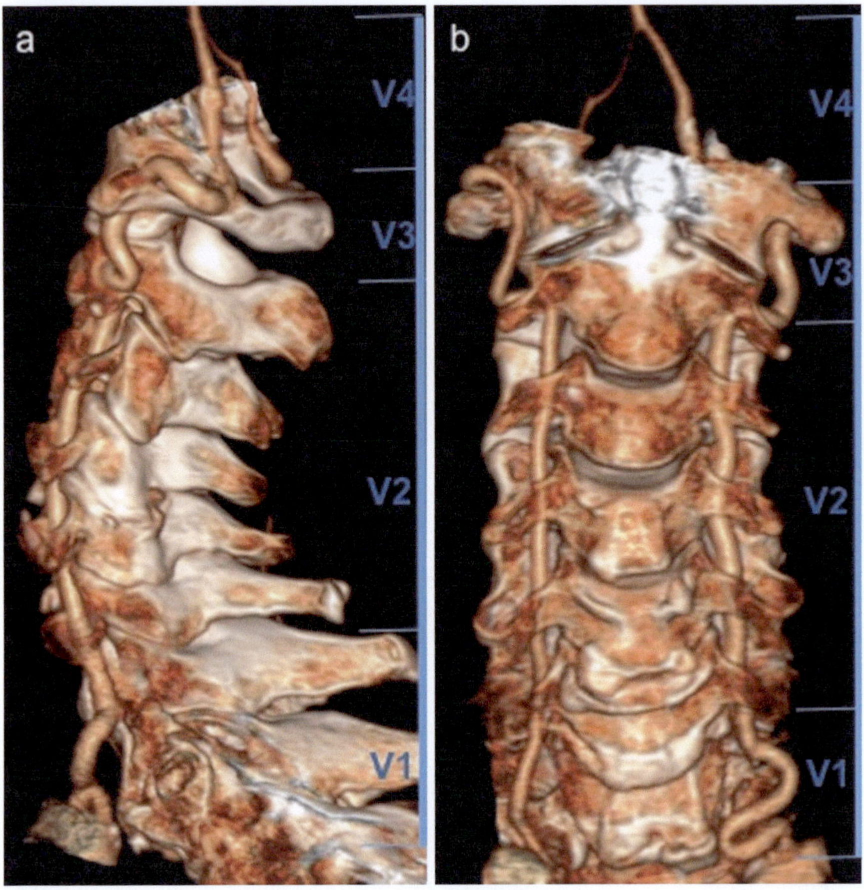

Fig. 3.7 Contrast-enhanced CT scan with 0.6 mm slice thickness, 3D reconstruction: standard vertebral artery segmentation in four parts in lateral (**a**) and anterior (**b**) view

Actually the radiological gold standard for the first approach evaluation in case of acute cervical trauma is represented by multiplanar CT imaging with almost 1.25 mm thickness [6]. The new viewer softwares allow radiologists to quickly modify the standard imaging acquisitions with different reformatting tools, such as MultiPlanar Reconstruction (MPR), Maximum Intensity Projection (MIP), and 3D imaging. MPR produces 2D images in any plane of the space in order to choose the best 2D visualization based on the lesion site; MIP is used to improve the sense of depth of the original data; 3D is a bit longer computational process, mainly applied to obtain a panoramic view of a district that will be faced by the surgeon; these softwares also allow to erase part of the imaging not of interest in order to highlight the target (e.g., deleting bony or vascular segments that cover an underlying lesion).

The second step is MR. This is required to detect soft tissue lesions, in particular spinal cord. Today, with high-field magnet (almost 1.5 Tesla) and thin slice acquisitions, it is also possible to assess the joint stability by evaluating the intrinsic ligaments:

dedicated protocols are required, especially applying T2-weighted and GRE sequences where normal ligaments appear as linear homogeneously hypointense structures and lesions are characterized by areas of heterogeneous signal intensity [7]. As for CT scan, MPR softwares are available for isometric thin slice MR acquisitions.

In the trauma scenario, the lesion pattern depends mainly on the following elements: the intensity and the direction of the force hitting the CCJ as well as the position of the junction itself; when available, these elements greatly support the radiologist in the diagnostic process. On the other hand, the radiologist can reconstruct the dynamic of the trauma on the basis of imaging findings [8].

3.2.1 Imaging in Joint Dislocations

3.2.1.1 Occipital-Atlas Dissociation

High energy trauma, especially occurring after motorbike accidents, frequently cause extreme hyperextension of the CCJ causing lesions of the tectorial membrane and alar ligaments. These kinds of lesions, presenting in approximately 30% of motor vehicle accidents, produce occipital-atlas dissociation which is a lesion with high mortality rate because of brainstem involvement [9]. Bone lesions may not be present because the occipital-atlas joint is stabilized mainly by ligaments rather than osseous contacts; however, sometimes condylar avulsion fractures can be associated because of alar ligaments traction.

Three types of occipital-atlas dissociation are classified:

- I. Ventral dislocation of the occipital bone, it is the most frequent.
- II. Longitudinal distraction of the occipital bone, it is more dangerous being more unstable.
- III. Posterior dislocation of the occipital bone.

The first evaluation is performed with CT in sagittal plane: an imaging accepted criteria to diagnose occipital-atlas dissociation is to measure a distance >10 mm between the anterior margin of the foramen magnum and the odontoid process [10]. Condylar fracture must be detected as well in the other planes.

After diagnosis at CT evaluation, MR is imperative in order to assess injuries of the spinal cord and lower cranial nerves; finally tectorial membrane and alar ligaments not appreciable at CT should be analyzed at MR. Indeed these evaluations may lead the surgeon to choose a treatment of internal fixation.

3.2.1.2 Atlas-Axis Distraction

This is a challenging condition to evaluate because of the heterogeneous spectrum that the radiologist can observe; indeed the distance between atlas and axis can amply vary on the basis of patient age [11]. Moreover, after trauma, the lesion can be symmetric and so more difficult to appreciate. It must be taken into account that the atlas-axial joint is the most mobile of the spine because of the flat morphology of the articular facet essential to allow wide movement excursion.

In case of trauma, especially secondary to hyperflexion and hyperotation, lesions of the alar ligaments can occur and lead to rotatory atlas-axial subluxation; it is prevalent in children because the facets are even more shallow.

Rotatory atlas-axial subluxation can occur even in nontraumatic conditions: this is named Grisel syndrome and occurs especially in children affected by pathological ligamentous laxity (e.g., Down or Marfan syndromes). In this case, to diagnose Grisel syndrome, CT evaluation is not enough, and clinical assessment is required.

3.2.2 Imaging in Fractures

3.2.2.1 Fractures of the Occipital Condyles

Fractures of the occipital condyles are distinguished according to two classifications: from Anderson and Montesano [12, 13] and from Tuli [14].

The classification from Anderson and Montesano presents three types of lesions (Fig. 3.8):

- I. Comminuted fracture of the condyle without foramen magnum involvement, related to compression injuries
- II. Linear fracture of the skull with the involvement of the occipital condyle, related to direct head injuries
- III. Fracture with avulsion of the occipital condyle, related to alar ligaments injuries.

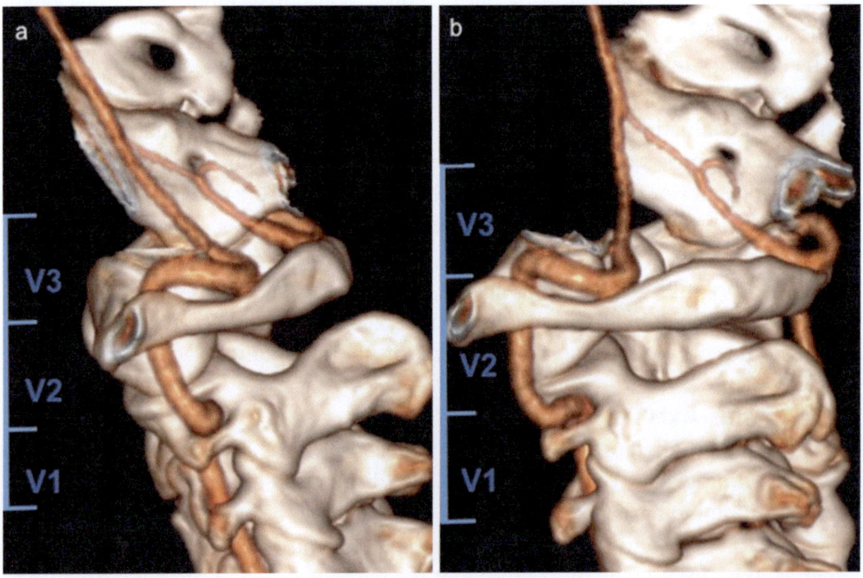

Fig. 3.8 Contrast-enhanced CT scan with 0.6 mm slice thickness, 3D reconstruction: vertebral artery segmentation in relationship to C1–C2 vertebrae from C3 transverse foramina to the point of its dural entry according to Cacciola et al. in lateral (**a**) and posterolateral (**b**) view

The classification from Thuli presents two types:

- I. Fractures without fragment displacement
- II. Fractures with fragment displacement, to be distinguished in stable (IIa) and unstable (IIb) according to ligaments involvements.

The benefit from Thuli classification is that it clearly indicates the treatment strategy: types I and IIa fractures are managed with a rigid collar, and type IIb fractures require surgery.

In all these conditions, CT is required to detect condyle fractures; in Anderson and Montesano type III as well as Thuli type II injuries, MR is essential to investigate ligaments involvement and assess joint stability/instability.

3.2.2.2 Fractures of Atlas (C1)

Atlas is a ring-shaped bone with paired lateral masses and thin anterior and posterior arches; therefore, the arches are the more fragile structures and more frequently ruptured in case of trauma. Because of the morphology, the fractures occur in more than one point.

These lesions are also called Jefferson fractures, according to the classification that this author proposed into four types (Fig. 3.9):

- I. Anterior arch fracture, related to hyperflexion injuries
- II. Posterior arch fracture, related to hyperextension injuries
- III. Lateral mass fracture, related to lateral hyperflexion injuries
- IV. Burst fractures with the involvement of anterior and/or posterior arches and lateral masses, related to excessive axial load to the skull

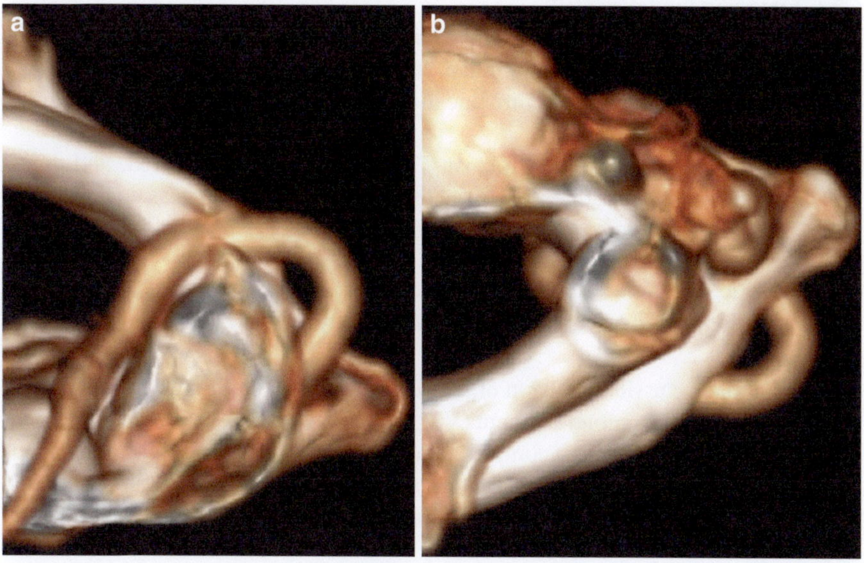

Fig. 3.9 Contrast-enhanced CT scan with 0.6 mm slice thickness, 3D reconstruction: vertebral artery loop in relation to the transverse foramina and posterior arch of C1 (**a**) and C2 (**b**)

While anterior and posterior isolated fractures are stable, lateral mass and burst fractures are frequently unstable because these lesions may involve the transverse ligament; if the transverse ligament is injured, the odontoid process is free to displace posteriorly with consequent pressure on the thecal sac and injury of the encephalic trunk [15].

As well as in the case of condyle fractures, CT must be performed in the first instance in order to detect the fracture lines; a quick way to assess lateral mass involvement is to reconstruct thin slice CT in the coronal plane and search for external dislocation of atlas lateral mass compared to the axis body.

Then MR in case of lateral mass or burst fractures must be acquired in order to detect transverse ligament involvement and direct patient to surgery.

3.2.2.3 Fractures of Axis (C2)

An overflow of classifications of axis fractures is present in literature [16]. To approach this issue in a schematic and practical way, three main groups of lesions depending on the anatomical area involved can be considered: the odontoid process, the Hangman's fracture (both pedicles), and miscellaneous (non-odontoid and non-Hangman's fractures).

The traditional classification of odontoid fractures is the one proposed by Anderson and D'Alonzo into three types [17]: (I) apical dens fracture, (II) base of the dens fracture, and (III) fracture involving any part of the dens and extending into the body of the axis. These may be due to different kind of trauma, related to hyperflexion, hyperextension, and axial load. Type II has been subdivided by Roy-Camille according to the inclination of the fracture line into four more subtypes [18]: (II1) anterior, (II2) posterior, (II3) lateral, and (II4) rotational.

The Hangman's fracture presents three injury patterns with increasing severity: displacement of C2 over C3, angulation of C2 over C3, and involvement of the C2-C3 intervertebral disc [19].

The non-odontoid and non-Hangman's fractures include a wide range of lesions affecting the body, lateral mass, laminae, and spinous processes. Body fractures are classified on the basis of the fracture line in three types [20]: (I) coronal, (II) sagittal, and (III) transverse.

All these lesions require multiplanar CT imaging to be recognized, and this is crucial for subsequent treatment: displaced and angulated fractures as well fractures with C2-C3 disc disruption require surgery.

3.3 Imaging in Vascular Anatomy: The Vertebral Artery

According to the classical division of the vertebral artery into four parts (Fig. 3.10), the last portion of the second segment (V2) and the third segment (V3) show serpentine flow in CCJ and present a complex relation with atlas and axis. Detailed knowledge of the anatomy and course of this artery before attempting surgery at the posterior fossa and CCJ is mandatory, especially when approaching with a lateral access; indeed an injury of vertebral artery would represent a catastrophic event.

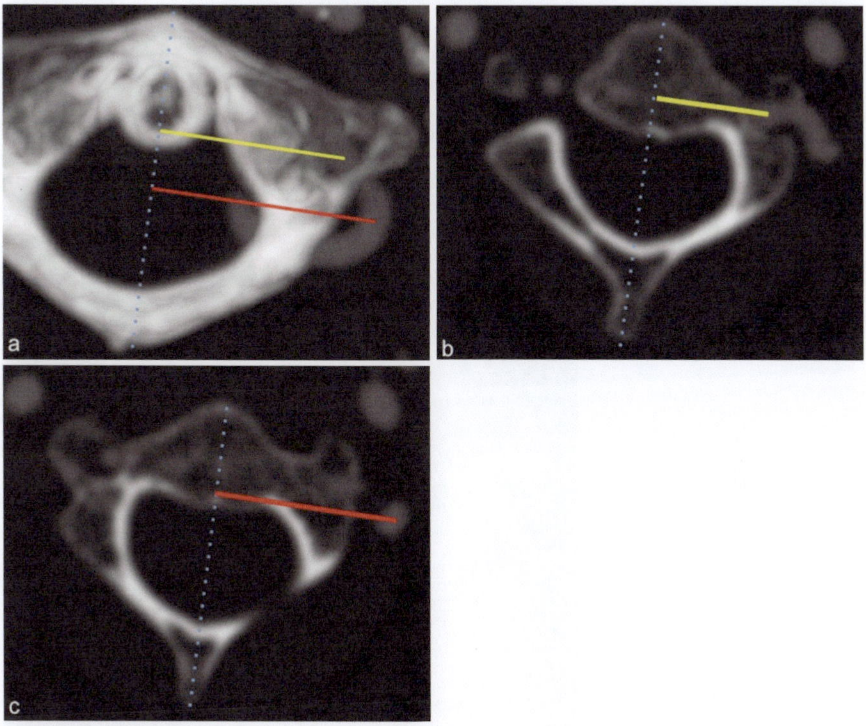

Fig. 3.10 Contrast-enhanced CT scan with 0.6 mm slice thickness, axial MIP reconstruction (**a**), and standard axial imaging (**b**, **c**): distances from the point of vertebral artery transverse foramen exit (yellow line in **a** and **b**) and from the midpoint of vertebral artery V2 segment loop (red line in **a** and **c**) to the midline (blue dotted line in **a**, **b**, and **c**)

Furthermore, vertebral artery injuries associated with cervical trauma occur in V2 and V3 in more than 80% of the cases [21].

A recent classification of this vascular area detailed the vertebral artery from its course from the C3 transverse foramen to the C2 transverse foramina as V1, the artery during its course from C2 transverse foramina to C1 transverse foramina as V2, and the artery in its course from the transverse foramen of C1 to the point of its dural entry as V3 segment (Fig. 3.11) [22].

Reliable landmarks could facilitate safe exposure and identification of the artery and the role of the radiologist should support the surgeon in analyzing these aspects (Fig. 3.12).

Certainly CT angiography images has rapidly improved in the last two decades, especially thanks to fast acquisitions and postprocessing techniques, including maximal intensity projection, multiplanar reconstruction, and three-dimensional volume rendering; as already mentioned above, CT allows even an optimal evaluation of the bone structures, and because of this, it is considered the radiological technique of choice in this issue to analyze bony and arterial structures together.

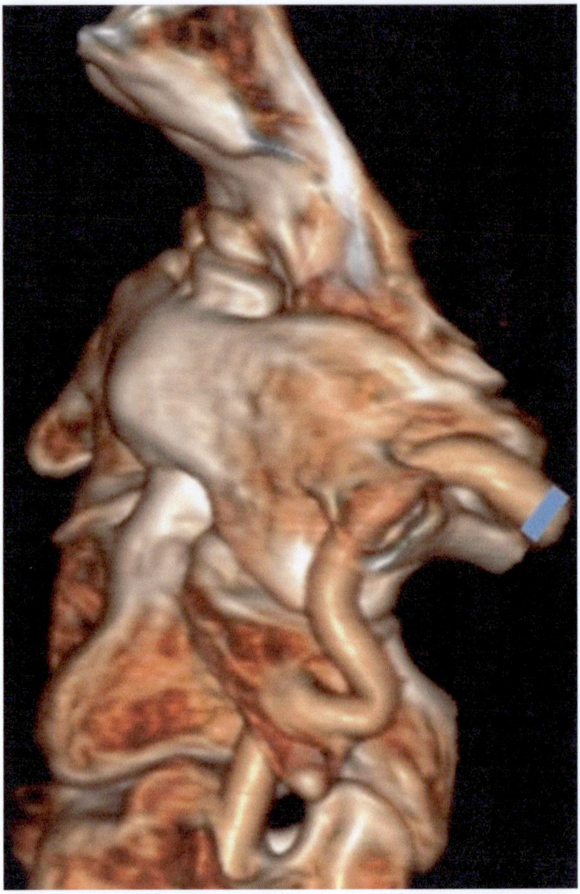

Fig. 3.11 Contrast-enhanced CT scan with 0.6 mm slice thickness, 3D reconstruction: vertebral artery course in relation to C1 and C2 in lateral view; the blue line shows the maximum width of the arterial loop

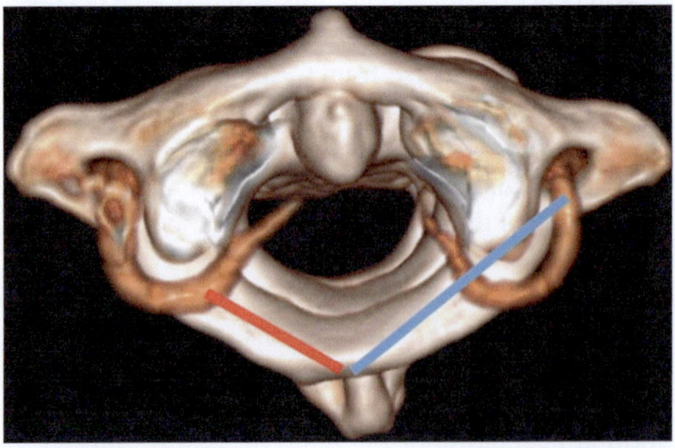

Fig. 3.12 Contrast-enhanced CT scan with 0.6 mm slice thickness, 3D reconstruction: distance from the central point of the posterior arch of C1 to the point of vertebral artery intersecting the C1 vertebra most laterally (blue line) and most medially (red line)

Optimal imaging requires patient head standing in neutral position without rotation or flexion-extension and correct intraluminal contrast enhancement regulating the acquisition time with bolus-tracking technique; 100 mL of contrast agent is enough and slice thickness of almost 1 mm is necessary, possibly even 0.75 mm [21].

To clarify the relationship of the vertebral artery loops with atlas and axis bones, transverse foramens and foramen magnum, especially to drill the bone tissues safely, is fundamental (Figs. 3.13, 3.14 and 3.15).

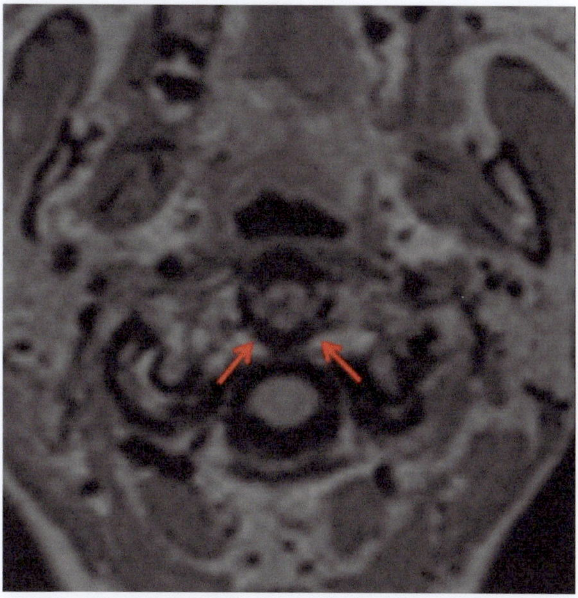

Fig. 3.13 T2-weighted FLAIR MR in axial plane with 1 mm slice thickness; transverse ligament (red arrows) spanning from the lateral masses of the atlas

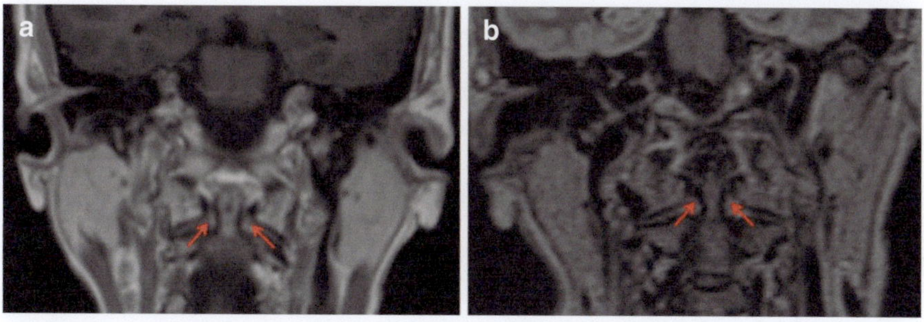

Fig. 3.14 T1-weighted (**a**) and T2-weighted FLAIR (**b**) MR in coronal plane with 1 mm slice thickness; alar ligaments (red arrows) spanning from the tip of the odontoid process to the medial margin of the occipital condyles

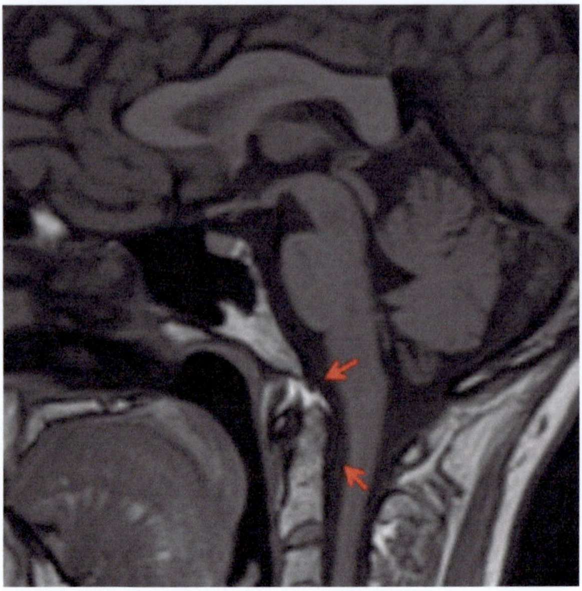

Fig. 3.15 T1-weighted MR in sagittal plane with 1 mm slice thickness; red arrows indicate the tectorial membrane

The loop formation of the atlas-axis part of the vertebral artery has been classified into four types according to Lang and Kessler [23], but many variations have been described in literature [24, 25]; therefore, a dedicated vertebral artery evaluation with CT angiography before CCJ surgery could prevent serious complications.

3.4 Bone Anomalies at the CCJ

The CCJ anomalies usually become symptomatic by compressing neural or vascular structures. A detailed knowledge of bone abnormalities and syndromes associated with craniovertebral pathology is critical for radiologists and surgeons in order to promptly diagnose and treat these complex conditions and to prevent potential long-term complications.

In this section, we discuss the most common congenital bone anomalies and syndromes involving the CCJ.

3.4.1 CCJ Craniometry

Pathology at the CCJ can show slight imaging abnormality and can be insidious to diagnose for radiologists. Familiarity with the main lines and angles used to evaluate CCJ craniometry is essential in order to correctly recognize congenital as well as acquired diseases.

Some basic remarks of the most commonly used measure in clinical practice are presented below (Fig. 3.16) [2].

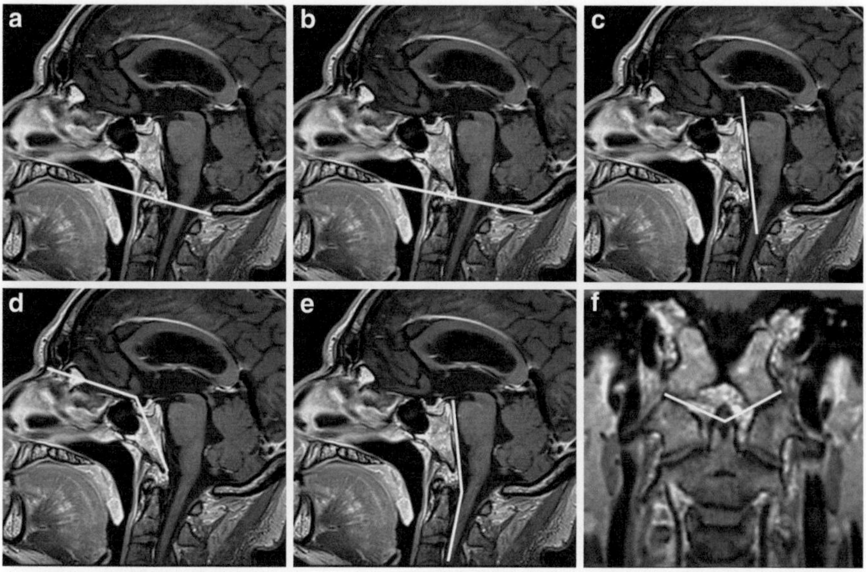

Fig. 3.16 T1 sagittal (**a**, **b**, **c**, **d**, and **e**) and coronal MR images (**f**). Chamberlain's line (**a**), McGregor's line (**b**), Wackenheim's clivus baseline (**c**), basal angle (**d**), clivus-canal angle (**e**), and atlanto-occipital joint angle (**f**)

- **Chamberlain's line**: From the posterior margin of the hard palate to the opisthion. The tip of the odontoid process should normally be below or just tangent to the line. The basilar impression can be diagnosed if the tip of the odontoid projects more than 5 mm above Chamberlain's line.
- **McGregor's line**: From the posterior margin of the hard palate to the lowest point of the occipital squamosal surface. This line is used on plain radiographs instead of Chamberlain's line. The tip of the odontoid process should normally be above this line no more the 6 mm in females and 7 mm in males.
- **Wackenheim's clivus baseline**: Line along the clivus and extending inferiorly into the upper cervical spinal canal. This line should normally be tangent to the posterior aspect of the odontoid tip. The abnormal findings are whether the line is too posterior to the odontoid (posterior craniocervical dislocation may be present) and whether the line intersects the body or base of the odontoid (anterior craniocervical dislocation may be present).
- **The basal angle**: Intersection of nasion–midsella and midsella–basion tangents. A different version of this angle is with the use of tuberculum sella rather than midsella (nasion–tuberculum and tuberculum–basion tangents). There variation between these two methods is about 2–3°. The average value is 134–135°, the minimum is 121°, the maximum is 148–149°, and a platybasia can be diagnosed if the angle is >150° [2].
- **The clivus-canal angle**: Intersection of Wackenheim's line and a line along the posterior margin of the dens and axis body. The angle normally should be between 150° in flexion and 180° in extension. The abnormal finding is if the angle is less than 150°, in these cases ventral spinal cord compression may be present.

- **The atlanto-occipital joint angle:** Formed by the intersection of tangents drawn parallel to the atlanto-occipital joints. If the condyles are symmetric, these tangents intersect at the center of the odontoid process. The average value is 124°–127°. If the angle is more obtuse, an occipital condylar hypoplasia may be present (>180° in severe cases).
- **Atlantodental interval (ADI):** Anterior atlantodental interval should be <5 mm. If is more than 5 mm, atlanto-axial instability may be present.

3.4.2 Bone Anomalies

3.4.2.1 Occipital Bone

- Basiocciput hypoplasia

  In basiocciput hypoplasia (or short clivus), the tip of the odontoid process and the anterior arch of C1 are above the Chamberlain's line, the clivus-canal angle can be decreased, and Wackenheim's clivus baseline may be normal or abnormal.

  This condition is associated with basilar invagination and can be associated to condyle hypoplasia and to Chiari I malformation. Basiocciput hypoplasia frequently results in compression of the cervicomedullary junction (Fig. 3.17).
- Occipital condyle hypoplasia

  In occipital condyle hypoplasia, the occipital condyles show an abnormal shape, length, width, or orientations. The abnormality can be unilateral or bilateral and usually asymmetric. The odontoid process and the anterior arch of C1 are above Chamberlain's line with decreased skull base height and basilar invagination, atlanto-occipital joint axis angle is increased, and Wackenheim's clivus baseline may be normal or abnormal (Fig. 3.18).

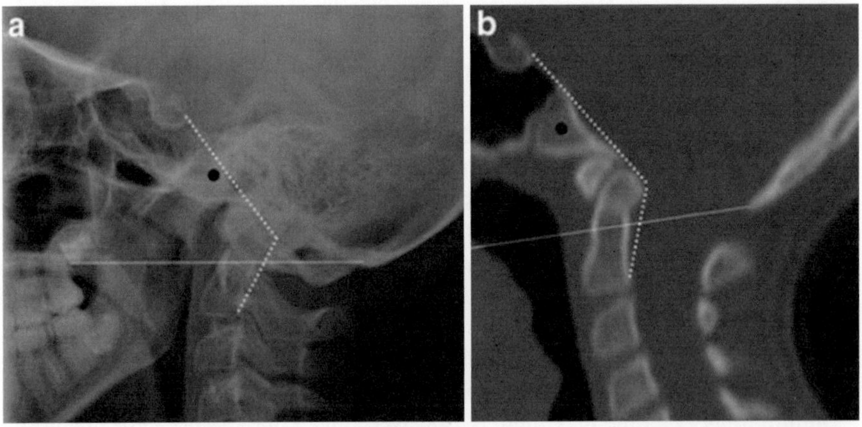

Fig. 3.17 Plain radiograph (**a**); sagittal CT scan (**b**); and sagittal MR images (**c**, **d**). Hypoplastic appearance of the basiocciput in the four patients (dots in **a**, **b**, **c**, and **d**). The tip of the odontoid process and the anterior arch of C1 are above Chamberlain's line in the four cases. The clivus canal angle is abnormal in patients **a** and **c**. There is associated Chiari I malformation and C2–C3 nonsegmentation in patient **d**. (Reprinted with permission from Smoker and Khanna 2008 [2])

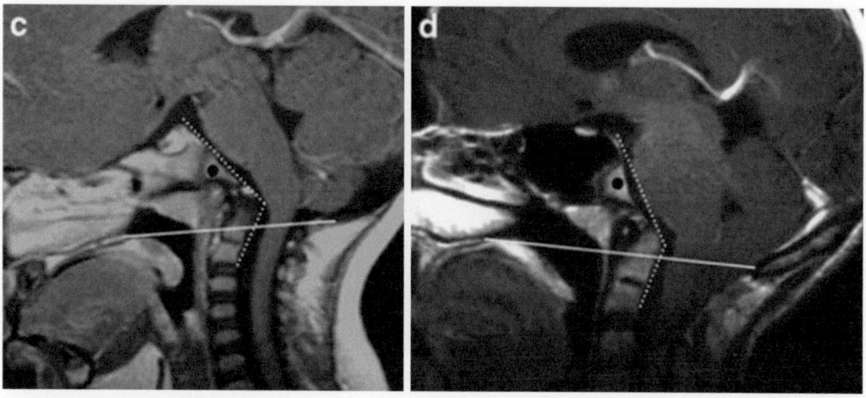

Fig. 3.17 (continued)

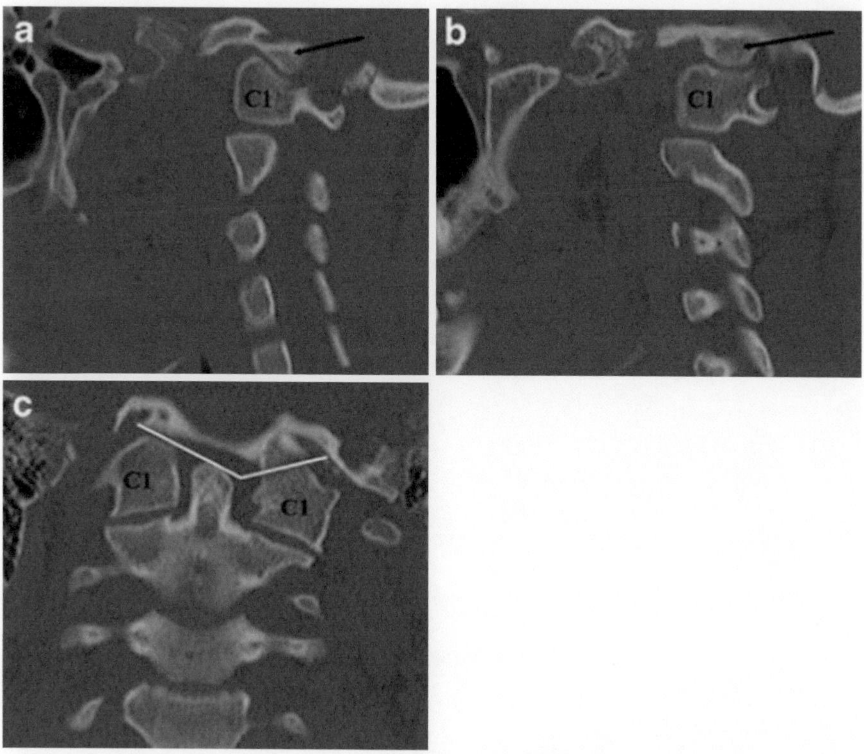

Fig. 3.18 Parasagittal CT images showing bilateral occipital condyle hypoplasia (**a** and **b** arrow), severe on the right side (**a**). Coronal CT image demonstrating abnormal atlanto-occipital joint axis angle (140°); (**c**) in round graft, after 140°, white lines. (Modified with permission from Smoker and Khanna 2008 [2])

Occipital condyles hypoplasia, due to third occipital sclerotome hypoplasia or aplasia, is frequently associated with hypoplasia of the exoccipital bone and jugular tubercles.

Condylar hypoplasia may reduce the mobility of the atlanto-occipital joint or cause articular instability potentially resulting in compression of the vertebral artery [26].

– Atlanto-occipital non-segmentation

The atlanto-occipital non-segmentation (or occipitalization of the atlas) is characterized by a failure of segmentation between the fourth occipital sclerotome and the first cervical sclerotome. This abnormality may involve the anterior arch, the posterior arch, the lateral masses, or a combination [27] (Fig. 3.19). Instability

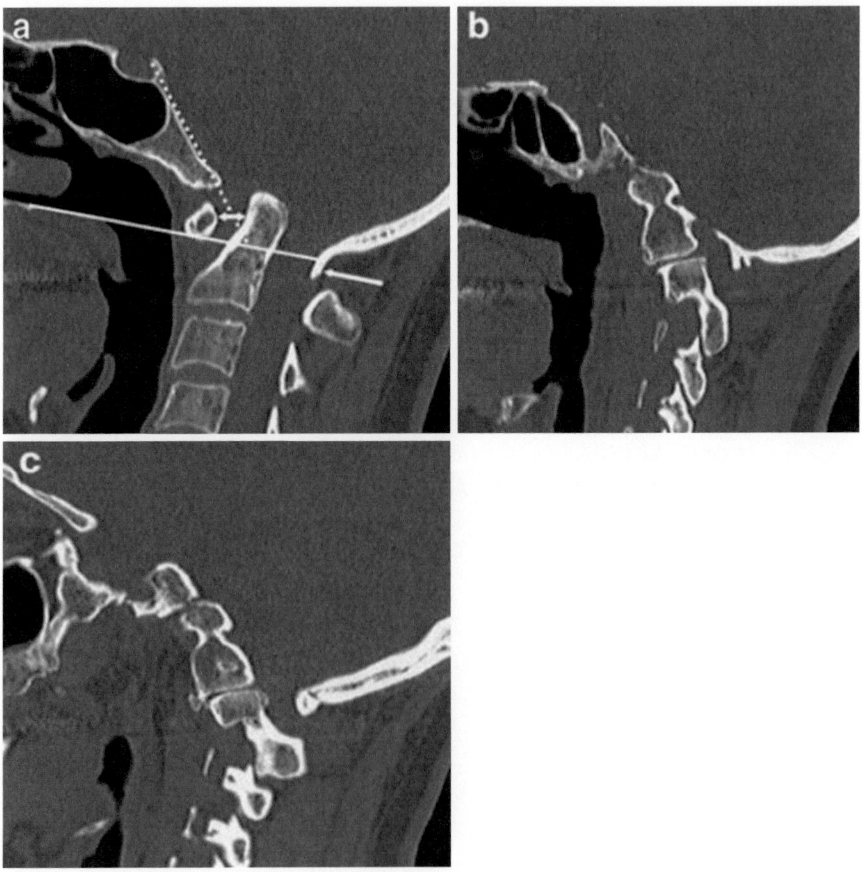

Fig. 3.19 Sagittal CT image showing posterior atlanto-occipital nonsegmentation (arrow in **a**). Widening of the anterior atlantodental interval (double arrow in **a**). Basilar invagination with the odontoid process and the anterior arch of C1 above Chamberlain's line (**a**). Abnormal Wackenheim's clivus baseline (dotted line in **a**). Right (**b**) and left (**c**) parasagittal CT images indicative of lateral atlas masses non-segmentation. (Modified with permission from Smoker and Khanna 2008 [2])

at C1–C2 is associated in half of patients due to increased mechanical stress consequent to the reduction of mobility at the atlanto-occipital junction. Non-segmentation at C2–C3 is associated in up to 70% of patients [28].

If the non-segmentation is between the anterior atlas arch and the anterior portion of the foramen magnum, a "comma-shaped" appearance of the clivus tip can be observed (Fig. 3.20). In these cases, there is association with basilar invagination, dorsal displacement of the odontoid process, stenosis of the foramen magnum, and compression of the cervicomedullary junction.

Clinically, patients might often have a low hairline, short neck, and restriction of neck movement. In about 20% of patients, other congenital abnormalities may be present, including incomplete clefting of the nasal cartilage, cleft palate, external ear deformities, cervical ribs, hypospadias, and urinary tract anomalies [29].

3.4.2.2 Atlas

The lateral masses and superior portion of the posterior atlas arch derive from the caudal division of the neural arch of the proatlas and the atlas vertebra from the first spinal sclerotome [30]. The posterior arch anomalies represent the most common anomalies of the atlas and include complete aplasia, Keller-type aplasia with the persistence of the posterior tubercle, aplasia with a unilateral or bilateral remnant, midline rachischisis and hemiaplasia or partial hemiaplasia of the posterior arch.

- Rachischisis

  Among the posterior arch anomalies, the posterior arch rachischisis is the most common, reported to be present in 4% of the autopsy [31]. The vast majority of them (97%) are arch *cleft* of the midline; only 3% are lateral clefts through the sulcus of the vertebral artery [2]. Posterior atlas arch rachischisis can be diag-

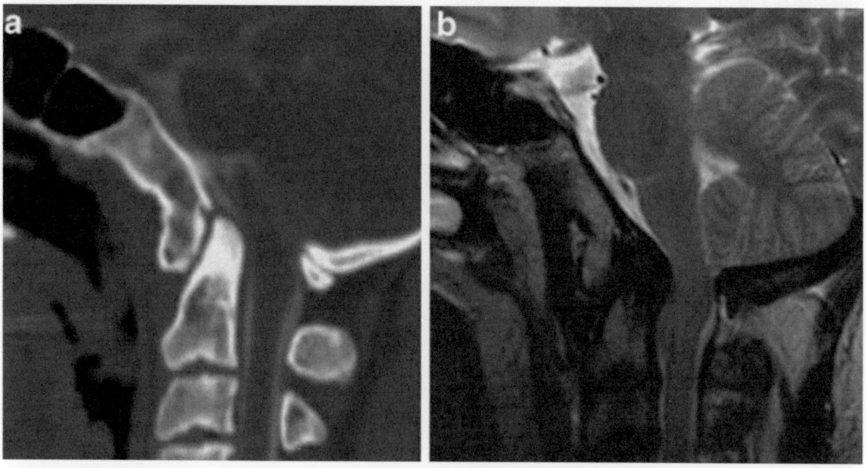

Fig. 3.20 Sagittal CT-myelogram (**a**) and T2-weighted MR (**b**) images. A complete anterior atlanto-occipital non-segmentation with "comma" configuration is depicted. (Reprinted with permission from Smoker and Khanna 2008 [2])

nosed with plain lateral radiographs as two separate hemiarches (Fig. 3.21). This condition could mimic a vertical fracture, especially in trauma setting, requiring a CT scan.

Anterior arch rachischisis is a rare entity, reported in only 0.1% of the autopsy [32]. On a plain lateral radiograph, when rachischisis is present, the anterior arch assumes a "rounded" or "plump" shape, overlapping the odontoid process and the anterior atlantodental interval. On sagittal MR images, there is anterior arch hypointensity due to fibrous tissue replacing the normal marrow signal intensity, a condition known as anterior arch pseudotumor (Fig. 3.22).

Anterior arch rachischisis is often associated with rachischisis or aplasia/hemiaplasia of the posterior arch known as "split atlas" and may cause atlas instability.

– Aplasia-hypoplasia
  Partial hemiaplasias and aplasia of the posterior arch are usually asymptomatic, although anterior atlanto-axial subluxation and bilateral atlanto-axial offset can be associated. On plain radiographs, these conditions could simulate fractures (Fig. 3.23). Complete posterior hypoplasia may cause a spinal canal stenosis and high cervical myelopathy and become symptomatic with Lhermitte's phenomenon, transient quadriparesis, and chronic neck pain [2, 33].

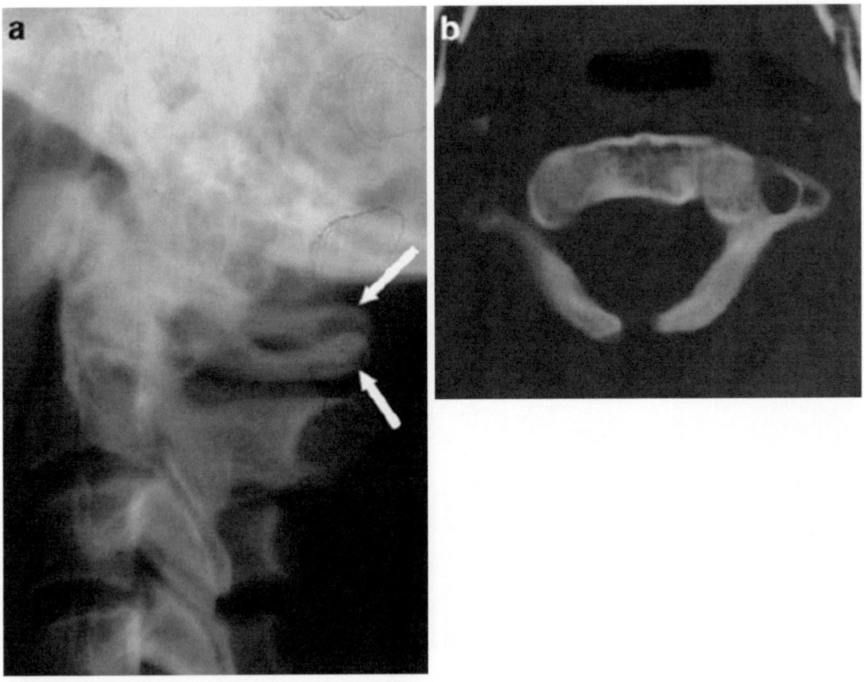

Fig. 3.21 Lateral radiograph (**a**) and axial CT (**b**) images, demonstrating posterior atlas arch rachischisis. (Reprinted with permission from Smoker and Khanna 2008 [2])

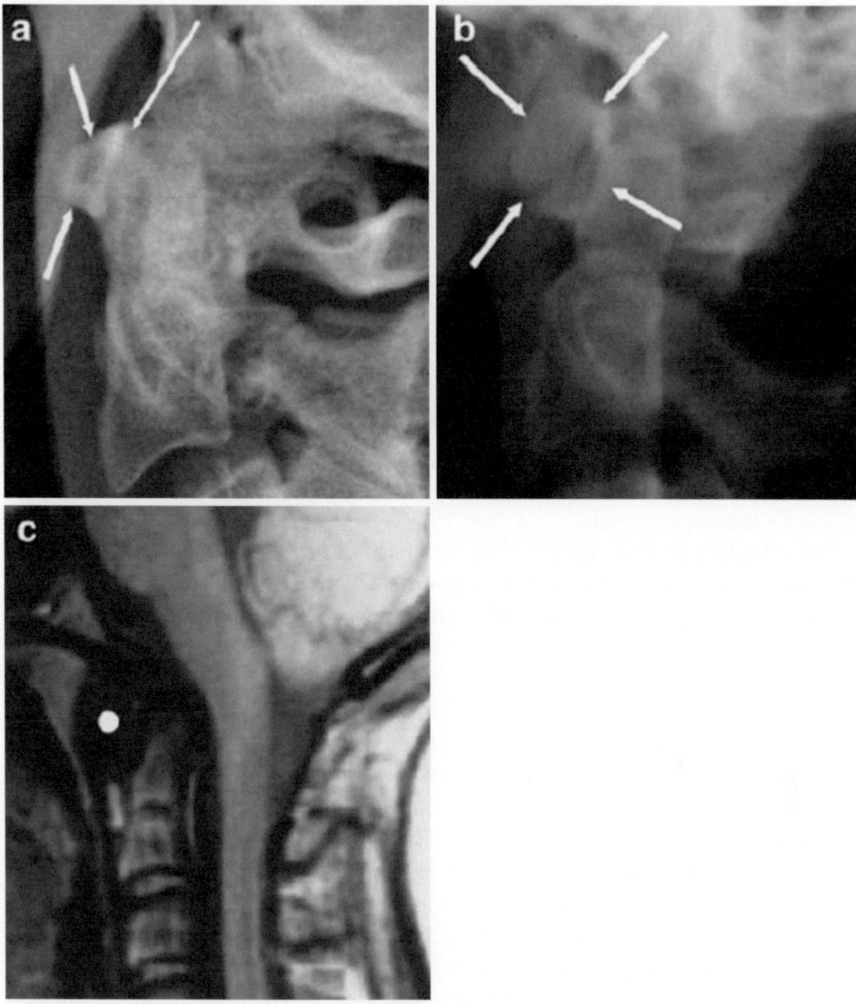

Fig. 3.22 Lateral radiograph (**a**) of a normal anterior atlas arch with well-corticated margins (short arrows) and normal anterior atlantodental interval (long arrow). Lateral radiograph (**b**) showing abnormally rounded and hypertrophic anterior atlas arch without cortex (arrows). Sagittal T1-weighted MR image (**c**) shows a rounded, low signal intensity, midline fibrous tissue (dot). (Reprinted with permission from Smoker and Khanna 2008 [2])

3.4.2.3 Axis

The odontoid process derives from the centrum of the first spinal sclerotome, the C1 arch from the neural arch of this sclerotome. The axis body originates from the centrum of the second spinal sclerotome and the facets and posterior axis arch form from the neural arch of this sclerotome. The terminal portion of the dens derives from the proatlas.

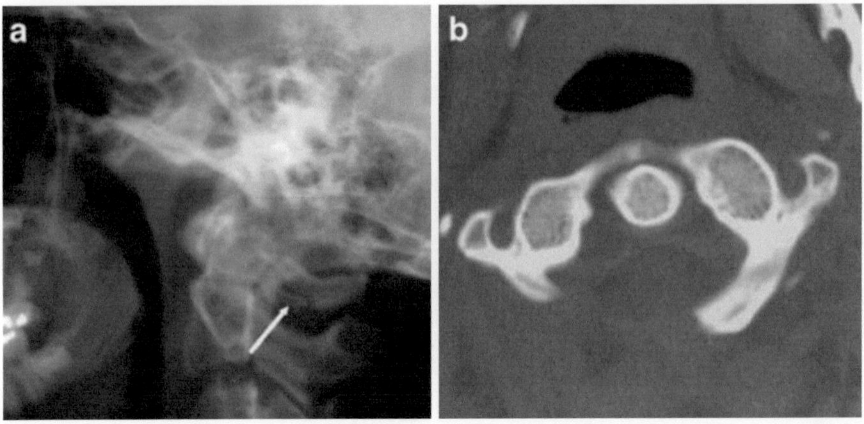

Fig. 3.23 Lateral radiograph (**a**) and axial CT images (**b**) showing posterior atlas arch aplasia. (Reprinted with permission from Smoker and Khanna 2008 [2])

The odontoid is separated from the axis body at birth by the neural central synchondrosis that disappears about 8 years of age. The terminal ossicle usually ossifies in about 3 years of age and fuses with the rest of the dens by 12 years of age.

- Os odontoideum

  The term "os odontoideum" was introduced by Giacomini in 1886 [34].

  The most accepted theory about os odontoideum etiology states that it represents an acquired condition caused by a trauma between 1 and 4 years of age [2, 35].

  The os odontoideum appears as a rounded, well-corticated structure just below the basion that can be diagnosed with X-ray, CT, or MRI (Fig. 3.24). It is usually associated with a rounded, hypertrophic appearance at the anterior arch of the atlas that is in important feature, especially in trauma setting, to guide the differential diagnosis with type II odontoid fracture. Findings like flattened, sharp, and uncorticated upper margin of the axis body with half-moon crescentic appearance of the anterior C1 arch are indicative of type II odontoid fracture. Os odontoideum is often associated with atlanto-axial instability due to gap between the os and the axis body extending above the level of the superior articular facets with incompetence of the cruciate ligament; compression of the spinal cord is common. Thus, from an imaging standpoint, flexion and extension plain radiographs can give more information about atlanto-axial instability, CT can better study the osseous relationships and anatomy and MRI is as essential technique to rule out cord compression and myelopathy.

  Patients with os odontoideum can be asymptomatic or may experience neck pain, paresis or myelopathic symptoms with or without history of trauma. Os odontoideum can be associated with congenital syndromes such as Down syndrome, Morquio syndrome, spondyloepiphyseal dysplasia, Klippel–Feil anomaly and Laron syndrome [2].

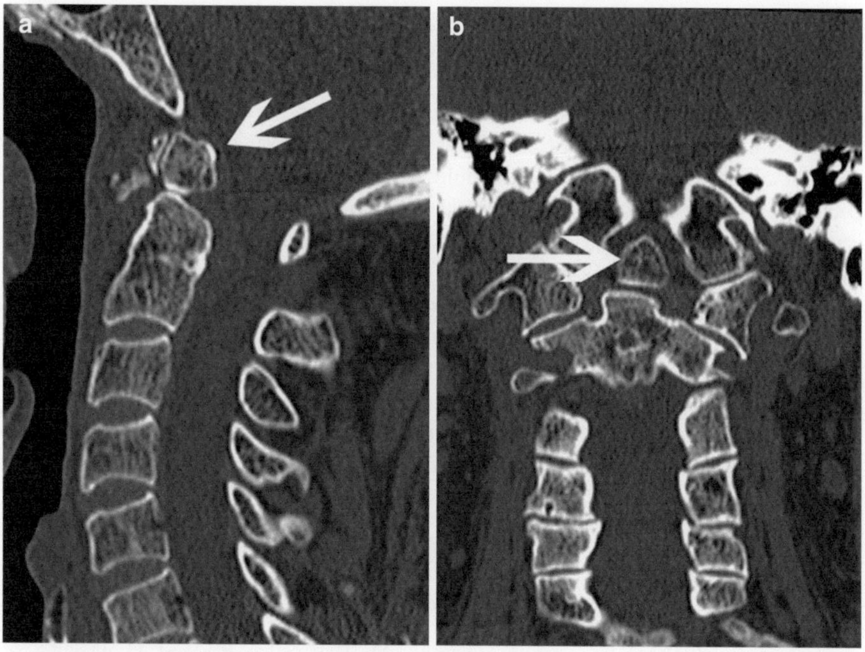

Fig. 3.24 Sagittal (**a**) and coronal CT images (**b**). A 57-year-old woman with os odontoideum (arrows in **a** and **b**)

- Persistent ossiculum terminale

  Persistent ossiculum terminale (or Bergman's ossicle) is the result of an absent fusion of the proatlas to the rest of the odontoid process.

  The presence of a cortical bone in persistent ossiculum terminale can guide the differential diagnosis with a type I odontoid fracture.

  Persistent ossiculum terminale, if not associated with other anomalies, is usually stable and of poor clinical significance.
- Odontoid hypoplasia and aplasia

  Odontoid hypoplasia and aplasia are rare conditions. There is a predisposition to atlanto-axial instability and consequent cord compression in both hypoplasia and aplasia, due to the absent attachments for the apical and alar ligaments.

  Odontoid hypoplasia can be associated with syndromes including spondylo-epiphyseal dysplasia, the mucopolysaccharidoses, and metatropic dwarfism [2].

3.5 Conclusions

In the last two decades, technology has produced significant progresses in medical imaging, especially in CT and MR apparels development.

Fast acquisitions, thin slice thickness, postprocessing reconstructions, high-field magnets, and dedicated MR sequences are the weapons in the hands of the twenty-first-century radiologist.

In the CCJ district, a deepen radiological evaluation is possible regardless of the clinical scenario, no matter if trauma, vascular, pre-surgery, or anatomical variants.

Thin-section multidetector CT should be the primary screening study for suspected cervical spine injury, with sagittal and coronal multiplanar reconstruction to improve identification and characterization of fractures and subluxations. In the same way, MR imaging is essential for detecting soft-tissues injuries, especially ligaments disruption and encephalic trunk in accordance with the clinical data.

CT angiography represents an accurate tool to assess the vertebral artery relationship with atlas and axis and planning the surgical strategy.

In this context, a detailed knowledge of anatomy, basic craniometric measurements, as well as bone abnormalities associated with craniovertebral pathology is essential in order to promptly diagnose and treat these complex conditions and to prevent potential long-term complications.

References

1. Riascos R, Bonfante E, Cotes C, Guirguis M, Hakimelhai R, West C. Imaging of AtlantoOccipital and atlantoaxial traumatic injuries: what the radiologist needs to know. Radiographics. 2015;35:2121–34.
2. Smoker WRK, Khanna G. Imaging the craniocervical junction. Childs Nerv Syst. 2008;24:1123–45.
3. Kiresi D, Gumus S, Cengiz SL, Cicekcibasi A. The morphometric analysis of the V2 and V3 segments of the vertebral artery: normal values on MDCT. Comput Med Imaging Graph. 2009;33:399–407.
4. Griffen MM, Frykberg ER, Kerwin AJ, et al. Radiographic clearance of blunt cervical spine injury: plain radiograph or computed tomography scan? J Trauma. 2003;55(2):222–7.
5. Holmes JF, Akkinepalli R. Computed tomography versus plain radiography to screen for cervical spine injury: a meta-analysis. J Trauma. 2005;58(5):902–5.
6. Daffner RH, Hackney DB. ACR appropriateness criteria on suspected spine trauma. J Am Coll Radiol. 2007;4(11):762–75.
7. Lummel N, Schöpf V, Bitterling H, et al. Effect of magnetic resonance imaging field strength on delineation and signal intensity of alar ligaments in healthy volunteers. Spine. 2012;37(17):E1062–7.
8. Izzo R, Ambrosanio G, Cigliano A, Cascone D, Gallo G, Muto M. Biomechanics of the spine III. The cranio-cervical junction. Neuroradiol J. 2007;20:209–17.
9. Labler L, Eid K, Platz A, Trentz O, Kossmann T. Atlanto-occipital dislocation: four case reports of survival in adults and review of the literature. Eur Spine J. 2004;13(2):172–80.
10. Rojas CA, Hayes A, Bertozzi JC, Guidi C, Martinez CR. Evaluation of the C1-C2 articulation on MDCT in healthy children and young adults. Am J Roentgenol. 2009;193(5):1388–92.
11. Gonzalez LF, Fiorella D, Crawford NR, et al. Vertical atlantoaxial distraction injuries: radiological criteria and clinical implications. J Neurosurg Spine. 2004;1(3):273–80.
12. Theodore N, Aarabi B, Dhall SS, et al. Occipital condyle fractures. Neurosurgery. 2013;72(Suppl 2):106–13.
13. Leone A, Cerase A, Colosimo C, Lauro L, Puca A, Marano P. Occipital condylar fractures: a review. Radiology. 2000;216(3):635–44.

14. Tuli S, Tator CH, Fehlings MG, Mackay M. Occipital condyle fracture. Neurosurgery. 1997;41(2):368–77.
15. Marcon RM, Cristante AF, Teixeira WJ, Narasaki DK, Oliveira RP, de Barros Filho TE. Fractures of the cervical spine. Clinics (Sao Paulo). 2013;68(11):1455–61.
16. Brotis AG, Paraskevi TM, Tsitsopoulos P, Tasiou A, Fotakopoulos G, Fountas KN. An evidence-based approach towards the cranio-cervical junction injury classifications. Eur Spine J. 2015;24:931–9.
17. Anderson LD, D'Alonzo RT. Fractures of the odontoid process of the axis. J Bone Joint Surg Am. 1988;56:1663–74.
18. Roy-Camille R, Saillant G, Judet T, De Botton G, Michel G. Factors of severity in the fractures of the odontoid process. Rev Chir Orthop Reparatrice Appar Mot. 1980;66:183–6.
19. Francis WR, Fielding JW, Hawkins RJ, Pepin J, Hensinger R. Traumatic spondylolisthesis of the axis. J Bone Joint Surg Br. 1981;63:313–8.
20. Benzel EC, Hart BL, Ball PA, Baldwin NG, Orrison WW, Espinosa M. Fractures of the C2 vertebral body. J Neurosurg. 1994;81:206–12.
21. Alterman DM, Heidel RE, Daley BJ, Grandas OH, Stevens SL, Goldman MH, Freeman MB. Contemporary outcomes of vertebral injuries. J Vasc Surg. 2013;57:741–6.
22. Cacciola F, PhalkeU GA. Vertebral artery in relationship to C1–C2 vertebrae an anatomical study. Neurol India. 2004;52:178–84.
23. Lang J, Kessler B. About the suboccipital part of the vertebral artery and the neighboring bone-joint and nerve relationships. Skull Base Surg. 1991;1:64–72.
24. Bruneau M, Cornelius JF, Marneffe V, Triffaux M, George B. Anatomical variation of the V2 segment of the vertebral artery. Neurosurgery. 2006;59:20–4.
25. Macchi C, Giannelli F, Catini C. The measurement of the calibers of the branches of the aortic arch: a statistical investigation of 430 living subjects using ultrasonic tomography. Ital J Anat Embryol. 1993;98:69–79.
26. Bernini FP, Elefante R, Smaltino F, Tedeschi G. Angiographic study on the vertebral artery in cases of deformities of the occipitocervical joint. Am J Roentgenol. 1969;107:526–9.
27. Gholve PA, Hosalkar HS, Ricchetti ET, Pollock AN, Dormans JP, Drummond DS. Occipitalization of the atlas in children. Morphologic classification, associations, and clinical relevance. J Bone Joint Surg Am. 2007;89:571–8.
28. McRae DL, Barnum AS. Occipitalization of the atlas. Am J Roentgenol. 1953;70:23–46.
29. Hensinger RN. Anomalies of the atlas. In: Cervical Spine Research Society Editorial Committee, editor. The cervical spine. 2nd ed. Philadelphia: JB Lippincott; 1989. p. 244.
30. Menezes AH. Craniocervical developmental anatomy and its implications. Clin Neurosurg. 2005;52:5364.
31. Gehweiler J, Daffner R, Roberts LJ. Malformations of the atlas vertebra simulating the Jefferson fracture. Am J Roentgenol. 1983;149:1083–6.
32. VonTorklus D, Gehle W. The upper cervical spine. Regional anatomy, pathology and traumatology. In: Georg Theime Verlag, editor. A systemic radiological atlas and textbook. New York: Grune & Stratton; 1972. p. 1–9.
33. Currarino G, Rollins N, Diehl JT. Congenital defects of the posterior arch of the atlas: a report of seven cases including an affected mother and son. Am J Neuroradiol. 1997;15:249–54.
34. Giacomini C. Sull'esistenza dell' "os odontoideum" nell'uomo. Gior Acad Med Torino. 1886;49:24–8.
35. Fielding JW, Hensinger RN, Hawkins RJ. Os odontoideum. J Bone Joint Surg Am. 1980;62:376–83.

Biomechanics of the CVJ

4

Francesco Signorelli and Massimiliano Visocchi

4.1 CVJ Motion

Spinal movements are characterized by two types of motion: angular (rotation) and linear (translations). Each type of motion is described relative to each of the three axes of motion on a three-dimensional Cartesian coordinate system (x, y, and z) [1]. Rotation about the x-axis is referred to as flexion/extension, y-axis rotation is referred to as axial rotation, and z-axis rotation is referred to as lateral bending (Fig. 4.1). Clinically, most translations are referred to as subluxations.

Both types of movement, rotations and translations, are important for understanding normal and pathological spinal behaviors.

Different spinal movements are coupled together. Coupling refers to simultaneous motions (rotation and\or translation) that occur secondarily and in combination to a main motion (rotation and\or translation) [2, 3].

4.2 Biomechanics Flexibility Testing

Most of biomechanical information concerning the CVJ has been derived from the experimental method known as *Flexibility Testing*. It uses, in vitro, cadaveric spinal segments of two or more vertebrae that have been deprived of muscle tissue, leaving the ligaments and the bone structures intact. Torsional forces (bending moments), lateral forces, or combined loads are applied to the spinal segments, and the spinal movement thus obtained are then misurated [4]. Analysis of load-deformation responses reveals parameters such as stiffness, flexibility, range of motion, rotation,

F. Signorelli
Institute of Neurosurgery, Fondazione Policlinico A. Gemelli IRCCS, Rome, Italy

M. Visocchi (✉)
Cranio Cervical Junction Surgery Operative Unit, Institute of Neurosurgery, Catholic University of Rome, Rome, Italy

E. Tessitore et al. (eds.), *Surgery of the Cranio-Vertebral Junction*,
https://doi.org/10.1007/978-3-030-18700-2_4

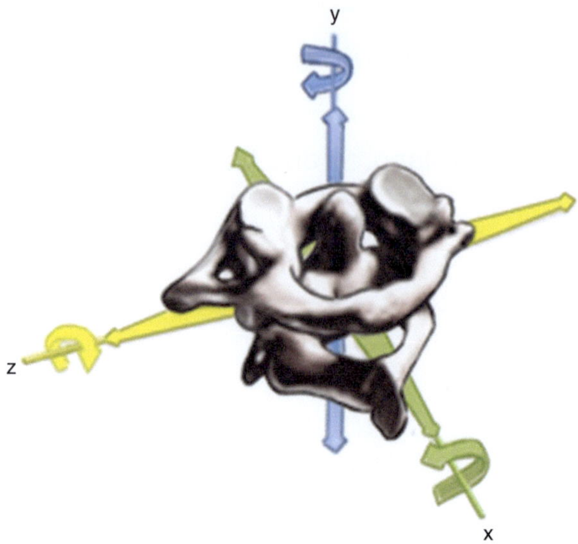

Fig. 4.1 Cartesian coordinate system for analyzing CVJ motions

translation, neutral zones, elastic zones, and axes of rotation. These biomechanical parameters are different and unique for each single spinal segment and are sensitive indices of spinal instability. The information obtained through the flexibility test “in vitro” represents the total contributions provided by bone joints and the ligamentous apparatus between each motion segment.

4.3 Load-Deformation Response of the CVJ

Several parameters can be calculated from the load-deformation curve.

Flexibility represents the amount of deformation in response to a unit load [5, 6]. *Stiffness* is the opposite of flexibility. It is the amount of resistance to a unit increment of displacement in the specimen.

Range of motion (ROM) is defined as the displacement between the neutral or resting position of the motion segment and the limit of its physiological motion. The *neutral position* is defined as the posture where minimal joint stresses occur and where minimal muscular effort is required to maintain the spatial orientation. This neutral position is best approximated by the midpoint of the bilateral *neutral zone* (NZ) [7].

The NZ is the portion of the ROM where the ligaments are lax and small forces produce large vertebral displacements. The *elastic zones* (EZ) is the steep portion of the load-deformation curve where the ligaments become stretched and stiffness increases, causing resistance to any further movement.

The motion characteristics of the different levels of the CVJ are due to the geometry of the vertebrae and skull base, the shapes of the joints, and the arrangements of the ligaments.

Neither the C0-C1 nor the C1-C2 joints have an intervertebral disc. The spherical shape (concave-convex) of C0-C1 joint allows slightly more flexion and extension than the other levels of the cervical spine, although these are quite rigid in axial rotation and lateral bending. The biconvex articular surfaces of the C1-C2 joints allow wide rotation of C1 around the dens. The atlantoaxial motion segment is the most flexible of the entire spine with respect to axial rotation, allowing a bilateral ROM of 80° or more. More than half of all cervical axial rotations occur at the atlantoaxial motion segment. Both C0-C1 and C1-C2 allow less lateral bending than the subaxial cervical motion segments, which average approximately 8° unilaterally [3] (Figs. 4.2 and 4.3).

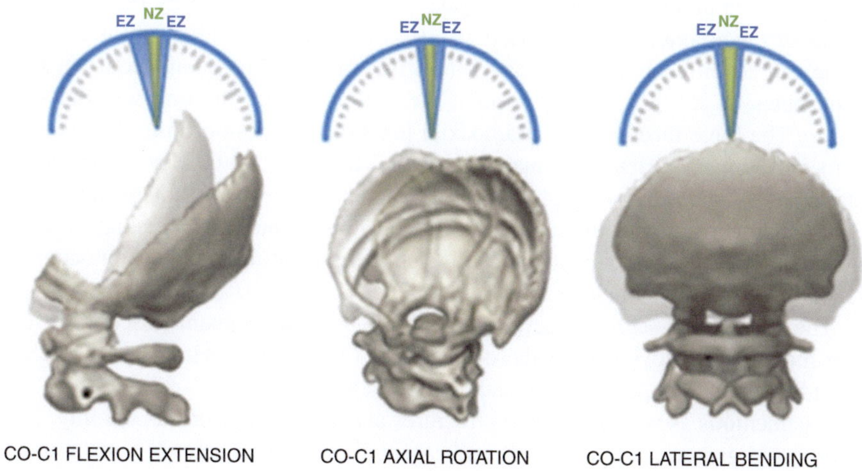

Fig. 4.2 Representation of the normal angular motions at the occipitoatlantal motion segments

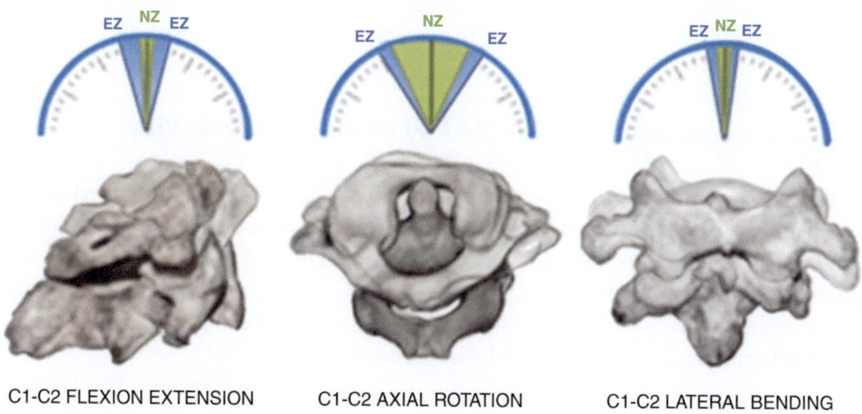

Fig. 4.3 Representation of the normal angular motions at the atlantoaxial motion segments

4.4 Physiological Biomechanics

The cervical spine's range of motion is approximately 80°–90° of flexion, 70° of extension, 20°–45° of lateral flexion, and up to 90° of rotation on both sides. However, movement of the cervical spine is complex and movement into any range is not the simple sum of equal motion from one vertebra to the next.

The occipitoatlantal junction contributes to 23°–24.5° of flexion/extension of the skull and the atlantoaxial joint provides an additional 10.1°–22.4° [6]. At the occipitoatlantal junction, the abutment of the dens against the foramen magnum prevents supraphysiologic flexion, whereas odontoid contact with the tectorial membrane has been proposed to limit extension. The transverse ligament prevents pathological flexion of the atlantoaxial segment while extension is inhibited by the bony elements of the atlantoaxial joint facets [8–10]. Physiological motion of the cervical spine can accomplish 90° of rotation from the midline. The atlantoaxial junction contributes to 25°–30°, at which point the motion occurs through subaxial segments. The bone facets of the atlantoaxial junction will permit up to 40° rotation before locking, contributing a major restriction to over rotation. The contralateral alar ligament and the ipsilateral transverse ligament also resist pathological rotation with support from the joint capsules of the occipitoatlantal and atlantoaxial junctions [11, 12]. The occipital condyles restrict lateral bending of the occipitoatlantal junction to 3.4°–5.5° in either direction.

The atlantoaxial segment reaches 6.7° before the alar ligaments discourage further motion [6]. Movement in the other planes of motion is minimal at the CVJ, including translation, distraction, and compression.

Ligamentous as well as osseous structures are responsible for this stability. The transverse ligament, alar ligaments, and capsular joints resist anterior translation in the sagittal plane while the occipital condyles and the contact of the dens with the atlas and foramen magnum constitute bone barriers against posterior translation [10, 11, 13, 14].

The capsular joints of the occipital condyles and the atlantoaxial zygapophyseal joints resist compression. Distraction is not a physiological motion of the CVJ [14].

4.5 Biomechanics of Simple CVJ Pathology: Overview

In response to trauma, the CVJ exhibits predictable patterns of failure based on the mechanism of injury [15]. The most commonly encountered traumas occur during motor vehicle accidents, falls, diving accidents, and gunshot wounds [16]. Fracture-dislocation or occipitocervical dissociation at the CVJ is a leading cause of death in motor vehicle accidents [16]. Multiple mechanisms have been proposed to explain these patterns, such as whiplash and flexion-distraction injury.

Pathological flexion increases tension on the transverse ligament, resulting in failure of either the cruciate ligament or the odontoid waist [16]. Failure of the tectorial membrane has also been associated with flexion in front-end motor vehicle collisions [17] and may lead to dural tears. Isolated tectorial membrane failure contributes minor instability in flexion and extension [18–20].

Hyperextension may lead to fracture of the atlas at the posterior ring or fracture of the axis at the pars interarticularis or the odontoid. Shearing injury may occur to the ligaments of the anterior CVJ, including the alar ligaments, accessory atlantoaxial ligaments, cruciform ligament, and tectorial membranes. Supraphysiologic rotation at the atlantoaxial junction can predict, or even diagnose, alar ligament disruption.

Traumatic compression of the CVJ commonly causes osseous pathology at the occipitoatlantal junction. Axial loading has been associated with burst fractures of the atlas and with occipital condyle fractures. When evaluating trauma to the CVJ, current guidelines recommend initial evaluation by CT followed by MRI to assess ligamentous injury [21]. T2-weighted MRI obtained within 72 h of injury is the preferred modality for diagnosing soft-tissue injury. After 72 h, decreased tissue edema may lead to overlooked ligamentous damage [22]. Disruption of the ligamentous structures is sufficient to cause instability at the CVJ; additionally, these ligaments are irreparable once torn [23]. The most critical ligaments to evaluate for stability in the CVJ are the transverse ligament of the cruciform complex, the alar ligaments, and the tectorial membrane [9, 17, 24, 25].

4.6 Alar Ligament Failure

Failure of one alar ligament results in modest rotatory atlantoaxial instability. This instability is manifested as an increase in the C1-C2 ROM during the axial rotation, mostly through an increase in the NZ [26, 27]. The EZ and the flexibility, however, do not change significantly.

The bilateral transection of the alar ligaments determines considerably more extensive alterations of C0-C1-C2 motion than unilateral alar ligament disruption. The NZ and ROM during axial rotation, lateral bending, and flexion-extension are all increased significantly. The pivotal function of the alar ligaments is to stabilize the spine during flexion and extension and to limit axial rotation and lateral bending [3]. Failure of an alar ligament most likely occurs near the condylar insertion [25] and introduces instability in rotation and an increase in flexion, extension, and lateral bending [9]. Isolated rupture of the alar ligament is rare but has been associated with hyperflexion paired with rotation in all reported cases. Unfortunately, evaluation of the alar ligaments by MRI is complicated by their size and anatomical conformation [28, 29].

4.7 Transverse Ligament Failure

The transverse atlantal ligament is the thickest (1 cm) and strongest ligament of the entire spine. It is the most important stabilizer of the atlas, constraining C1 around the dens. Extremely high loads with anteriorly directed vectors at C1 are required to disrupt the transverse ligament. The mechanisms leading to failure of the transverse ligament have been extensively evaluated in vitro [30]. The accessory ligaments at C1-C2 are relatively weak and stretch with ease after the transverse ligament is rendered incompetent. This feature has important clinical consequences. The transverse ligament tears suddenly with a principle of "all or nothing" because it is stiff and inelastic. This ligament does not tear partially or gradually. When torn, the transverse ligament is incapable of repair. Because the transverse ligament injury renders the articulation of C1 enormously unstable, stabilization (fusion) of the C1-C2 complex must be performed.

4.8 Capsular Ligament Failure

Failure of the C1-C2 joint capsular ligament primarily slightly increases the ROM during axial rotation but has a minimal effect on lateral bending or flexion and extension [31]. Most of the increase in ROM is due to an increase in the EZ. Injury to the capsular ligaments is an important mechanism associated with rotatory C1-C2 subluxation.

Avulsion of a synovial joint capsule causes only a mild increase in rotatory motion; however, a rupture of the joint capsule warrants investigation of the more critical ligaments as it has been associated with the disruption of the transverse atlantal and alar ligaments.

4.9 Biomechanics Effects of Atlas Fractures

Experimental laboratory studies regarding atlas injuries indicate that burst fractures of the atlas outbreak derive from compressive injuries [32, 33]. Atlas burst fractures result in instability that is manifested as increases in the NZ and the ROM during flexion, extension, and lateral bending. In these studies, "in vitro" compressive injury caused a 90% increase in the flexion\extension NZ, a 44% increase in the flexion\extension ROM, and a 20% increase in lateral bending NZ and ROM. However, no significant changes were seen in axial rotation NZ or ROM.

References

1. Panjabi MM, Whithe AA III, Brand RA Jr. A note on defining body parts configurations. J Biomech. 1974;7(4):385–7.
2. Goel VK. Three-dimensional motion behavior of the human spine—a question of terminology. J Biomech Eng. 1987;109(4):353–5.
3. White AA III, Panjabi MM. Clinical biomechanics of the spine. 2nd ed. Philadelphia, PA: JB Lippincott; 1974.
4. Panjabi MM. Biomechanical evaluation of spinal fixation devices: a conceptual framework. Spine. 1988;13(10):1129–34.

5. Dickman CA, Crawford NR, Tominga T, et al. Morphology and kinematics of the baboon upper cervical spine. A model of the atlantoaxial complex. Spine. 1994;19(22):2518–23.
6. Panjabi MM, Dvorák J, Duranceau J, et al. Three–dimensional movements of the upper cervical spine. Spine. 1988;13(7):726–30.
7. Panjabi MM. The stabilizing system of the spine. Part II. Neutral zone and instability hypothesis. J Spinal Disord. 1992;5(4):390–6.
8. Dvorak J, Panjabi MM, Novotny JE, Antinnes JA. In vivo flexion/extension of the normal cervical spine. J Orthop Res. 1991;9:828–34.
9. Dvorak J, Schneider E, Saldinger P, Rahn B. Biomechanics of the craniocervical region: the alar and transverse ligaments. J Orthop Res. 1988;6:452–61.
10. Ghanayem AJ, Zdeblich TA, Dvorak J. Functional anatomy of joints, ligaments, and discs. In: Clark CR, Ducker TB, Cervical Spine Research Society Editorial Committee, editors. The cervical spine. 3rd ed. Philadelphia: Lippincott-Raven; 1998. p. 45–52.
11. Dvorak J, Panjabi MM. Functional anatomy of the alar ligaments. Spine (Phila Pa 1976). 1987;12:183–9.
12. Iai H, Moriya H, Goto S, Takahashi K, Yamagata M, Tamaki T. Three-dimensional motion analysis of the upper cervical spine during axial rotation. Spine (Phila Pa 1976). 1993;18:2388–92.
13. Fielding JW, Gv C, Lawsing JF III, Hohl M. Tears of the transverse ligament of the atlas. A clinical and biomechanical study. J Bone Joint Surg Am. 1974;56:1683–91.
14. Wolfla CE. Anatomical, biomechanical, and practical considerations in posterior occipitocervical instrumentation. Spine J. 2006;6(6 Suppl):225S–32S.
15. Debernardi A, D'Aliberti G, Talamonti G, Villa F, Piparo M, Collice M. The craniovertebral junction area and the role of the ligaments and membranes. Neurosurgery. 2011;68:291–301.
16. Clark CR, White AA III. Fractures of the dens. A multicenter study. J Bone Joint Surg Am. 1985;67:1340–8.
17. Krakenes J, Kaale BR, Moen G, Nordli H, Gilhus NE, Rorvik J. MRI of the tectorial and posterior atlanto-occipital membranes in the late stage of whiplash injury. Neuroradiology. 2003;45:585–91.
18. Harris MB, Duval MJ, Davis JA Jr, Bernini PM. Anatomical and roentgenographic features of atlanto occipital instability. J Spinal Disord. 1993;6:5–10.
19. Oda T, Panjabi MM, Crisco JJ III, Oxland TR. Multidirectional instabilities of experimental burst fractures of the atlas. Spine (Phila Pa 1976). 1992;17:1285–90.
20. Werne S. Studies in spontaneous atlas dislocation. Acta Orthop Scand Suppl. 1957;23:1–150.
21. Como JJ, Diaz JJ, Dunham CM, Chiu WC, Duane TM, Capella JM, et al. Practice management guidelines for identification of cervical spine injuries following trauma: update from the eastern Association for the Surgery of Trauma Practice Management Guidelines Committee. J Trauma. 2009;67:651–9.
22. Mirvis SE, Shanmuganathan K. Trauma radiology: part V. Imaging of acute cervical spine trauma. J Intensive Care Med. 1995;10:15–33.
23. Frank C, Amiel D, Woo SL, Akeson W. Normal ligament properties and ligament healing. Clin Orthop Relat Res. 1985;(196):15–25.
24. Heller JG, Amrani J, Hutton WC. Transverse ligament failure: a biomechanical study. J Spinal Disord. 1993;6:162–5.
25. Saldinger P, Dvorak J, Rahn BA, Perren SM. Histology of the alar and transverse ligaments. Spine (Phila Pa 1976). 1990;15:257–61.
26. Panjabi MM, Dvorák J, Crisco JJ III, et al. Effects of alar ligament transection on upper cervical spine rotation. J Orthop Res. 1991;9(4):584–93.
27. Panjabi MM, Dvorák J, Crisco JJ III, et al. Flextion, extension, and lateral bending of the upper cervical spine in response to alar ligament transections. J Spinal Disord. 1991;4(2):157–67.
28. Borchgrevink G, Smevik O, Haave I, Haraldseth O, Nordby A, Lereim I. MRI of cerebrum and cervical column within two days after whiplash neck sprain injury. Injury. 1997;28:331–5.

29. Ronnen HR, de Korte PJ, Brink PR, van der Bijl HJ, Tonino AJ, Franke CL. Acute whiplash injury: is there a role for MR imaging?—a prospective study of 100 patients. Radiology. 1996;201:93–6.
30. Fielding JW, Cochran GVB, Lawsing JF III, et al. Tears of the transverse ligament of the atlas. A clinical and biomechanical study. J Bone Joint Surg Am. 1974;56(8):1683–91.
31. Crisco JJ, Oda T, Panjabi MM, et al. Transection of the C1–C2 joint capsular ligaments in the cadaveric spine. Spine. 1991;16(10 suppl):474–9.
32. Panjabi MM, Oda T, Crisco JJ, et al. Experimental study of atlas injuries. I. Biomechanical analysis of their mechanisms and fracture patterns. Spine. 1991;16(10 suppl):460–5.
33. Oda T, Panjabi MM, Crisco JJ III, et al. Experimental study of atlas injuries. II. Relevance to clinical diagnosis and treatment. Spine. 1991;16(10 suppl):466–73.

Sagittal Balance Concept Applied to the Craniovertebral Junction

5

Ibrahim Obeid and Derek T. Cawley

5.1 Comparative Anatomy and Evolution of Balance

The acquisition of vertical posture and bipedal locomotion represents the most important transformation in the history of the *Hominidae*, including the change in relationship between the foramen magnum orientation and cervical spine [1].

With the evolution of our species has come significant change in the function and alignment of the cervical spine, defined by adaptive abilities to feed, move, and breath. The amphibian typically has a singular cervical vertebra with a non-mobile craniovertebral joint (CVJ), and it may possess a long extensible tongue to eat its prey. While the reptile has a less constrained CVJ, it is constrained by the force required to lift a relatively heavy head; the tetrapod can rapidly project and retract the mouth, armed with teeth, toward its prey or aggressor.

Sagittal alignment of the CVJ has evolved in synchrony with our progression from quadruped to biped posture [2]. The center of gravity of the head in quadrupeds is located quite anterior of the CVJ due to the development of the splanchnocranium, the horizontality of the base of the skull, and the posterior position of the occipital condyles, so that the occipito-atlantal (OC1) joint alignment is almost vertical. In primates and even more markedly in humans, basicranial flexion is observed in the sphenoid, with the clivus then forming an angle with the anterior part of the base of the skull. This process, probably related to the development of the cerebral hemispheres and the reduction of the facial mass, coincides with the anterior migration of the occipital condyles, which has the effect of considerably reducing the bending moment of the center of gravity of the head. In humans, the OC1 articulation is horizontal, and the center of gravity of the head vertical line passes right in front of the dens. Head posture is governed by the ability to maintain horizontal gaze, hearing, equilibrium, nasorespirational function, and even psychological condition (Fig. 5.1).

I. Obeid (✉) · D. T. Cawley
Spine Unit, Bordeaux University Hospital, Bordeaux, France

E. Tessitore et al. (eds.), *Surgery of the Cranio-Vertebral Junction*,
https://doi.org/10.1007/978-3-030-18700-2_5

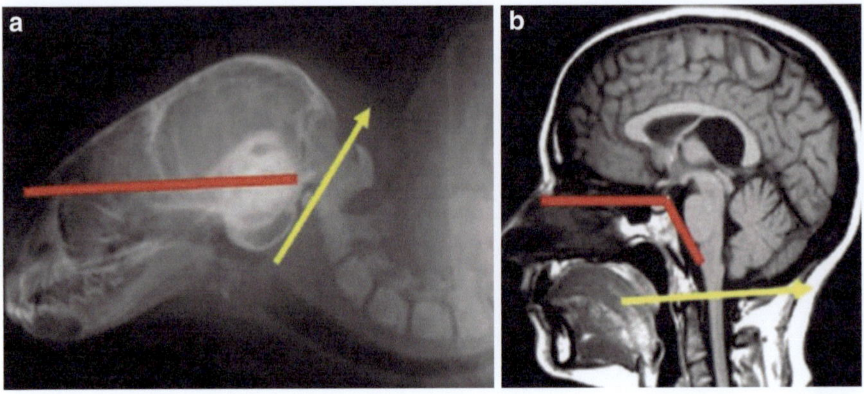

Fig. 5.1 In quadrupeds (**a**) the skull base is horizontal (platybasia), the occipital condyles are located at the back of the skull and the foramen magnum is tilted back and top. In humans (**b**) basicranial flexion is more important between the anterior floor of the skull base and clivus, the occipital condyles are almost under the skull and the foramen magnum is horizontal. (With permission from Vital JM, Anatomie de la Colonne Vertebrale)

5.2 Functional Anatomy

The CVJ functions primarily in rotation of the head and secondarily in flexion and extension. At the outset, slightly more flexion/extension occurs at the OC1 joint, and most axial rotation occurs at the C1C2 complex. Adult OC1 motion includes approximately 25° of flexion–extension, 5° of lateral bending, and 5° of rotation. C1C2 motion includes approximately 20° of flexion–extension, 5° of lateral bending, and 40° of rotation [3]. There should be no translation at the OC1 junction.

Compared with the sub-axial spine (SAS), the ratio of lordosis of OC2 to C2-C7 is 77%:23% [4]. Cranial dimensions vary significantly, but the natural head position is constant [5]. As mentioned, the center of gravity of the head sits almost directly over the centers of C1 and C2 vertebrae, as reflected by the external auditory meatus (EAM) so the associated short radii may explain why most cervical spine lordosis occurs between C1 and C2 [6]. This anatomic feature also allows assessment of *EAM tilt*, a global alignment assessment of the cervical spine, represented by the angle between the vertical and the line joining the center of C7 and the EAM.

Given the intimate relations of the occiput, atlas, and axis bones, the optimal angle for portraying alignment of the CVJ is the *occipitocervical angle*, the OC2 angle between McGregor's line (external occipital cortex to hard palate) and the lower end plate of C2 [7, 8]. Its mean value is 14° (±7°) in asymptomatic subjects over 18 years, 12° (±6°) in those over 60 years and significantly greater in females [8, 9]. The *C1C2 angle* is defined as the angle between the horizontal axis of C1 and the lower end plate of C2, found to be 29° (±7°) [10]. OC2 is always lordotic in an asymptomatic normal population, whereas C2C7 may be neutral or sinusoid or kyphotic in up to a third of the normal population [10].

Sagittal alignment of the CVJ with respect to overall vertical sagittal balance has only recently been described using data from EOS imaging, a new low-dose radiographic system that images the upright skeleton. The system therefore relies on the depiction of one's natural posture. As described by Morvan et al., the individual is required to place one's fingertips on their clavicles and look straight ahead at the mirror mounted in front of them [11]. A higher C7 slope is associated with a higher lordosis in the SAS and a lower slope means a lower lordosis, but this does not affect the sagittal orientation of the CVJ. Le Huec et al. found that the median C7 slope value was 20°. They evaluated the OC2 of two groups—those with a value less than, and greater than 20°—finding that the C2C7 values were −2.5° and 11.5°, respectively, but that the OC2 value was 15.8° in both the groups. Despite significant variations in cervical spine lordosis or the slope of the C7 vertebra, the OC2 angle displayed constant values [10].

Both the OC1 and the C1C2 articulations have the capacity to contribute to sagittal alignment of the cervical spine, 25% and 20%, respectively. There are two basic postures of the neck (retraction-protraction) in primates including humans (Figs. 5.2 and 5.3). Retraction refers to an active position when the OC1C2 joints are flexed under the effect of the posterior musculature, such as in the "military tuck" position. Protraction corresponds to a passive rest position when the OC2 joint is extended (as in reading or sleep in a sitting position). This would increase the SVA, the horizontal offset distance from C2C7 causing flexion of C2C7 segments and hyperextension of C0C2 segments to maintain horizontal orientation of the head [12]. This is in fact a "push-forward with the head attitude" which one observes through efforts

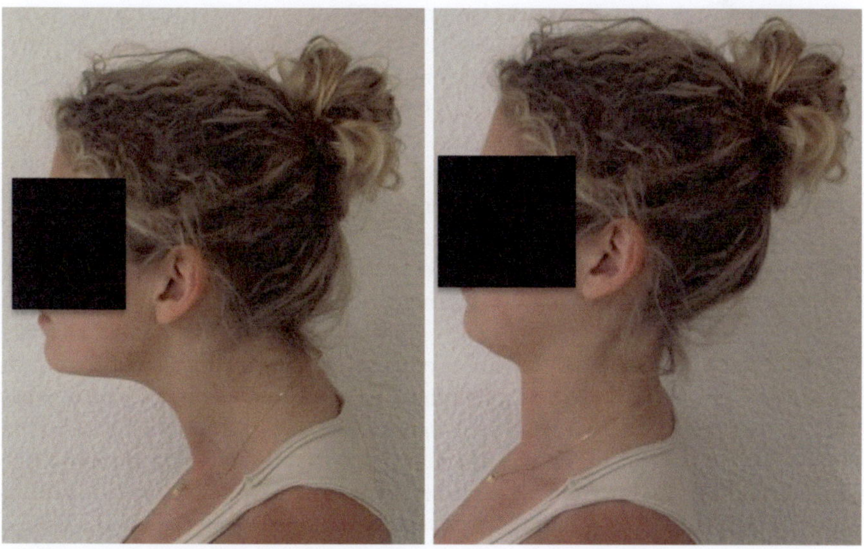

Fig. 5.2 Clinical photographs of protraction (protrusion) and retraction ("military tuck") of the neck

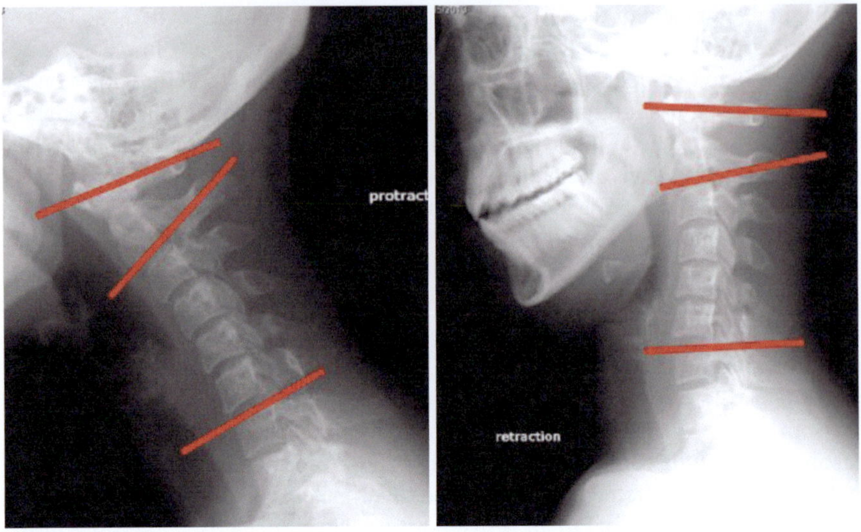

Fig. 5.3 Radiographs (lateral view) of protraction and retraction of the neck, demonstrating the reverse behaviors of the CVJ and SAS

of pushing (as in collision sports). It is in this posture that the CVJ reaches its maximum amplitude in extension [2].

The only constant variable in this context is gaze direction. A *coupling mechanism* is evident to achieve it: flexion of the subaxial cervical spine induces extension at the craniovertebral junction and vice versa [13].

What is further relevant to the CVJ is the effect that distal curves have on the cervical spine (Fig. 5.4). Given the fixed relationship between the pelvis and spine (pelvic incidence) and stiffness of the thoracic spine, the more mobile lumbar and cervical spinal articulations compensate for this as required. As thoracic kyphosis increases, cervical lordosis increases. In young adults with thoracic hyperkyphosis, for example, patients have a lordosis of 27° at C1C2 compared with 20° in the normal population [14], despite similar head positions and craniofacial morphology [15]. Furthermore, a reversal of the kyphosis induces a reduction in cervical lordosis (Fig. 5.5).

While the OC2 parameters of asymptomatic subjects remain constant despite the variables of C7 slope and C2C7 lordosis, compensatory abilities with increasing age and deformity include the CVJ as well as other mechanisms. If the global alignment predisposes to a head forward position, the CVJ can contribute to horizontal positioning of the head and gaze. This *"fine tuning" concept* is a representative feature of the CVJ, an adaption to changing alignment characteristics as required throughout both the cervical and thoracic/lumbar spine. These principles are evident in Figs. 5.2, 5.3, and 5.5 in both normal physiological functioning and as an adaptive feature in pathological conditions.

While our understanding of the compensatory alignment features of the CVJ are known in the sagittal context, we can assume that the CVJ can function to adapt to maintain a horizontal position of the head in coronal and rotatory planes as well.

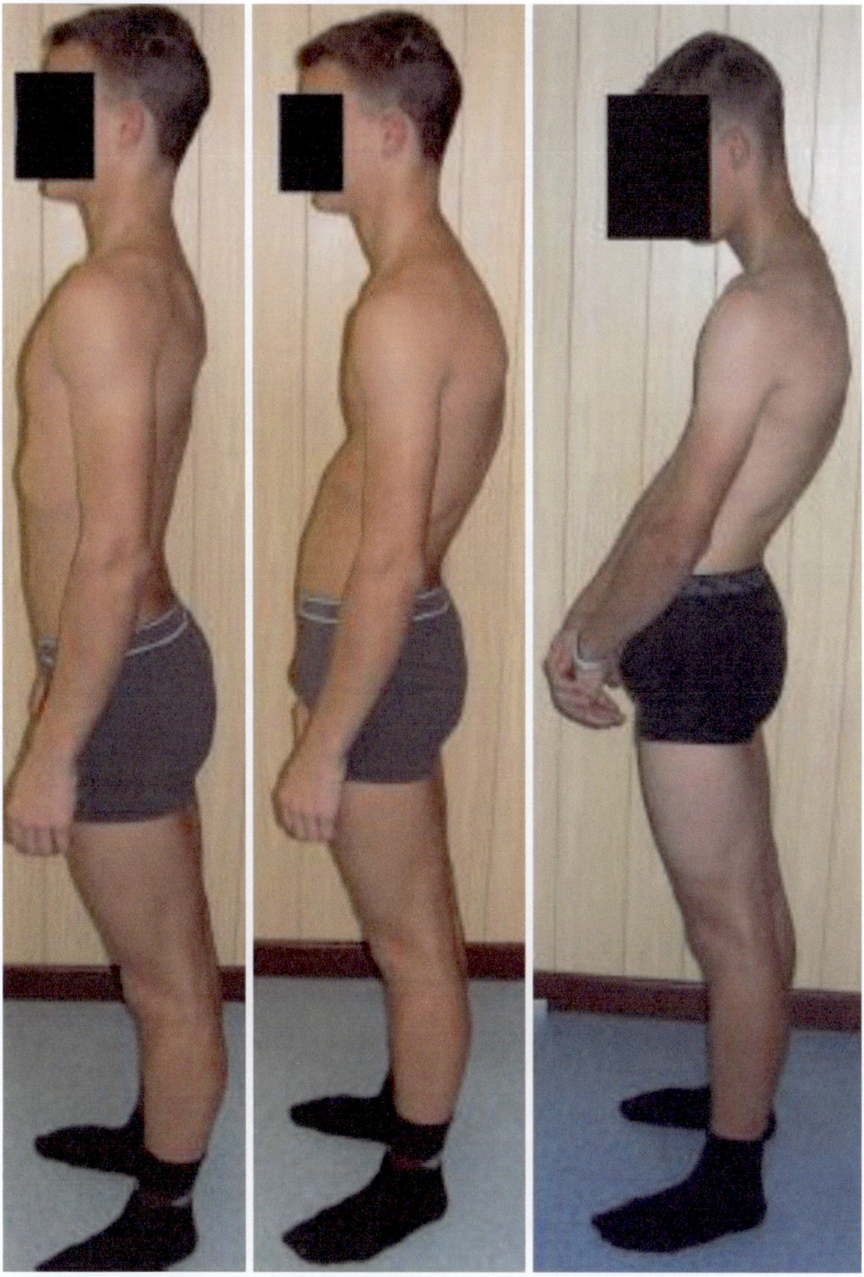

Fig. 5.4 Three poses in profile with the evidence of compensation along the entire spine from the CVJ to the pelvis (erect-relaxed-slouched)

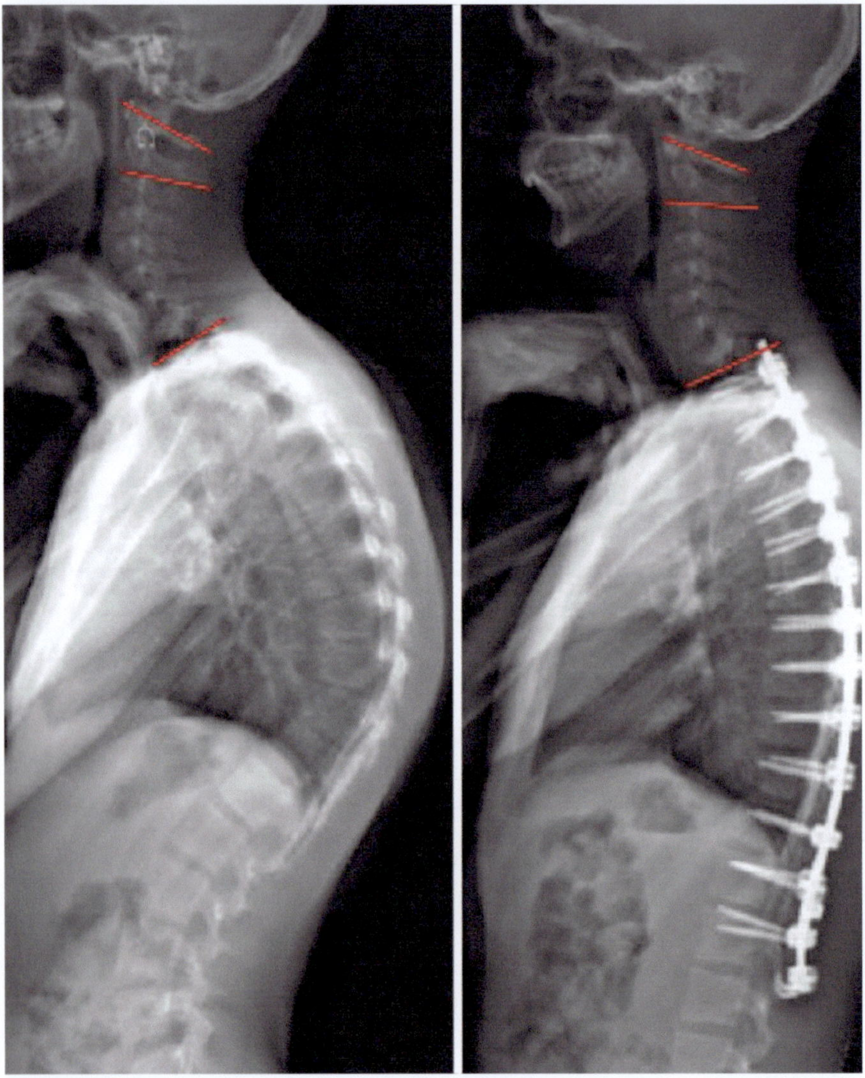

Fig. 5.5 Scheuermann's kyphosis pre- and post-deformity correction with the evidence of reduction of thoracic kyphosis and reduction of cervical lordosis

5.3 Degenerative Conditions

The most accurate method of assessing C2C7 alignment is the *Harrison method* of comparison between the tangents of each posterior wall along the subaxial cervical spine [16, 17]. It has been suggested that the Cobb C1C7 angle overestimates cervical lordosis, that the Cobb C2C7 angle underestimates cervical lordosis, and that the Harrison method (C2C7) may provide the best estimate of lordosis. Thus, little is

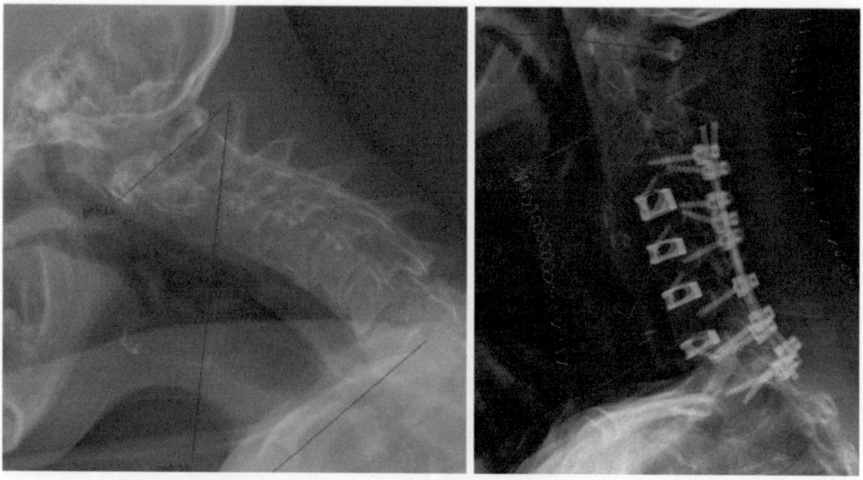

Fig. 5.6 Preoperative EOS radiograph of a degenerative cervical spine with a history of dropped-head syndrome with anterior multilevel autofusions. Postoperative radiograph with anterior osteotomies and cage placement (first stage) and posterior construct with pedicle and lateral mass screws (second stage). Notably there is a significant increase in SAS lordosis (from −44° to +1°) and decrease in CVJ lordosis (from 43° to 32°)

known on the contributions of the CVJ in cervical disc degeneration. Furthermore, despite the roles of OC1 and C1C2 articulations are quite different, their contributions are mostly quoted summarily as OC2.

Normal lordosis at the C4C7 levels only accounts for 6° (15%) of that of the cervical spine and includes the levels that undergo most degenerative change. Degenerative changes of the cervical spine are commonly associated with a reduction or loss of the segmental or global lordosis [17]. The net effect of loss of lordosis at distal levels contributes proportionally to a greater loss of sagittal alignment. This is compensated for by an increase at the CVJ, particularly OC1, to maintain horizontal gaze [18]. Appropriate correction of lordosis will reverse this (Fig. 5.6).

Traditionally, posterior-based approaches for posterior-based stenotic pathology with laminectomies of the cervical spine have been implicated in causing postoperative kyphosis and neck pain (Fig. 5.7). This is mostly due to the detachment of subaxial deep extensor muscles from the C2 or C7 spinous processes. Laminoplasty of C3 and at levels caudal to it results in less kyphosis than a dome-shaped laminotomy or especially C2 laminectomy [19]. C4–C7 laminoplasty with C3 laminectomy preserving the semispinalis cervicis insertion into C2 can reduce postoperative axial symptoms compared with C3–C7 laminoplasty and reattaching the muscle to the C2 spinous process [20]. The range of motion across OC1C2 has been shown to increase over time post-laminoplasty and is thought to represent a compensation for increasing stiffness from C2C7 [21].

Resection of C3 spinous process is thought to reduce the incidence of C2C3 spinous process autofusion post-laminoplasty which may otherwise occur in up to 53% [22]. Potentially some of what is described as neck pain may alternatively be

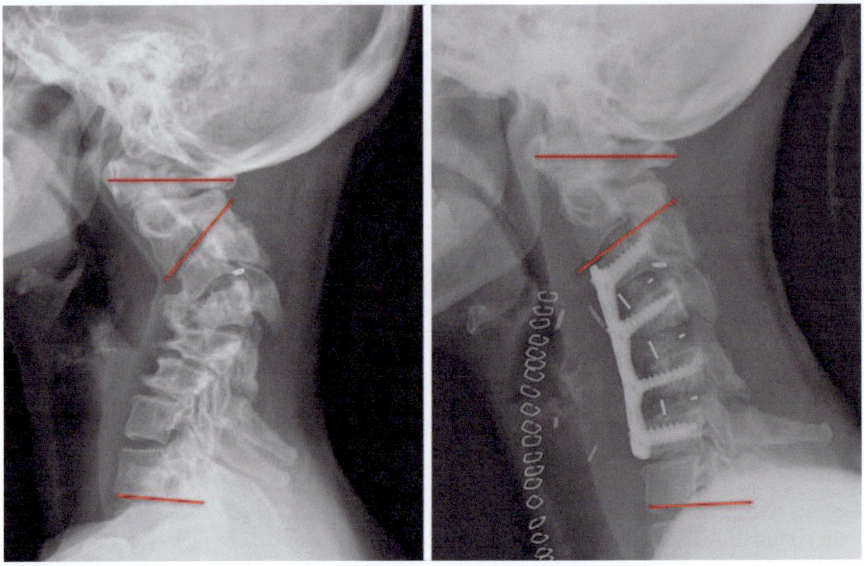

Fig. 5.7 Preoperative EOS radiograph of degenerative cervical spine with a history of a previous posterior laminectomy/laminoplasty and loss of extensor muscle action with the evidence of compensatory OC2 hyperlordosis. Postoperative radiograph with SAS lordosis increases and CVJ lordosis decreases

OC2 extension with occipital neuralgia and warrants consideration when evaluating sagittal images on MRI.

Decompensation of cervical sagittal balance can be represented as an increase in *chin brow vertical angle (CBVA)*, a reliable clinical measure of horizontal gaze. This angle reflects activities of daily living and quality of life. It is commonly used as a reference for ankylosing spondylitis and has been identified in many studies as an important parameter when correcting cervical deformity. It should be close to 0° in asymptomatic individuals. This may not be as apparent on lateral cervical spine radiographs, thus the C2 slope may be used to correlate with one's ability to maintain a horizontal gaze. Therefore, the C2 slope should be close to 15° for a comfortable horizontal gaze. What is often apparent on clinical examination are other adaptive features of compensation to maintain sagittal balance, such as thoracic extension, pelvic retroversion, and knee flexion.

Normalization of cervical spine alignment has been demonstrated after lumbar deformity correction (Fig. 5.8). A review of 31 lumbar pedicle subtraction osteotomy (PSO) cases was taken by the author with the evaluation of spinopelvic parameters [23]. A pattern resembling previous compensatory mechanisms emerged: there was a significant decrease of C7 slope, a decrease in distal C2C7 lordosis, and an increase in proximal cervical lordosis and OC2 angle. There was no significant difference between global cervical lordosis angle and EAM tilt (Fig. 5.9). The decrease in C7 tilt was caused by the corrective lumbar surgery, so the distal cervical lordosis manifested because there was no longer a requirement for compensation at this level. The

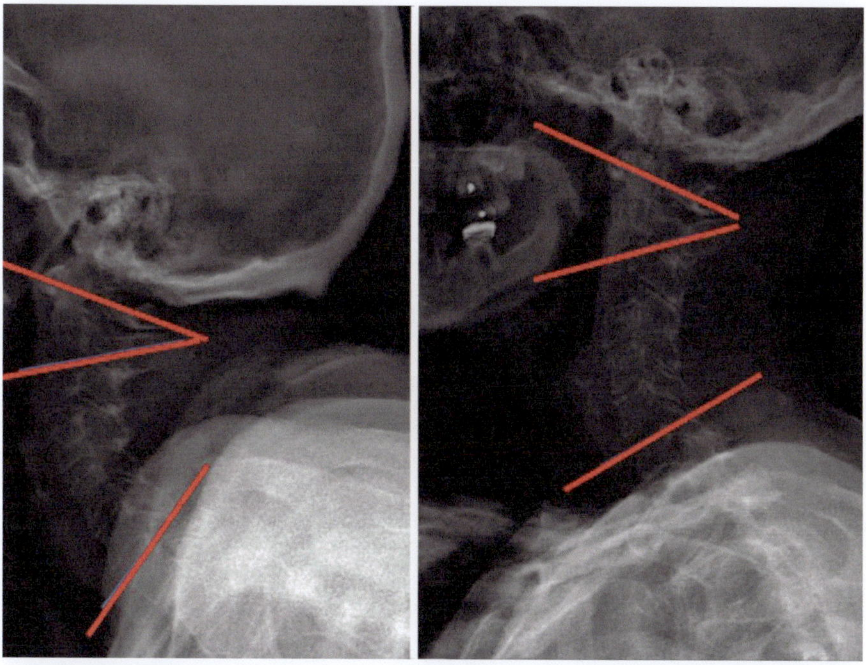

Fig. 5.8 Post-lumbar pedicle subtraction osteotomy with horizontalization of C7 and increase in C1C2 lordosis

proximal cervical spine readjusted to adapt a slightly flexed position to maintain horizontal sight. In effect, the adaptive features of the cervical spine maintained its global angulation and position relative to vertical balance.

5.4 Other CVJ Alignment Considerations

Bony malformations of the CVJ are best divided into malformations of the central pillar such as odontoid or basioccipital dysgeneses or of the surrounding rings such as pro-atlas or C1 sclerotome anomalies. Thus, relevant malformations are mostly associated with decreased skull-based height (platybasia as described in quadrupeds, Fig. 5.1) and/or, to a lesser extent, increased vertebral column height. In practical terms, structural anomalies mostly involve the occiput, including condylus tertius (third occipital condyle), basiocciput hypoplasia and atlanto-occipital assimilation. As malalignment may extend intracranially, both primary cranial angles (basal and Boogard's) and craniovertebral angles (Wackenheim clivus-canal, McGregor-C2, and OC1 joint axis angle) are relevant [24]. Platybasia may manifest as a short or horizontal clivus causing lordotic tilt of the foramen magnum and occipital condylar plane. Frequently with this condition, the odontoid is retroflexed, pointing toward the brainstem, often associated with cerebellar herniation, a syringomyelia and hypolordosis in the SAS.

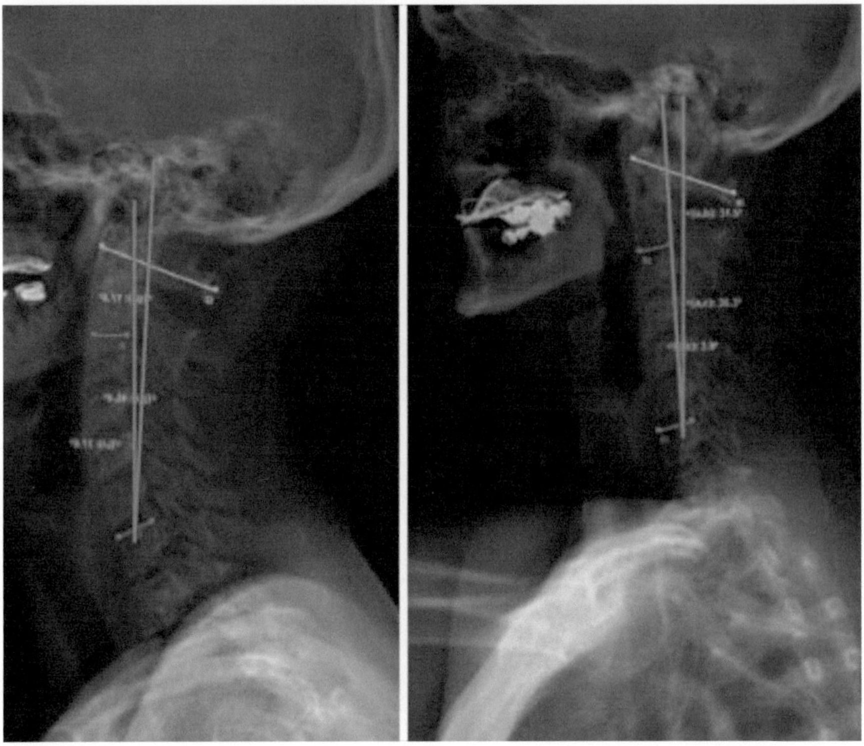

Fig. 5.9 Pre- and post-lumbar deformity measurement of cervical parameters. EAM tilt remains close to 0°, upper and lower cervical curvature changes are significant

Alignment pathology associated with trauma to the CVJ mostly involves type II fractures of the odontoid process of C2. Most of these fractures have either an oblique posterior or transverse orientation, almost half occur in combination with a fracture of C1, and 60% are posteriorly displaced [25]. Halo vest immobilization is an accepted form of treatment but not well tolerated in the elderly. Whether using halo vest or operative fixation, one must check for fracture reduction and alignment on intraoperative imaging. Displaced fractures perform poorly regardless of treatment. In attempts to reduce the fracture, one can immobilize the cervical spine in an abnormal alignment. Particularly with posteriorly displaced fractures, patients develop kyphosis of C2C7 with anterior displacement of the proximal cervical spine, in what has been described as a "Geier" or *vulture-like deformity* [26]. The underlying pathomechanism may be disequilibrium of the anterior load and posterior muscle forces in the upper cervical spine, thus posterior C1C2 stabilization may be the optimal treatment in those with osteoporosis. Forced hyperextension causes fracture of the C2 pars, as the odontoid process and cephalad structures displace anteriorly while the posterior aspect of C2 remain aligned with the caudal structures. Levine and Edwards types II and III display increasing displacement, kyphotic angulation, and instability, with increased indication for operative stabilization, including anterior, posterior, or combined approaches. Posterior approaches for operative fixation of either of these types of fractures will usually involve dissection of the C2 process and loss of extensor muscle function. This may lead to significant kyphosis at the CVJ.

5.5 Alignment Considerations When Operating on the CVJ

Preventative measures must be taken when instrumenting the CVJ to maintain a normal sagittal alignment. Using a Halo frame or Mayfield clamp for posterior cervical surgery serves to optimize three-dimensional positioning of the head as close to neutral as possible. Patients are frequently placed in a slight reverse Trendelenburg position to diminish venous congestion and bleeding. Therefore the position of the head must match that of the body. Head position is best imaged to ensure optimal CVJ alignment which in more recent times involves a trend toward intraoperative CT. Similar to fluoroscopy, the 2D facility can be used to check this. Longer occipito-cervical constructs placed in extension can be disabling, and one should err slightly toward flexion [27]. A hyperkyphotic angle at the CVJ can predispose to a higher incidence of postoperative dysphagia, dyspnea, and decreased oropharynx volumes [28]. As the trajectory of transarticular screws or pars screws is orientated cephalad, one may need to drape as far caudally as T3 to allow for this. Thus, obesity, a short neck or a hyperkyphotic thorax may compromise screw trajectory, particularly for Magerl transarticular fixation.

Multiple reports have shown that an excessive lordosis at the CVJ through surgical correction leads to compensatory kyphotic changes of the subaxial cervical spine. Yoshimoto et al. demonstrated that in a series of patients with C1C2 fixation, mean lordotic angles increased from 18° preoperatively to 26° postoperatively [29]. The fixation techniques in this series were diverse, but the authors felt that bone graft compression between the posterior elements of C1 and C2 from such techniques as Brooks (interlaminar graft) wiring or a Halifax clamp led to a C1C2 hyperlordosis with a resultant C2C7 postoperative kyphosis. The C1C7 angle did not change significantly given the segmental compensation mechanisms within the cervical spine as mentioned previously.

Likewise, in a series of mostly rheumatoid patients, corrective surgery with fusion at the CVJ has shown that restoration of lordosis at OC2 leads to a decrease in lordosis at C2C7 [26]. This has also been shown in patients with congenital atlanto-axial dislocations [30]. Distraction arthrodesis is a helpful technique at C1C2 for C2 root compression or between O-C1-C2 to disengage the odontoid process with basilar invagination. Ding et al. reported disengaging the odontoid process in congenital malformations using the application of the combined forces of extension and distraction between the occipital plate and the cervical pedicle screws [31]. Parallelism must be maintained with distraction so as not to cause kyphotic deformity. C1C2 intervertebral cages may also be used to achieve this.

When treating pathology at the CVJ, the most caudal aspect of the fixation may extend to the distal cervical spine. Sagittal balance between the proximal and distal segments of the cervical spine should be checked on imaging before the rods are secured.

5.6 Conclusions

The proximal OC2 and distal C2C7 segments of the cervical spine work synergistically to ensure that the head remains balanced over the pelvis. Within a functional range of motion, deformities of each can be compensated for by the other. The "fine-tuning" features of the CVJ allow for obtaining horizontal gaze despite the variations in relative positions of the head and spine. Furthermore, this compensatory mechanism is especially important in pathological conditions.

Correction of deformities of the subaxial C2C7 cervical, thoracic, and lumbar spine can reduce lordosis at the CVJ, so that the head and gaze remain horizontal. Surgical objectives when operating on the CVJ must include normalization of the CVJ which relies on several factors including positioning, anatomy-specific instrumentation, instrument placement, and the use of intraoperative imaging or navigation.

Glossary

CVJ Craniovertebral junction including occiput to axis (O-C1-C2, OC2)
SAS Subaxial spine, including C2-C7
OC1 Occipito-atlantal joint
C1C2 Atlanto-axial joint
SVA Sagittal vertical alignment

References

1. Roussouly P, Pinheiro-Franco JL. Biomechanical analysis of the spino-pelvic organization and adaptation in pathology. Eur Spine J. 2011;20(5):609–18.
2. Vital, Jean Marc, Cawley, Derek T (Eds.). Spinal Anatomy: Modern Concepts. © 2020. ISBN 978-3-030-20924-7.
3. White AA III, Panjabi MM. The clinical biomechanics of the occipitoatlantoaxial complex. Orthop Clin North Am. 1978;9(4):867–78. (no abstract available).
4. Lee SH, Kim KT, Seo EM, Suk KS, Kwack YH, Son ES. The influence of thoracic inlet alignment on the cranio-vertebral sagittal balance in asymptomatic adults. J Spinal Disord Tech. 2012;25:E41–7.
5. Akçam MO, Köklü A. Investigation of natural head posture in different head types. J Oral Sci. 2004;46(1):15–8.
6. Beier G, Schuck M, Schuller E, et al. Determination of physical data of the head I. Center of Gravity and Moments of Inertia of Human Heads: Office of Naval Research; 1979. p. 44.
7. Moussellard H. Osteosynthese du rachis cervical superieur. In: Masson, editor. Conference d'enseignement; 2009. p. 364–83.
8. Kuntz C, Shaffrey CI, Ondra SL, Durrani AA, Mummaneni PV, Levin LS, Pettigrew DB. Spinal deformity: a new classification derived from neutral upright spinal alignment measurements in asymptomatic juvenile, adolescent, adult, and geriatric individuals. Neurosurgery. 2008;63:25–39.
9. Matsunaga S, Onishi T, Sakou T. Significance of occipitoaxial angle in sub axial lesion after occipitocervical fusion. Spine. 2001;26:161–5.

10. Le Huec JC, Demezon H, Aunoble S. Sagittal parameters of global cervical balance using EOS imaging: normative values from a prospective cohort of asymptomatic volunteers. Eur Spine J. 2015;24(1):63–71.
11. Morvan G, Mathieu P, Vuillemin V, Guerini H, Bossard P, Zei- toun F, Wybier M. Standardized way for imaging of the sagittal spinal balance. Eur Spine J. 2011;20:602–8. https://doi.org/10.1007/s00586-011-1927-y.
12. Patwardhan AG, Havey RM, Khayatzadeh S, Muriuki MG, Voronov LI, Carandang G, Nguyen NL, Ghanayem AJ, Schuit D, Patel AA, Smith ZA. Postural consequences of cervical sagittal imbalance: a novel laboratory model. Spine. 2015;40(11):783–92.
13. Ordway NR, Seymour RJ, Donelson RG, Hojnowski LS, Edwards WT. Cervical flexion, extension, protrusion, and retraction: a radiographic segmental analysis. Spine. 1999;24:240–7.
14. Fort D, Tassin JL, Chatelain G, Paysant J. Comparative radiological study of the sagittal spinal alignment of 240 adolescents with Scheuermann disease with 100 healthy teenagers. Pediatrie. 2013;56(S1):e281.
15. Zepa I, Hurmerinta K, Kovero O, Nissinen M, Könönen M, Huggare J. Associations between thoracic kyphosis, head posture, and craniofacial morphology in young adults. Acta Odontol Scand. 2000;58(6):237–42.
16. Harrison DD, Troyanovich SJ, Harrison DE, Janik TJ, Murphy DJ. A normal sagittal spinal configuration: a desirable clinical outcome. J Manipulative Physiol Ther. 1996;19(6):398–405.
17. Grob D, Frauenfelder H, Mannion AF. The association between cervical spine curvature and neck pain. Eur Spine J. 2007;16(5):669–78.
18. Hayashi T, Daubs MD, Suzuki A, Scott TP, Phan K, Aghdasi B, Ruangchainikom M, Hu X, Lee C, Takahashi S, Shiba K. The compensatory relationship of upper and subaxial cervical motion in the presence of cervical spondylosis. Clin Spine Surg. 2016;29(4):E196–200.
19. Takeshita K, Seichi A, Akune T, Kawamura N, Kawaguchi H, Nakamura K. Can laminoplasty maintain the cervical alignment even when the C2 lamina is contained? Spine. 2005;30(11):1294–8.
20. Takeuchi K, Yokoyama T, Aburakawa S, Saito A, Numasawa T, Iwasaki T, Itabashi T, Okada A, Ito J, Ueyama K, Toh S. Axial symptoms after cervical Laminoplasty with C3 laminectomy compared with conventional C3–C7 Laminoplasty: a modified Laminoplasty preserving the Semispinalis Cervicis inserted into axis. Spine. 2005;30(22):2544–9.
21. Aita I, Wadano Y, Yabuki T. Curvature and range of motion of the cervical spine after laminaplasty. J Bone Joint Surg Am. 2000;82(12):1743.
22. Iizuka H, Iizuka Y, Nakagawa Y, Nakajima T, Toda N, Shimegi A, Tsutsumi S, Takagishi K. Interlaminar bony fusion after cervical laminoplasty: its characteristics and relationship with clinical results. Spine. 2006;31(6):644–7.
23. Obeid I, Boniello A, Boissiere L, Bourghli A, Pointillart V, Gille O, Lafage V, Vital JM. Cervical spine alignment following lumbar pedicle subtraction osteotomy for sagittal imbalance. Eur Spine J. 2015;24(6):1191–8.
24. Botelho RV, Ferreira ED. Angular craniometry in cranio-vertebral junction malformation. Neurosurg Rev. 2013;36(4):603–10.
25. Reinhold M, Bellabarba C, Bransford R, Chapman J, Krengel W, Lee M, Wagner T. Radiographic analysis of type II odontoid fractures in a geriatric patient population: description and pathomechanism of the "Geier"-deformity. Eur Spine J. 2011;20(11):1928–39.
26. Matsubayashi Y, Shimizu T, Chikuda H, Takeshita K, Oshima Y, Tanaka S. Correlations of cervical sagittal alignment before and after occipitocervical fusion. Global Spine J. 2016;6(04):362–9.
27. Allen RT, Decker R, Hong JT, Sasso R. Complications of occipitocervical fixation. Seminars in Spine Surgery, vol. 21. Philadelphia: WB Saunders; 2009. p. 167–76.
28. Miyata M, Neo M, Fujibayashi S, et al. Oc-C2 angle as a predictor of dyspnea and/or dysphagia after occipitocervical fusion. Spine. 2009;34:184–8.
29. Yoshimoto H, Ito M, Abumi K, et al. A retrospective radiographic analysis of subaxial sagittal alignment after posterior C1-C2 fusion. Spine. 2004;29:175–81.

30. Passias PG, Wang S, Kozanek M, Wang S, Wang C. Relationship between the alignment of the occipitoaxial and subaxial cervical spine in patients with congenital atlantoaxial dislocations. J Spinal Disord Tech. 2013;26(1):15–21.
31. Ding X, Abumi K, Ito M, Sudo H, Takahata M, Nagahama K, Iwata A. A retrospective study of congenital osseous anomalies at the cranio-vertebral junction treated by occipitocervical plate-rod systems. Eur Spine J. 2012;21(8):1580–9.

Part II

Perioperative Considerations

Surgical Positioning

6

Claudio Schonauer and Enrico Tessitore

6.1 Introduction

Proper patient positioning for upper cervical surgery is crucial for the correct execution of the surgical procedure and, if not applied correctly, can give rise to dangerous complications. We can compare the surgical patient positioning to the alignment of military troops before a battle: if strategically correct, it can influence the result, if applied improperly it can lead to disaster.

Key to success are the several adjustments that can be made during surgery and that must be taken into account beforehand. Neuromonitoring, navigation and fluoroscopy can be difficult to plan in such a small anatomic area i.e. everything should be planned and checked before. As a rule, these adjustments should be carried out preoperatively, whilst the patient is still awake, verifying the possible ranges of neck hyperflexion–hyperextension to simulate what will be [1, 2].

Planning the position of the Mayfield's blocks before draping enables us to adjust the neck flexion during surgery while fixing the patient safely to the table, making possible to tilt the table safely.

Supine and prone positions are the most commonly used for the anterior transoral approach and posterior fusion/decompression procedures, respectively. Lateral positioning is also used when a combined anterior-posterior approach is required, minimizing the risk of a double positioning procedure and reducing operating times [3].

C. Schonauer
Neurosurgical Unit, ASL Napoli 2 Nord, Naples, Italy

E. Tessitore (✉)
Neurosurgical Unit, Geneva University Hospitals, Geneva, Switzerland
e-mail: enrico.tessitore@hcuge.ch

E. Tessitore et al. (eds.), *Surgery of the Cranio-Vertebral Junction*,
https://doi.org/10.1007/978-3-030-18700-2_6

6.2 Supine Position

Supine position is mainly used for anterior endoscopic endonasal or transoral approaches to the CVJ. Positioning is similar to the one used for anterior cervical discectomy (ACDF). Usually a flexible armoured nasotracheal tube is used. Retractors and endoscopic holder are fixed to the table contralateral to the surgeon, as well as the monitors (Fig. 6.1).

6.2.1 The Body

The body remains in dorsal decubitus. This is the easiest positioning, and attention should be focused in fixing the patient safely to the table and to elevate the legs slightly (7–10°) to allow a correct venous backflow to the heart [4].

The so-called lawn chair (contoured) position is a variation of the horizontal position adding a 15° flexion at the trunk and hips. A blanket or soft (gel) pillow can be placed under the knees to keep them slightly flexed. This position provides more physiological positioning of the lumbar spine, hips, and knees. The other advantages of the lawn chair position include a slight head elevation improving venous drainage from the brain, and a slight elevation of the legs, that improves venous return to the heart [5]. The head-up tilt or reverse Trendelenburg position usually involves a 10–15° repositioning from the horizontal axis in order to provide optimal venous drainage from the brain [6].

6.2.2 The Head

In case of concomitant spinal stenosis and cervical cord compression, the patient is usually transferred to theatre with a Philadelphia collar that is held in place during intubation, so that the anaesthesist can safely perform awake fibre-optic intubation.

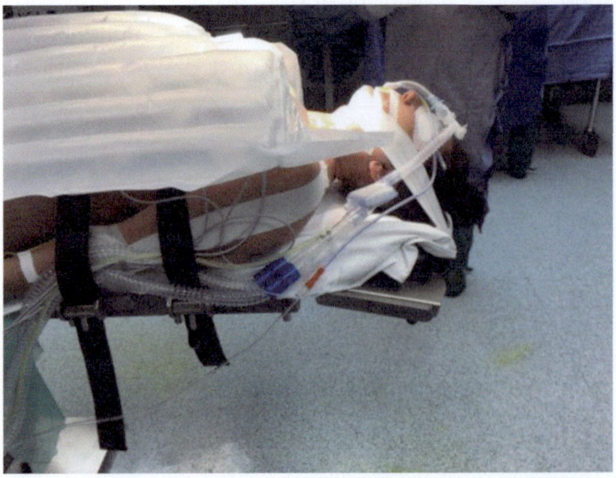

Fig. 6.1 Supine positioning with cervical and shoulders taping

With regards to the head position in supine patients, we have two options.

In the first one, the patient's head is extended backward and downward with the surgeon standing at the back of it. The microscope will be at 90° on the operative field. Head extension will allow a wider exposure of the skull base. When instability and/or potentially cord compressing lesions are present, the head will be initially positioned in neutral position, and only once satisfactory decompression is achieved, the suregon will be able to change the degrees of head extension. When anterior instrumentation is required, is mandatory to achieving neutral position before fixing the spine.

The second option is mainly used in endoscopic assisted surgery, with the surgeon facing the patinet [7]. In this case the head is placed on a horseshoe headrest and may not be fixed allowing multiple minimal adjustements intraoperatively.

Whichever of these positions is chosen, care must be taken in planning in advance the position of the fluoroscopic arm, should it be used during surgery, as the arm of the Mayfield clamp might interfere with AP views. To avoid this, the patient should be positioned on a Jackson table. If a Jackson table is not available, the head clamp could be secured on the arch used for sitting position. The arch is secured anteriorly with the head clamp in the centre (Fig. 6.2).

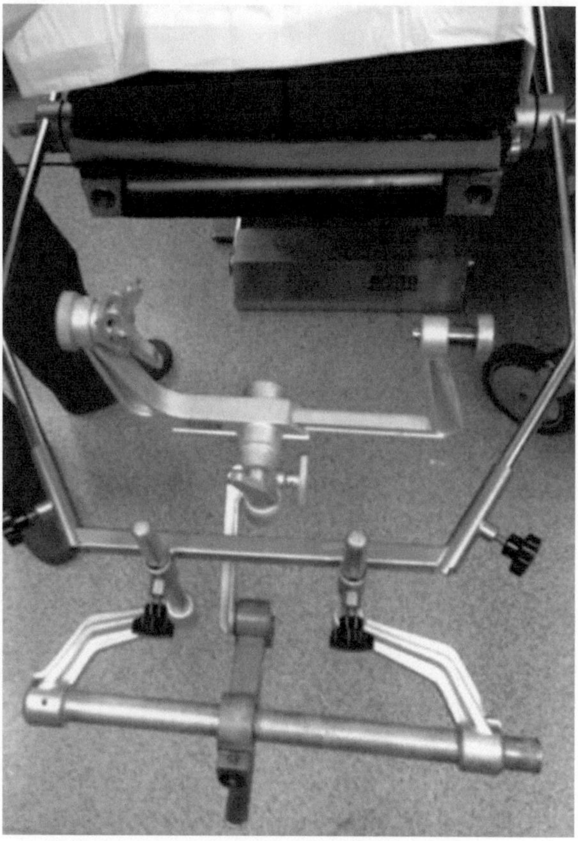

Fig. 6.2 Head clamp positioning when fluoroscopic AP projections are required: note that the area under the patient's neck is completely free of metal structures that could interfere with the imaging

Even if the supine position is the most physiological one, it is not risk free. Peripheral nerve compression injuries are the most common complications of this position although are less frequent than in the prone one. Other complications of the supine position include pressure alopecia (for long procedures), backache, and tissue ischemia [8].

6.3 The Prone Position

The so-called Concorde or landing Concorde position (Fig. 6.3) is the most common prone position for posterior or posterolateral approaches to the CVJ. It is used for posterolateral approaches to the CVJ. The principle is that the head is flexed to better expose the C0–C2 region, and elevated higher than the right cardiac atrium to achieve better venous return.

6.3.1 The Body

The patient is intubated in supine position and then carefully turned on a square soft pillow to allow release of the abdominal pressure both arms are secured along the body to allow secure table tilting. Shoulders are gently pulled downwards with tape to visualize C7 vertebral body during intraoperative lateral X-rays when necessary. When taping acre must be paid to avoid excessive stretching of the brachial plexus. Knees are flexed with the feet slightly elevated to obtain a better venous flow gradient. A pneumatic leg compression machine or alternatively leg wrapping with compression bandages are also applied.

6.3.2 The Head

For the posterior approach, neck flexion is helpful to obtain the proper trajectory for drills and screws whose direction is almost parallel to the bone surface of the spine. The so-called military tuck position is often required in CVJ surgery, in order to increase the surgical exposure between the occiput and C2. The patient is positioned with the head put in the Mayfield clamp. Mayfield pins are positioned in a way to keep the posterior fossa area completely free.

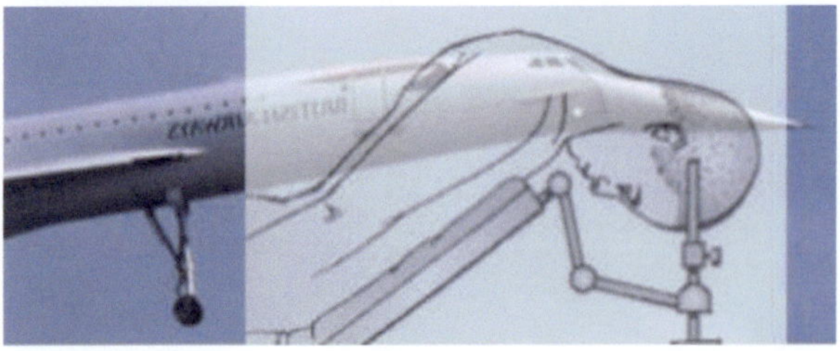

Fig. 6.3 Author's illustration of Concorde position

Some degrees (20°–30°) of anti-Trendelenburg are applied to the cranial part of the table in order to raise the head and to facilitate venous outflow, which is extremely important in order to avoid eye complication and perivertebral venous plexus bleeding. In this way we can obtain an operative site that is parallel to the floor [6].

When draping, one should consider the possibility of extra stub incisions, which are often necessary to keep the right trajectory of drill and screws.

If a Jackson table is used, the head clamp could be directly connected to the table.

Specific complications include necrosis of the chin and an obstruction of cerebral venous outflow.

6.4 Lateral Position

Lateral position can be used for one stage anterior transoral decompression surgery and posterior fixation. The rationale is to avoid repositioning e redraping the patient after the decompression and before performing stabilization. With the head secured in the Mayfield clamp, the patient's neck is absolutely stable throughout the whole surgery. The difficulty is to provide a position that can also be comfortable for the surgeon and for the instrumentation [3, 9]. Lateral positioning leads to gravitational changes in the ventilation–perfusion relationship in the lung. Lung tissue above 18 cm from bed level is not perfused. During general anaesthesia and positive pressure ventilation, the non-dependent lung zones are ventilated better with respect to the dependent zones, worsening ventilation–perfusion mismatch.

6.4.1 Park Bench Position

The Park Bench is a modification of the lateral position. It gives the surgeon a more comfortable operative position with better access to the posterior fossa, as compared to the lateral position. The upper arm is positioned along the lateral trunk and the upper shoulder is taped towards the table. Special attention is required for positioning the patient's dependent (lower) arm because of the potential danger of axillary artery compression and brachial plexus injury [2, 10]. The dependent arm can be positioned in hanging or ventral position and may be rested on a low padded arm board, inserted between the table and head fixator. Alternatively, the forearm can be hung on a pillow and towels wrapped over the arm and forearm. The shoulder should be abducted, and the elbow flexed. An axillary roll, inflatable pillow or a gel pad should be placed under the upper chest (not directly in the axilla) in order to take pressure off the dependent shoulder and prevent arm ischemia, brachial plexus injury and compartment syndrome. It is also critical to support the patient's head with a pillow or gel pad to minimize angulation of the cervical spine, which can be achieved with the simultaneous inflation of both inflatable pillows under head and chest [6].

The lower extremities should be slightly flexed, and a pillow should be placed between the legs (particularly the knees). Reverse Trendelenburg and marked flexion of the legs at hips and knees should be avoided, as it can lead to lower extremity venous stasis and decrease of venous return to the heart. Leg wrapping with compression bandages can be used to prevent venous pooling [1].

References

1. Robertson JT, Coakham HB, Robertson JH. Cranial base surgery. London: Churchill Livingstone; 1999.
2. Bambakidis NC, Dickman CA, Spetzler RF, VKH S, editors. Surgery of the craniovertebral junction. Stuttgart: Thieme; 2012.
3. Mouchaty H, Perrini P, Conti R, Di Lorenzo N. Craniovertebral junction lesions: our experience with the transoral surgical approach. Eur Spine J. 2009;18(Suppl 1):13–9.
4. Rozet I, Vavilala MS. Risks and benefits of patient positioning during neurosurgical care. Anesthesiol Clin. 2007;25(3):631–5.
5. Schonauer C, Bocchetti A, Barbagallo G, Albanese V, Moraci A. Positioning on the surgical table. Eur Spine J. 2004;13(Suppl 1):S50–5.
6. Miller RD. Miller's Anesthesia. London: Churchill Livingstone; 2006. p. 1151–70.
7. Lin ZK, Chi YL, Wang XY, Yu Q, Fang BD, Wu LJ. The influence of cervical spine position on the three anterior endoscopic approaches to the craniovertebral junction: an imaging study. Spine J. 2014;14(1):80–6.
8. Warner MA. Positioning in anesthesia and surgery. 3rd ed. Philadelphia: W. B. Saunders; 1997. p. 39–46.
9. Suchomel P, Choutka O. Reconstruction of upper cervical spine and craniovertebral junction. Berlin: Springer; 2011.
10. Goel A, Cacciola F. The craniovertebral junction. Diagnosis, pathology, surgical techniques. Stuttgart: Thieme; 2011.

7 Neuroanesthetic Considerations for Patients Undergoing Posterior Fossa and Craniovertebral Junction Surgery

Dominic J. Nardi, Shamik Chakraborty, and Amir R. Dehdashti

Surgical conditions treated at the craniovertebral junction include tumors, cerebral vascular malformations, aneurysms, congenital craniovertebral anomalies, often with accompanying instability, and major trauma [1]. Anesthesia for such surgeries is also appropriately recognized as complex and presents unique challenges for the anesthesiologist as well.

For craniovertebral instability, maintaining proper cervical alignment is key during intubation and positioning. Patients who have suffered traumatic injury or chronic stenosis of the cervical spine are particularly at risk for neurologic sequelae when extending the head and neck during intubation. Congenitally lax joints resulting in subluxation and cord compression can also be present in patients with known Chiari malformation, Klippel–Feil syndrome, and Morquio's syndrome, just to mention a few [2]. Preoperative inquiry should be made as to the severity of nerve root or spinal cord impingement. If the patient shows significant signs and symptoms of myelopathy or cord compression, an awake fiberoptic intubation should be considered. A well conducted awake intubation need not be traumatic to the patient, and it would allow for post-intubation clinical assessment of upper and lower extremity function prior to the induction of general anesthesia and patient positioning. In all such cases, a member of the surgical team should be present during intubation to help assure neutrality of neck alignment as well as for the post-intubation evaluation.

If an awake fiberoptic intubation is indicated, preoperative patient education as to the necessity for the procedure and as to what is to be expected are key elements to ensure the successful cooperation of the patient. Major obstacles to awake intubation are language barriers and extremes of anxiety. However, with proper

D. J. Nardi (✉) · S. Chakraborty · A. R. Dehdashti
Department of Anesthesiology, Zucker School of Medicine, Hofstra University/Northwell Health, Hempstead, NY, USA

Department of Neurosurgery, Zucker School of Medicine, Hofstra University/Northwell Health, Hempstead, NY, USA
e-mail: DNardi@northwell.edu

E. Tessitore et al. (eds.), *Surgery of the Cranio-Vertebral Junction*,
https://doi.org/10.1007/978-3-030-18700-2_7

preoperative preparation and adequate topicalization of the oropharyngeal airway, intubation can be accomplished with minimal sedation. For an excellent example of technique, I would recommend viewing the following YouTube video: Dr. Michael Bailin demonstrates an awake endotracheal intubation at the Massachusetts General Hospital [3]. Following adequate pharyngeal-tracheal topicalization, awake intubation can be accomplished with a variety of fiberoptic devices including a number of newer video laryngoscopes. Post-intubation, the awake patient should be able to voluntarily cooperate in a clinical assessment of extremity strength, thus providing real-time monitoring of their function. Additionally, for patients considered to be at risk during positioning, the awake intubated patient may be allowed to self-position, thereby allowing for an awake post-position assessment of extremity strength and function prior to the induction of general anesthesia.

An alternative approach to the management of the airway for patients with less severe craniovertebral instability, or patients considered poor candidates for an awake technique, has been the use of an asleep fiberoptic intubation technique. This can be accomplished following the induction of general anesthesia with a fiberoptic scope through an intubating laryngeal mask device, such as an iGel, or with the use of a video laryngoscope. If an asleep technique is used, a member of the surgical team should be present to help confirm neutrality of neck position during the intubation. Successful intubation should be immediately followed by neurophysiologic monitoring, such as SSEPs and MEPs, to confirm integrity of cord function prior to patient positioning. The anesthesiologist must carefully consider his choice of induction of anesthesia so as to allow for post-intubation neurophysiological monitoring. So as to allow for post-intubation MEPs, a muscle relaxant free induction with the use of a combination of propofol, ketamine, and remifentanil is frequently used, immediately followed by a TIVA anesthetic for the remainder of the surgical procedure. Once the procedure is underway, it is not uncommon for our surgeons to request muscle relaxants while working on the surgical exposure so as to minimize muscular contraction during the use of electrocautery.

Obtaining post-intubation neurophysiological monitoring baseline data can prove invaluable prior to surgical positioning of the patient. Clinical experience has shown that the most common cause for neurophysiological degradation of potentials occurs during positioning of the patient, particularly the prone position. Vigilance and frequent communication between the anesthesiologist, surgeon, and neurophysiological monitoring personnel is particularly critical during this time. If significant changes are detected, the anesthesiologist should immediately assess his anesthetic choice and blood pressure so as to maximize perfusion of the cord. Should the neurophysiologic changes persist, the indication for a "wake-up" test should be considered, either while still in the surgical position or upon returning the patient to the supine position. In extreme situations where the degeneration of potentials persist, the surgical procedure may have to be aborted.

Positioning of the patient for posterior fossa and craniovertebral junction surgery has evolved significantly over the last several decades. Prior to the 1990s, the sitting position was the position of choice for the majority of posterior fossa and posterior cervical procedures. Venous air emboli (VAE) was a known and respected possibility as a result of the positioning, but the anesthesiologist and surgical team felt that the benefits far outweighed the risks. Surgical exposure was considered far superior to the alternative positioning options, and bleeding was significantly less secondary to the lower venous pressure. However, with the realization in the 1980s that over 25–30% of the general population are known to have "probe-patent" foramen ovale, the fear of paradoxical air emboli resulting in possible strokes, MI, or even death resulted in the sitting position being all but abandoned [3, 4]. This is important not only from an historical perspective, but also from the observation that positioning for such patients appears to have come full circle, with the return of the sitting position regaining popularity once again [4, 5].

Presently, the most commonly used position for the majority of posterior fossa and craniovertebral junction operations is a variation of the prone position, ranging from straight prone to three-quarter prone or full lateral. Unlike the sitting position, this positioning is associated with anegligible incidence of venous air embolism. However, it does have a number of downsides for the surgeon. The main one is a result of the increase in intrathoracic pressure associated with the prone or lateral position. The increased intrathoracic pressure is transmitted to the intracranial and cervical venous system resulting in venous bleeding during the operation. Another consideration to be contended with by the anesthesiologist is the inherent limitations in the case of an airway or cardiac emergency. Emergency airway management and performing CPR and chest compressions are next to impossible without flipping the patient onto another bed or stretcher. For these reasons, when in the prone or lateral position, the tolerance for placing external pacing electrodes on patients susceptible to cardiac events should be low, and a stretcher should always be made readily available with a sign indicating "PRONE POSITION—DO NOT REMOVE".

Patients positioned prone for extended periods of time are also susceptible to a number of position- related complications. Unless the patients head is secured in pins, a brasions or skin tears of the face, particularly the pressure areas of the cheek bones, are not uncommon. This is particularly true if the patient's face is placed in a dry foam or padded headrest. Applying a lubricant to the patient's cheeks or foam headrest at the pressure points prior to positioning can minimize such risk. If a foam headrest is used, one in which the face and eyes can be easily visualized throughout the procedure by way of a mirror or video monitoring system is preferred. Avoiding compression of the eyes and maintaining patency of the airway and endotracheal tube throughout the case must be assured. The presence of conjunctival or airway edema postoperatively may warrant the patient remaining intubated for the swelling to subside. On rare occasions, patients have been reported to develop blindness secondary to retinal artery thrombosis and/or retinal venous hypertension while in the prone position [1]. However, most patients who undergo posterior fossa or craniovertebral junction surgery are placed in head-pins for additional stability, thereby minimizing the pressure on the eyes and face. In either case, the judicial management of fluid administration and constant vigilance as to the face and eye positioning should mitigate such risks.

As mentioned previously, the sitting position has been long known to provide excellent exposure and access to the posterior fossa and craniovertebral junction [6]. The superior drainage of cerebral spinal fluid as well as blood from the intracranial veins and sinuses allows for better access to anatomical structures by the surgeon, resulting in less manipulation of surrounding tissues and nerves. By avoiding the more commonly used prone position, the anesthesiologist has better visualization and access of the face and airway should an emergency arise. However, despite these obvious advantages, the potential risk of VAE in the sitting position continues to limit its adoption in most neurosurgical centers [6–8].

In one retrospective study of 4806 patients, the overall rate of venous air embolism during neurosurgery in sitting position, as detected by transesophageal echocardiogram (TEE), was 39% for posterior fossa surgery and 12% for cervical surgery [9]. These numbers, however, can be misleading in that TEE monitoring is known to be exquisitely sensitive at detecting venous air embolization that is of no physiologic consequence. In one such study using TEE for detection of venous air embolization in patients undergoing laparoscopic hysterectomy, the incidence of detected air was reported to be 100% [10]. Despite the high incidence of detected air, none of the cases of VAE resulted in hemodynamic changes or were found to be of clinical significance [10]. More recent reviews consider the risks of the sitting position to be relatively low: between 1 and 2% at high volume centers with experienced personnel [11, 12]. The highest risk of VAE complications are associated with suboccipital craniotomy and craniectomy, with a complication rate of 2.8%, and the lowest are cervical spine cases with complications of approximately 0.7% [11, 12]. It is important to note that air embolism has been reported in a variety of less likely neurosurgical procedures, including burr holes for deep brain stimulation as well as awake craniotomies in the supine position [13–15]. A common denominator in many of these cases was that the patient was breathing spontaneously, thereby facilitating the potential for entrainment of air. The possibility of VAE should always be on the anesthesiologists differential when hemodynamic instability of unknown origin occurs.

If the sitting position is to be used, it is highly recommended that the patients have a preoperative workup for the presence of a patent foreman ovale (PFO). However, recent evidence suggests that the decision to avoid the sitting position based solely on the presence of a diagnosed PFO should be reconsidered [9, 16]. The relationship between a PFO and the risk of a paradoxical air embolism is not existent [16]. In all patients at risk of VAE, the sensitivity of the device used for early detection of air, the experience of the anesthesia team in caring for such patients, and the rapid response by the anesthesiologist and surgical team in response to air detection is paramount in avoiding serious complications.

Over the years, there have been many methods advocated for the detection of VAE intraoperatively, ranging from the gasp reflex in the spontaneously breathing patient, to the detection of a mill-wheel murmur using an esophageal or precordial stethoscope, precordial dopplers and most recently by the use of intraoperative TEE [1, 17]. Although the relative sensitivity of the techniques used for the detection of air should be considered, it should not be the only factor in the choice of monitoring technique used. For example, the use of TEE, though exquisitely sensitive in the detection of VAE, has been shown to be more of a hindrance due to the resultant frequent and unnecessary interruption of the surgery whenever air is detected. Furthermore, the availability of a TEE device and the skill required for proper insertion and positioning of the probe can also be limiting factors.

The early detection and termination of VAE when it occurs is critical. The surgical team should communicate when they believe the patient to be at risk of VAE based not only on positioning but on the proximity of critical structures, such as major intracranial sinuses or venous plexuses. The anesthesia team must maintain constant vigilance during such cases for the possibility of VAE by the application and use of appropriate monitors and constant communication with the surgeons during the progression of the case.

A precordial Doppler is likely to be the most commonly used method of monitoring for air embolism, used in conjunction with end tidal CO_2 ($ETCO_2$) [1, 18]. A properly positioned precordial Doppler is more sensitive to the detection of VAE then a drop in the $ETCO_2$ by a factor of 10. When used together, the precordial Doppler should be considered a qualitative device, indicating the early detection of VAE, and the $ETCO_2$ a more quantitative device, indicating the beginning of physiological changes due to the presence of air in the right ventricle and pulmonary circulation. Unless a large amount of air is entrained into the venous system quickly, the precordial Doppler will detect the presence of VAE long before a drop in $ETCO_2$ is noted. This early detection should allow the anesthesiologist ample time to alert the surgeon of the VAE, terminate the use of N_2O, and provide 100% oxygen to the patient. The surgical team should consider applying bone wax or flooding the surgical field with fluid, depending on the point of surgery, so as to stop further VAE. A systematic search for the source of air embolization should be immediately conducted. The anesthesiologist can assist the surgeon by applying gentle compression to the jugular veins if needed. This maneuver will not only raise the venous pressure in the cerebral venous vasculature, frequently allowing the surgeon to identify the source of the air but will also result in an attenuation of the entrainment of air [1]. The application of a Valsalva maneuver to increase cerebral venous pressure should be avoided as it may result in a rise in the right atrial pressure and theroetically promote a right to left intra-atrial shunt, possibly resulting in a paradoxical arterial embolization [5]. If the source of the VAE is not detected and air continues to accumulate in the lungs, the $ETCO_2$ will begin to drop. This is the result of the air accumulating in the pulmonary circulation and an increase in physiologic pulmonary dead space. At this point, every effort should be made to identify and stop further VAE, lest the patient become hemodynamically unstable or worse [3, 11]. As a last resort, if the source of air remains undetected, the patient's head should be lowered below the level of the heart to stop further entrainment of air and allow the surgeon to identify the source. There has been much debate as to the usefulness of central-line aspiration during VAE, with some evidence that aggressive aspiration may actually result in a lowering of central venous pressure, and resultant worsening of VAE. Should central-line aspiration be considered, it is essential that the placement of the tip of the line be verified as being at the atrial-SVC junction prior to the beginning of the surgical procedure [1, 5]. At our institution, a central line is reserved for those patients with medical issues warranting central pressure monitoring intraop and for patients with known patent foramen ovale, though we consider the last to be a soft indication.

Anesthesiologists caring for patients undergoing posterior fossa and craniovertebral junction surgery must be aware of the potential for the sudden onset of cardiac arrhythmias, acute hemodynamic changes, or respiratory pattern alterations in the spontaneously breathing patient. Such hemodynamic and respiratory changes may be centrally mediated by the surgical manipulation of the brainstem or the traction of intracranial nerves. It is imperative that the anesthesiologist communicate these changes immediately to the surgeon before the initiation of intervention. As intracranial anatomy can be obscured by lesions, the surgeon often views the report of such physiologic changes as important information as to the proximity and location of important anatomical structures. The use of pharmacologic interventions by the anesthesiologist, such as atropine to block bradycardia, should ideally be conveyed and discussed with the surgeon prior to administration less he lose this valuable feedback.

Also, the anesthesiologist should be alert to the possible intraoperative manipulation and/or damage to the ninth and tenth cranial nerves responsible for the patient's gag and swallow reflexes, either unilaterally or bilaterally. If it is suspected that the nerve may have been either compromised or injured during the surgery, then prior to extubation an assessment of the patient's gag reflex of the posterior pharynx should be tested bilaterally with the use of a suction catheter. If there is any doubt as to the integrity of the gag and swallow reflex postop, consideration should be given to the patient remaining intubated. This problem has been minimized recently, however, by the monitoring of the cranial nerves intraoperatively when indicated.

Neurophysiologic monitoring has become an integral part of many neurosurgical procedures, and nowhere is this more true than during procedures of the posterior fossa. The most commonly used neuromonitoring modalities for patients having surgery of the posterior fossa and craniovertebral region include somatosensory evoked potentials (SSEP), motor evoked potentials (MEP), brainstem auditory evoked response or potentials (BAER/BAEP), and EMG monitoring of various cranial and cervical nerves. A thorough discussion must be had between the anesthesiologist, surgeon, and neuromonitoring personnel as to what is being monitored and at what phase of the surgery it is being monitored. Only by being fully appraised as to the proposed monitoring can a plan for a safe and complementary anesthetic be devised. It is important that the anesthesiologist be fully knowledgeable and conversant as to the type of anesthesia to be provided so as to allow for the monitoring to be maximally predictive of neurologic compromise. BAERs are the least sensitive to anesthetic interference allowing for the use of any anesthetic technique and muscle relaxants. Ideal anesthesia for SSEP monitoring requires the use of no more than one half MAC of inhalation agent with propofol supplementation, no N_2O, and the use of muscle relaxants as needed. MEPs are the most susceptible to inhalation effects. As such, a pure TIVA anesthetic is frequently administered, without the use of muscle relaxants. EMGs of cranial nerves require the absence of muscle relaxants during the monitoring phase. During the course of the surgical procedure, it may be necessary for the anesthesiologist to adjust his technique to accommodate the monitoring modality in use during that particular phase of surgery [19]. The author appreciates, however, that the accepted anesthetic technique used during neurophysiologic monitoring may vary considerably from one institution to another, so it is important for the anesthesiologist to have a thorough discussion with the monitoring team and surgeon prior to the commencement of anestheisa.

With the advent of intraoperative neurophysiological monitoring, the monitoring of spontaneous breathing under anesthesia as an indicator of brainstem function has become increasingly rare. That having been said, there are certain lesions for which the monitoring of spontaneous ventilation as a complement to BAERs may be requested by the surgeon as the preferred intraoperative monitoring technique [20, 21]. Monitoring of spontaneous ventilation has been shown to provide additional information while operating on lesions located at the base of the fourth ventricle, adjacent to the respiratory center, as well as during vertebrobasilar circulation surgery requiring temporary or permanent blood vessel occlusion [20, 22].

The anesthesiologist must be open to all positioning and monitoring modalities that will allow the surgeon to perform the most definitive procedure and ultimately provide the best possible outcome for the patient. More than perhaps in any other type of surgery, communication between the anesthesiologist, surgeon, and neurophysiologic monitoring personnel is imperative. Only with intimate knowledge of the risks and benefits associated with each requested technique, as well as a thorough understanding of the physiologic and anesthetic challenges posed, can the neuroanesthesiologist best devise a plan for the optimal anesthetic care of the patient.

References

1. Smith DS. Anesthetic management for posterior fossa surgery. In: Cottrell JE, Young WL, editors. Cottrell and Young's neuroanesthesia. Amsterdam: Elsevier; 2010. p. 203–17.
2. Geetha L, Radhakrishnan M, Raghavendra BS, Rao GSU, Indira Devi B. Anesthetic management for foramen magnum decompression in a patient with Morquio syndrome: a case report. J Anesth. 2010;24:594–7.
3. YouTube. "Dr. Michael Bailiin demonstrates an awake endotracheal intubation at the Massachusetts General Hospital: December 21, 2009." Online video clip.
4. Engelhardt M, Folkers W, Brenke C, Scholz M, Harders A, Fidorra H, Schmieder K. Neurosurgical operations with the patient in sitting position: analysis of risk factors using transcranial Doppler sonography. Br J Anaesth. 2006;96:467–72.
5. Feigi GC, Decker K, Wurms M, Krischen B, Ritz R, Unerti K, Tatagiba M. Neurosurgical procedures in the semisitting position: evaluation of the risk of paradoxical venous air embolism in patients with a patent foramen ovale. World Neurosurg. 2014;81(1):159–64.
6. Dilmen OK, Akcil EF, Tureci E, Tunali Y, Bahar M, Tanriverdi T, Aydin S, Yentur E. Neurosurgery in the sitting position: retrospective analysis of 692 adult and pediatric cases. Turk Neurosurg. 2011;21:634–40.
7. Albin MS, Carroll RG, Maroon JC. Clinical considerations concerning detection of venous air embolism. Neurosurgery. 1978;3:380–4.
8. Gottdiener JS, Papademetriou V, Notargiacomo A, Park WY, Cutler DJ. Incidence and cardiac effects of systematic venous air embolism. Echocardiographic evidence of arterial embolization via noncardiac shunt. Arch Intern Med. 1988;148:795–800.
9. Fathi AR, Eshtehardi P, Meier B. Patent foramen ovale and neurosurgery in the sitting position: a systematic review. Br J Anaesth. 2009;102:588–96.
10. Chang SK, Ji YK, Ja-Young K, Seung HC, Sungwan N, et al. Venous air embolism during total laparoscopic hysterectomy: comparison to total abdominal hysterectomy. Anesthesiology. 2009;111:50–4.
11. Himes BT, Mallory GW, Abcejo AS, et al. Contemporary analysis of the intraoperative and perioperative complications of neurosurgical; procedures performed in the sitting position. J Neurosurg. 2016:1–7.
12. Saladino A, Lamperti M, Mangraviti A, Legnani FG, Prada FU, Casali C, Caputi L, Borrelli P, DiMeco F. The semisitting position: analysis of the risks and surgical outcomes in a contemporary series of 425 adult patients undergoing cranial surgery. J Neurosurg. 2016:1–10.

13. Edelman JD, Wingard DW. Air embolism arising from burr holes. Anesthesiology. 1980;53(2):167–8.
14. Hooper AK, Okun MS, Foote KD, Haq IU, Fernandez HH, Hegland D, Robicsek SA. Venous air embolism in deep brain stimulation. Sterotact Funct Neurosurg. 2009;87(1):25–30.
15. Blake M, Manninen PH, McGuire GP, El-Beheiry H, Bernstein M. Venous air embolism during awake craniotomy in a supine patient. Can J Anesth. 2003;50(8):835–8.
16. Marshall WK, Bedford RF. Use of a pulmonary-artery catheter for detection and treatment of venous air embolism: a prospective study in man. J Neurosurg. 1980;55:610–4.
17. Standefer M, Bay JW, Trusso R. The sitting position in neurosurgery: a retrospective analysis of 488 cases. Neurosurgery. 1984;14:649–58.
18. Gildenberg PL, O'Brien RP, Britt WJ, Frost EA. The efficacy of Doppler monitoring for the detection of venous air embolism. J Neurosurg. 1981;54:75–8.
19. Watabnabe E, Schramm J, Strauss C, Fahlbusch R. Neurophysiologic monitoring in posterior fossa surgery. II. BAEP-waves I and V and preservation of hearing. Acta Neurochir. 1989;98:118–28.
20. Schramm J, Watanabe E, Strauss C, Fahlbusch R. Neurophysiologic monitoring in posterior fossa surgery. I. Technical principles, applicability and limitations. Acta Neurochir. 1989;98:9–18.
21. Radtke RA, Erwin CW, Wilkins RH. Intraoperative brainstem auditory evoked potentials: significant decrease in postoperative morbidity. Neurology. 1989;39:187–91.
22. Radtke RA, Erwin CW. Intraoperative monitoring of auditory and brain-stem function. Neurol Clin. 1988;6:899–915.

8 Perioperative Management: Surgical Site Infection Prevention, DVT Prophylaxis, and Blood Loss Management

Granit Molliqaj, Matthias Robin, Christoph Czarnetzki, Marie-Josée Daly, Americo Agostinho, and Enrico Tessitore

8.1 Prevention of Surgical Site Infections in Spine Surgery

The risk of surgical site infection (SSI) in spine surgery is approximately 1–3% in elective and clean surgery [1].

SSIs are the health-associated infections with the most influence in terms of morbidity, mortality, and expenses for hospitals and society [2]. They can cause major suffering for the patients and families, increase the consumption of antibiotics and antimicrobial resistances, and cause the consumption of health and societal resources (hospitalization, loss of production, and salary support).

There are several risk factors for SSIs (endogenous and exogenous to the patient) and numerous measures to correct them, but there is a lack of evidence for real benefit for a part of them [3, 4].

In this chapter, we resume some of the most important measures based on the best level of evidence (IA and IB), which provide a real protection to prevent SSIs and to be necessarily applied.

G. Molliqaj
Department of Neurosurgery, Geneva University Hospitals, Geneva, Switzerland

M. Robin · C. Czarnetzki · M.-J. Daly
Department of Anesthesiology, Pharmacology and Intensive Care Medicine, Geneva University Hospitals, Geneva, Switzerland

A. Agostinho
Infection Control Program and WHO Collaborating Centre on Patient Safety, Geneva University Hospitals, Geneva, Switzerland

E. Tessitore (✉)
Neurosurgical Unit, Geneva University Hospitals, Geneva, Switzerland
e-mail: enrico.tessitore@hcuge.ch

E. Tessitore et al. (eds.), *Surgery of the Cranio-Vertebral Junction*,
https://doi.org/10.1007/978-3-030-18700-2_8

8.1.1 Preoperative Phase [5]

In the preoperative phase, adjustment of concomitant morbidities of the patient (infections, diabetes, overweight, alcohol, and tobacco) is the first important step to improve. A shower or a full body bath using soap the evening before and the day of surgery is recommended.

8.1.2 Perioperative Phase [5]

Concerning the perioperative phase, surgical hand preparation with an antimicrobial soap or suitable, using an alcohol-based hand-rub solution is required [6]. An adequate surgical antimicrobial prophylaxis (SAP) has the best strong evidence in the prevention of SSI [1]. The goal is to obtain a minimum inhibitory concentration (MIC) of the appropriate molecule in the operative and circular tissues throughout the operation, but especially at the time of incision and closure. For that reason, there is evidence showing that intravenous administration is imperative and SAP should be done as a single shot [7, 8]. A single dose should be properly administered (rules of the 4R—see Table 8.1) before the incision.

Table 8.1 Surgical antimicrobial prophylaxis: recommendations for spine surgery and rule of 4R [1]

	First choice (and second)	If MRSA carriage	If allergies to cephalosporins
1. Right antimicrobial			
Antibiotic	Cefazolin (2nd = cefuroxime)	Vancomycin	Clindamycin
2. Right dose			
Patient <120 kg or BMI <35 kg/m^2	2 g	1 g	600 mg
Patient >120 kg or BMI >35 kg/m^2	3 g	1.5 g	900 mg
3. Right timing for administration [9, 10]			
SAP administration starts…Before skin incision	60–15 min	90–60 min (slow administration)	60–15 min (slow administration)
After first of SAP administration, if operation begins >2 h later	Re-administration of a ½ dose	–	Re-administration of a ½ dose
4. Right redosing, if operation still ongoing (or blood loss >1500 mL) [11]			
Each 4 h after previous administration or blood loss	Re-administration of a ½ dose	–	Re-administration of a ½ dose
Each 8 h after previous administration or blood loss		Re-administration of a ½ dose	

The use of an electric clippers for shaving with a single-use head as close as possible to the operation site is superior to shaving with a standard razor blade [12]. Then, skin antiseptic preparation must be done with povidone-iodine alcohol-based on three successive applications. Chlorhexidine is not recommended for spine surgery because of its cytotoxic effect on the meninges. Consequently, iodophor-impregnated incise drape can be used unless the patient has an iodine allergy. At the moment, there is no strong evidence for the use of vancomycin powder put directly in the surgical site prior to closure, as well as antimicrobial skin sealants should not be used with the objective of reducing SSI (conditional recommendations) [13]. Double-gloving or glove-changing during surgery is recommended [14], as well as maintaining patient temperature and optimal tissue oxygenation during the surgery [15]. Finally, the use of a surgical safety checklist can improve communication and reduce infection complication rates [16].

8.1.3 Postoperative Phase

For the postoperative phase, regular follow-up with wound care and disinfection by a specialized nursing team is necessary. An active post-discharge surveillance of SSI with feedback is essential.

8.2 Deep Vein Thrombosis and Pulmonary Embolism Prophylaxis

Deep vein thrombosis (DVT) and subsequent pulmonary embolism (PE) can occur following spinal surgery, leading to potential increased morbidity and mortality.

The content of the literature on DVT and PE is extensive. It is well known that these complications may occur spontaneously or may be precipitated by risk-increasing factors such as long bone fractures or spinal procedures. Other factors such as the extent and duration of surgery, postoperative immobilization, or ethnicity hereby suggesting a genetic susceptibility may influence the risk of thromboembolic disease. Literature analysis with regard to the natural risk of DVT after spinal surgery is complex, because few studies have measured the risk of DVT without any prophylactic therapies. The rate of DVT and PE is, respectively, 0.8% and 0.4% in a large cohort of 22,434 patients undergoing spinal surgery between 2006 and 2010 [17]. In the same paper, the authors developed a VTE risk score, taking into consideration a total of 13 factors identified as relevant after a multivariate regression. The factors were operation time $\geq$4 h, dependent functional status, paraplegia, emergency presentation, ASA score $\geq$III, sepsis, disseminated cancer, inpatient status, hypertension, quadriplegia, history of ischemic attack, postoperative sepsis, and African American race. Patients were assigned a total score, with scores ranging from 0 to 13. The VTE risk score showed high predictability of VTE, with the incidence rate of 0.1% for patients with a score of 0 and 11.7% for those with a score $\geq$7 [17].

Furthermore, according to the implemented diagnostic method, the rate of postoperative DVT or PE diagnosed can vary widely. For example, in a prospective study of 134 patients, Oda et al. obtained a DVT rate of 15.5% by venography, whereas none of these patients showed any clinical symptoms [18].

8.2.1 Diagnostic Methods for DVT and PE

Deep vein thrombosis of the lower extremity is subdivided into either distal (calf vein) or proximal (thigh) vein thrombosis [19, 20].

The clinical diagnostic signs to be looked for are the presence of a palpable cord, pain, and tenderness along the course of major veins, ipsilateral edema, heat, and superficial venous dilatation [21, 22]. However, these clinical signs are not specific and a clinical examination alone is not a reliable method to confirm the diagnosis of DVT. A useful measure is the D-dimers. This test has a high sensibility but lacks specificity for the diagnosis of DVT and is therefore only useful when negative (i.e., cut-off value <500 ng/mL) [23].

Nowadays, thrombosis without apparent clinical signs may be diagnosed thanks to evolving technologies. Noninvasive tests as ultrasound or impedance plethysmography, with nearly equivalent diagnostic accuracy, have replaced venography [24]. Magnetic resonance (MR) venography is almost as accurate as contrast venography for the diagnosis of DVT [25, 26]. This MR imaging technique relies on the detection of thrombosis due to the formation of methemoglobin [27].

Pulmonary embolism (PE) has a large variety of clinical manifestations, going from a lack of symptoms to sudden death. The most frequently encountered presenting symptom is dyspnea followed by pleuritic chest pain and cough [28]. Patients with suspected PE might present electrocardiogram (ECG) abnormalities such as tachycardia, nonspecific ST-segment, and T-wave changes [28]. Computed tomographic pulmonary angiography (CTPA) is the first-choice diagnostic imaging modality because it is sensitive and specific for the diagnosis of PE [29]. Contrast-enhanced pulmonary angiography (i.e., digital subtraction angiography) was the historical gold standard for the diagnosis of PE [30]. With the emergence of CTPA, it has become usually reserved for patients with suspected PE in whom CTPA or V/Q scanning has not a diagnostic value.

8.2.2 Recommendations for Appropriate Antithrombotic Prophylaxis

8.2.2.1 Mechanical Prophylaxis

Mechanical pumps or compressive stockings are the first-line of prevention routinely and widely used after spinal surgery [31, 32]. Rokitko et al. in their prospective randomized study reported a 0.3% (1/329) rate of DVT after spine procedures, by using compression stockings alone, compression stocking with pneumatic compression boots, or Coumadin prophylactic anticoagulation. Nevertheless, they also found that 5.7% of patients treated with Coumadin presented bleeding complications [32].

Thus, according to the low rate of DVT associated with spinal surgery (ranging from 0.9 to 14% literature), using pneumatic compression boots with graduated compression stockings seems to be the best option of antithrombotic prophylaxis in patients going for a posterior spinal approach [32]. Use of stockings may be combined with acetylsalicylic acid (ASA) in elective spinal surgery to decrease the incidence of thromboembolic complications [33]. According to NASS guidelines, initiation of mechanical compression just prior to or at the beginning of surgery and continuation until the patient is fully ambulatory is a reasonable practice [33]. The risk for DVT/PE also depends on the type of spinal procedure. According to the large retrospective analysis of 4377 patients published by Sebastian et al. in 2016, VTE rates were higher in patients undergoing corpectomy, or at high risk for thromboembolic disease, such as multiple trauma, malignancy, or a hypercoagulable state [34].

8.2.2.2 Chemical Prophylaxis

Chemoprophylaxis by low molecular weight heparin (LMWH) or low-dose warfarin may be used postoperatively to decrease the risk of thromboembolic complications for patients at risk or undergoing anterior-posterior (circumferential) spine surgery. According to expert reviews, intravenous heparin should be preferred to other anticoagulants as a bridging therapy in patients already treated prior to surgery for a non-spinal condition (e.g., atrial fibrillation, valve replacement, or other), because of an easier management and more predictable effects [33].

A number of pharmacologic agents are now available for VTE prevention in surgical patients, including unfractionated heparin (UFH), the low molecular weight heparins (LMWH), fondaparinux (Arixtra®), vitamin K antagonists as warfarin, and the new oral antithrombotic agents as rivaroxaban, dabigatran, and apixaban. Subcutaneous UFH for prophylaxis of VTE seems to reduce the incidence of fatal PE in patients undergoing major surgical procedures from 0.7 to 0.1% compared with controls [35]. Low molecular weight heparin have the advantage that they can be given subcutaneously once or twice daily at a constant dose without laboratory monitoring of therapeutic effect. The anticoagulant effect of the vitamin K antagonists is not achieved until the third or fourth day of treatment, making these agents a poor choice for immediate postoperative preventive anticoagulation. New anticoagulants as rivaroxaban, apixaban, and dabigatran are superior to placebo but their benefits compared with other anticoagulants remain uncertain [36].

With regard to the duration of thromboembolic prophylaxis after surgery, the NASS clinical guidelines recommend thromboembolism prophylaxis until the patient is discharged, although specific evidence for spinal surgery is lacking [33].

8.3 Blood Loss Management

8.3.1 Management of Preoperative Anemia

Anemia is a common finding before elective surgery, especially in the case of associated comorbidities. It is proved that preoperative anemia and its underlying predisposal to blood transfusion is associated with a rise in cardiac, respiratory, and infectious complications and an increase of mortality and morbidity in the perioperative period, as well as the length of hospital stay [37, 38].

Preoperative anemia is detected during the anesthesiological preoperative assessment. However, this preoperative screening is usually only available for elective spinal procedures.

The European Society of Anaesthesiology (ESA) recommends anesthesiological preoperative assessment of patients 4–8 weeks before elective surgery [39].

The etiology of anemia must be investigated, in particular anemia due to iron deficiency. It should be orally or intravenously substituted in case of oral intolerance or inflammatory origin. It increases the hemoglobin rate and decreases the risk for perioperative transfusion [40].

In anemic patients without iron deficiency, preoperative administration of erythropoietin is efficient and reduces need for blood transfusion [41]. However, the literature has shown an increase in the risk of venous thromboembolic events in particular in spinal surgery patient cohorts [42]. Autologous blood transfusion is no longer appropriate, leading to an increased blood transfusion rate and increasing the risk of intraoperative anemia [43].

8.3.2 Preoperative Management of Antiplatelet Aggregation

It is known that antiplatelet drugs' use increases the risk of hemorrhage [44]. Therefore, when scheduled, spinal interventions preferably require the discontinuation of all antiplatelet therapy, after a multidisciplinary discussion between surgeons, anesthetists, and cardiologists.

Aspirin should be discontinued between 3 and 5 days before surgery depending on the patient's platelet count. The effects of aspirin disappear completely after 7 days, but it is assumed that 10% of the platelet pool is regained each day, which allows the recovery of a sufficient platelet function 3 days after the interruption if the platelet count is normal. Other antiplatelet agents should be systematically discontinued before surgery, at least 5 days for clopidogrel and ticagrelor and 7 days for prasugrel.

In case of emergency surgery on patients under antiplatelet therapy, the only possibility is to administer platelet transfusion, whose efficacy is still debated [45, 46].

8.3.3 Preoperative Management of Anticoagulants

In the same way as antiplatelet therapy, all anticoagulant and fibrinolytic treatments must be discontinued before a neurosurgical intervention. Thus, anti-vitamin K (AVK) drugs should be discontinued at least 3 days before surgery associated with high hemorrhagic risk. In cases where anticoagulation must be pursued because of a high thrombotic risk, the AVK should be interrupted 5 days before and replaced by heparin or LMWH. At curative dose, heparin should be discontinued 6 h before surgery and LMWH 24 h before surgery.

In emergencies, they can also be antagonized by the administration of vitamin K or activated prothrombin complex.

Oral new anticoagulants are also increasingly used. They are classically interrupted 3 days before surgery. In emergencies, their effect is reduced by the administration of vitamin K or activated prothrombin complex. Oral anticoagulants do not allow routine biological monitoring. Plasma assays are available however.

At present, in emergency situations, only dabigatran can be reversed specifically by the administration of an antidote, the idarucizumab [47].

8.3.4 Fluid Administration and Fluid Challenge

In the perioperative phase of an elective surgery, normovolemic hemodilution may be performed. It consists of taking from the induction of anesthesia, a quantity of blood bringing the hematocrit to 28–30% and simultaneously replacing this loss with crystalloid or colloid solutions in order to maintain normovolemia. The objective is to reduce the amount of erythrocytes lost during surgery in the operative field and to restore this volume at the end of the procedure [48]. The decrease in oxygen transport capacity is physiologically compensated by increased cardiac output and increase in tissue oxygen extraction. The tolerable limit value of hemodilution is the hematocrit to which oxygen consumption (VO_2) becomes dependent on the transport of O_2 (DO_2). Normovolemic hemodilution is thus considered only in case of high hemorrhagic risk neurosurgical act [49]. It is contraindicated in patients with high cardiovascular risk.

Fluid administration is the first treatment of acute hemorrhage, in order to maintain a blood volume and avoid early organ failure. However, before bleeding control, it is recommended to limit fluid administration in order to avoid the dilution of the coagulation factors [50].

Perioperative fluid intake should be guided by a fluid challenge strategy with systematic evaluation of preload dependence. Several modalities are accessible to the operating room such as the esophageal Doppler or the Lidco-type hemodynamic monitoring based on blood pressure.

To date, there is insufficient data suggesting that the use of colloid solutions improves the prognosis of patients in hemorrhagic shock. On the other hand, adverse effects associated with their use have been reported, some of which may be severe: renal insufficiency and coagulation disorders especially with hydroxyethyl starches or allergic with fluid gelatins. Renal toxicity is also suspected [51]. Crystalloids appear to be the first choice in resuscitation of hemorrhagic shock because of their clinical efficacy, moderate toxicity, and low cost.

8.3.5 Blood Recovery Systems

In a simple manner, blood recovery systems (cell savers) via surgical aspiration allow to collect part of the lost blood volume. This blood is then treated and concentrated in order to proceed to blood transfusion. This technique reduces the need for labile blood products transfusion, if recovery of a minimum of blood volume is achieved. A previous history of infection or tumor is a contraindication to the use of cell saver.

Blood recovery systems cause hemodilution and loss of clotting factors. Therefore, they need to be associated with transfusion of fresh frozen plasma. The presence of coagulopathy is also one of the main contraindications.

8.3.6 Pharmacological Strategy: Antifibrinolytics

Tranexamic acid is an analog of lysine that inhibits fibrinolysis. It is the most widely used antifibrinolytic agent in current practice and the most widely studied in the literature. A meta-analysis of 65 studies showed that tranexamic acid reduced the relative risk of transfusion by 32% in cardiac surgery and 51% in orthopedic surgery (total knee or hip prosthesis, spine surgery) [52]. Numerous studies converge and have demonstrated the benefit of tranexamic acid on the reduction of blood loss and blood transfusion especially for spinal surgery [53]. Antifibrinolytic agents expose to an increased risk of arterial or venous thrombosis. However, no study has yet demonstrated an increased risk of thrombotic events, especially in spinal surgery.

8.3.7 Intraoperative Direct Control of Bleeding

As well as any type of surgery, spinal surgery is associated with a risk of bleeding in connection with handling of small (e.g., epidural veins) or large vessel (e.g., iliac veins or arteries). Thus, bleeding control is essential to achieve a safe spinal procedure.

8.3.7.1 Mechanical Compression and Thermal Coagulation

Hemostasis of the subcutaneous adipose tissue and the muscular layer is done by bipolar coagulation and maintained by mechanical compression from spreaders. Spreaders should be occasionally released to ensure muscles' vascularization and oxygenation during the entire surgery. Subperiostal dissection is performed using the monopolar electric coagulation. The use of a rolled compress inserted using a Cobb during subperiosteal preparation is a very useful technique to ensure good hemostasis. Hydrogen peroxide solution may also be useful for hemostasis. Bipolar coagulation can also be used to control deeper bleeding on the spinal venous plexus. However, use of bipolar can be harmful to nervous tissue. Heat dissipation from the ends of the bipolar forceps can induce thermal damage to neighboring neural structures [54].

8.3.7.2 Local Pro-Hemostatic Methods

Different hemostatic agents exist for the control of bleeding during surgery. One of them used since a long time is bone wax. It is composed of bees' wax (70%) and

Vaseline (30%), and it is used for stopping bleeding from bone surfaces. It is a non-absorbable material, becoming soft and malleable in the hand when warmed. Bone wax can cause allergic reaction and infections complications [55].

Absorbable gelatin sponges (Gelfoam, Spongostan) are a water-insoluble, non-elastic, porous, pliable product prepared from animal skin gelatin. When applied directly to bleeding surfaces, they stop bleeding by forming an artificial clot and by producing a mechanical matrix that facilitates clotting. While its mode of action is not fully understood, its effect appears to be more physical, but some authors suggested that this clotting effect might be due to release of thromboplastin from platelets in contact with the sponge [56].

Microfibrillar collagen fleece (Avitene®) adhere tightly to bloody surfaces, provide a surface to which thrombocyte can adhere, and undergo their release reaction and activation of coagulation factors. In an experimental study on rats, it was found that oxidized regenerated cellulose in fibrillar form (ORC) and microfibrillar collagen fleece (CF) have a similar effect in reducing bleeding time [57]. ORC permits activation of the initial coagulation phase by the contact effect. It also seems to confer hemostasis by decreasing the pH, which adds an antimicrobial effect of ORC [55] and thus being superior to gelatin sponge from the standpoint of infection prevention [58].

An elaborate product is TachoComb®, which is composed of collagen coated with fibrinogen, thrombin, and aprotinin. A further development is TachoSil®, which does not contain aprotinin, thereby avoiding its known side effects as renal failure or anaphylactic reactions [55, 59, 60].

Fibrin sealants contain human fibrinogen, human thrombin, and some human factor XIII and bovine aprotinin. These agents all have a role in the coagulation cascade by forming a fibrin clot [61]. The Floseal® hemostatic matrix is a combination of the gelatinous matrix component and the reconstituted thrombin (human) component. Renkens et al. provided favorable results in spinal procedures [62].

Surgiflo™ is a sterile hemostatic matrix, corresponding to an absorbable porcine gelatin paste applied directly to a broad bleeding surface, very useful in difficult to reach areas and cavities. This paste might be mixed with sterile saline solution or with thrombin increasing its effectiveness. Landi et al. did not show any differences in terms of efficacy or ease of use between Surgiflo and Floseal [63].

Tissucol is fibrin glue, containing a highly concentrated solution of fibrinogen and other cryoglobulins derived from human plasma and prepared by cryoprecipitation. It contains coagulation factor XIII, which, in the presence of thrombin and calcium, makes it possible to produce highly adhesive filamentous precipitates of fibrin [64, 65].

8.3.8 Specific Concerns During CVJ Surgery

The craniovertebral junction is rich of vascular structures. The vertebral artery venous plexus (VAVP) is a well-developed network of venous channels covering the V2 and V3 segments of the vertebral artery. Manipulation of the VAVP may lead to troublesome bleeding during CVJ surgical procedures. The VAVP is potentially in danger during the dissection phase or during insertion of C1 or C2 screws. The dissection should be carefully done especially in the region lateral to the C2 lamina and isthmus and below the posterior arch of C1. A subperiosteal dissection is recommended at that level. Any bleeding during this phase may be easily controlled by cautious bipolar electrocautery or by packing with gelatin sponges.

The ideal entry point of C1 lateral mass screws is located in the mid-point of the lateral mass just below the posterior arch of C1. The medial and lateral borders of the lateral mass need to be identified in order to determine the entry point. Dissection is performed with a Penfield dissector and the C2 nerve root is downward displaced. Bleeding at this stage may be very abundant because of the redundancy of the VAVP. Bipolar electrocautery is often ineffective to stop the bleeding. Packing with gelatin sponges and cottonoids or using fibrin sealants is highly recommended. Furthermore, surgeon should quickly perform the screw insertion under fluoroscopic control.

Alternative methods have been developed to avoid excessive manipulation of the VAVP during C1 screw insertion. Garces et al. presented a novel approach to reduce bleeding from venous plexus during C1-C2 Harms instrumentation. They conducted a retrospective analysis of patients with atlantoaxial instability admitted and treated from August 2010 to December 2013. After having exposed C1 arch and C2 lamina, a Penfield n.1 instrument was used to carry a sub-periosteal dissection from the C2 lamina to the lateral mass and pars of C2 and upward toward the C1-C2 joint and the C1 lateral mass. This maneuver allowed for the surgeon to elevate the C2 nerve root along with the venous plexus without disruption. They observed an EBL going from 25 to 500 mL, the latter being related to a tumor resection at C1-C2 level. Thus, the C1 lateral mass screw insertion caudally from the C2 nerve root may become an alternate method for insertion of C1 screws, as shown in the paper from Wada K et al. [66]. Furthermore, insertion of the lateral mass screw via the posterior arch for C1 fixation is also possible, avoiding any manipulation of the VAVP, even in patients with a small posterior arch, ponticulus posticus, or persistent first intersegmental artery [67].

References

1. Bratzler DW, Dellinger EP, Olsen KM, Perl TM, Auwaerter PG, Bolon MK, et al. Clinical practice guidelines for antimicrobial prophylaxis in surgery. Surg Infect (Larchmt). 2013;14(1):73–156.
2. Broex ECJ, van Asselt ADI, Bruggeman CA, van Tiel FH. Surgical site infections: how high are the costs? J Hosp Infect. 2009;72(3):193–201.
3. Uçkay I, Harbarth S, Peter R, Lew D, Hoffmeyer P, Pittet D. Preventing surgical site infections. Expert Rev Anti Infect Ther. 2010;8(6):657–70.
4. Berríos-Torres SI, Umscheid CA, Bratzler DW, Leas B, Stone EC, Kelz RR, et al. Centers for Disease Control and Prevention guideline for the prevention of surgical site infection, 2017. JAMA Surg. 2017;152(8):784–91.
5. Mangram AJ, Horan TC, Pearson ML, Silver LC, Jarvis WR. Guideline for prevention of surgical site infection, 1999. Hospital Infection Control Practices Advisory Committee. Infect Control Hosp Epidemiol. 1999;20(4):250–78; quiz 279-280.

6. Widmer AF, Rotter M, Voss A, Nthumba P, Allegranzi B, Boyce J, et al. Surgical hand preparation: state-of-the-art. J Hosp Infect. 2010;74(2):112–22.
7. McDonald M, Grabsch E, Marshall C, Forbes A. Single- versus multiple-dose antimicrobial prophylaxis for major surgery: a systematic review. Aust N Z J Surg. 1998;68(6):388–96.
8. Allegranzi B, Zayed B, Bischoff P, Kubilay NZ, de Jonge S, de Vries F, et al. New WHO recommendations on intraoperative and postoperative measures for surgical site infection prevention: an evidence-based global perspective. Lancet Infect Dis. 2016;16(12):e288–303.
9. Zelenitsky SA, Ariano RE, Harding GKM, Silverman RE. Antibiotic pharmacodynamics in surgical prophylaxis: an association between intraoperative antibiotic concentrations and efficacy. Antimicrob Agents Chemother. 2002;46(9):3026–30.
10. Weber WP, Mujagic E, Zwahlen M, Bundi M, Hoffmann H, Soysal SD, et al. Timing of surgical antimicrobial prophylaxis: a phase 3 randomised controlled trial. Lancet Infect Dis. 2017;17(6):605–14.
11. Swoboda SM, Merz C, Kostuik J, Trentler B, Lipsett PA. Does intraoperative blood loss affect antibiotic serum and tissue concentrations? Arch Surg. 1996;131(11):1165–71; discussion 1171–1172.
12. Alexander JW, Fischer JE, Boyajian M, Palmquist J, Morris MJ. The influence of hair-removal methods on wound infections. Arch Surg. 1983;118(3):347–52.
13. Manniën J, Wille JC, Snoeren RLMM, van den Hof S. Impact of postdischarge surveillance on surgical site infection rates for several surgical procedures: results from the nosocomial surveillance network in The Netherlands. Infect Control Hosp Epidemiol. 2006;27(8):809–16.
14. Thomas S, Agarwal M, Mehta G. Intraoperative glove perforation—single versus double gloving in protection against skin contamination. Postgrad Med J. 2001;77(909):458–60.
15. Hovaguimian F, Lysakowski C, Elia N, Tramèr MR. Effect of intraoperative high inspired oxygen fraction on surgical site infection, postoperative nausea and vomiting, and pulmonary function: systematic review and meta-analysis of randomized controlled trials. Anesthesiology. 2013;119(2):303–16.
16. Lübbeke A, Hovaguimian F, Wickboldt N, Barea C, Clergue F, Hoffmeyer P, et al. Effectiveness of the surgical safety checklist in a high standard care environment. Med Care. 2013;51(5):425–9.
17. Piper K, Algattas H, DeAndrea-Lazarus IA, Kimmell KT, Li YM, Walter KA, et al. Risk factors associated with venous thromboembolism in patients undergoing spine surgery. J Neurosurg Spine. 2017;26(1):90–6.
18. Oda T, Fuji T, Kato Y, Fujita S, Kanemitsu N. Deep venous thrombosis after posterior spinal surgery. Spine. 2000;25(22):2962–7.
19. Galanaud J-P, Sevestre-Pietri M-A, Bosson J-L, Laroche J-P, Righini M, Brisot D, et al. Comparative study on risk factors and early outcome of symptomatic distal versus proximal deep vein thrombosis: results from the OPTIMEV study. Thromb Haemost. 2009;102(3):493–500.
20. Galanaud JP, Quenet S, Rivron-Guillot K, Quere I, Sanchez Muñoz-Torrero JF, Tolosa C, et al. Comparison of the clinical history of symptomatic isolated distal deep-vein thrombosis vs. proximal deep vein thrombosis in 11 086 patients. J Thromb Haemost. 2009;7(12):2028–34.
21. Hirsh J, Hull RD, Raskob GE. Clinical features and diagnosis of venous thrombosis. J Am Coll Cardiol. 1986;8(6 Suppl B):114B–27B.
22. Browse NL. The painful deep-vein syndrome. Lancet. 1970;1(7659):1251–3.
23. Wells PS, Anderson DR, Bormanis J, Guy F, Mitchell M, Gray L, et al. Application of a diagnostic clinical model for the management of hospitalized patients with suspected deep-vein thrombosis. Thromb Haemost. 1999;81(4):493–7.
24. Kearon C, Julian JA, Newman TE, Ginsberg JS. Noninvasive diagnosis of deep venous thrombosis. McMaster diagnostic imaging practice guidelines initiative. Ann Intern Med. 1998;128(8):663–77.
25. Fraser DGW, Moody AR, Morgan PS, Martel AL, Davidson I. Diagnosis of lower-limb deep venous thrombosis: a prospective blinded study of magnetic resonance direct thrombus imaging. Ann Intern Med. 2002;136(2):89–98.

26. Carpenter JP, Holland GA, Baum RA, Owen RS, Carpenter JT, Cope C. Magnetic resonance venography for the detection of deep venous thrombosis: comparison with contrast venography and duplex Doppler ultrasonography. J Vasc Surg. 1993;18(5):734–41.
27. Moody AR, Pollock JG, O'Connor AR, Bagnall M. Lower-limb deep venous thrombosis: direct MR imaging of the thrombus. Radiology. 1998;209(2):349–55.
28. Stein PD, Beemath A, Matta F, Weg JG, Yusen RD, Hales CA, et al. Clinical characteristics of patients with acute pulmonary embolism: data from PIOPED II. Am J Med. 2007;120(10):871–9.
29. Raczeck P, Minko P, Graeber S, Fries P, Seidel R, Buecker A, et al. Influence of respiratory position on contrast attenuation in pulmonary CT angiography: a prospective randomized clinical trial. Am J Roentgenol. 2016;206(3):481–6.
30. Wittram C, Waltman AC, Shepard J-AO, Halpern E, Goodman LR. Discordance between CT and angiography in the PIOPED II study. Radiology. 2007;244(3):883–9.
31. Hartman JT, Pugh JL, Smith RD, Robertson WW, Yost RP, Janssen HF. Cyclic sequential compression of the lower limb in prevention of deep venous thrombosis. J Bone Joint Surg Am. 1982;64(7):1059–62.
32. Rokito SE, Schwartz MC, Neuwirth MG. Deep vein thrombosis after major reconstructive spinal surgery. Spine. 1996;21(7):853–8.. discussion 859
33. Bono CM, Watters WC, Heggeness MH, Resnick DK, Shaffer WO, Baisden J, et al. An evidence-based clinical guideline for the use of antithrombotic therapies in spine surgery. Spine J. 2009;9(12):1046–51.
34. Sebastian AS, Currier BL, Kakar S, Nguyen EC, Wagie AE, Habermann ES, et al. Risk factors for venous thromboembolism following thoracolumbar surgery: analysis of 43,777 patients from the American College of Surgeons National Surgical Quality Improvement Program 2005 to 2012. Glob Spine J. 2016;6(8):738–43.
35. Kakkar VV, Corrigan TP, Fossard DP, Sutherland I, Thirwell J. Prevention of fatal postoperative pulmonary embolism by low doses of heparin. Reappraisal of results of international multicentre trial. Lancet. 1977;1(8011):567–9.
36. Kim S-M, Moon Y-W, Lim S-J, Kim D-W, Park Y-S. Effect of oral factor Xa inhibitor and low-molecular-weight heparin on surgical complications following total hip arthroplasty. Thromb Haemost. 2016;115(3):600–7.
37. Clevenger B, Richards T. Pre-operative anaemia. Anaesthesia. 2015;70(Suppl 1):20–8, e6–8.
38. Musallam KM, Tamim HM, Richards T, Spahn DR, Rosendaal FR, Habbal A, et al. Preoperative anaemia and postoperative outcomes in non-cardiac surgery: a retrospective cohort study. Lancet. 2011;378(9800):1396–407.
39. Kozek-Langenecker SA, Ahmed AB, Afshari A, Albaladejo P, Aldecoa C, Barauskas G, et al. Management of severe perioperative bleeding: guidelines from the European Society of Anaesthesiology: first update 2016. Eur J Anaesthesiol. 2017;34(6):332–95.
40. Kumar A. Perioperative management of anemia: limits of blood transfusion and alternatives to it. Cleve Clin J Med. 2009;76(Suppl 4):S112–8.
41. Laupacis A, Fergusson D. Erythropoietin to minimize perioperative blood transfusion: a systematic review of randomized trials. The International Study of Peri-operative Transfusion (ISPOT) Investigators. Transfus Med Oxf Engl. 1998;8(4):309–17.
42. Stowell CP, Jones SC, Enny C, Langholff W, Leitz G. An open-label, randomized, parallel-group study of perioperative epoetin alfa versus standard of care for blood conservation in major elective spinal surgery: safety analysis. Spine. 2009;34(23):2479–85.
43. Henry DA, Carless PA, Moxey AJ, O'Connell D, Forgie MA, Wells PS, et al. Pre-operative autologous donation for minimising perioperative allogeneic blood transfusion. Cochrane Database Syst Rev. 2002;(2):CD003602.
44. Burger W, Chemnitius J-M, Kneissl GD, Rücker G. Low-dose aspirin for secondary cardiovascular prevention—cardiovascular risks after its perioperative withdrawal versus bleeding risks with its continuation—review and meta-analysis. J Intern Med. 2005;257(5):399–414.

45. Downey DM, Monson B, Butler KL, Fortuna GR, Saxe JM, Dolan JP, et al. Does platelet administration affect mortality in elderly head-injured patients taking antiplatelet medications? Am Surg. 2009;75(11):1100–3.
46. Washington CW, Schuerer DJE, Grubb RL. Platelet transfusion: an unnecessary risk for mild traumatic brain injury patients on antiplatelet therapy. J Trauma. 2011;71(2):358–63.
47. Pollack CV, Reilly PA, Bernstein R, Dubiel R, Eikelboom J, Glund S, et al. Design and rationale for RE-VERSE AD: a phase 3 study of idarucizumab, a specific reversal agent for dabigatran. Thromb Haemost. 2015;114(1):198–205.
48. Monk TG. Acute normovolemic hemodilution. Anesthesiol Clin N Am. 2005;23(2):271–81.. vi
49. Parasa SK, Bidkar PU, Parida S. Acute normovolemic hemodilution to avoid blood transfusion during intracranial aneurysm surgery in a patient with atypical antibodies. Anesth Essays Res. 2016;10(1):136–8.
50. Bickell WH, Wall MJ, Pepe PE, Martin RR, Ginger VF, Allen MK, et al. Immediate versus delayed fluid resuscitation for hypotensive patients with penetrating torso injuries. N Engl J Med. 1994;331(17):1105–9.
51. Zarychanski R, Abou-Setta AM, Turgeon AF, Houston BL, McIntyre L, Marshall JC, et al. Association of hydroxyethyl starch administration with mortality and acute kidney injury in critically ill patients requiring volume resuscitation: a systematic review and meta-analysis. JAMA. 2013;309(7):678–88.
52. Henry DA, Carless PA, Moxey AJ, O'Connell D, Stokes BJ, Fergusson DA, et al. Anti-fibrinolytic use for minimising perioperative allogeneic blood transfusion. Cochrane Database Syst Rev. 2011;(1):CD001886.
53. Winter SF, Santaguida C, Wong J, Fehlings MG. Systemic and topical use of tranexamic acid in spinal surgery: a systematic review. Glob Spine J. 2016;6(3):284–95.
54. Gazzeri R, De Bonis C, Galarza M. Use of a thrombin-gelatin hemostatic matrix (Surgiflo) in spinal surgery. Surg Technol Int. 2014;25:280–5.
55. Schonauer C, Tessitore E, Barbagallo G, Albanese V, Moraci A. The use of local agents: bone wax, gelatin, collagen, oxidized cellulose. Eur Spine J. 2004;13(Suppl 1):S89–96.
56. Jenkins HP, Senz EH. Present status of gelatin sponge for the control of hemorrhage; with experimental data on its use for wounds of the great vessels and the heart. JAMA. 1946;132(11):614–9.
57. Tessitore E, Schatlo B, Schaller C, Schonauer C. Fibrillary structure is key for hemostasis: a similar effect of collagen fleece and oxidized cellulose on experimental hemorrhagic brain injury. J Neurol Surg Part Cent Eur Neurosurg. 2012;73(2):89–92.
58. Scher KS, Coil JA. Effects of oxidized cellulose and microfibrillar collagen on infection. Surgery. 1982;91(3):301–4.
59. Agger P, Langhoff J, Smerup MH, Hasenkam JM. Comparison between TachoComb and TachoSil for surgical hemostasis in arterial bleeding: an animal experimental study. J Trauma. 2010;68(4):838–42.
60. Szpalski M, Gunzburg R, Aebi M, Weiskopf R. Research and evidence about blood sparing in spine surgery. Eur Spine J. 2004;13(Suppl 1):S1–2.
61. Jackson MR. Fibrin sealants in surgical practice: an overview. Am J Surg. 2001;182(2 Suppl):1S–7S.
62. Renkens KL, Payner TD, Leipzig TJ, Feuer H, Morone MA, Koers JM, et al. A multicenter, prospective, randomized trial evaluating a new hemostatic agent for spinal surgery. Spine. 2001;26(15):1645–50.
63. Landi A, Gregori F, Marotta N, Efficacy DR. Security, and manageability of Gelified hemostatic matrix in bleeding control during thoracic and lumbar spine surgery: FloSeal versus Surgiflo. J Neurol Surg Part Cent Eur Neurosurg. 2016;77(2):139–43.
64. Arnautović KI, al-Mefty O, Pait TG, Krisht AF, Husain MM. The suboccipital cavernous sinus. J Neurosurg. 1997;86(2):252–62.

65. San Millán Ruíz D, Gailloud P, Rüfenacht DA, Delavelle J, Henry F, Fasel JHD. The craniocervical venous system in relation to cerebral venous drainage. Am J Neuroradiol. 2002;23(9):1500–8.
66. Wada K, Tamaki R, Yui M, Numaguchi D, Murata Y. C1 lateral mass screw insertion caudally from C2 nerve root—an alternate method for insertion of C1 screws: a technical note and preliminary clinical results. J Orthop Sci. 2017;22(2):213–7.
67. Yeom JS, Kafle D, Nguyen NQ, Noh W, Park K-W, Chang B-S, et al. Routine insertion of the lateral mass screw via the posterior arch for C1 fixation: feasibility and related complications. Spine J. 2012;12(6):476–83.

9 Surgery of the Cranio-Vertebral Junction: Image Guidance, Navigation, and Augmented Reality

Philippe Bijlenga and Max Jägersberg

9.1 Introduction

Safety, efficacy, and accessibility of surgery are major aims identified by the World Health Organization to improve global care. Safety is the power to avoid injury. Efficacy is the power to cure. Accessibility is the power of being within reach that may take different dimensions being affordable, timely, frequently mastered, and easy to perform. Quality of surgery relies mostly on adequate human resources (trained and accredited surgical staff and anesthesia professionals) as well as processes optimizing the exploitation of material resources (operating rooms and equipment). Management formalization and checklists will help institutions and surgeons to optimize resources and better adhere to best clinical practice. Image guidance, navigation, and augmented reality should assist surgeons to better deal with frequent patient-specific anatomical variations (personalized care) and master a larger spectrum of diseases as well as better modify strategies on the fly. It is expected but not yet formally demonstrated that image guidance, navigation, and augmented reality assist surgeons in achieving the objectives in line with the Safe Surgery WHO guidelines to avoid excessive blood loss, minimize surgical site infection by reducing open skin intervention time, skin incision size and traction, and potentially improve communication of critical patient information between members of the team. It may also improve efficacy by assisting surgeons to more precisely access the disease, more precisely implant devices or remove diseased tissues. Despite limitations associated with the cost of the equipment and the

P. Bijlenga (✉)
Department of Clinical Neurosciences, Geneva University Hospital and Faculty of Medicine, Geneva University, Geneva, Switzerland
e-mail: philippe.bijlenga@hcuge.ch

M. Jägersberg
Department of Neurosurgery, University of Mainz Medical Center, Mainz, Germany
e-mail: max.jaegersberg@unimedizin-mainz.de

E. Tessitore et al. (eds.), *Surgery of the Cranio-Vertebral Junction*,
https://doi.org/10.1007/978-3-030-18700-2_9

complexity of its handling, image guidance, navigation and augmented reality should soon be widely accessible, accelerate the training learning curve, and broaden the surgical field of each surgeon.

Improving surgical accuracy and safety by means of navigation is of special interest for cervical and craniocervical spine procedures, where demands for precision are extremely high to place long and resilient screws [1]. The anatomical complex relations of the vertebral artery and the spinal cord leave only narrow bony corridors available for screw placement in the lateral masses (C1), the pedicles (C2-C7), articular facets (C1-C2), or the lamina (C2). In many locations, precision tolerances are less than 1 mm in translation and 5° in angulation [2]. Neoplastic, traumatic, or inflammatory diseases alter anatomy and can increase these topographical challenges.

In spite of precision needs, the introduction of navigation for cervical spine procedures had to overcome more obstacles than cranial or lumbar spine surgeries [3]. Accuracy is affected when images are acquired preoperatively and in a different position to that required during the intervention. The size of the operation field, the geometrical access corridors, and size of instruments increase the complexity to optimally position the reference object for accurate navigation during the whole procedure. Constant accuracy checks and registration corrections at the single vertebra scale are considered too time-consuming by many surgeons.

9.2 Definitions

Image-guided surgery is a generic term used to characterize any surgery performed using pre- or intra-operative patient-specific images to guide the operation as opposed to interventions performed according to generic procedures or anatomical landmarks. **Imaging-tracked surgery** are interventions where images are specifically acquired to track the progression of the intervention. A procedure is navigated (**navigated surgery**) when instruments are tracked in real-time and their location and orientation projected on patient-specific pre- or intra-operative acquired images. An operation is performed using **augmented reality (AR)** when images are presented to the surgeon's eye field as a transparent overlay adjusted to the operative field. Augmented reality can be either direct when the surgeons look at the operative field or remote when the operative field and overlays are projected on a screen.

Besides improving the perception of the operating field and overall context, surgery may also be improved by more gentle manipulation of tissues, increased degrees of freedom, precision, and stability of movements that can be provided by robotics. Surgery can be performed as freehand (**freehand surgery**) when surgeons directly manipulate surgical tools or be **robot-assisted** (RAS).

As an example, pedicle screws can be inserted using (1) only anatomical landmarks to identify the entry point and standard reference angles to approximate the insertion trajectory [4, 5]; (2) intra-operative image guidance using a C-arm fluoroscopy to visualize the screw location relative to the bone structures [6]; (3) navigation by tracking the position of the screw relative to a fixed reference previously registered and by displaying the extrapolated location of the screw relative to earlier acquired images [7]. (4) A virtual semitransparent representation of the vertebra and pedicle is visualized as an overlay on the anatomical structures of the operative field with the optimal entry point and trajectory. The surgeon then inserts the screw following the projected images [3]. (5) A robot is fixed on the spinous process of the targeted vertebra. Two orthogonal fluoroscopic images are acquired including the spine and a reference marker to allow registration with a high-resolution CT scan obtained preoperatively. The screw trajectories are programed, and the robot arm orients a cannula that is used for the drilling. Robot-assisted screw implantation is nowadays frequently used in the lumbar spine but to our knowledge has so far only been tested on cadavers and on a single case regarding cervical spine screws [8, 9].

9.3 Basic Principles

9.3.1 Matching the Resolution and Precision to the Needs

Precision of freehand motion is at best when using microsurgical techniques in the range of one tenth of a millimeter. It is heavily affected by the force to be applied, fatigue, and distance to any pivot point. Visual feedback is essential to allow precise manipulations, and proprioceptive feedback is relevant when the hand or manipulated instrument is out of the visual field. It can be easily experimented performing simple tasks with and without a binocular operative microscope. A normal eye can at best distinguish a 0.07 mm size object. Operative microscopes usually provide a 10× to 60× magnification, reducing the resolution to 1 μm. As a general rule the visual feedback should be 10 times sharper than the required movement precision. The difference between the needed perception resolution and the resulting manipulation precision can be reduced when using micromanipulators or robots. Such a high precision required when operating in the medulla is nevertheless not necessary in most craniocervical surgeries where mechanical constraints are the limiting factors to keep precision within the range of ±0.5 mm and ± 2°.

The precision and limitation of image-guided surgery, navigation, and augmented reality are affected by multiple factors that need to be well understood by the users.

1. Resolution of acquired data set
2. Distortion of the data set, perspective, parallax, special field heterogeneities
3. Co-registration accuracy
4. Structures' motion and deformation

9.3.2 Data Set Acquisition Resolution

The resolution of any imaging data set still remains at least one order of magnitude lower than what can be provided by an operative microscope. The highest resolution reaches 50 µm when using flat panel detectors but standard thin-sliced CT scan images have a resolution of 0.1 mm, O-arm 0.41 mm in the axial plane, and 0.83 mm in z axis, Ziehm FD Vario 3D 0.375 mm, Arcadis Orbic 3D 0.475 mm, and standard MRI 0.5 mm. The spatial resolution further decreases when using particular imaging protocols such as fiber tracking or functional imaging. The precision of any guidance system will be at best equivalent to the resolution of the most refined data set available. It is therefore recommended to use the data set with the highest resolution as the reference data set to which all others will be registered.

9.3.3 Imaging Distortion

Users need to be aware that 2D images are subject to projection distortions. Most of the intra-operative imaging is acquired using C-arm-mounted fluoroscopic equipment. Here the X-ray source is projecting toward a detector array, and the X-ray beam has a cone shape (Fig. 9.1a). Objects closer to the X-ray source will

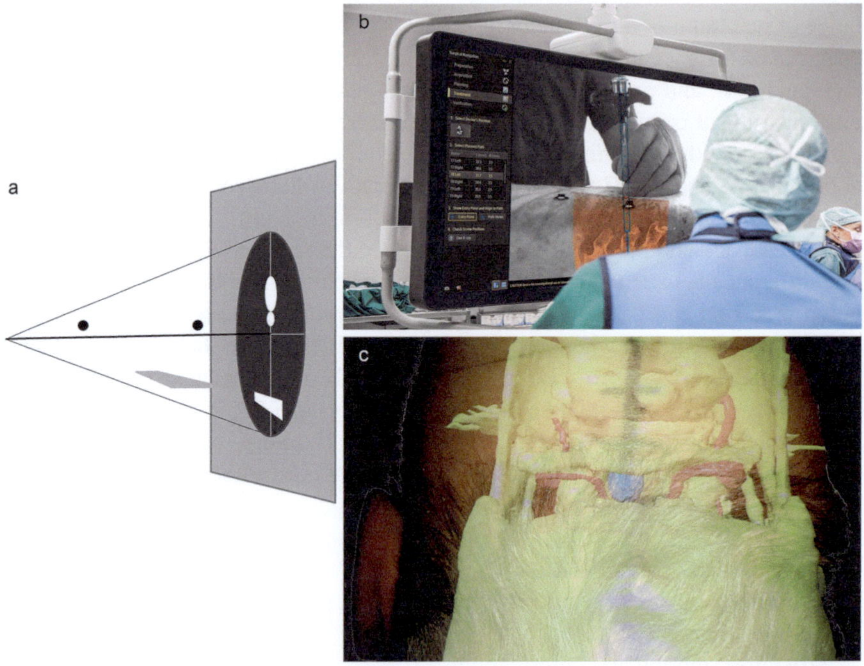

Fig. 9.1 Projection deformation, parallax, and augmented reality. (**a**) Illustration of deformation and relative displacement of objects induced by the projection from a point to a surface. (**b**) Indirect augmented reality. A calibrated video of the intervention field is overlaid on the radiological image (Courtesy Philips Best Netherlands). (**c**) Direct augmented reality. A 3D computer-generated surface rendering of different structures of interest and corresponding to the surgeon's line of sight is projected as an overlay on the microscope head-up display when looking at the patient. Bone is presented in yellow, arteries in red, and lesion in blue

be projected on the detector larger than objects more distant. A surface parallel to the axial beam (beam centered on the source and orthogonal to the detector) will appear progressively more oblique as shifted off center. To minimize errors resulting from inadequate correction of distortion by surgeons, it is recommended to center the axial beam on the target and orient the beam if possible along the surgical axis or as second choice orthogonally. This requires frequent C-arm displacement. Those distortions are avoided when using devices acquiring multiple projections and generating volumetric data displayed as either orthogonal slices or 3D-rendered volumes.

Now, users are faced with another pitfall which is the parallax. Parallax is the apparent relative displacement of objects when viewed from different lines of sight. This commonly tricks surgeons when drawing projections of structures on the surface of the skin. The drawing then only applies when using the line of sight initially used. For deep seated targets, only very small shifts from the initial line of sight can induce great shifts. Errors can be minimized by avoiding to draw on the skin surface and by displaying projections or 3D-rendered image overlays that update continuously for the appropriate line of sight. The overlays can either be projected on a screen and on top of a video image of the operating scene (indirect augmented reality, Fig. 9.1b) or on a head-up display allowing the surgeon to directly look at the operating field and visualize the target as if he could see through the skin of the patient (Fig. 9.1c). Stereoscopic 3D display of the scenery and overlays greatly improve the perception.

Finally users need to be aware that in contrast to X-ray-based imaging, magnetic resonance imaging (MRI) may be significantly distorted because of magnetic field heterogeneities during image acquisition. MRI geometric distortions are reduced as much as possible by calibration and sometimes by imaging post processing. The calibration tolerance for geometrical distortion is less than 2 mm over a 30 cm field of view. When imaging patients, the magnetic field can be extremely deformed (centimeters) by any ferromagnetic object close to the imaging field of view. When head images are acquired, deformation may be induced by ferromagnetic dental material, ventriculoperitoneal shunt valves, or clips. Earrings and piercings, another common source of imaging distortion, are normally removed before performing imaging.

9.3.4 Registration Accuracy

The co-registration accuracy may be affected at multiple levels, but the most vulnerable step is the physical co-registration of the patient with the virtual model when performing a navigated intervention. Navigation relies on recording the relative position of points (identified both on the surface of the skin of the patient and in the virtual model) according to a reference object visible to the navigation system. Most frequently this co-registration process is performed using multiple points to surface-matching the exposed vertebrae. This technique is rapid, easy, and reliable for standard patients positioned in prone decubitus.

The development of intra-operative imaging has helped to overcome some of the registration shortcomings. Based on fluoroscopy, intra-operative imaging acquisition is performed after surgical exposure with the navigation reference-object in position. Initially based on orthogonal 2D image acquisitions, progress in engineering led to the development of devices that isocentrically rotate around the patient. Such devices allow the reconstruction of 3D data sets from images acquired in multiple projections (O-Arm, Medtronic Surgical Technologies, Louisville, USA; Airo Mobile Intraoperative CT, Brainlab, Munich, Germany; Ziehm FD Vario 3D, Ziehm Imaging GmbH, Nuremberg, Germany; Arcadis Orbic 3D, Siemens Medical Solutions, Erlangen, Germany; see Fig. 9.2). 3D navigation of instruments can hence be used immediately without further accuracy-decreasing point matching (StealthStation, Medtronic Surgical Technologies, Louisville, USA; VectorVision[2], Brainlab, Munich, Germany). The gain in precision derived from this in situ and navigation-referenced acquisition allows fixing a larger reference object via an attachment to the head holder instead of a clamp fixed on cervical bone. It reduces the problem of interference between surgical and navigation instruments.

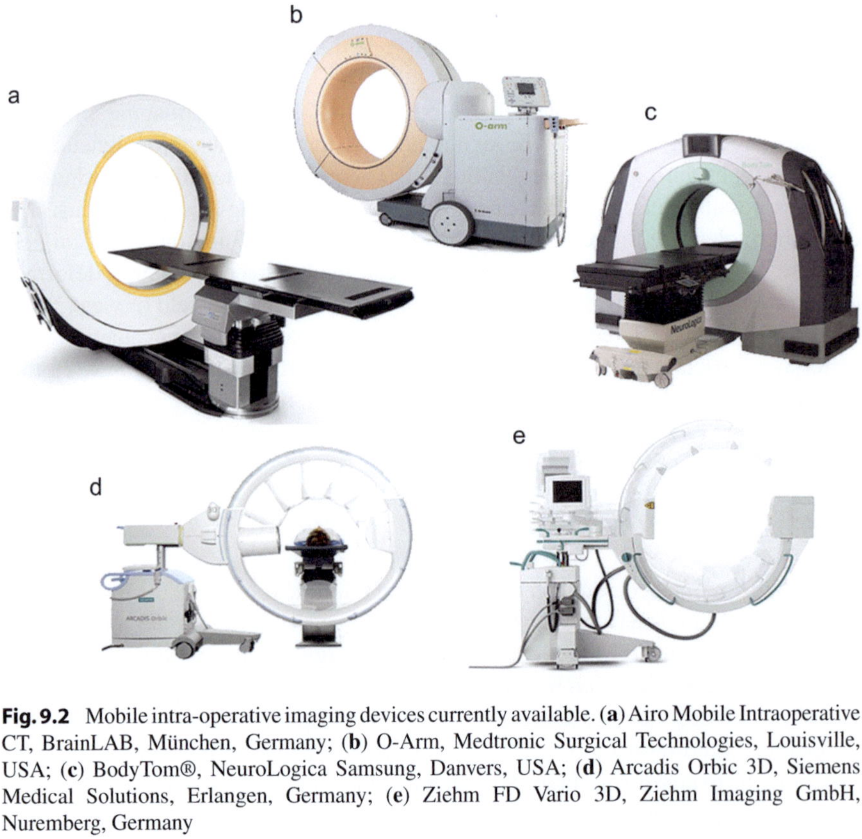

Fig. 9.2 Mobile intra-operative imaging devices currently available. (**a**) Airo Mobile Intraoperative CT, BrainLAB, München, Germany; (**b**) O-Arm, Medtronic Surgical Technologies, Louisville, USA; (**c**) BodyTom®, NeuroLogica Samsung, Danvers, USA; (**d**) Arcadis Orbic 3D, Siemens Medical Solutions, Erlangen, Germany; (**e**) Ziehm FD Vario 3D, Ziehm Imaging GmbH, Nuremberg, Germany

The accuracy of the registration may be affected by the distance between the reference object and the navigation camera, as well as by the distance between the reference object and the operating field. To improve accuracy, distances should be minimized. The reference object should be placed as close as possible to the operating field but should not disturb or enter in collision with instruments. It should be avoided placing the reference object between the surgeon and the scrub nurse. The maximum recommended distance between the operating field and the reference object should be below 30 cm. The identification of navigated instruments and of the reference object and their relative positions are calculated based on relative angle measurements between infrared-reflecting fiducials fixed on the objects and detected by two stereoscopic cameras. The optimal distance is usually between 1.5 and 2 m. Most of the systems use infrared light sources and camera and require direct line of sight between cameras, reference object, and instruments.

Some navigation systems use electromagnetic field generators to localize instruments. Those systems do not require line of sight. They allow not only to track the instrument as a rigid object but also to track the tip of flexible tools like stylets and catheters. A drawback that users have to be aware of is that the electromagnetic field may be distorted by other sources of electromagnetic fields such as coagulation generators or ferromagnetic objects.

The registration process is a major step subject to the highest risk of inaccuracy. It is therefore mandatory to check the accuracy. Most navigation systems prompt surgeons to point on easily identifiable structures on both sides of the patient to check the overall orientation and accuracy.

Using augmented reality, the microscope or head-up display need to be registered and calibrated. It is then easy to verify the overall registration accuracy by projecting a model of the patient's skin surface on the head-up display and verify the perfect adjustment of the model with reality (Fig. 9.3). It is recommended to check the registration accuracy at least in two planes, typically the coronal plane using the face (nose, eyes, and eyebrow) and the sagittal plane using the nose and ears. In prone position, mastoid processes and ears as well as the inion and upper neck skinfolds may be used.

Once the registration accuracy is checked, it is recommended to mark four points and record their position with the navigation system in case either the reference object or the patient is inadvertently moved during draping, trephination, or drilling. This process can be repeated when bone is exposed. Four small holes can be drilled just to allow the tip of the pointer to be stabilized. This is the most accurate method to verify the registration all along the procedure.

9.3.5 Structures' Motion and Deformations

When working on soft tissues or on the spine, structures may move. It is unlikely that the patient will lie in the operating room exactly in the same position as during imaging acquisition. Furthermore manipulations during the operation will most probably change the relative position of mobile structures of interest. During

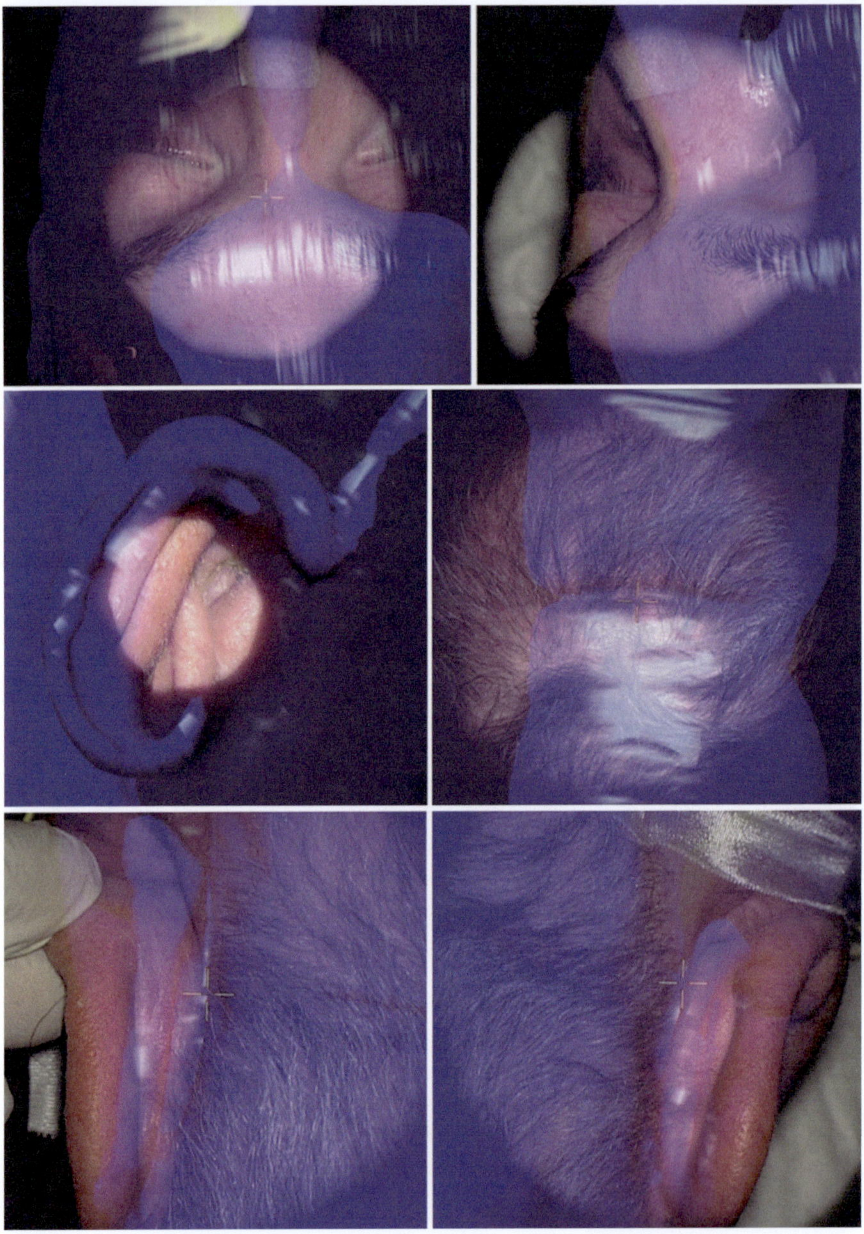

Fig. 9.3 Co-registration accuracy check. The accuracy of the registration process is verified by visually assessing how the virtual model of the patient head (blue) matches the real anatomy. If the patient's face is accessible, the nose (lateral registration and sagittal plane rotation assessment) and forehead (vertical registration and axial plane rotation assessment) are excellent landmarks. The depth registration (anteroposterior registration and coronal plane rotation assessment) is verified by scanning up and down, visualizing the plane of focus moving over the facial 3D anatomy (upper left and right). In prone position the ear anatomy, the mastoid, and the inion are the major landmarks. Care must be taken during image acquisition to avoid excessive deformation of the concha when immobilizing the patient's head

cerebral surgery, removal of craniospinal fluid, opening of fissures, and resection of tissue may lead to brain shifts ranging up to tens of millimeter. In the craniocervical junction C0-C1 and C1-C2 may rotate by 15° each in the flexion/extension axis and a few degrees in lateral flexion but up to 70° between C1 and C2 in rotation. Errors due to structure motion can be prevented by repeating registration for each mobile structure.

During spine surgery navigation based on preoperative imaging, it is recommended to fix the reference object on the spinous process of the vertebra that will be operated on to maximize precision. When performing cervical spine surgery, navigation based on intra-operative imaging, a metallic head holder, and head holder table attachment provide better fixation than radiolucent head holder systems and can be used without problematic radiologic artifacts if placed with a rostral angle [10]. Care must be taken that the attachment of the head holder to the table allows the required space for the applied radiologic device allowing the cervical spine to be placed into the C-arm iso-center (see Fig. 9.4). Table systems allowing the head fixation from the rostral table extremity (e.g. Jackson Table System, Mizuho OSI, Union City, USA; Maquet Alphamax with extension, Maquet Cardiovascular LLC, New Jersey, USA) are advantageous but not mandatory. The acquisition should be performed under apnea and with the wound retractors left in situ since their repositioning can alter the positions between vertebrae [11]. The wound cavity should be filled with saline solution to enhance image quality.

If avoidable, the operation table should not be moved until instrumentation is accomplished. Other movements that can alter intervertebral position must be avoided or left to the end of the procedure. It is hence suggested that entry points and pressure-free trajectory drilling should be accomplished for all planned screws before tapping and screw placing is performed. It is advantageous to start the procedure at the most caudal vertebra which has the greatest distance to the reference arc

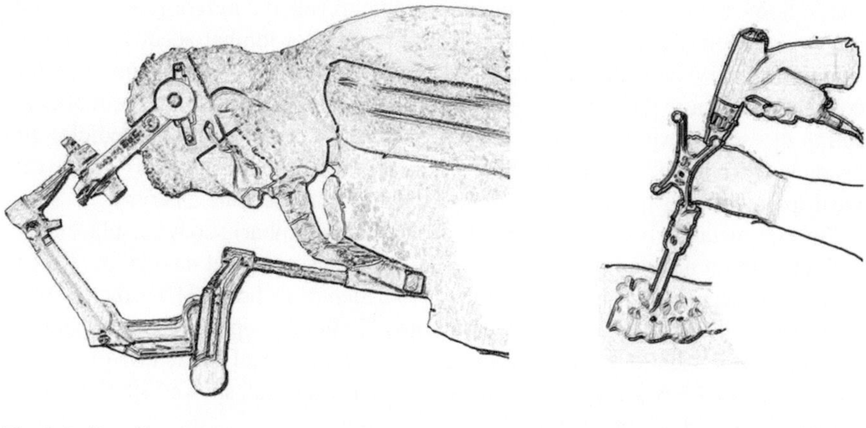

Fig. 9.4 Specific equipment and adjustments to optimize craniocervical junction surgeries using intra-operative imaging and navigation. Positioning of the patient, head clamp, and support extension (left). Navigated drill guide (right)

and to advance in the rostral direction, this way the increasing loss of precision with surgery time is not adding to the loss of precision due to distance to the reference arc. The use of a navigated drill guide (Fig. 9.4) is recommended in order to reduce pressure on the vertebrae. Then, a bone trajectory is performed with a 2.7 or 2.9 mm drill which is inserted through the guide. A screw is then inserted following a k-wire into the performed trajectory. If occipital fixation is necessary, these screws will accordingly be the last screws to place, since the reference arc is directly fixed to C0, and since these screws do not require precise navigation.

An analogous setup can be used for anterior instrumentation in the supine position; however, usually only one type of screw, the odontoid screw, is of interest for navigation, and not all considerations mentioned above are hence of importance for this surgery [12].

Augmented reality allows a better perception and correction by surgeons of inadvertent displacement of structures from original position. When using augmented reality, it is recommended to segment each mobile structure that could be used as a reference and all target structures. It is then easy for the surgeon to see how well the reference structure fits the projected overlay model, correct for the misalignment, and extrapolate where the target structure or desired trajectory is. The process of local registration using a reference structure is crucial for precise navigation at the millimetric scale which is important when operating in the craniocervical junction. The process is illustrated in the case description below.

9.4 Spinal Navigation: Current Status

The majority of studies about spinal navigation and implant accuracy address the lumbar spine, and misplacement classification systems (e.g., the often-mentioned Gertzbein-Robins classification [13]) have the shortcoming that their thresholds have been chosen with regard to lumbar spine morphometry and respective tolerances. Some authors consider minor misplacements (up to 2 mm or grade 1 according to Gertzbein-Robins) as correctly placed screws for lumbar accuracy analysis. In contrast, cervical spine pedicle screw misplacements of 2 mm in any direction could already cause damage. Some authors therefore apply a misplacement classification of "screw exposure" (less than 50% of the screw outside the pedicle) and "pedicle perforation" (more than 50% of the screw outside the pedicle) for the cervical spine which is more suitable in the context of this delicate anatomy.

Several meta-analyses report the rates of (mainly lumbar) screw misplacements with or without navigation and show an advantage using spinal navigation. Mason et al. analyzed 30 publications including 1973 patients in whom 9310 pedicle screws were inserted. With conventional fluoroscopy, 2D fluoroscopic navigation, and 3D fluoroscopic navigation, accuracy (absence of pedicle wall breaches) of 68.1%, 84.3%, and 95.5% was respectively achieved [14]. Tian et al. showed similar results in their meta-analysis of 43 studies [15].

In the cervical spine, special interest for navigation addresses the placement of pedicle screws in subaxial levels C3-C6. These screws are far more resilient than the less challenging lateral mass screws, but highest possible precision is crucial because of the challenging pedicle dimensions immediately adjacent to sensitive neurovascular structures. Yukawa et al. reports a series of fluoroscopy assisted insertions of 620 cervical pedicle screws with 3.9% (95%CI 2.5% to 5.8%) rate of perforation (>50% of screw outside pedicle) and 9.2% (95%CI 7% to 12%) rate of "screw exposure" (<50% of screw outside pedicle) [16]. Abumi et al. report a cervical screw misplacement rate of 4.7% with conventional fluoroscopy in their collective of 26 patients [17]. A multicenter study led by Nagoya University and including 84 patients reports a rate of screw exposure of 15.4% and pedicle perforation of 4.1% [18]. Richter et al. prospectively enrolled 52 patients in their comparative study and observed 8.6% and 3% for conventional and navigated surgery, respectively [19]. Using spinal navigation, according to Kotani et al., the misplacement rate can be reduced to 1.2% [20]. On the other hand, Uehara et al. who analyzed the misplacement rates in their collective of 359 patients along the cervical to lumbar spine, all operated under navigation, report higher misplacement rates, especially of subaxial pedicle screws (5.0% for C2, 11.4% for C3–5, and 7.0% for C6–7, [21]). Lateral mass screws in C1 and pars screws in C2 are less critical when placed conventionally under fluoroscopy. Tessitore et al. who analyzed 111 of these screws found 3% misplacement, all less than 2 mm [22]. Those rates increase in the presence of anatomy-altering disease [21, 23]. Misplacement, including "screw exposures," can potentially cause devastating complications in the cervical spine. The cited data shows that accuracy improvement by means of navigation significantly lowers the risk of screw misplacement and thereby enhances patient safety.

Furthermore, 3D navigation device has been used to safely insert odontoid screws in case of dens fracture [12, 24]. Another valuable advantage in the intraoperative 3D radiological control of implants is the possibility to correct misplaced screws within the same session. Finally, the exposure of surgical teams to irradiation is drastically reduced [25, 26].

9.5 Case Description

A 78-year-old patient complaining of neck pain, limited motion when turning the head clockwise, and long-lasting right-sided headaches sought medical advice. An unsuccessful infiltration of the second cervical nerve on the right side was performed. The patient then benefitted of a head and neck magnetic resonance imaging that led to the discovery of a right-sided and anterior intradural extramedullary cystic lesion at the craniocervical junction typical of a neuro-enteric cyst. A resection of the lesion was recommended to the patient.

A CT scan of the cervical spine was obtained. T2-weighted MRI images 1.4 mm in thickness, time-of-flight (TOF) sequence 1.2 mm in thickness, and bone windowed CT scan images 1.25 mm in thickness were merged and fused on the navigation planning station (iPlan Netnet®, Brainlab, Germany). Virtual objects were segmented using gray scale thresholding. The skin surface of the head and the bone surface of the skull and vertebra were segmented from the CT scan, the vertebral arteries from the TOF imaging, the brain stem, and medulla from the T2 MRI imaging (Fig. 9.5).

The patient was installed in prone position and the head fixed in a head clamp. The reference stars with reflecting fiducials were fixed on the head holder and microscope. The patient's position was registered using skin surface matching with the Softouch® (Brainlab, Germany) starting with the guide option using both lateral canthus and inion and then multiple points on both lateral aspects of the perioccular skin surface and both concha cymba and cavum as well as mastoid processes. The microscope calibration was checked and recalibrated on the reference star as a standard procedure. Both microscope and patient registration were checked by projecting the virtual head skin surface on the real patient using the microscope head-up display and orienting the microscope. The microscope was first oriented perpendicular to the sagittal plan and aiming toward the ears both sides to capture possible mismatches in the superoinferior and anteroposterior axis and finally perpendicular to the coronal plan and aiming to the inion to

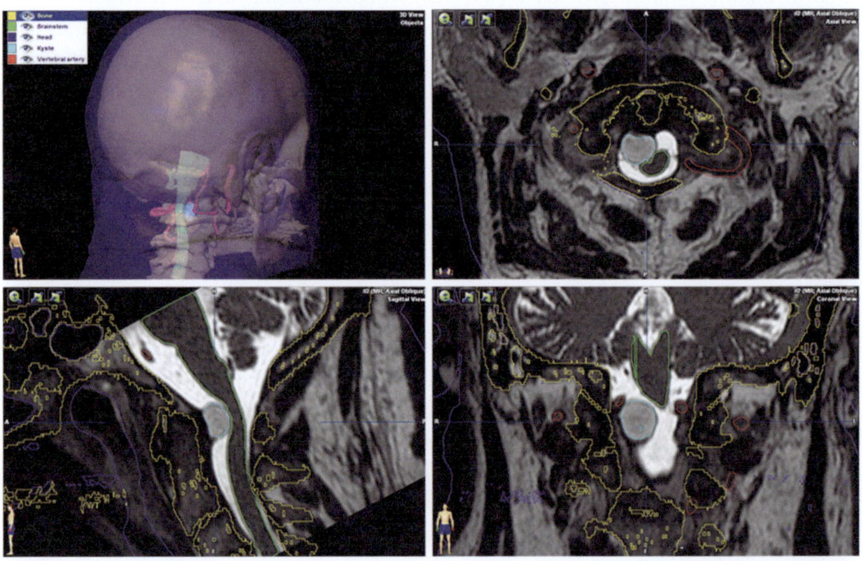

Fig. 9.5 Neuronavigation screenshot illustrating segmented objects: skin surface of the patient's head (blue), bone (yellow), brainstem (green), arteries (red), and lesion (light blue). 3D semitransparent surface rendering projection (upper left), axial slice (upper right), sagittal plane (lower left), and coronal plane (lower right)

capture possible mismatches in the lateral axis and superoinferior axis on the midline (Fig. 9.3).

Once the accuracy was checked, the bone structures, vertebral arteries, the cyst, and the medulla were projected as overlays on the head-up display and the optimal intervention trajectory defined. Skin incision was drawn on the skin accordingly.

After exposure of the skull and C1 vertebra the virtual bone surface was overlaid in the microscope head-up display to verify the accuracy of the registration, and no significant displacement of the vertebra was induced by the patient positioning. If displacements are noticed, local point-based registrations on the bone surface can be performed. The vertebral artery was then projected to be formally localized before proceeding to the C1 vertebra drilling (Fig. 9.6a, b).

Once the C1 right-sided lamina and inferior aspect of the foramen magnum were drilled, the accuracy of the registration was assessed again and the cyst and medulla were projected before dura opening (Fig. 9.6c, d).

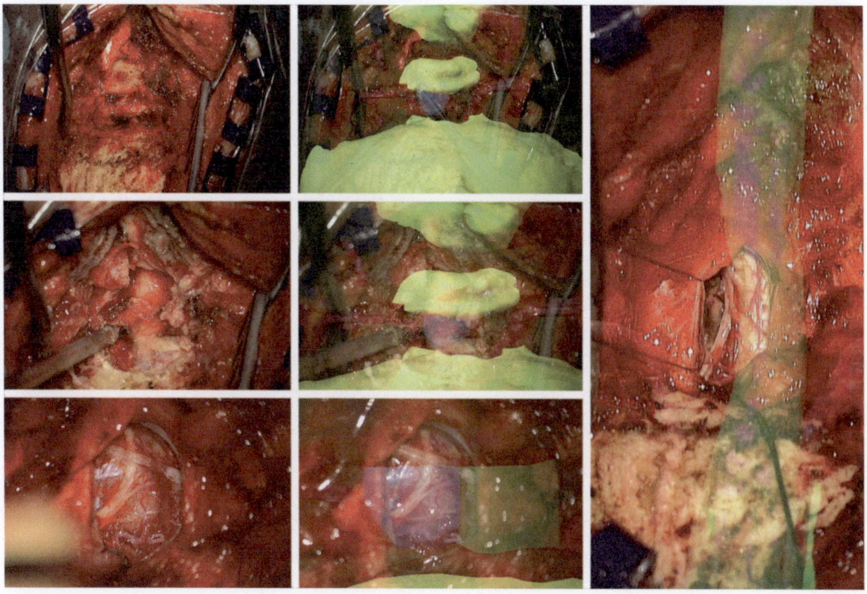

Fig. 9.6 Case illustration. Surgical field photographs without augmented reality taken before the drilling of C1 (upper left), before dura opening (middle left), before lesion resection (lower left), and with the addition of augmented reality (middle column). Surgical field overview illustration after lesion removal with the addition of augmented reality illustrating the deformation of the medulla. Notice how augmented reality facilitates the identification of the vertebral artery, how the anatomy is perfectly matched prior to the drilling, and how it has to be checked and corrected prior to dura opening (vertical shift induced by the pressure of the drill on the lamina)

After dura opening, the location of the cyst and medulla were confirmed by the projection of the virtual objects (Fig. 9.6e, f). Complete cyst removal was achieved laterally, and the most medial aspect of the cyst basis on the anterior aspect of the dura was coagulated. The overlap of the virtual and real medulla and its deformation by the cyst is illustrated (Fig. 9.6g).

9.6 Perspectives

For the purpose of demonstration, a pointer was positioned on the trajectory of a potential screw to be inserted in the C2 lateral mass on the right side and the projection in the head-up display switched to the 2D view. The image visualized corresponds to the CT scan image slice orthogonal to the optic axis of the microscope at the level of the microscope focus plane. The green cross shows the extended pointer tip and the line of the pointer trajectory. Here the surgeon can scan up and down using the focus to visualize all the structures along the pointer trajectory. Surgeons have two visualization options: either a semitransparent 3D representation of structures or a 2D image scrawling along the surgical path. Both views are complementary for a better understanding of the anatomy (Fig. 9.7).

In the future, computer vision and automatic anatomical co-registration should allow to avoid the use of the navigation cameras and reference objects. It should allow very accurate registration using marks (methylene blue marking of bone edges or other type of marks) to be aligned with the contour lines of the bone or vessels (Fig. 9.8). Direct image-based registration should allow accurate and updated 3D augmented reality overlays using the microscope or protection glasses avoiding most of the pitfalls and cumbersome registration and checks currently needed.

Such assistance, associated with continuous and regular education, regular practice, case-specific preparation, and formalizing each step from initial evaluation to final assessment using structured care pathways, may both increase efficiency and quality.

Fig. 9.7 Perspective using augmented reality for screw insertion. The stereoscopic image of the skull and cervical spine is projected in the microscope head-up display. A pointer is used to identify the entry point and trajectory angle (upper inset). The surgeon switches to a 2D representation of the imaging showing a slice orthogonal to the line of sight at the level of the focus plane. The surgeon can easily scan up and down to visualize the relationship between the trajectory path and surrounding structures. The trajectory is expanded from the skin to the depth using the tip extension tool. The green cross shows the tip of the pointer. The red cross shows the tip of the virtual extension located in the middle of the pedicle and in the focal plane (middle insert). 3D volume rendering projection of the structures with planned trajectory. The surgeon can adjust the pointer orientation to the optimal trajectory and check the accuracy by verifying the collocation of the virtual image of the spinous processes of C1 and C2 with their actual location by palpation (lower inset)

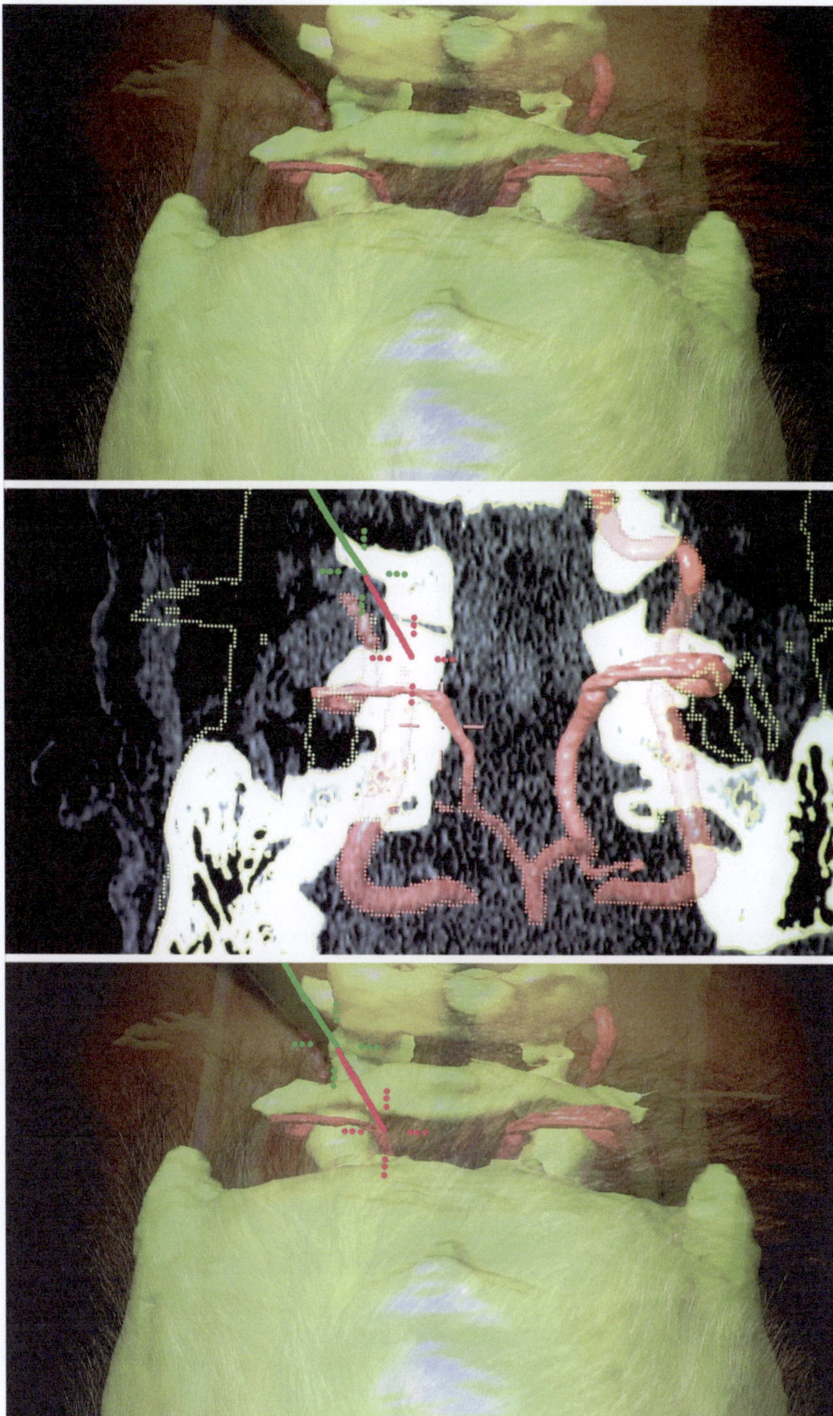

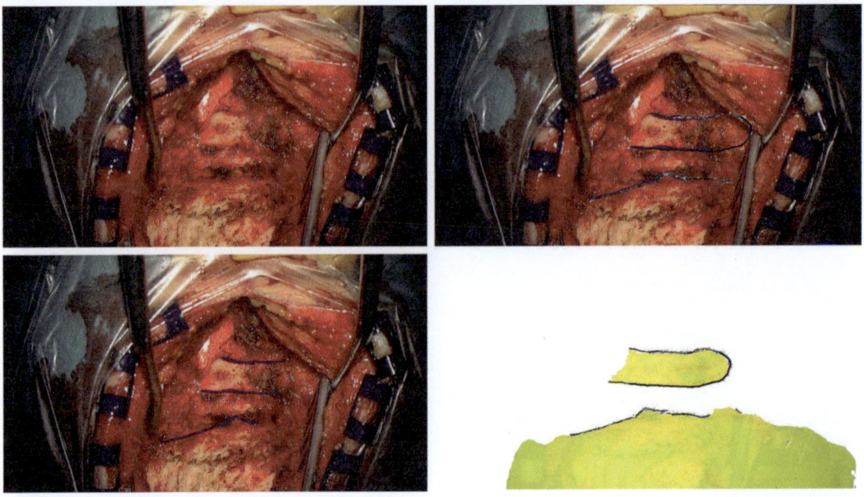

Fig. 9.8 Example of possible solution to facilitate image-based re-registration and computer vision life registration correction. Signature bone edges are identified from the computer reconstruction of the operative field (lower right). The signature bone edges are exposed in the operative field (upper left) and marked using methylene blue ink (lower left). The computer adjusts the virtual image to reality by overlapping the signature shape of the calculated bone edges with the methylene blue marking. Vertebra and skull being independent objects with specific signature edges, the computer should be able to track and correct for relative motion of different rigid objects

Acknowledgments I would like to thank Nadja Heindl and Valentin Elefteriu for their careful review of the manuscript.

References

1. Ogihara N, et al. Long-term results of computer-assisted posterior occipitocervical reconstruction. World Neurosurg. 2010;73(6):722–8.
2. Rampersaud YR, Simon DA, Foley KT. Accuracy requirements for image-guided spinal pedicle screw placement. Spine (Phila Pa 1976). 2001;26(4):352–9.
3. Elmi-Terander A, et al. Surgical navigation technology based on augmented reality and integrated 3D intraoperative imaging: a spine cadaveric feasibility and accuracy study. Spine (Phila Pa 1976). 2016;41(21):E1303–11.
4. King D. Internal fixation for lumbosacral fusion. J Bone Joint Surg Am. 1948;30A(3):560–5.
5. Roy-Camille R, Saillant G, Mazel C. Internal fixation of the lumbar spine with pedicle screw plating. Clin Orthop Relat Res. 1986;(203):7–17.
6. Odgers CJt, et al. Accuracy of pedicle screw placement with the assistance of lateral plain radiography. J Spinal Disord. 1996;9(4):334–8.
7. Kalfas IH, et al. Application of frameless stereotaxy to pedicle screw fixation of the spine. J Neurosurg. 1995;83(4):641–7.
8. Tian W. Robot-assisted posterior C1–2 transarticular screw fixation for atlantoaxial instability: a case report. Spine (Phila Pa 1976). 2016;41(Suppl 19):B2–5.
9. Kostrzewski S, et al. Robotic system for cervical spine surgery. Int J Med Robot. 2012;8(2):184–90.

10. Nottmeier EW, Young PM. Image-guided placement of occipitocervical instrumentation using a reference arc attached to the headholder. Neurosurgery. 2010;66(3 Suppl Operative):138–42.
11. Guppy KH, Chakrabarti I, Banerjee A. The use of intraoperative navigation for complex upper cervical spine surgery. Neurosurg Focus. 2014;36(3):E5.
12. Pisapia JM, et al. Navigated odontoid screw placement using the O-arm: technical note and case series. J Neurosurg Spine. 2017;26(1):10–8.
13. Gertzbein SD, Robbins SE. Accuracy of pedicular screw placement in vivo. Spine (Phila Pa 1976). 1990;15(1):11–4.
14. Mason A, et al. The accuracy of pedicle screw placement using intraoperative image guidance systems. J Neurosurg Spine. 2014;20(2):196–203.
15. Tian NF, et al. Pedicle screw insertion accuracy with different assisted methods: a systematic review and meta-analysis of comparative studies. Eur Spine J. 2011;20(6):846–59.
16. Yukawa Y, et al. Cervical pedicle screw fixation in 100 cases of unstable cervical injuries: pedicle axis views obtained using fluoroscopy. J Neurosurg Spine. 2006;5(6):488–93.
17. Abumi K, et al. Posterior occipitocervical reconstruction using cervical pedicle screws and plate-rod systems. Spine (Phila Pa 1976). 1999;24(14):1425–34.
18. Nakashima H, et al. Complications of cervical pedicle screw fixation for nontraumatic lesions: a multicenter study of 84 patients. J Neurosurg Spine. 2012;16(3):238–47.
19. Richter M, Cakir B, Schmidt R. Cervical pedicle screws: conventional versus computer-assisted placement of cannulated screws. Spine (Phila Pa 1976). 2005;30(20):2280–7.
20. Kotani Y, et al. Improved accuracy of computer-assisted cervical pedicle screw insertion. J Neurosurg. 2003;99(3 Suppl):257–63.
21. Uehara M, et al. Screw perforation rates in 359 consecutive patients receiving computer-guided pedicle screw insertion along the cervical to lumbar spine. Eur Spine J. 2017;26(11):2858–64.
22. Tessitore E, et al. Accuracy of freehand fluoroscopy-guided placement of C1 lateral mass and C2 isthmic screws in atlanto-axial instability. Acta Neurochir. 2011;153(7):1417–25; discussion 1425.
23. Uehara M, et al. Perforation rates of cervical pedicle screw insertion by disease and vertebral level. Open Orthop J. 2010;4:142–6.
24. Zou D, et al. Three-dimensional image navigation system-assisted anterior cervical screw fixation for treatment of acute odontoid fracture. Int J Clin Exp Med. 2014;7(11):4332–6.
25. Mendelsohn D, et al. Patient and surgeon radiation exposure during spinal instrumentation using intraoperative computed tomography-based navigation. Spine J. 2016;16(3):343–54.
26. Villard J, et al. Radiation exposure to the surgeon and the patient during posterior lumbar spinal instrumentation: a prospective randomized comparison of navigated versus non-navigated freehand techniques. Spine (Phila Pa 1976). 2014;39(13):1004–9.

Part III

Surgical Techniques

Open Transoral Approach

10

David Choi

10.1 Indications for Open Transoral Surgery

Transoral surgery is ideally suited for ventral midline pathologies. The approach may be extended superiorly, inferiorly, or laterally depending on the specific indication of surgery.

The standard transoral approach [1] was originally developed to treat anterior compression of the cervicomedullary junction due to rheumatoid pannus and vertical translocation of the odontoid peg in congenital conditions of the skull base. Indications for the approach have changed over recent decades, in response to changes in epidemiology and pathology [2]. The standard technique involves a modified Boyd-Davis or Crockard retractor, which opens the mouth, depresses the tongue, and elevates the soft palate, affording access to the posterior pharyngeal wall. If additional superior access is required, then the soft palate may be split by a midline vertical incision, deviating to one side of the uvula at its inferior extent. The standard approach is suitable for gaining access to the inferior clivus, C1 anterior arch and C2 odontoid peg (Fig. 10.1).

For greater superior exposure, the maxilla may be opened with an "open door maxillotomy" [3–5] or le Fort 1 osteotomy, to access the superior clivus to the pituitary fossa (Fig. 10.2).

Lateral exposure via maxillotomy is limited by the medial pterygoid plates and the internal carotid artery at the skull base. Endoscopic transnasal approaches have largely replaced the need of maxillotomy for accessing the superior clivus, and thereby minimizing the complications of maxillotomy and the need for gastrostomy and tracheostomy in the perioperative period [4].

Inferior extension of the standard transoral approach is possible by mandibulotomy, with or without glossotomy (Fig. 10.3). This approach requires the

D. Choi (✉)
The National Hospital for Neurology and Neurosurgery, Queen Square, London, UK
e-mail: david.choi@nhs.net

E. Tessitore et al. (eds.), *Surgery of the Cranio-Vertebral Junction*,
https://doi.org/10.1007/978-3-030-18700-2_10

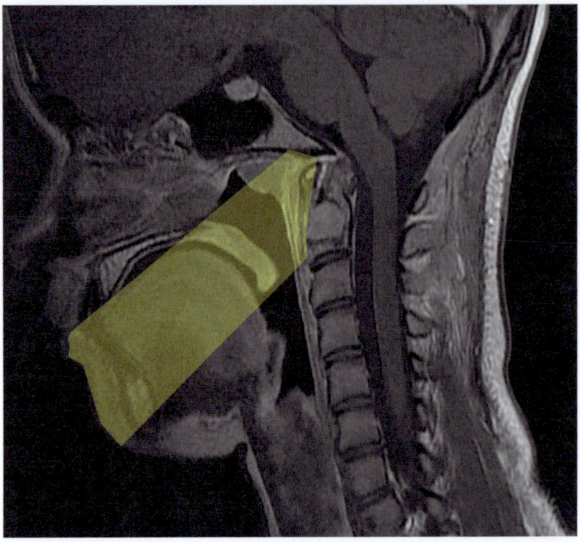

Fig. 10.1 Access by the standard transoral approach

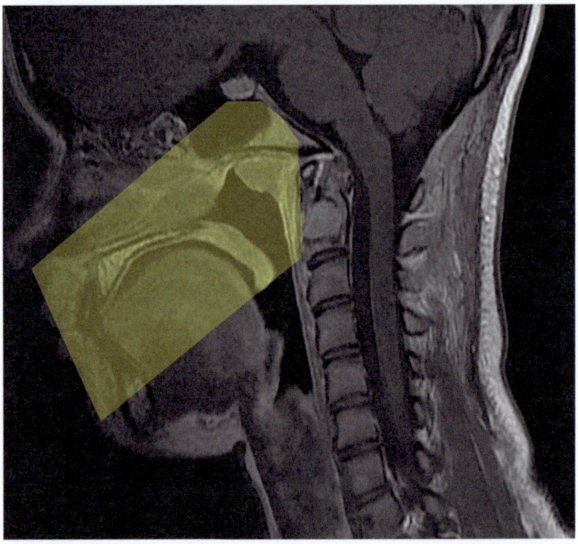

Fig. 10.2 Access by the open door maxillotomy approach

preoperative insertion of tracheostomy and gastrostomy feeding tube. It is useful for inferior midline access down to the C4 vertebral body.

Lateral exposure is possible to access the lateral masses of the vertebrae and the vertebral artery if required. A paramedian mucosal incision and a door-shaped flap can help achieve additional paramedian access when required.

The open transoral approaches may also be combined with additional staged approaches, particularly for the resection of complex primary tumors. A posterior approach may be used to insert occipitocervical fixation and also resect

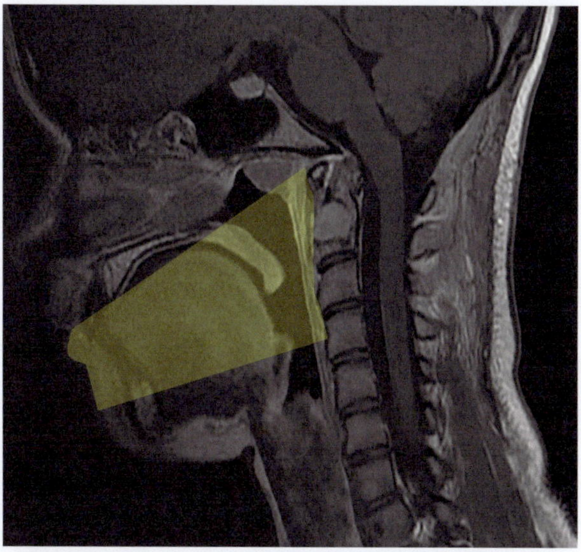

Fig. 10.3 Access by the mandibulotomy approach

additional tumor and mobilize the vertebral artery as required. The far lateral approach is a useful staged approach to access the lateral aspects of C1 and C2, and endoscopic transnasal surgery may be performed for pathologies extending above the hard palate, intracranial extension, or into the apex of the medial petrous temporal bone.

Previously the open transoral approach was more commonly used for the removal of odontoid pannus in rheumatoid disease, in conjunction with occipitocervical stabilization. With the advent of disease modifying drugs and immunotherapies, however, the technique is now more commonly used for the excision of primary bone sarcomas and tumors, in particular, chordomas and chondrosarcomas, and for congenital conditions of basilar invagination. The technique is also suitable for anterior stabilization of C1 and C2 fractures, decompression of degenerative pseudotumor of the odontoid peg, and less commonly for debridement of infection.

Present common indications for the open transoral approach include midline tumors, particularly chordomas, chondrosarcomas, other primary bone and soft tissue tumors, acute neurological deterioration due to degenerative odontoid pseudotumor, or diagnostic biopsy of infection. Contraindications include oral sepsis, limited mouth opening, or fixed flexion deformity of the cervical spine ("chin-on-chest deformity").

10.2 Pathologies and Trends

In the 1980s to 1990s, the driving force for the development of open transoral techniques was the large number of rheumatoid patients with C1-C2 instability and odontoid pannus or translocation of the odontoid peg [2].

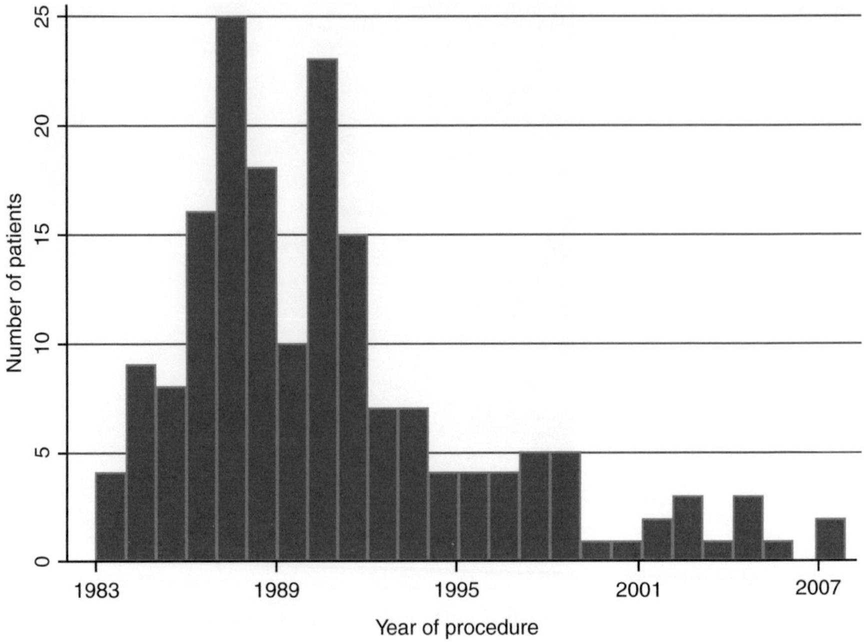

Fig. 10.4 Decreasing numbers of patients with rheumatoid arthritis undergoing transoral surgery over the past few decades

Over recent decades, there have been fewer patients with advanced rheumatoid arthritis presenting for surgery, due to a combination of more effective medical treatments and change in disease epidemiology, resulting in a decreased requirement for the open transoral operation [6–8] (Fig. 10.4).

However, it remains a very useful approach for tumors of the craniovertebral junction, particularly chordomas and chondrosarcomas, which often transgress several surgical tissue planes in this region and are challenging to remove. Although transnasal endoscopic surgery can access down to C2, the open transoral approach affords a wider surgical avenue, greater lateral exposure, and the ability to close the posterior pharynx and effectively deal with potential leakage of cerebrospinal fluid (CSF) if the dura has been opened.

The modern skull base surgeon needs to be familiar with both endoscopic and open approaches. The standard transoral approach is associated with a surprisingly low infection rate of 0.6% due to the inherent immunity of the mucosa and a low CSF leak rate of 0.3% [2]. With a greater exposure of the posterior pharyngeal wall, it is possible to close the defect with a sutured two-layer closure involving the longus colli muscles and the pharyngeal mucosa separately. The transnasal endoscopic approach to the C1-C2 region is a useful technique, developed in the last decade [9], which has the advantage of shorter hospital stay, quicker recovery for the patients, and lower rates of postoperative velopharyngeal incompetence. The endoscopic technique is better suited for pathologies above the level of the hard palate, for

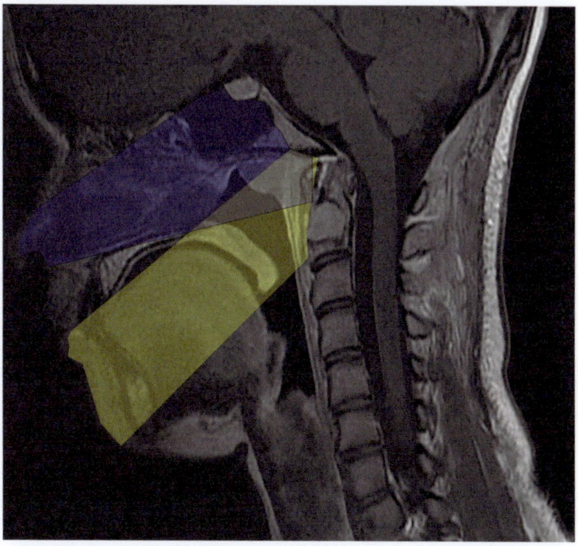

Fig. 10.5 Comparison of transnasal (blue) and transoral (yellow) approaches

example, congenital platybasia and basilar impression or vertical translocation of the odontoid peg causing brainstem compression [10]. The endoscopic approach may be more acceptable to patients, avoids tongue swelling, and delays in oral feeding, dysphagia, and dysphonia, and therefore leads to quicker recovery. However, the endoscopic and open transoral approaches are not always interchangeable, and in general, pathologies of the C1-C2 region and below are often better served by the transoral approach (Fig. 10.5).

Alternative surgical approaches include the subfrontal transbasal or transethmoid approaches to the sphenoid sinus, the preauricular infratemporal fossa approach to the clivus and infratemporal fossa, far lateral and extreme lateral approaches to the C1-C2 region, and the anterolateral submandibular approach to the C1-C2 upper cervical spine.

Advances in radiotherapy have also changed the indications for open transoral surgery. Although the mainstay of treatment for chordomas and chondrosarcomas is maximal safe resection and adjunctive radiation treatment, small tumors may be treated primarily with proton beam or carbon ion therapy, although long-term outcome data is awaited. Stereotactic beam radiation, Gamma knife radiation, and intensity modulated radiotherapy have also been used to treat craniovertebral junction chordomas and chondrosarcomas, but generally do not achieve the high radiation dose that is possible with heavy particle therapies. The combined use of surgery and radiation has led to the concept of "separation surgery" in which the aim of surgery is to provide at least 3 mm clearance of the tumor margin from the brainstem, and 5 mm from the optic chiasm and optic nerves, to allow dose escalation in subsequent postoperative radiation treatment [11]. However, longer tumor-free survival is associated with maximal tumor resection from the outset.

10.3 Preoperative Assessment

For the standard open transoral approach, a minimum of 2.5 cm of mouth-opening is required in the midline. Additional exposure can be obtained if required by the division of the mandible for inferior exposure or by maxillotomy for superior exposure.

Stability of the craniovertebral junction should be assessed with cervical X-rays in flexion and extension, and MRI assessment of ligamentous integrity. Occipitocervical fusion is required to supplement transoral surgery if the odontoid peg is resected, together with apical and alar ligaments, or if the transverse ligament is incompetent.

Magnetic resonance imaging (MRI) is important to assess the degree of compression of the brain stem or spinal cord, location of skull base tumors, extent of rheumatoid pannus formation, integrity of ligaments, and discs. The relationship of the hard palate with the level of the pathology is important. The hard palate should be above the tumor or pathology for resection, for successful transoral surgery.

Computed tomography (CT) scans are useful for assessing bone involvement of tumors, integrity of joints and facets, size and position of pedicles and lateral masses for fixation, and the relative position of the foraminae transversarii. CT angiography can also be performed to view the vertebral artery positions and, in particular, the relations in the C2 vertebra for safe placement of C2 pedicle screws, although often sufficient information may be obtained by observing the foraminae on a standard CT cervical spine images with bone windows.

Usually fixation is required by inserting rods from an occipital plate to C2, C3, or C4 lateral masses, using standard 3.5 mm diameter polyaxial screws in the lateral masses of the cervical vertebrae and pedicle screws in C2 vertebra. If surgery is performed for chordomas and chondrosarcomas, it is important to minimize the use of cross-links and metalwork at the level of tumor resection, to allow accurate planning of postoperative radiotherapy or proton beam therapy [11].

Airway assessment should be performed by the anesthetic team. Fiber optic nasotracheal intubation is required, with in-line spine stabilization during the anesthetic induction.

Nasal and oral microbiological swabs are taken preoperatively, in case of postoperative infection.

10.4 Consent for Surgery

Open transoral surgery is technically demanding and therefore should be performed in specialist centers with sufficient numbers of operations to maintain competencies. The intended benefits of surgery should be determined for the particular condition and clearly explained to the patient before surgery. Potential complications should be discussed before informed consent is provided by the patient.

Standard transoral surgery has a low complication rate, with up to 1.1% CSF leak rate, 10% respiratory complications such as chest infection, 2–3% dysphagia, 1%

pharyngeal wound infection rate, 1% neurological deterioration, 3% meningitis, and a risk of coma and mortality which varies depending on the presenting pathology and patient factors [2].

The procedures of mandibulotomy and maxillotomy have higher complication rates, including 10–20% risk of velopharyngeal incompetence and dysphagia, 30% respiratory complications, and 10% mortality [2].

Operations to decompress the spinal cord intend to prevent deterioration and may not be associated with improved neurological function. If surgery is performed for tumor resection, the small chance of incomplete tumor resection, or tumor recurrence in the future, should be mentioned to the patient prior to surgery.

10.5 Technique

There are several methods of transoral surgery described in the literature, using specific transoral retractor systems [12–14]. We routinely perform the Crockard technique [15]. The patient is placed in a Mayfield three-pin headrest, in supine position with the extension of the neck to aid access to the superior cervical spine and brain. Reverse Trendelenburg position will also aid access and minimize bleeding and soft tissue swelling. Image guidance can be provided by neuronavigation systems and preoperative imaging or by real-time X-ray imaging with an intraoperative image intensifier. Neurophysiological monitoring by somatosensory evoked potentials is routinely used. It is not possible to monitor motor potentials due to the risk of mouth closure and damage to the teeth and tongue.

A right-handed surgeon would normally stand on the patient's right side, and vice versa for a left-handed surgeon. A standard operating microscope is used, with 300–400 mm focal length.

The oral cavity is cleaned with swabs and 0.5% aqueous chlorhexidine, and topical 1% hydrocortisone ointment is smeared on the tongue to minimize intraoperative and postoperative swelling.

A Codman Crockard transoral retractor (Codman, Raynham, MA) is used to hold the mouth open, retract the tongue inferiorly, and elevate the soft palate (Figs. 10.6 and 10.7).

The anterior tubercle of C1 arch can be palpated, or if not obvious may be confirmed using the image intensifier or navigation system. Other useful midline markers are the pharyngeal tubercle of the clivus and the midline tubercle of the C2 vertebral body. Once the retractor is in place, the posterior pharyngeal mucosa should be incised, either with a midline linear incision through the back of the mouth or by a crescentic incision. The straight incision is ideally suited to midline pathologies such as for odontoidectomy, whereas for tumors which may extend more laterally, a crescentic or door-shaped mucosal opening allows wider exposure. The mucosal layer is elevated and retracted laterally using a Howarth elevator, and then the longus colli muscles are divided in the midline using diathermy cauterization and the Howarth elevator. Lateral exposure is improved by using the self-retaining toothed retractors.

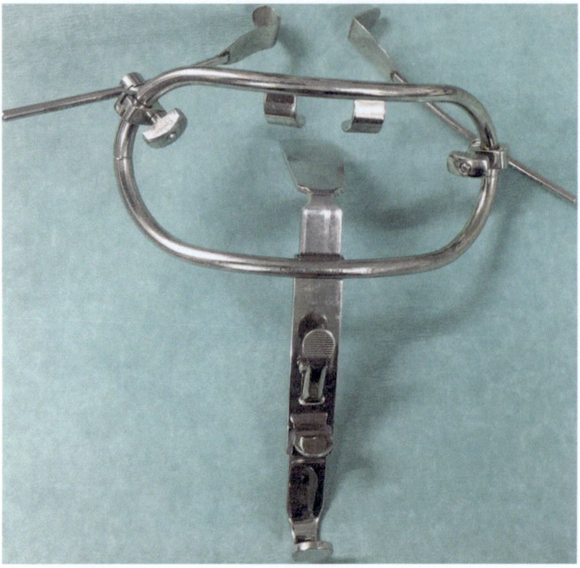

Fig. 10.6 The Crockard transoral retractor is a modified Boyd-Davis Gag, with ratcheted tongue blade and "L"-shaped and "J"-shaped soft palate retractors fitted

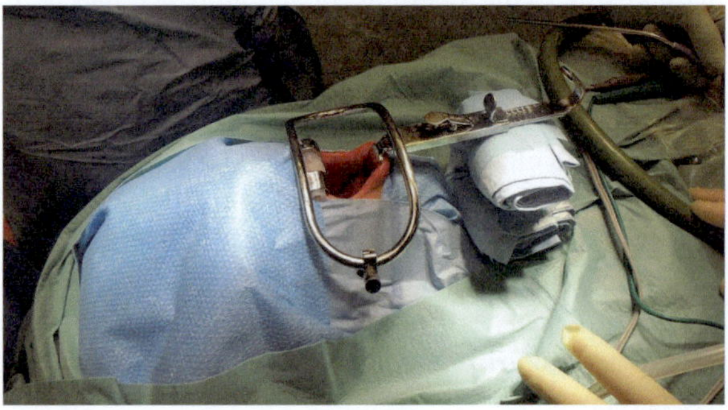

Fig. 10.7 Operative setup for transoral surgery with retractor in place

For more superior exposure, the soft palate may be divided in the midline, deviating inferiorly to one side of the uvula.

When resecting a tumor, it is important to work on the capsule and stay outside the tumor as much as possible. Although en bloc excision is difficult to achieve, understanding the anatomy and relations of the tumor capsule will allow a more complete excision to be performed.

The vertebral arteries are distant from the midline at the C1 arch level (approximately 24 mm laterally) but closest to the midline at the C2/C3 disc level (about 11 mm from the midline) which is where damage might occur with inadvertent drilling of the C2 vertebral body.

After surgical resection and decompression of the brainstem and spinal cord, reconstruction can commence. If the patient will receive adjuvant radiotherapy after tumor resection, then reconstruction should use minimal metal components. Posterior craniocervical fixation will be required using titanium occipital plate, lateral mass screws, and rods. Anterior cages and plates should be made of carbon fiber or PEEK to minimize radiotherapy planning artifacts, beam scattering, or shielding.

It is essential to achieve a robust two layer closure of the posterior oropharynx to minimize the risk of wound breakdown, infection, or fistula formation. The longus colli muscle layer is closed using interrupted 2/0 absorbable sutures (Vicryl™, Ethicon, New Jersey) and then the pharyngeal mucosa is closed as a separate second layer using 3/0 absorbable sutures. The soft palate is closed in two layers (deep and superficial mucosal layers).

10.6 Perioperative Management

At the time of anesthetic induction, prophylactic doses of cephalosporin and metronidazole antibiotics should be given and continued for 24 h after surgery.

Patients should be managed in the intensive care unit after surgery, with sedation to maintain the position of the nasotracheal tube. Due to the possibility of postoperative pharyngeal swelling, extubation is usually performed the day after surgery. Prior to extubation, the cuff of the nasotracheal tube is deflated to assess if the pharyngeal swelling has subsided sufficiently to allow air to bypass around the sides of the nasotracheal tube; extubation can proceed if the air leak test is positive.

The patient should be nil-by-mouth for 5 days after surgery, and nutrition should be given by nasogastric feeding tube for 5 days. Visual inspection of the posterior pharynx and soft palate will determine the quality of mucosal healing, and if satisfactory, then oral feeding may re-commence 5 days after surgery.

If the surgery was performed for tumor excision, an MRI scan with and without contrast injection should be performed the day after surgery. The contrast will demonstrate peripheral enhancement around the postoperative hematoma cavity, and this is very useful for determining whether there is any significant residual tumor (Fig. 10.8).

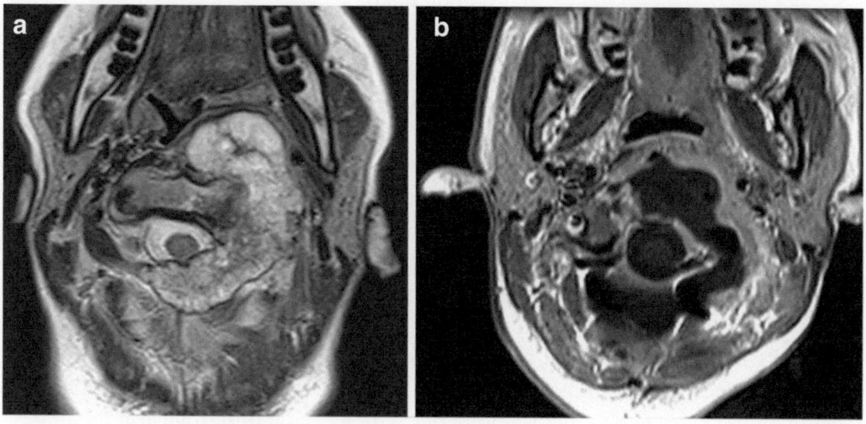

Fig. 10.8 Preoperative axial MRI of extensive C1 chondrosarcoma (**a**) and postoperative MRI with contrast, 24 h after surgery showing contrast enhancement in the margins of the normal hematoma cavity (**b**)

10.7 Management of Complications

Potential early local complications include infection, CSF leak, hematoma formation, and wound breakdown.

10.7.1 Infection

The risk of mucosal infection is less than 1% after simple transoral surgery [2]. Preoperative microbiological swabs are taken, and significant cultures and sensitivities can be evaluated to guide appropriate microbiological therapy if required. If the patient has clinical features of possible meningitis, then lumbar puncture should be performed for CSF evaluation and culture.

Posterior neck infections can occur in 2.1% of patients and can usually be managed with wound lavage and intravenous antibiotic treatment [2, 16]. Persistent infection may require removal of colonized metalwork and application of a halo-jacket, but this is rarely necessary.

10.7.2 CSF Leak

CSF leak should be distinguished from mucosal secretions by the identification of beta-transferrin or tau proteins. MRI or CT cisternogram can be useful to determine the site of possible fistula. If a positive CSF leak is found, then surgical revision of the pharyngeal wound should be performed with standard two later closures. Parallel releasing incisions may be performed in the pharyngeal mucosa if the mucosa does not approximate without undue tension. Lumbar drainage of CSF may be required for large or persistent fistulae, and CSF drainage of between 5 and 15 mL per hour maintained for 5 days. During this period, the patient should be fed by nasogastric tube and maintained nil by mouth to allow healing.

10.7.3 Wound Breakdown and Hematoma

Coexistent infection or CSF leak should be excluded as causes of wound breakdown. Re-suture of the pharyngeal wound under general anesthetic should be performed, with care to approximate the mucosa without tension by undermining the mucosal layer and using releasing incisions if required.

Hematoma causing neurological deterioration should be identified by MRI scans unless there is rapid neurological deterioration which should be treated by prompt re-exploration of the wound. If an anterior cage or bone graft has been used, occasionally this needs to be removed to allow adequate wound healing and minimize tension on the pharyngeal mucosa, together with a period of nasogastric feeding.

10.7.4 Delayed Complications

Other complications include meningitis, palatal dehiscence, nasopharyngeal regurgitation, nasal speech due to velopharyngeal incompetence, abscess or fistula formation, failure of fixation or fusion, delayed neurological consequences, and chest infection.

References

1. Crockard HA, Pozo JL, Ransford AO, Stevens JM, Kendall BE, Essigman WK. Transoral decompression and posterior fusion for rheumatoid atlanto-axial subluxation. J Bone Joint Surg Br. 1986;68(3):350–6.
2. Choi D, Crockard HA. Evolution of transoral surgery: three decades of change in patients, pathologies, and indications. Neurosurgery. 2013;73(2):296–303.
3. Anand VK, Harkey HL, Al-Mefty O. Open-door maxillotomy approach for lesions of the clivus. Skull Base Surg. 1991;1(4):217–25.
4. Choi D, Subramanian A, Elwell V, Andrews P, Roberts D, Gleeson M. Endoscopic transnasal surgery as a replacement for maxillotomy techniques to approach the central skull base: fewer complications and more acceptable to patients? J Neurol Surg B Skull Base. 2014;75(3):165–70.
5. James D, Crockard HA. Surgical access to the base of skull and upper cervical spine by extended maxillotomy. Neurosurgery. 1991;29(3):411–6.
6. Choi D, Casey AT, Crockard HA. Neck problems in rheumatoid arthritis—changing disease patterns, surgical treatments and patients' expectations. Rheumatology (Oxford). 2006;45(10):1183–4.
7. Hamilton JD, Gordon MM, McInnes IB, Johnston RA, Madhok R, Capell HA. Improved medical and surgical management of cervical spine disease in patients with rheumatoid arthritis over 10 years. Ann Rheum Dis. 2000;59(6):434–8.
8. Ward MM. Decreases in rates of hospitalizations for manifestations of severe rheumatoid arthritis, 1983-2001. Arthritis Rheum. 2004;50(4):1122–31.
9. Snyderman CH, Kassam AB. Endoscopic techniques for pathology of the anterior cranial fossa and ventral skull base. J Am Coll Surg. 2006;202(3):563.
10. Liu JK, Patel J, Goldstein IM, Eloy JA. Endoscopic endonasal transclival transodontoid approach for ventral decompression of the craniovertebral junction: operative technique and nuances. Neurosurg Focus. 2015;38(4):E17.
11. Matloob SA, Nasir HA, Choi D. Proton beam therapy in the management of skull base chordomas: systematic review of indications, outcomes, and implications for neurosurgeons. Br J Neurosurg. 2016;30(4):382–7.
12. Mouchaty H, Perrini P, Conti R, Di Lorenzo N. Craniovertebral junction lesions: our experience with the transoral surgical approach. Eur Spine J. 2009;18(Suppl 1):13–9.
13. Spetzler RF, Hadley MN, Sonntag VK. The transoral approach to the anterior superior cervical spine. A review of 29 cases. Acta Neurochir Suppl (Wien). 1988;43:69–74.
14. Menezes AH, VanGilder JC. Transoral-transpharyngeal approach to the anterior craniovertebral junction. Ten-year experience with 72 patients. J Neurosurg. 1988;69(6):895–903.
15. Crockard HA. The transoral approach to the base of the brain and upper cervical cord. Ann R Coll Surg Engl. 1985;67(5):321–5.
16. Choi D, Melcher R, Harms J, Crockard A. Outcome of 132 operations in 97 patients with chordomas of the cranio-vertebral junction and upper cervical spine. Neurosurgery. 2010;66(1):59–65; discussion.

Endoscopic Transnasal Approach

11

Felice Esposito, Fabio Cacciola, Domenico Solari, Rosa Maria Gerardi, Filippo Flavio Angileri, Oreste de Divitiis, Antonino Germanò, and Paolo Cappabianca

11.1 Introduction

Anterior approach to the craniovertebral junction (CVJ) and, particularly, to the odontoid process of the second cervical vertebra has classically been performed, in neurosurgical settings, via a transoral route. Such technique is still considered the gold standard treatment for odontoid process diseases.

However, the advent of endoscopy in neurosurgery and the development and the refinement of the endonasal approaches to the entire midline skull base [1–5] have meant that also this field, once dominated by microsurgery, has become territory of exploration for neurosurgeons who have dedicated clinical and scientific efforts is this direction. As a matter of fact, the endoscopic endonasal approach (EEA) to the craniocervical junction, and to the odontoid process, is among the areas of most interest to which endoscopic technique is developed.

Indeed, several studies either anatomical or clinical have been reported showing the interest of approaching the CVJ through the nasal corridor [6, 7]. In fact, the availability of new technologies, such as endoscopes, high-definition endoscopic cameras, navigation systems, ultrasound micro-Doppler, dedicated endonasal instruments, and bipolar forceps have opened new horizons to manage pathologies

F. Esposito · F. Cacciola · F. F. Angileri · A. Germanò
Department of Neurosurgery, University of Messina, Messina, Italy

D. Solari (✉) · R. M. Gerardi · O. de Divitiis · P. Cappabianca
Division of Neurosurgery, Department of Neurosciences, Reproductive and Odontostomatological Sciences, Università degli Studi di Napoli Federico II, Naples, Italy
e-mail: domenico.solari@unina.it; paolo.cappabianca@unina.it

E. Tessitore et al. (eds.), *Surgery of the Cranio-Vertebral Junction*,
https://doi.org/10.1007/978-3-030-18700-2_11

involving this complex region using the natural nasal corridors; this way/approach has demonstrated a remarkable improvement of the quality of disease resection as well of the functional outcome with a lower morbidity.

The endonasal route provides a direct access to the surgical field, minimizing the mucosal and the neurovascular manipulation: it follows a natural path road that goes from the nostrils to the mucosa covering the rhynopharynx, the rhinopharyngeal muscles, the anterior arch of C1, and finally the odontoid process. As a consequence, the surgical invasiveness of the endoscopic endonasal approach is lower than traditional transoral approach, and it does not require additional surgical maneuvers, such as mouth retraction, tongue compression or even splitting, possible injury to the teeth, injury to the uvula and/or the soft palate and velupendulum, or neurovascular manipulation through the oropharynx. Theoretically, such facts imply a lower rate of postoperative complications related to invasiveness with a lower rate of postoperative dysphagia and respiratory complications, which are due to the possibility that, with the endoscopic approach, extubation coincides with the end of the procedure. All this involves, consequently, a more rapid mobilization and a reduction of recovery times for natural feeding, which then is reflected, of course, on hospitalization time. Seen in this light, the endoscopic endonasal approach offers a viable alternative to the more established transoral approach, especially for the clear advantages that the endoscopic technique offers in cases where there is full indication to execute it. On the other hand, in case of dural opening, there will be an important risk of CSF leak and meningitis; as a consequence, the endonasal approach may be associated with a difficult dural closure with the related higher risk of postoperative CSF leakage and meningitis.

11.1.1 Anterior Versus Posterior Approach

The decision-making between an anterior or a posterior approach depends on different particular aspects: (1) the direction of the compression and (2) the surgeon's confidence and experience with the approaches and, thus, the possibility to perform the reduction of the compression with anterior, posterior, or a combined approach. In general, unreducible anterior subluxation associated with spinal cord compression requires anterior approach, whereas a reducible posterior compression requires a posterior surgical route. However, different complex diseases, acquired or congenital, can cause an alteration of atlanto-axial relationships and anterior cervicomedullary junction compression. In these cases, a fixation or a posterior stabilization could not be sufficient to resolve the ventral compression. As a matter of fact, in these last years, the option of a combined, anterior and posterior, approach has become the best choice for many authors.

11.1.2 Transoral Versus Transnasal Approach

During the last decades, the transoral approach with microscopic assistance has been proposed as the standard procedure to perform the anterior odontoidectomy, considering the etiology of the disease, the mechanism of compression, and finally its reducibility [8–11]. Specifically, in the absence of spinal cord contusion or progressive myelopathy, the posterior decompression and fusion are sufficient alone to achieve an acceptable outcome. Odontoidectomy is necessary when there is a non-reducible bony compression of spinal cord or soft tissue pannus, causing severe ventral compression and resulting in progressive myelopathy.

The risk of bacterial contamination, prolonged postoperative intubation, naso-gastric tube feeding, tongue swelling, and nasopharyngeal incompetence after transoral surgery have led authors to identify alternative routes to approach this region.

The anterior aspect of the craniocervical region can be exposed also via a transnasal despite the fact that some anatomical limits exist. In the transnasal route, the exposure of the C2 body below the odontoid process is limited by the posterior part of the hard palate; however, angled endoscopes, drills, and dedicated instruments provide access downwards to the lower edge of the C2 body [12–15]. On the other hand, the transoral approach is limited by the degree of mouth opening, the size of the patient's tongue, and the position of the uvula and the soft palate. The inferior limit of the access, usually the C_3 vertebra, is determined by the degree of mouth opening, the size of the patient's oral cavity, and the prominence of the incisors. However, also for the transoral approach, the use of angled endoscopes and instruments directs the approach superiorly increasing the rostral access above the anterior arch of the atlas to the lower clivus and C2 [16, 17]. One of the main anatomical landmarks to consider, especially in transoral route, is the course of vertebral artery (VA). The VA, after ascending through the transverse foramen of the axis and atlas, approximately 15 mm from the midline, courses medially along the upper surface of the posterior arch of the atlas to reach its dural entrance. It is mandatory to preserve the segment of the vertebral artery ascending between the C1 and C2 transverse processes.

Once the anterior arch of C1 is exposed, its drilling is necessary to expose the odontoid process of C2. Another difference between transoral and transnasal approach is the visualization of the ligamentous complex. For instance, the apical ligament is easily visualized directly straight ahead of the endoscope in the transnasal route but is seen later, after removal of the odontoid, in the transoral approach. The main step of the anterior odontoidectomy is represented by the drilling of the dens. In the transnasal approach, the dens is seen directly ahead. The anterior cortical surface and core of the dens is drilled, whereas the cortical shell is removed. On the other hand, the base of the dens is more easily accessed for drilling by the transoral route. In addition, a different view is offered by these two approaches regarding the exposure of the upper, middle, or lower clivus. The standard endoscopic transnasal transsphenoidal approach allows to reach the upper clivus, which corresponds to the posterior wall of the sphenoid sinus. Thus the middle and lower clivus are viewed directly straight ahead in the transnasal approach. The access to the middle and lower clivus generally does not require opening the sphenoid sinus. On the other hand, in the transoral approach the middle and the upper clivus are not easily accessible and soft and hard palates opening is required along with the splitting of the tongue and mandible to achieve an upward trajectory. However, certain maneuvers such as using an angled endoscope, retracting sufficiently the uvula, and widely opening the mouth provide a safe access to the lower clivus (Figs. 11.1 and 11.2).

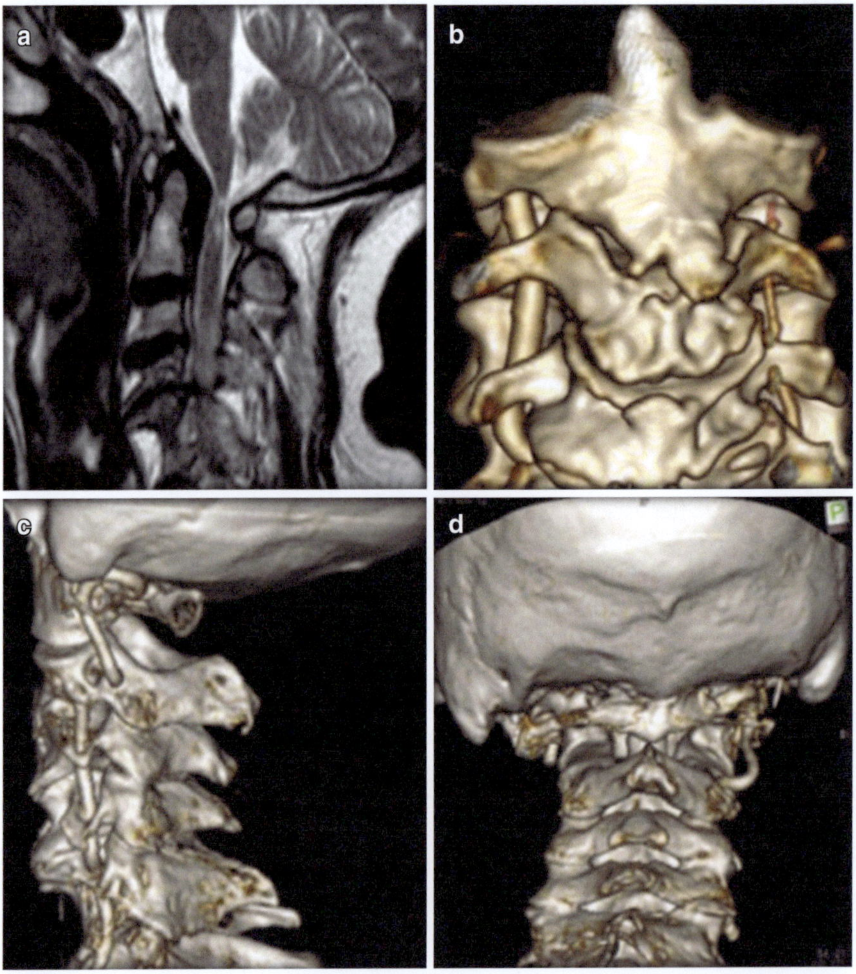

Fig. 11.1 Preoperative neuroimaging study of a cse of rheumatoid disease of CVJ. (**a**) T2-weighted sagittal MRI scan showing bulbo-medullary compression caused by an extradural inflammatory lesion at the level of the odontoid process, i.e. a rheumatoid pannus. (**b-d**) 3D reconstruction of an angio-CT of the patient

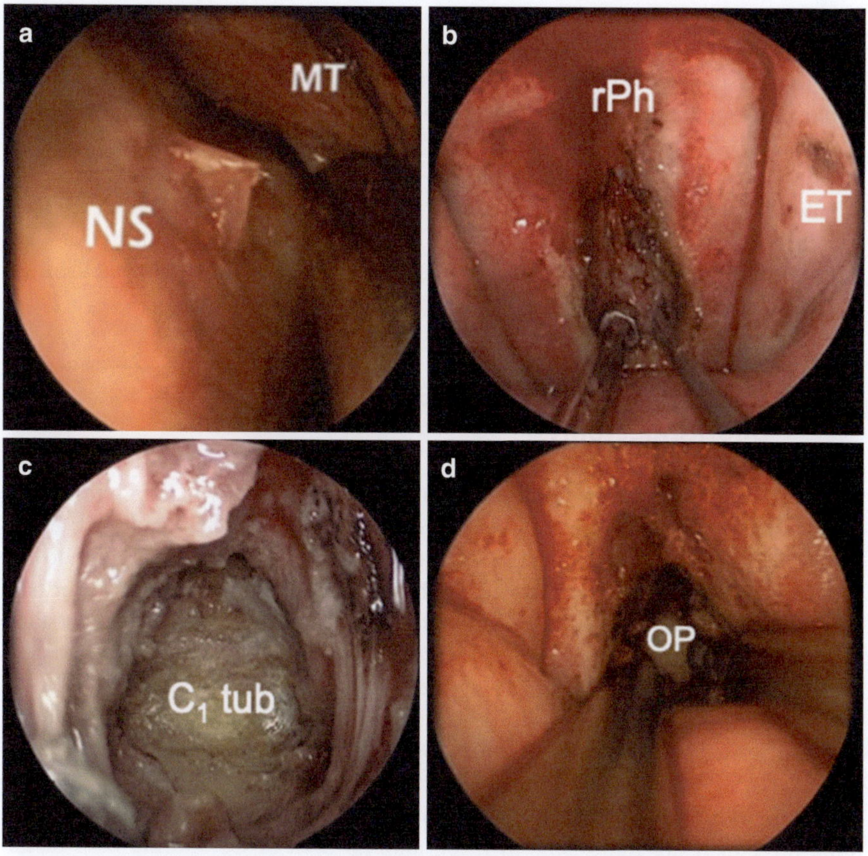

Fig. 11.2 Intraoperative pictures of the endoscopic endonasal approach. (**a**) Definition of the nasal corridor pushing laterally the middle turbinate in the left nostril; (**b**) incision into the rhinopharynx; (**c**) drilling of the anterior arch of C1; (**d**) drilling of the odontoid process of C2 and removal of the bony shell off the ligaments. *NS*: Nasal septum; *MT*: Middle turbinate; *rPh*: rhinopharynx; *ET*: Eustachian tubes; *C1 tub*: Anterior tubercle of C1; *OP*: Odontoid process

11.2 Indications

Odontoidectomy is the most common indication to the use of EEA to CVJ. It is a procedure that is necessary in all cases in which there is an impairment of the nervous structures of the CVJ due to an irreducible alteration of the relations that the odontoid process contracts with neighboring neurovascular structures.

The irreducibility is a crucial concept in the path that leads to the indication for surgery. In fact, several studies confirmed that, when feasible, the reduction of the compression by putting in traction the craniocervical junction and the subsequent fixation, as well as, in cases of compression due to the rheumatoid pannus, posterior stabilization of the craniocervical junction leads, in some cases, the improvement or even the resolution of the ventral compression.

Therefore, the indications for the odontoidectomy arise in all those cases in which there is irreducible atlanto-axial subluxation, associated with severe brainstem and/or spinal cord compression causing progressive neurological dysfunction. In most cases, the pathological process can be due to: (1) irreducible basilar impression [18–23]; (2) ventral compression, as in the cases of rheumatoid pannus, not resolved after posterior stabilization [24–26]; (3) significant retroflexion of the odontoid process or basilar invagination associated with Chiari disease; [27] (4) presence of *os odontoideum* [28–30]; (5) posttraumatic pseudoarthrosis or misalignment; (6) intradural lesions (several recent experiences have enlarged the indications of endoscopic endonasal odontoidectomy [3, 5, 31–33]).

11.3 Feasibility of the Endoscopic Endonasal Odontoidectomy

The goal of the surgical operation is to completely remove the odontoid process of C2 and obtain a sufficient decompression of the ventral brainstem and CVJ. In the debate between microsurgery and endoscopic technique, a remark is done to the eventuality, in the endonasal approach, to have difficulty in reaching the lower portion of the craniocervical junction and, namely, the base of the dens. To understand this aspect, numerous studies on cadavers and on radiological images were performed, with the purpose of delimiting the limits and then the indications to endoscopic approach to the odontoid process pathology. However, leading authors widely reported the feasibility of the endoscopic endonasal approach (EEA) to the CVJ [3, 6].

In case of low junction, located far below the level of the hard palate, it could be quite difficult if not impossible to reach anterior arch of C1 and the base of the odontoid process. Such cases can represent still an indication for the transoral approach. On the other hand, in a higher junction, the dens is more easily reachable and removable by the nasal route (Figs. 11.3 and 11.4).

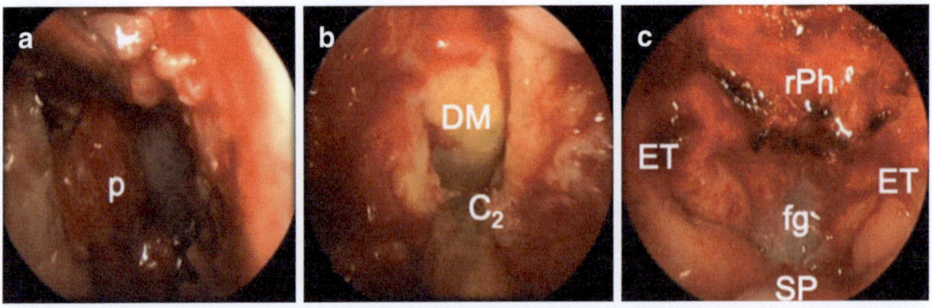

Fig. 11.3 Intraoperative pictures of the endoscopic endonasal approach. (**a**) removal of the pannus causing the compression; (**b**) dura mater of the CVJ; (**c**) closure of the muscle and mucosa with fibrin glue. *p*: Pannus; *C2*: Base of the dens (body of C2); *DM*: Dura mater of the CVJ; *ET*: Eustachian tube; *rPh*: rhinopharynx; *fg*: Fibrin glue; *SP*: Soft palate

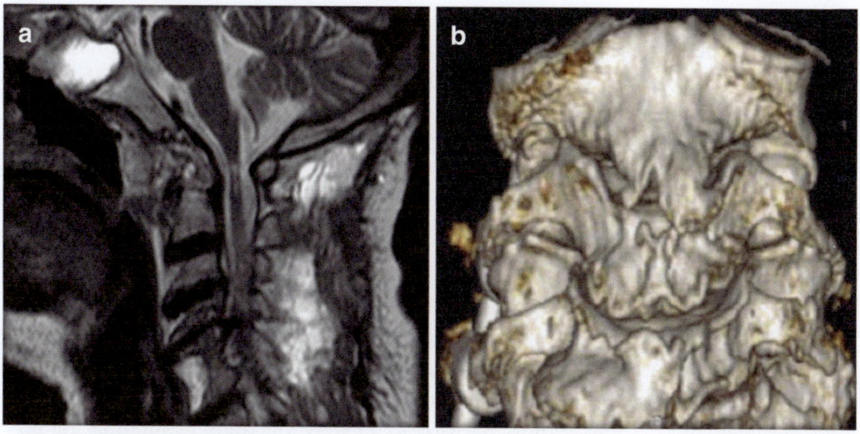

Fig. 11.4 Postoperative neuroimaging pictures: (**a**) T2-weighted sagittal MRI of the CVJ shows the decompression of the bulbo-medullary junction and (**b**) the 3D reconstruction of CT confirms the removal of the odontoid process

In order to preoperatively assess the feasibility of the odontoidectomy via an endoscopic endonasal route, in a midline sagittal CT slice with bone window, it is possible to draw four lines representing possible paths, to depart from piriform aperture of the nasal bones, which target the odontoid process and lead to assess the inferior limit for surgical exposure. Predicting the inferior limit of the CVJ is crucial to choose the appropriate approach in an area which is considered a transitional area between endonasal and transoral route.

11.3.1 Nasopalatine Line

One of the criticisms of the EEA to the upper cervical spine is the limited exposure inferiorly. Endonasal dissection of the upper cervical spine is limited superiorly by the nasal bones and soft tissues of the nose and inferiorly by the hard palate and soft palate [34, 35]. The line created by connecting the most inferior point of the nasal bone to the posterior edge of the hard palate in the midsagittal plane is defined the naso-palatine line (NPL) and considered a limitation of caudal dissection with straight endoscopic instruments. The angle created by this line and the plane of the hard palate, the nasopalatine angle (NPA) provides the window of exposure to the skull base and upper cervical spine. The mean nasopalatine angle is 27.1 ± 0.7°. The mean point of intersection between the nasopalatine line and the vertebral column is reported to be 8.9 ± 1.8 mm above the base of the C2 vertebral body. The NPL is considered by several authors, a controversial predictor of the maximal extent of inferior dissection in endoscopic endonasal resection of odontoid process [34], considering that the inferior limit predicted by the NPL was found by a mean value of 12.7 mm, below the real inferior extent of surgical dissection. Various pathologic (basilar invagination) and physiologic factors (head positioning) affect the point of intersection of the NPL with the cervical spine. In order to improve caudal exposure, the use of angled instruments or drills may be of value. Additionally, the retraction of the soft palate and drilling the posterior edge of the hard palate may improve the exposure but may increase the risks of palatal dehiscence and velopharyngeal insufficiency.

11.3.2 Naso-Axial Line

The naso-axial line (NAxL) is defined as the line constructed in the midsagittal plane using a starting point that corresponds to the midpoint of the distance from the rhinion to the anterior nasal spine of the maxillary bone and a second point at the tip of the posterior nasal spine of the palatine bone. It is extended posteriorly and inferiorly to the cervical spine. Some authors performed a cadaveric study evaluating the predictive value of NAxL. Their findings supported the close correspondence between the NAxL, drawn in preoperative CT images, and the anatomic surgical extent [36].

11.3.3 Hard-Palate Line

The hard-palate line (HPL) is defined as the line that passes through the anterior and posterior edges of the hard palate (anterior nasal spine of the maxillary bone and posterior nasal spine of the palatine bone, respectively) and intersects the craniovertebral junction posteriorly. This line represents the long axis of the hard palate [37]. It is considered a reliable marker of the inferior extension of CVJ especially in congenital abnormalities, such as platybasia with associated basilar invagination, where the tip of odontoid is often above the plane of the hard palate [38].

11.3.4 Rhinopalatine Line

The rhinopalatine line is defined as the line constructed in the midsagittal plane using a starting point that corresponds to the two-thirds point of the distance from the rhinion to the anterior nasal spine of the maxillary bone and a second point at the posterior nasal spine of palatine bone. The line is extended posteriorly and inferiorly, ending at the cervical spine. There have been great efforts from different groups to study the inferior limit of the endoscopic endonasal approach (EEA). De Almeida et al. [34] described the nasopalatine (NPL) as a good and accurate predictor of the inferior limit of the EEA, but in their study, the NPL resulted always below the inferior extent of surgical dissection with a mean value of 12.7 mm. Consequently, the naso-axial line was reported to predict more accurately and reliably the inferior caudal exposure of the EEA to the CVJ. Similarly, it was been found that the NAxL also overestimated the lower limits of the approach [37]. The rhino-palatine line (RPL) seemed to be a most accurate predictor in several studies.

This predictor accounts also for patient anatomical variability, such as the presence of nasal and palatal osseous and soft structures, together with the direction and length of the hard palate, which represent the most significant factors that limit the inferior extension of the EEA. The RPL cannot be used to predict the lateral limits of the EEA to the CVJ.

11.3.4.1 Operative Technique

According to different pathologies, we perform an endoscopic endonasal odontoidectomy followed by posterior decompression and fusion in a single-stage surgery.

In order to accurately choose the correct approach, we consider on sagittal CT scan the relationship between naso- and rhino-palatine line and the upper cervical spine.

We routinely use the neuronavigation system (StealthStation S7, Medtronic, Minneapolis [MN], USA), based on contrast-enhanced MR with angiographic TOF sequences merged with a 1 mm layer CT of the brain and cervical spine in unique volume. Generally, we use the optical tracking of the StealthStation S7® in order merged with the angiographic TOF sequences in order to provide feasible preoperative images regarding the relationship between bone CVJ and vascular structures such as vertebral and carotid arteries. Somatosensory evoked potential neuromonitoring is routinely used.

11.3.5 Patient Positioning and Preparation

Following general anesthesia and oro-tracheal intubation, the patient is placed in supine position with the trunk elevated to about 20°.The head is slightly turned on the right of, maximum 10°, not flexed, and fixed in a radiolucent Mayfield-Kees three-pin head clamp. The head is kept parallel to the floor and maintained without flexion or extension during the posterior fusion when the patient is turned by supine to prone position. In all cases we used the O-arm® system (Medtronic, Minneapolis [MN], USA) in the phase of posterior fusion. On this, the optical reference of the neuronavigation is mounted, should the optical system be used. On the contrary, the magnetic reference is positioned on the patient's head, in case the electromagnetic system is employed. We use antibiotic prophylaxis with Cefazolin 2 g 1 h before the procedure.

11.3.6 Nasal Phase

The nose is prepped with cottonoids soaked with diluted iodopovidone 5% solution inside the two nostrils. A 0-degree angled lens and 18 cm endoscope associated with an HD camera (Karl Storz, Tuttlingen, Germany) is introduced inside the right nostril. The identification of usual anatomical nasal landmarks is performed (inferior turbinate laterally and nasal septum medially). As a standard endoscopic endonasal procedure, above the inferior turbinate, the middle turbinate is identified and luxated laterally putting cottonoids soaked with diluted adrenaline between middle turbinate and nasal septum, to prevent bleeding of the nasal mucosa. The same maneuvers are carried out in the left nostril. The endoscope advances parallel to the floor of the nasal cavity until the choana is reached. With the aid of the neuronavigation system, the anatomical landmarks are verified. The mucosa over the posterior and inferior aspect of the nasal septum is cauterized with monopolar coagulation or, better, with bipolar forceps. We do not routinely perform the removal of the anterior wall of the sphenoid sinus since a transsphenoidal corridor is rarely needed, unless a higher exposure should be required in case of the tip of the dens goes quite high or when more space is required for the surgical maneuvers, due to patient's individual anatomy. Afterwards, an inferior septectomy is performed, removing sufficiently the vomer bone and extending inferiorly, down to the hard palate. The most superior limit reached is the clivus-nasal septum junction. At this stage few important anatomical landmark should be identified, which guide the surgeons to stay oriented: (1) the clivus-septum junction superiorly, (2) the Eustachian tubes laterally, (3) the nasal floor/soft palate inferiorly as marked by the hard and soft palate. The neuronavigation will confirm the position of such surgical landmarks and give the correct direction for the subsequent surgical steps.

11.3.7 Nasopharynx Phase

The key points of the nasal phase allow the widest exposure of the rhinopharynx and to avoid any conflict among the instruments during the next surgical steps. The nasopharynx mucosa is incised on the midline, and the muscles are dissected bilaterally in order to expose the anterior arch of C1. Several authors reported a reverse "U"-shaped flap of nasopharyngeal prepared with monopolar electrocautery, elevated and reflected caudally to the level of the soft palate in order to improve the surgical field. The craniocaudal extension of the flap involves the inferior third of the clivus superiorly, the C2 vertebral body inferiorly, and the lateral margin of the operative exposure included the lateral masses of the C1 vertebra. The U-shaped nasopharynx flap extends the surgical corridor laterally, but on the other hand increases the risk of injuries to parapharyngeal carotids which are located laterally to the superior pharyngeal constrictor muscle. We prefer doing a straight midline opening of the nasopharynx because of guarantees a sufficient exposure and a lower risk of vascular damage. Then, we proceed with skeletonizing of the anterior arch of C1 and of the odontoid process in a subperiosteal fashion.

11.3.8 C1 Anterior Arch Preservation in Selected Cases

Recently, several authors reported their experience in the matter of endoscopic endonasal odontoidectomy, focusing on the preservation of C1 anterior arch during the craniovertebral junction phase, avoiding the posterior fixation [32, 39]. Particularly, in case of rheumatoid arthritis or other inflammatory diseases, the anterior arch of the atlas is preserved by drilling the odontoid base, weakening its apical, and leading to the pulling downward of the dens in the working area. The following removal of the axis with other remaining compressive inflammatory lesions is performed using a combination of high-speed drill, ultrasonic bone curette, and standard Kerrison's rongeurs [32, 39]. According to such authors, working above and below the C1 anterior arch and its preservation not only represent an element of stability but also give an important opportunity for reconstruction and to reinforce the closure. Additionally, the same groups, in case of inveterate D'Alonzo type II fractures or in the combination of odontoid fracture associated with fracture of anterior arch of C1, proposed their technique of anterior fixation and anterior C1 arch reconstruction [40].

11.3.9 Craniovertebral Junction Phase and Closure

In our technique, the anterior arch of the atlas is exposed and removed through the high-speed drill with diamond burrs and Kerrison's rongeurs. Posteriorly, the odontoid process of C2 is exposed, separated from the alar and apical ligaments, dissected from the transverse ligament, thinned using the microdrill, and finally removed. At this point, a wide surgical corridor is created. The odontoidectomy is performed carefully by using high-speed drill, Kerrison's, and in case of lesions with soft consistency, curettes, and punches or ultrasound aspiration. When the removal is complete, the dural plane appears pulsating and indicates an optimal decompression of the brainstem.

After having obtained a satisfying hemostasis, the closure is guaranteed with a layer of fibrin glue only in the absence of a possible dural tearing. In case of CSF leak, a packing with gelfoam/surgicel and fibrin glue is realized to reinforce the closure. In these cases we consider the possibility to position and extended lumbar drain (ELD) at the end of the operation. We close the nasopharynx mucosa by a single stich because of the median opening allows a faster closure of the muscles at the end of endoscopic time. Generally, we position a nasogastric tube under endoscopic control.

11.3.10 Posterior Fusion

The second step of the operation is characterized by the posterior occipito-cervical fusion. The patient, already fixed to the Mayfield-Kees three-pin carbon fibers radiolucent head-holder, is turned by supine to prone position with the head parallel to the floor and with a slight degree of extension. This position considers the C0-C2 angle which is formed by the posterior extension of the hard palate and the vertical line passing through the dens and avoids the breath impairment related to the flexion. A midline incision is performed starting from the inion to the spinous process of C6. The fascia is exposed and incised on the midline with monopolar cautery. The muscle dissection is performed along the raphe in a subperiosteal fashion from the basiocciput to the posterior complex of C5. The bone landmarks are clearly visible: (1) the occipital bone; (2) posterior arch and lateral masses of C1; (3) posterior complex from C1 to C5.

Generally, we remove the posterior arch of C1, because, in most of our cases, it contributed to the bulbo-pontine compression. The lateral masses of C3 and C4 are identified and verified through the O-arm® system. The fixation system we used in all cases was the Vertex titanium system (Medtronic, Minneapolis [MN], USA). The high-speed drill is used to prepare the position of the screws within the lateral masses of C3 and C4. The polyaxial screws are inserted according to Magerl technique [41] in order to avoid vascular injuries. Differently, in the basiocciput the monoaxial screws are positioned 2 cm from the inion on both sides and 1 cm above the sinuses. The length of the screws we use is 8 mm. After screws are positioned, the two rods are pulled to obtain the correct alignment of the cervical spine and finally fixed through the wrench of wing nuts. The bone fusion is improved with the addition of bone substitutes. The last verification with the O-arm® system is done at the end of the procedure. At the discharge we recommend the use of cervical collar for 2 months.

11.4 Case Series

In the Neurosurgical Clinic of the University of Messina, a series of five endonasal endoscopic odontoidectomies have been performed. Demographic, clinical, and management details are summarized in Tables 11.1 and 11.2.

All patients were female, ranging between 62 and 82 years (mean age 68.8 years). Four patients were admitted with a neurological onset characterized by tetraparesis; in one patient, motor deficits were prevalent on the right arm. Urinary incontinence

Table 11.1 Demographic, etiological, and clinical data

N	Age (years)	Sex	Etiology	Symptoms	Postoperative outcome
1	62	F	Rheumatoid pannus	Right arm weakness Tetrahyperreflexia Urinary incontinence	Improved, oral feeding
2	64	F	Odontoid process misalignment in patient with previous type II Anderson-D'alonzo fracture (not stabilized)	Tetraparesis Tetrahyperreflexia Urinary retention	Improved, oral feeding
3	82	F	Rheumatoid pannus	Tetraparesis	Improved, oral feeding
4	63	F	CVJ malformation	Tetraparesis Severe dysphagia Dysphonia	Improved, dysphagia not completely resolved
5	73	F	Rheumatoid pannus	Tetraparesis	Improved, oral feeding

Table 11.2 Management details

N°	Procedures	OR setup	Postoperative hospital stay (days)
1	Endoscopic endonasal odontoidectomy and occipitocervical stabilization at the same stage	StealthStation S7® with optical tracking + O-arm®	17
2	Endoscopic endonasal odontoidectomy and occipitocervical stabilization at the same stage	StealthStation S7® with optical tracking + O-arm®	13
3	Endoscopic endonasal odontoidectomy and occipitocervical stabilization at the same stage	StealthStation S7® with optical tracking + O-arm®	19
4	Endoscopic endonasal odontoidectomy	StealthStation S7® with optical tracking	9
5	Endoscopic endonasal odontoidectomy and occipitocervical stabilization at the same stage	StealthStation S7® with optical tracking + O-arm®	7

was present in two patients. One patient presented severe dysphagia for either solids or liquids. In three patients, symptoms were related to the presence of a rheumatoid synovial pannus, while the other two cases showed signs and symptoms due to a complex malformation of the craniocervical junction and to a misalignment of the odontoid process following a previous non-fused Anderson-D'Alonzo type II fracture, respectively. Interestingly, the patient affected by the complex CVJ malformation underwent previously to aoccipital-cervical stabilization to another institution. Subsequently, she underwent an attempt of transoral odontoidectomy, which failed due to the higher position of the dens. She was referred in our clinic for an anterior decompression performed through an endoscopic endonasal odontoidectomy. In the remaining three patients, in the same single-stage surgery, anterior decompression and posterior stabilization were performed during the same operation.

The length of stay ranges from 9 to 19 days (including the first period of rehabilitation). In all patients, there was an improvement of the neurological conditions, compared to the preoperative one. In one patient the swallowing dysfunction resolved, allowing an early oral feeding. In two cases an implementation with parenteral nutrition was necessary for a few days.

11.5 Postoperative Management

In our practice, according to the general clinical condition of patient and the length of sedation, we preferred leaving the patient in our intensive care unit for 24 h. This occurred in two of the four cases treated. As a matter of fact, the primary aim is the early mobilization of the patient, to lower the risks of an extended bed rest. In addition, the use of the nasogastric tube may be required in cases when the patient has some preoperative swallowing difficulties, but we do not use it routinely, since a normal velo-pharyngeal function guarantees the separation of the oropharynx from the rhinopharynx during the swallowing. We perform at least two endoscopic postoperative controls: one in the first 24 h and one before the discharge. During such checks, we verified the proper closure of the surgical wound and the possible presence of CSF leak, and thus we removed the nasogastric tube, if any, under endoscopic control. This maneuver can be performed only after testing the functions of lower cranial nerves. A CT scan of the head and cervical spine documents the degree of the odontoidectomy and the correct position of screws and rods of the posterior fusion, and an MRI evaluates the decompression of the neurovascular structures. A further control was performed after 3 months. All patients start a physical rehabilitation program, which also continues after discharge.

References

1. Cappabianca P, Cavallo LM, Esposito F, de Divitiis O, Messina A, de Divitiis E. Extended endoscopic endonasal approach to the midline skull base: the evolving role of transsphenoidal surgery. In: Pickard JD, Akalan N, Di Rocco C, Dolenc VV, Lobo Antunes J, Mooij JJA, Schramm J, Sindou M, editors. Advances and technical standards in neurosurgery. Wien, New York: Springer; 2008. p. 152–99.
2. Cavallo LM, De Divitiis O, Aydin S, Messina A, Esposito F, Iaconetta G, Talat K, Cappabianca P, Tschabitscher M. Extended endoscopic endonasal transsphenoidal approach to the suprasellar area: anatomic considerations—part 1. Neurosurgery. 2008;62:ONS-24.
3. Cavallo LM, Messina A, Cappabianca P, Esposito F, de Divitiis E, Gardner P, Tschabitscher M. Endoscopic endonasal surgery of the midline skull base: anatomical study and clinical considerations. Neurosurg Focus. 2005;19(1):E2.
4. Esposito F, Becker DP, Villablanca JP, Kelly DF. Endonasal transsphenoidal transclival removal of prepontine epidermoid tumors: technical note. Neurosurgery. 2005;56(2 Suppl):E443.
5. Kassam A, Snyderman CH, Mintz A, Gardner P, Carrau RL. Expanded endonasal approach: the rostrocaudal axis. Part II. Posterior clinoids to the foramen magnum. Neurosurg Focus. 2005;19(1):E4.
6. Cavallo LM, Cappabianca P, Messina A, Esposito F, Stella L, de Divitiis E, Tschabitscher M. The extended endoscopic endonasal approach to the clivus and cranio-vertebral junction: anatomical study. Childs Nerv Syst. 2007;23(6):665–71.
7. Messina A, Bruno MC, Decq P, Coste A, Cavallo LM, de Divittis E, Cappabianca P, Tschabitscher M. Pure endoscopic endonasal odontoidectomy: anatomical study. Neurosurg Rev. 2007;30(3):189–94.. discussion 194
8. Crockard HA. The transoral approach to the base of the brain and upper cervical cord. Ann R Coll Surg Engl. 1985;67(5):321–5.
9. Crockard HA, Pozo JL, Ransford AO, Stevens JM, Kendall BE, Essigman WK. Transoral decompression and posterior fusion for rheumatoid atlanto-axial subluxation. J Bone Jt Surg Br. 1986;68(3):350–6.
10. Perrini P, Benedetto N, Guidi E, Di Lorenzo N. Transoral approach and its superior extensions to the craniovertebral junction malformations: surgical strategies and results. Neurosurgery. 2009;64:ons331. https://doi.org/10.1227/01.NEU.0000334430.25626.DC.
11. Perrini P, Benedetto N, Di Lorenzo N. Transoral approach to extradural non-neoplastic lesions of the craniovertebral junction. Acta Neurochir. 2014;156(6):1231–6.
12. Cappabianca P, Cavallo LM, Esposito F, de Divitiis E. Endoscopic endonasal transsphenoidal surgery: procedure, endoscopic equipment and instrumentation. Childs Nerv Syst. 2004;20(11–12):796–801.
13. Cappabianca P, de Divitiis O, Esposito F, Cavallo LM, de Divitiis E. Endoscopic skull base instrumentation. In: Anand VK, Schwartz TH, editors. Practical endoscopic skull base surgery. San Diego: Plural Publishing; 2007. p. 45–56.

14. Cappabianca P, Esposito F, Cavallo LM, Corriero OV. Instruments. Cranial, craniofacial skull base surgery; 2010. p. 7–15.
15. Esposito F, Di Rocco F, Zada G, Cinalli G, Schroeder HWS, Mallucci C, Cavallo LM, Decq P, Chiaramonte C, Cappabianca P. Intraventricular and skull base neuroendoscopy in 2012: a global survey of usage patterns and the role of intraoperative neuronavigation. World Neurosurg. 2013;80(6):709–16.
16. de Divitiis O, Conti A, Angileri FF, Cardali S, La Torre D, Tschabitscher M. Endoscopic transoral-transclival approach to the brainstem and surrounding cisternal space: anatomic study. Neurosurgery. 2004;54(1):125–30; discussion 130.
17. Visocchi M, Doglietto F, Della Pepa GM, Esposito G, La Rocca G, Di Rocco C, Maira G, Fernandez E. Endoscope-assisted microsurgical transoral approach to the anterior craniovertebral junction compressive pathologies. Eur Spine J. 2011;20(9):1518–25.
18. Goel A, Bhatjiwale M, Desai K. Basilar invagination: a study based on 190 surgically treated patients. J Neurosurg. 1998;88(6):962–8.
19. Karam YR, Menezes AH, Traynelis VC. Posterolateral approaches to the craniovertebral junction. Neurosurgery. 2010;66:A135. https://doi.org/10.1227/01.NEU.0000365828.03949.D0.
20. Menezes AH. Craniocervical developmental anatomy and its implications. Childs Nerv Syst. 2008;24(10):1109–22.
21. Menezes AH, VanGilder JC. Transoral-transpharyngeal approach to the anterior craniocervical junction. Ten-year experience with 72 patients. J Neurosurg. 1988;69(6):895–903.
22. Smoker WR. Craniovertebral junction: normal anatomy, craniometry, and congenital anomalies. Radiographics. 1994;14(2):255–77.
23. Smoker WRK, Khanna G. Imaging the craniocervical junction. Childs Nerv Syst. 2008;24(10):1123–45.
24. Joaquim AF, Appenzeller S. Cervical spine involvement in rheumatoid arthritis—a systematic review. Autoimmun Rev. 2014;13(12):1195–202.
25. Pare MC, Currier BL, Ebersold MJ. Resolution of traumatic hypertrophic periodontoid cicatrix after posterior cervical fusion: case report. Neurosurgery. 1995;37(3):531–3.
26. Sandhu FA, Pait TG, Benzel E, Henderson FC. Occipitocervical fusion for rheumatoid arthritis using the inside-outside stabilization technique. Spine (Phila Pa 1976). 2003;28(4):414–9.
27. Klekamp J. Chiari I malformation with and without basilar invagination: a comparative study. Neurosurg Focus. 2015;38(4):E12.
28. Arvin B, Fournier-Gosselin MP, Fehlings MG. Os Odontoideum: etiology and surgical management. Neurosurgery. 2010;66:A22. https://doi.org/10.1227/01.NEU.0000366113.15248.07.
29. Matsui H, Imada K, Tsuji H. Radiographic classification of Os odontoideum and its clinical significance. Spine (Phila Pa 1976). 1997;22(15):1706–9.
30. Vargas TM, Rybicki FJ, Ledbetter SM, MacKenzie JD. Atlantoaxial instability associated with an orthotopic os odontoideum: a multimodality imaging assessment. Emerg Radiol. 2005;11(4):223–5.
31. Cappabianca P, Cavallo LM, Esposito F, de Divitiis O, Messina A, de Divitiis E. Extended endoscopic endonasal approach to the midline skull base: the evolving role of transsphenoidal surgery. In: Pickard JD, editor. Advances and technical standards in neurosurgery. Wien: Springer-Verlag; 2007. p. 1–48.
32. Iacoangeli M, Gladi M, Alvaro L, Di Rienzo A, Specchia N, Scerrati M. Endoscopic endonasal odontoidectomy with anterior C1 arch preservation in elderly patients affected by rheumatoid arthritis. Spine J. 2013;13(5):542–8.
33. Kassam AB, Gardner PA, Snyderman CH, Carrau RL, Mintz AH, Prevedello DM. Expanded endonasal approach, a fully endoscopic transnasal approach for the resection of midline suprasellar craniopharyngiomas: a new classification based on the infundibulum. J Neurosurg. 2008;108(4):715–28.
34. De Almeida JR, Zanation AM, Snyderman CH, Carrau RL, Prevedello DM, Gardner PA, Kassam AB. Defining the nasopalatine line: the limit for endonasal surgery of the spine. Laryngoscope. 2009;119(2):239–44.

35. Kassam AB, Snyderman C, Gardner P, Carrau R, Spiro R. The expanded endonasal approach: a fully endoscopic transnasal approach and resection of the odontoid process: technical case report. Neurosurgery. 2005;57(1 Suppl):E213.
36. Aldana PR, Naseri I, La Corte E. The naso-axial line: a new method of accurately predicting the inferior limit of the endoscopic endonasal approach to the craniovertebral junction. Neurosurgery. 2012;71:ons308. https://doi.org/10.1227/NEU.0b013e318266e488.
37. La Corte E, Aldana PR, Ferroli P, Greenfield JP, Hartl R, Anand VK, Schwartz TH. The rhinopalatine line as a reliable predictor of the inferior extent of endonasal odontoidectomies. Neurosurg Focus. 2015;38(4):E16.
38. El-Sayed IH, Wu J-C, Ames CP, Balamurali G, Mummaneni PV. Combined transnasal and transoral endoscopic approaches to the craniovertebral junction. J Craniovertebr Junct Spine. 2010;1(1):44–8.
39. Gladi M, Iacoangeli M, Specchia N, Re M, Dobran M, Alvaro L, Moriconi E, Scerrati M. Endoscopic transnasal odontoid resection to decompress the bulbo-medullary junction: a reliable anterior minimally invasive technique without posterior fusion. Eur Spine J. 2012;21:55. https://doi.org/10.1007/s00586-012-2220-4.
40. Re M, Iacoangeli M, Di Somma L, Alvaro L, Nasi D, Magliulo G, Gioacchini FM, Fradeani D, Scerrati M. Endoscopic endonasal approach to the craniocervical junction: the importance of anterior C1 arch preservation or its reconstruction. Acta Otorhinolaryngol Ital. 2016;36(2):107–18.
41. Suchomel P, Stulik J, Klezl Z, Chrobok J, Lukas R, Krbec M, Magerl F. Transarticular fixation of C1-C2: a multicenter retrospective study. Acta Chir Orthop Traumatol Cech. 2004;71(1):6–12.

Odontoid Screw Fixation and Anterior C1-C2 Fixation Techniques

12

Andrea Brunori, Daniele Marruzzo, Valentina Russo, and Alberto Delitala

12.1 Introduction

The axis (C2 vertebra) is the strongest cervical vertebra while the dens is the superior process of C2, articulating the anterior arch of C1 and providing about half rotation in the cervical spine. Strong ligaments, including the transverse, alar, and apical, hold the odontoid in close approximation with the atlas (Fig. 12.1). Odontoid fractures have been classified according to the fracture line by Anderson and D'Alonzo in 1974 [1] and represent about 12% of cervical fractures.

Anderson and D'Alonzo provide three fractures typologies (Fig. 12.2):

- Type I fracture line is commonly located in the apex of odontoid process (above the level of the transverse band of cruciform ligament).
- Type II fracture line occurs at the base of odontoid process (below the level of transverse band of cruciform ligament); type II A is a result of a fracture due to a splinters detachment on dens base.
- Type III fracture line is extended through the body of the axis (C2).

Type II fractures are usually unstable, at high risk of nonunion especially in elderly patients, and furthermore, they can be associated with the atlas fracture, influencing prognosis and therapeutic titer. Fractures involving both vertebrae can cause atlanto-axial instability. This can be managed by a variety of different techniques in order to achieve stability of the C1-C2 junction: among them the anterior C1-C2 transarticular fixation has proved safe and successful as the posterior fixation approaches, although less used by most spine surgeons. The supine vs prone positioning and minimal soft

A. Brunori · D. Marruzzo (✉) · V. Russo · A. Delitala
Neurosurgery, Department of Neuroscience "G.M. Lancisi", San Camillo-Forlanini Hospital, Rome, Italy
e-mail: delitala@sinch.it

E. Tessitore et al. (eds.), *Surgery of the Cranio-Vertebral Junction*,
https://doi.org/10.1007/978-3-030-18700-2_12

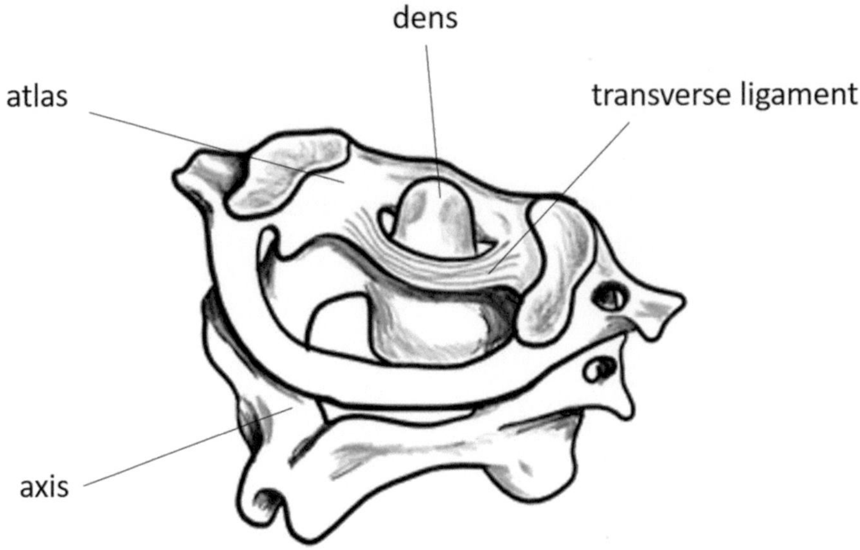

Fig. 12.1 Atlas-axis complex. Transverse ligament holds the dens to the anterior arch of the atlas

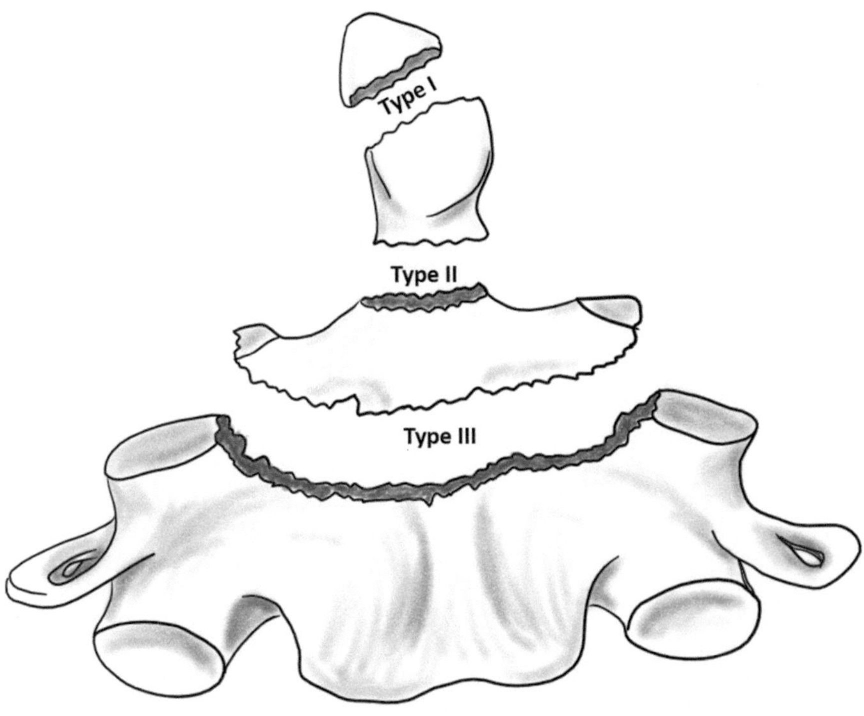

Fig. 12.2 Fractures of C2 according to Anderson and D'Alonzo classification. Type I fracture line is commonly located in the apex of odontoid; type II fracture line occurs at the base of odontoid process (below the level of transverse band of cruciform ligament); type III fracture line extends through the body of the axis (C2)

tissue dissection make the anterior approach less traumatic. In this chapter we describe two surgical techniques that can be performed through an anterior approach: odontoid screw fixation and C1-C2 transarticular fixation.

12.2 Odontoid Screw Fixation Technique

12.2.1 Treatment Indications

External cervical orthosis immobilization may be considered as a starting recourse in all types of mentioned fractures of odontoid. Type I and III fractures can be stabilized through cervical collar or Halo-Vest stabilization, obtaining notable results and the recovery in the following 12 weeks. Type II fractures (Fig. 12.3) are generally treated using surgery as considered unstable due to the high probability of the dens dislocation and the consequent cervical spine injury. The Halo-Vest initial treatment may be unable to fully stabilize the C1-C2 spine, and it may be associated, especially in elderly population, with pins' infection or loosening, while external orthosis may lead to pressure sores in occipital region related to dorsal recumbency [2].

Imaging studies are warranted on evaluating the fracture, the dens dislocation rate and the ligament complex integrity (CT scan with multiplanar reformatting and MRI with T1- and T2-weighted and STIR sequences). CT scan enables to measure the odontoid peg diameter and length in order to choose the appropriate screw dimension (Fig. 12.4).

Anterior odontoid screw placement for type II fractures was first introduced by Bohler in 1981 [3]. The mentioned treatment yields better results on increasing the final recovery outcome and healing time and reducing myelopathy onset.

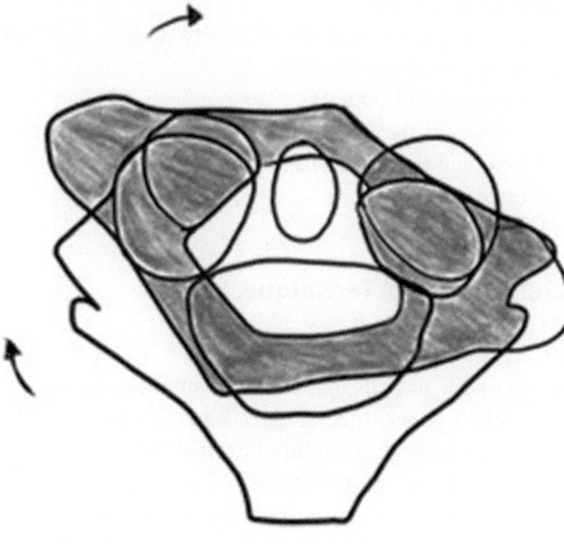

Fig. 12.3 Type II fractures have been reproduced by axially rotating the head and force in the lateral or oblique directions

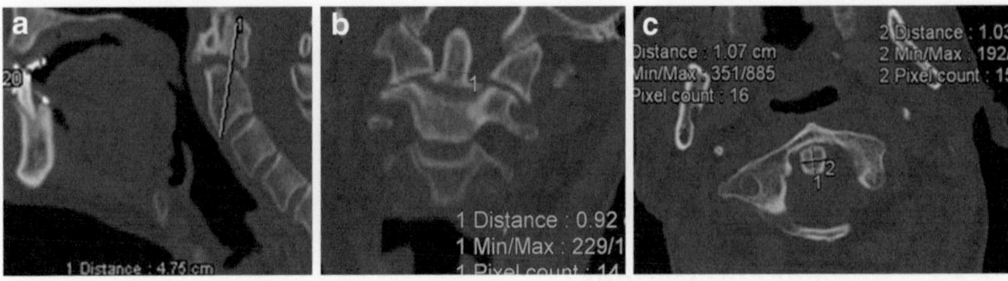

Fig. 12.4 (**a**, **b**, **c**) Preoperative CT scan allows to plan the right screw, measuring in sagittal the length (**a**) and the diameter of the screw (**b**, **c**)

Advantages of anterior screw fixation technique:

- Improved fracture alignment
- Preservation of atlantoaxial rotation
- Immediate fragments stabilization through a cannulated screw
- Easy access to the surgical site
- Reduction in length of stay
- Faster mobilization compared to Halo-Vest
- Improved quality of life

Indications:

- Transversal atlantal ligament (TAL) integrity
- Odontoid dislocation fracture >5 mm
- More than 10° angulation
- Failure of closed reduction and orthosis treatment

Contraindications:

- Unfavorable fracture line obliquity (oblique anterior line) (Fig. 12.5) [4]
- Osteoporosis/osteopenia
- Comminuted fractures
- Diastasis of the fragments, non-reducible fractures
- Prominent thorax (Barrel's chest)
- Cervical kyphosis

12.2.2 Surgical Technique

12.2.2.1 Patient Positioning

We routinely place the patient in the supine position. Due to the commonly advanced age of the patient, special care is paid to proper padding of an X-ray transparent surgical bed; legs are slightly flexed at the knee to avoid stretching of sciatic nerve. Correct positioning of the head is the key for a successful odontoid screwing: a pad at the inter-scapular region and the occiput resting in a gel donut allow for a suitable extension of the neck. The head is secured in a sharp neutral 0° position by lateral

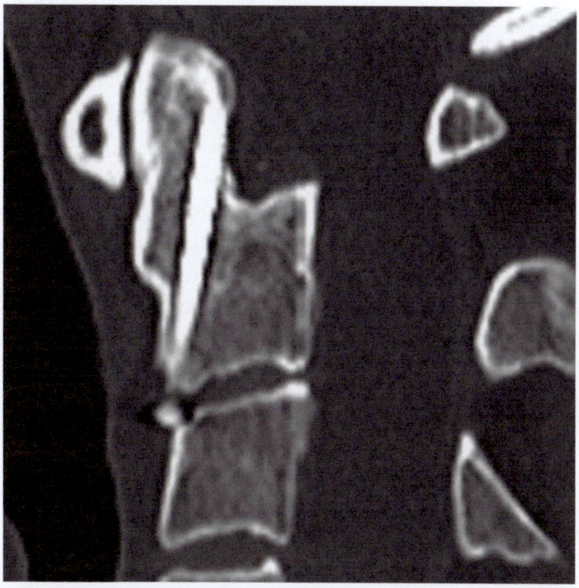

Fig. 12.5 When the fracture line obliquity is unfavorable (oblique anterior line), the anterior screwing of the dens is not recommended: the figure shows how the screw carries the fragment forward

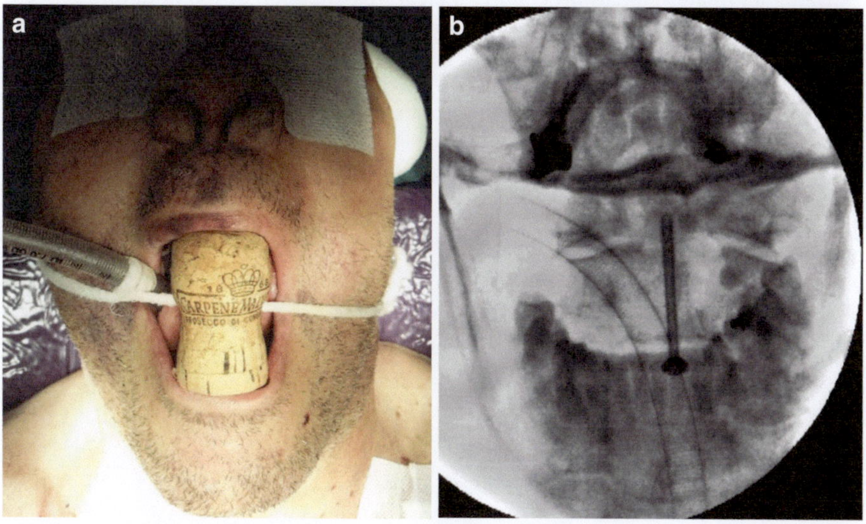

Fig. 12.6 (**a**, **b**) The mouth is kept opened with a guttered cork (**a**) to facilitate the visualization of the dens in intraoperative X-ray AP view (**b**)

pads if available or by soft bandaging of the forehead. Based on our experience we consider a transparent Mayfield headrest as unnecessary, time consuming, and invasive. The endotracheal tube is displaced laterally based on the surgeon's hand dominance an italian Prosecco sparkling wine guttered cork has just the right size and consistency to allow mouth opening; X-ray being transparent, AP views are not affected by any means (Fig. 12.6).

12.2.2.2 Operating Theater Set-Up

Extreme importance is attributed in this process to machines equipment in relation to the surgical team location (surgeons, anesthesiologist, and scrub nurse). This is especially true when the theater room is small.

A double fluoroscopy for simultaneous AP/LL projections is not an option and should be the standard for two reasons: (a) length procedure is reduced by at least 50%; (b) manual rotation of "C arm" requires a trained and compliant technician during whole procedure; even variation of a few degrees to compliance with the initial adjustment implied and repeated AP to LL projections changes could result an unfortunate surgical failure. Figure 12.7 shows the recommended theater setup. The two fluoroscopies are positioned at 45°, respectively, where fluoroscopy monitor must be in the vision line of the main surgeon, i.e., at 30–40° with respect to the main axis of the surgical bed, slightly rotated. It is very important that both pedals are operated by the surgeon himself, virtually setting to zero the dependency from the radiology technician.

The theater setup for odontoid screwing can be depicted, as a clock dial being the bed on the 12/6 axis, C-arm 1 on the 9/3, C-arm 2 on the 10/4, the scrub nurse at 7, surgeon at 8, anesthesiologist and respirator at 12, and monitors at 2. A scrubbed assistant is stand by and ready to join the procedure in case of need.

Being an image-guided procedure, a clear visualization of the odontoid process is mandatory. The AP view is usually more difficult to set because of the

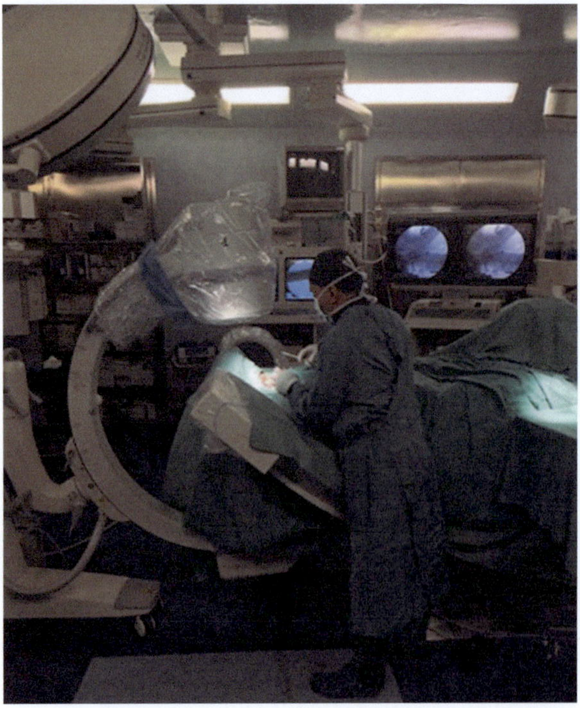

Fig. 12.7 Operating room setup: a double fluoroscopy for simultaneous AP/LL projections; the fluoroscopy monitor must be in the surgeon's line of view

superimposition of occipital plane and inferior dental arch; therefore, obtaining the best angle to outline the profile and odontoid tip is worth it. Lateral images are more valuable to observe the base, a correct alignment of fragments and the crossover line fracture by screw.

12.2.2.3 Incision and Exposure

We use a right transverse incision in a neck crease at the C4-C6 level running from the anterior sternocleidomastoid muscle up to the midline. A different approach can be performed by using a K-wire on lateral radiological monitoring to simulate the screw's path on the patient skin. Muscle planes are dissected in a blunt fashion as usual in the upper spine pre-carotid/retropharyngeal approach; a good application is visualizing directly the C3 body such as the longus colli insertion keeping strictly the midline, from both sides. Odontoid process visualization is not easy to achieve nor useful, but palpation with the fingertip is possible; in elderly patients, dissection is easier due to tissues laxity. A trocar retractor/cannula with pinned tip is then adopted to point the entrance of the K-wire guide, target estimated just few millimeter behind the anteroinferior tip of the C2-body where the C2-endplate is softer and there is less slippery of the anterior cortical layer. Sometimes drilling of the upper anterior portion of C3 vertebral body is necessary in order to obtain the right obliquity of the screw. Failure on breaching cortical layer and K-wire slipping guide could result as injury of the pharynx; moreover, at the end of this procedure, the screw head will rest in a niche preventing soaring on the pharynx and possible dysphagia.

12.2.2.4 Odontoid Screw Insertion

Dens Access system from DePuy-Synthes and a K-wire mounted on a Colibri drill are adopted (Colibri drills are very light and comfortable to handle). In patients with prominent chest, it is advised to hold it in reverse fashion (i.e., grip upwards), avoiding bumping on the sternum. Drill's buttons (clock/counter clockwise rotation and K-wire release) can be operated with a single hand. Once planned trajectory is found by AP/LL, the guide wire is frequently advanced checking the direction. As K-wire is placed in the correct position, the appropriate screw length is chosen by using a similar K-wire and the sterile ruler. Cannulated screw inserted through the K-wire is screwed up to the cortical tip of dens. Supervision must be done, during screwing and after passing fracture line, avoiding possible caudocranial displacement of distal fragment; therefore, pressure onto the drill must be dosed, and drill speed needs to be homogeneous.

12.2.2.5 End of Procedure

Once the optimal positioning screw is obtained, K-wire is removed and screw head is checked by palpation. The procedure is usually bleeding less, and monitoring hemostasis at the end is granted by direct vision. Muscle and skin layers are then sutured, and cervical Philadelphia-like collar is put in position for 8–12 weeks to avoid stress on the fusion line (Fig. 12.8).

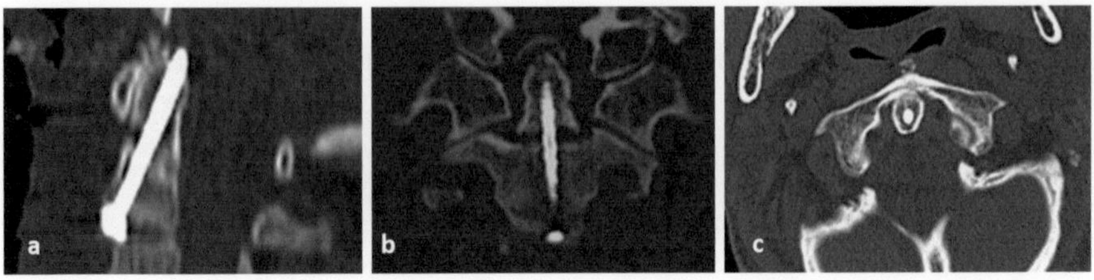

Fig. 12.8 (**a**, **b**, **c**) Postoperative CT scan in sagittal, coronal, and axial view (**a**, **b**, **c**) the screw is in the center of the dens in the three projections

12.3 Anterior C1-C2 Fixation Technique

12.3.1 Treatment Indications

Fractures of the axis are often associated with ligamentous injuries or other cervical fractures. C1 fractures in combination with odontoid fracture type II are considered unstable and it has to be managed with surgical stabilization and fusion. Surgical anterior techniques include C1-C2 fixation with transarticular screws and anterior odontoid screw fixation. This technique was first performed in 2003 by Reindl et al. [5, 6] as an alternative to posterior approaches technique known before.

Advantages:

- Prone positioning.
- Feasible in the presence of a thoracic kyphosis which would create problems for the posterior approach.
- Ideal for patients with severe trauma which may not tolerate the prone position.
- Reduces the trauma of muscles that normally occurs in posterior approaches.
- This technique can be performed with the standard Smith-Robinson approach.
- The possibility of vertebral artery damage is reduced because the vertebral artery foramen is close to the screw entry point; therefore, the artery can be well controlled.

12.3.1.1 Patient Positioning

The patient is in a supine position on a carbon fiber radiolucent operating table. Two image intensifiers are used to identify the dens in the AP and LL projections. The fracture is reduced under X-ray visualization meanwhile the patient's head is positioned in the extended position; this enables correct alignment and facilitates the screw insertion.

12.3.1.2 Incision and Exposure

A standard approach to the anterior cervical spine is performed, with a unilateral horizontal incision placed in correspondence with the projection of the intended direction of the screw and viewing on the image intensifier. Projection generally corresponds to the vertebral C4-C5 level.

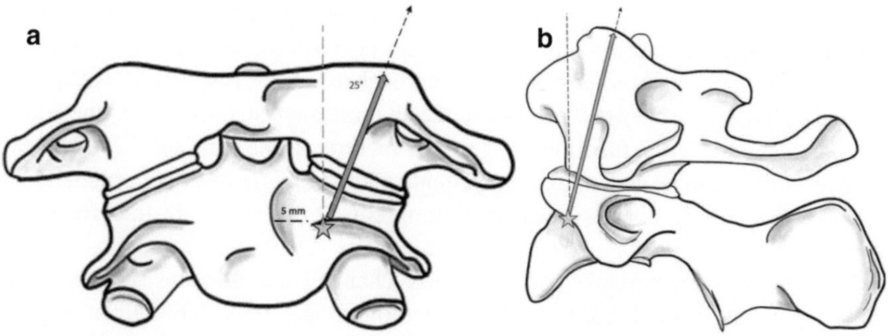

Fig. 12.9 Entry point. Anterior-posterior view (**a**) and lateral projection (**b**): At 5 mm from the lateral border of the base of C2, the screw follows a trajectory 25° cranially and laterally to target the lateral mass of C1

12.3.1.3 C1-C2 Screwing

Preoperative measurements on CT scan are strictly required to determine the correct screw length. The entry point, assigned for each side, is on the overhanging lip surface of C2 lateral mass: 5 mm laterally to the base of the dens and 25° lateral head oriented to it, in order to locate the screw in the C1 lateral mass (Fig. 12.9). As the entry point is identified on the C2 vertebra, an access is created to insert with a drill, the appropriate screw with the angled cannulated screwdriver. The use of tissue protectors is safely recommended, to avoid damaging vital structures, while drilling and tapping. It is essential to observe these procedures on the lateral image intensifier to ensure that guide wire does not advance cranially.

12.4 Risks and Complications

Besides the well-known risks and complications of anterior approach to the cervical spine (i.e., damage of neck vessels, laryngeal and autonomic nerves, upper respiratory and digestive tracts), most failures are due to screw malpositioning, injury of critical vascular, and neurological structures. In some cases screw loosening can occur especially in elderly patients due to poor quality of porotic bone [7, 8, 10, 11]. In a minority of cases, when dislocation is symptomatic, a surgical revision is recommended. Some studies report dysphagia following these procedures [7–9] probably related to impinging of the screw head on pharyngeal soft tissues.

12.5 Conclusions

In this chapter, the authors describe two surgical techniques performed for the treatment of odontoid fractures and C1-C2 vertebrae instability. The treatments of the mentioned pathologies, for a while, were approached with the posterior cerclage wiring [10, 11]. Afterwards with a better knowledge of anatomy and the coming of biomechanics principles, applied to the spinal column, surgical strategies have boosted, both with anterior approach and with posterior access, revising the treatment of mentioned pathologies. Anterior approach techniques avoid muscles trauma typical of posterior ones, and they guarantee an immediate stabilization of the odontoid process and C1-C2 functional segment. Fractures of the dens and C1-C2 vertebrae instability can be encountered in patients with severe trauma (as sternum or rib fracture, respiratory distress because of lung contusions or pelvic fractures) and with higher surgical risks in prone position.

The discussed techniques fundamentally changed the fractures approach for elderly patients. Type II fractures of the odontoid treated with immobilization represent, in patients over 50 years old, a high risk of nonunion 21 times greater than in younger patients [2]. Therefore, odontoid screw fixation is recommended for type II odontoid fractures in patients over 50 years.

Extreme importance is attributed to the theater room setup and to the imaging studies warranted during intervention, on evaluating the fracture and the visualization of the anatomic landmarks. Fluoroscopy projections have to be the standard routine before surgical incision to keep away from intraoperative complications.

Disclosure The authors report no conflict of interest concerning the materials or methods used in this study.

They also declare no funding has been allocated for this work.

References

1. Anderson LD, D'Alonzo RT. Fractures of the odontoid process of the axis. J Bone Joint Surg Am. 1974;56:1663–74.
2. TC R, Hadley MN, Aarabi B, Dhall SS, Gelb DE, Hurlbert RJ, Rozzelle CJ, Theodore N, Walters BC. Management of isolated fractures of the axis in adults. Neurosurgery. 2013;72(Suppl 2):132–50.
3. Bohler J. Screw-osteosynthesis of fractures of the dens axis (author's transl). Unfallheilkunde. 1981;84:221–3.
4. Roy-Camille R, de la Caffinière JY, Saillant G. Les traumatismes du rachis cervical supérieur. Paris: Masson et Cie; 1973.
5. Reindl R, Sen M, Aebi M. Anterior instrumentation for traumatic C1-C2 instability. Spine. 2003;28:E329–33.
6. MK S, Steffen T, Beckman L, Tsantrizos A, Reindl R, Aebi M. Atlantoaxial fusion using anterior transarticular screw fixation of C1-C2: technical innovation and biomechanical study. Eur Spine J. 2005;14(5):512–8.
7. Andersson S, Rodrigues M, Olerud C. Odontoid fractures: high complication rate associated with anterior screw fixation in the elderly. Eur Spine J. 2000;9(1):56–9.
8. Josten C, Jarvers JS, Glasmacher S, Heyde CE, Spiegl UJ. Anterior transarticular atlantoaxial screw fixation in combination with dens screw fixation for type II odontoid fractures with associated atlanto-odontoid osteoarthritis. Eur Spine J. 2016;25(7):2210–7.
9. Osti M, Philipp H, Meusburger B, Benedetto KP. Analysis of failure following anterior screw fixation of type II odontoid fractures in geriatric patients. Eur Spine J. 2011;20(11):1915–20. https://doi.org/10.1007/s00586-011-1890-7.
10. Gallie WE. Fracture and dislocations of the cervical spine. Am J Surg. 1939;46:495–9.
11. Brooks AL, Jenkins EB. Atlantoaxial arthrodesis by the wedge compression method. J Bone Joint Surg Am. 1978;60(3):279–84.

Atlanto-Axial Fixation Techniques

13

Surgery of the Craniovertebral Junction

Joseph A. Osorio, Markus Schomacher, and Christopher P. Ames

13.1 Introduction

The atlanto-axial region of the spine is a complex area of anatomical structures that consists of the upper two vertebrae of the cervical spine, their articular surfaces, several crucial ligaments, and the vertebral artery that courses along and within these bones. The nature of this junction allows for the movement of the cervical region in rotation, lateral bending, flexion, and extension [1]. Given the complexity of this region, stabilization of the atlanto-axial spinal column when it has become disrupted presents a unique set of challenges, which include higher complexity in screw placement (compared to the other cervical vertebrae), lack of fusion surface comparatively to other regions in the cervical spine, and avoidance of vertebral artery injury during screw placement. The high degree of mobility in this area also makes adequate fusion inherently problematic, and the rates of fusion at the C1-C2 level have been reported lower than the subaxial spine [1]. In addition, potential operative interventions are limited by the complex articular anatomy of this region and also the potential inconstant vertebral artery location [2, 3]. Until the past few decades, the mainstay of treatment for atlanto-axial complex instability was external immobilization. However, external immobilization is associated with high non-fusion rates and also increased morbidity; given these important pitfalls, an alternative to external immobilization was desired [1].

The first description of a surgical treatment for atlanto-axial instability appeared in 1910. Mixter and Osgood described wiring the posterior arch of the atlas to the spinous process of the axis with a heavy silk thread [1]. Since then, other wiring techniques have been developed. The use of posterior cervical wiring of the lamina of C1 and C2 dates to 1939 in a report by Gallie [1]. Brooks and Jenkins described

J. A. Osorio · M. Schomacher · C. P. Ames (✉)
Division of Neurovascular Surgery and Endovascular Neurosurgery, Department of Neurological Surgery, Thomas Jefferson University Hospital, Philadelphia, PA, USA
e-mail: Amesc@neurosurg.ucsf.edu

E. Tessitore et al. (eds.), *Surgery of the Cranio-Vertebral Junction*,
https://doi.org/10.1007/978-3-030-18700-2_13

an alternative method of posterior C1-C2 laminar wiring in 1978 [1]. In 1991, Dickman and Sonntag further modified the posterior wiring technique [1]. In the 1980's, the interlaminar clamp technique was published as an alternative method for posterior C1-C2 fixation [1]. The field continued to advance with Magerl introducing the transarticular screw; the C1-C2 rod-cantilever technique was introduced by Goel, and the C2 laminar screw technique were developed for fixation of the atlanto-axial complex [1–5]. In the last decade many of these traditional techniques were continuously further developed and refined. The goal of these latest techniques is to facilitate the surgical application and workflow, to enhance fusion rates and reduce potential risks and complications of surgical treatment in the atlanto-axial region [1–3].

13.2 Indications

Traumatic injuries that result in unstable fractures or ligamentous disruption are among the most frequent indications for posterior C1-C2 fixation. There are several classifications that exist to describe the types of fractures that exist in this region, and the reason for these classifications is largely to help navigate the various options that exist for their management [1].

The most commonly used classification system for fractures at the C2 level is the Anderson and D'Alonzo, which divides the dens fracture into three groups based on location. Type 1 fracture involves a fracture through the upper dens, specifically above the transverse ligament of the atlas; these fractures are considered stable. Type 2 fractures occur at the junction of the dens and the body of C2 and are associated with the disruption of the transverse ligament of the atlas, which results in an unstable fracture. Type 3 fractures extend into the C2 body [1].

Although type 2 odontoid fractures can be treated with either immobilization, posterior surgical instrumentation and fusion, or anterior odontoid screw fixation, some of the techniques for anterior fixation have limitations and contraindications [1]. The contraindications to anterior fixation of type 2 fractures include disruption of the transverse ligament of the atlas, having a comminuted fracture of one or both atlanto-axial joints, unstable type 3 fractures, atypical type 2 fractures with oblique or comminuted fracture lines, irreducible fractures, and those fractures with an associated thoracic kyphosis. Aside from traumatic type 2 fractures, contraindications to anterior fixation also exist in pathological fractures from neoplastic disease of the dens, where ventral fixation screws are contraindicated, a dorsal fusion technique is preferred and suggested in these circumstances [1].

Ligamentous laxity and associated ligamentous instability of C1 and C2 could be the result of a traumatic and/or a nontraumatic etiology that could require surgical correction. The ligamentous instability is evaluated by obtaining lateral X-ray views that allow a measurement of the atlanto-dental interval when the patient is in both flexion and extension. The interval measurement within this space should not exceed 2–4 mm [1]. When the atlanto-dental interval exceeds 5 mm in nonrheumatoid patients, and when it exceeds 8 mm in rheumatoid patients, instability of the C1 and

C2 complex and posterior atlanto-axial fixation is indicated. In congenital disorders (hypoplasia, aplasia of the odontoid process, or os odontoideum), instability of the C1 and C2 complex can also occur. Os odontoideum is the failure of the dens to fuse with the body of the axis. Both os odontoideum and odontoid agenesis may lead to incompetence of the cruciate ligament and subsequently C1 and C2 instability [1].

Rheumatoid arthritis is a systemic inflammatory disease that can affect the cervical spine at the dens and result in atlanto-axial subluxation or superior migration of the odontoid into the foramen magnum. When the result of this disease is compression of the brainstem and upper cervical spinal cord, often there is an indication for decompression. In these settings, posterior occipito-cervical decompression is often coupled with atlanto-axial instrumentation and fusion [1].

13.3 Techniques of C1-C2 Fusion

13.3.1 Dorsal Wiring Techniques

The techniques described below that utilized dorsal wiring of the atlanto-axial region for fusion have variations of wiring technique, but all of the techniques discussed have similarities in that they are wiring the posterior elements of the axis and atlas together. In order to achieve these wiring techniques, an intact posterior arch of C1 and posterior elements of C2 is necessary. These techniques are contraindicated when the posterior elements are disrupted or at risk of being disrupted, which include Jefferson's fracture, Hangman's fracture, significant osteoporosis, or posterior decompression of C1 and C2. Wiring techniques are technically less demanding than the more recent screw fixation of the atlanto-axial region, in particular as it relates to the intraoperative equipment, because surgical navigation or fluoroscopy is not necessary for wiring. To achieve successful fusion rates following wiring techniques in the postoperative period, all of the described techniques subsequently require rigid postoperative immobilization.

13.3.1.1 Gallie Fusion

In 1939, Gallie first described the use of a steel wire around the posterior elements of C1-C2 in the sublaminar space for fixation [6]. In the Gallie fusion, a dorsal midline bone graft is notched over the spinous process of C2, with a sublaminar wire placed around the posterior arch of C1 and looped around the spinous process of C2 to hold the graft in place. The Gallie fusion offers good stability in flexion and extension but provides little stabilization in rotation. The rate of C1-C2 nonunion with the Gallie-type fusion has been reported to be as high as 25% [1]. Given the limitations in rotational stabilization and nonunion rates, the Gallie fusion is used for the supplementation of other techniques.

13.3.1.2 Brooks-Jenkins Fusion

In the Brooks-Jenkins fusion technique, the posterior arch of the atlas and the lamina of the axis are exposed, and doubled 20-gauge wires are passed under the lamina of C1 and C2 bilaterally. Two posterolateral autologous iliac crest bone grafts are beveled to fit both interlaminar spaces and held in place by the overlying wire [7]. The Brooks-Jenkins wire fusion technique provides more rotational stability than the Gallie technique [1]. Fusion rates of 93% have been reported with the reports supporting improved fusion rates when subsequent halo immobilization is utilized [8].

13.3.1.3 Sonntag Posterior C1-C2 Technique

In 1991 Sonntag and colleagues modified the Gallie technique. The Sonntag technique involves the use of a sublaminar cable that is passed under the posterior C1 arch from inferior to the superior. This is followed by the placement of a notched iliac crest graft that is placed in between the spinous process of C2 and wedged underneath the posterior arch of C1. The superior aspect of the C2 spinous process and the inferior arch of C1 are decorticated prior to graft placement. The cable is then looped over the iliac crest autograft and placed into a notch created on the inferior aspect of the C2 spinous process. The cable is then tightened and crimped. Postoperatively, patients are recommended to stay in a halo for an immobilization period of 3 months, followed by a hard collar for 4–6 weeks. Fusion rates up to 97% have been reported by using this surgical technique together with postoperative immobilization [3].

13.3.2 Interlaminar Clamp Technique

The interlaminar clamp technique was published in the 1980s as an alternative method of posterior C1-C2 fixation. The clamps are used by placing hooks on the superior surface of the C1 lamina and hooks on the inferior surface of the C2 lamina. The hooks are tightened, and preferably a bone graft is placed between the C1 and C2 lamina. Biomechanical studies have shown that the interlaminar clamp technique provides excellent stability in flexion and extension movements. However, this technique lacks rotational stability and is felt to be even less successful than either the Brooks-Jenkins or the Margerl techniques [1, 9, 10]. Given that this technique also requires an intact arch of C1, the use of interlaminar clamps has the same contraindications as the wiring methods that are described above. An advantage to the postoperative management of this technique as compared to wiring techniques described earlier is that immobilization after surgery only requires a cervical collar, therefore allowing improved early mobilization for the patient.

13.3.3 C1-C2 Transarticular Screws

In 1979, Magerl and Jeanneret described the transarticular screw fixation technique for the treatment of odontoid fractures. The advantage of using the C1-C2 transarticular screw technique for atlanto-axial fusions is that there would be complete immobilization of rotational motion of the atlanto-axial joint, and the technique does not require that the posterior arch of C1 remains intact. However, the C1-C2 transarticular screw technique is technically more demanding because the margin for error is significantly reduced when compared to the other techniques described. Also, this technique requires the use of intraoperative fluoroscopy and/or surgical navigation tools in order to reduce injury to the neurovascular structures and to achieve the appropriate screw placement. There is the potential risk for serious complications to the neurovascular structures that could come as a result of an aberrant screw placement, which could result in spinal cord injury, dural tear, hypoglossal nerve injury, or injury to the vertebral artery. For safe preoperative planning, plain X-rays and fine-cut computed tomographic scans to exclude a high-riding vertebral artery or bone destruction at the side of intended screw placement are recommended [11]. Some surgeons advocate for preoperative fiber optic intubation and perioperative recording of somatosensory evoked potentials [1].

The technique involves placement of the patient in the prone position with the head fixed and in capital flexion of the head on the neck (military tuck position). An initial exposure of the posterior boney elements of C1, C2, and C3 is undertaken, which includes a view of the posterior arch of C1 and spinous processes C2. The dissection is carried laterally to expose the articular atlanto-axial processes. Additionally, the dissection is extended along the lamina of C2 into the joint space, and the adjacent neurovascular plexus containing the C2 nerve root is carefully retracted caudally or divided. The entry point for screw placement is about 3–4 mm rostral and 3–4 mm lateral to the medial aspect of the C2-C3 facet joint. The trajectory is approximately 15° medial with a steep superior angle, and it is visualized by fluoroscopy with the goal of aiming at the C1 anterior tubercle. While drilling along the correct trajectory, changes in resistance could be noticed as four cortical surfaces along the path are traversed. A K-wire technique could be used, and this is complimented with a cannulated screw that commonly will have a length of 36–46 mm in length. There have been several clinical and cadaveric studies that have shown a reliability in the strength and stability of the C1-C2 transarticular screw construct [1, 11]. Fusion rates have been described that range from 86.9% to 100%. Biomechanical cadaveric studies show that the transarticular C1-C2 construct is stable flexion, extension, and also in rotation [1, 10, 12]. Although the surgical technique is considered more demanding with an increase in surgical risk, compared to alternatives, complication rates for the transarticular C1-C2 fixation technique are not elevated, and range between 2% and 14% [9, 10, 12, 13]. There is a risk about 4% of vertebral artery injury, reported by Farey et al. Additionally, Dickman and Sonntag have documented a 2% risk of screw malpositioning with no neurological complications [1, 8]. The main limitation of the transarticular technique relates to anatomic variations that preclude safe screw placement. A cadaveric study by Abou Madawi et al. demonstrated that bilateral screws could not be placed in up to 20% of specimens because of anatomic variations in the location of the foramen transversarium, which placed the vertebral artery at risk during screw placement [1, 8].

13.3.4 C1 Lateral Mass Screw, C2 Pars-, Pedicle-, or Translaminar Screws

The technique of segmental atlantoaxial instrumentation and fusion using both C1 lateral mass and C2 pedicle mono-axial screws with plate fixation was first described by Goel et al. This technique provided 100% atlantoaxial fixation, and this technique also had a minimal rate of complications [14, 15]. The Goel technique was later modified to include C2 pars screws with C1 lateral mass screws connected by longitudinal bilateral titanium plates. Additionally, this technique was modified to address basilar invagination by the usage of customized titanium porous spacers placed in the atlantoaxial joint space to facilitate vertical reduction and load-bearing fusion (described in 2005) [16]. An advantage of the C1 lateral mass when used in combination with the C2 screw technique is that the anatomic alignment of the C1-C2 complex can be variable and does not need to be aligned prior to instrumentation. In addition, this technique can still be utilized in cases where there is an aberrant vertebral artery.

Harms and Melcher later introduced a technique modification for the stabilization of the atlantoaxial complex that utilized polyaxial screws placed in the C1 lateral mass and C2 pedicle connected by rods, in contrast to the mono-axial screws and small plates described above [11]. This technique did not rely on the integrity of the posterior elements of C1 or C2, and when compared to the very initial C1/C2 techniques, it avoided passing sublaminar wires. The path for the C2 pedicle screw can be selected independently of the location of the atlas. This technique also allows reduction or correction of any displacement or malalignment of the elements of the atlantoaxial complex by repositioning the patient's head or directly manipulating the C1 or C2 screws. For best preoperative planning, plain X-rays and fine-cut computed tomographic scans are recommended.

For the placement of C1 lateral mass screws, exposure of the vertebral artery on the superior aspect of the C1 arch is not recommended. Usually the C2 nerve root is either transected or mobilized caudally for C1 lateral mass exposure. Subsequently, a pilot hole can be made with a drill bit at the center of C1 lateral mass once the medial and lateral borders have been identified by either palpation or direct visualization. The screw trajectory is classically described as having 10° of medial angulation in the axial plane. A lateral fluoroscopic image is used to choose the direction in the cranial-caudal direction, and the drill is aimed toward the anterior tubercle of C1. After the hole has been drilled, the path is commonly tapped thereafter. The C1-lateral mass screw is then placed with common lengths measuring 30–36 mm in length. Review of preoperative CT scans provide planning for both screw trajectory and size, shown in Fig. 13.1.

The C2 pars screw is commonly described as having an entry point that is 3 mm rostral and 3 mm lateral to the inferior medial aspect of the inferior articular surface of C2. The trajectory of the pars in comparison to the pedicle screw at C2 is steep, and the trajectory is commonly described as being 45°–60°, with 10°–15° of medial angulation. The screw length is significantly shorter for C2 pars as compared to pedicle screws with typical screw lengths ranging from 12 to 16 mm. The C2 pedicle screw entry point is usually 2 mm lateral and 2 mm superior to the C2 pars screw

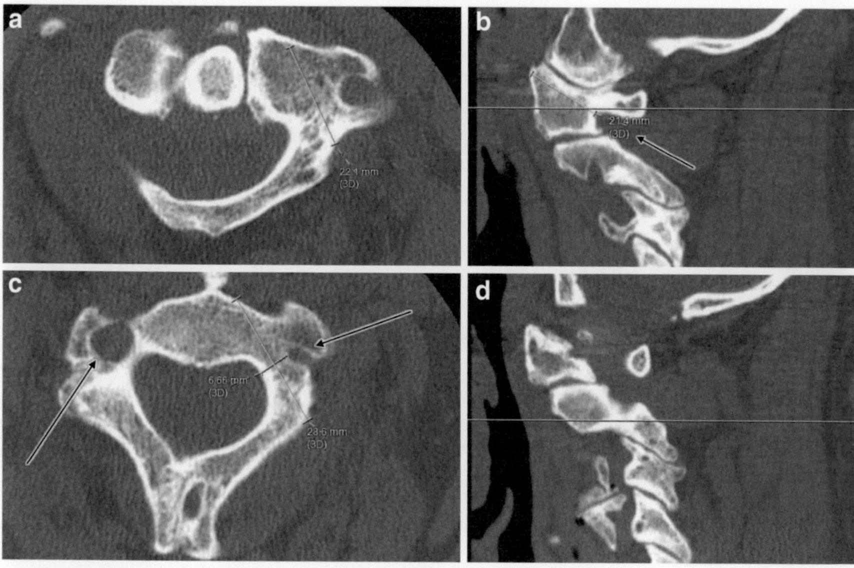

Fig. 13.1 A preoperative CT for a patient who was undergoing a C1-C2 fusion. In (**a**) you can appreciate adequate space for a C1 lateral mass screw, and a measure shown provides an initial assumption to the surgeon of a close approximation for potential screw length preparation. In (**b**) the trajectory for the C1 screw is shown, together with the measurement. In (**c**) the CT provides insight into the vertebral artery course and dominance; shown is a right-sided dominant vertebral artery and diminutive vertebral artery on the left. In (**d**) is the sagittal view CT that is often visualized preoperatively to get a sense of the pars trajectory into C2

entry point. For the placement of the C2 pedicle screw, a medial angulation of 15–25° with 20° upward trajectory is most commonly used; therefore, it requires more medial angulation than the pars screw at C2 but with less steep angulation. Review of preoperative CT scans provides planning for both screw trajectory and size, shown in Fig. 13.1.

The lamina at C2 can be cannulated with a shorter screw, a translaminar C2 screw, but this screw is not considered to have comparable strength to a pars or pedicle screw at C2. The translaminar screw can serve as salvage technique for C2 pars or pedicle screws, and particular for cases where a high-riding vertebral artery or thin pedicles exist. The entry point for the translaminar screw is the junction of the spinous process and the lamina, shown in Fig. 13.2. These screws are more commonly placed unilaterally, but they can be placed bilaterally. The trajectory is chosen to match the slope of the lamina.

The latest biomechanical studies have shown that the Goel-Harms technique is superior for the stabilization of the atlantoaxial segment. This technique provides the advantage that it can be utilized in very unstable cases, including those where the lamina of the C1 and C2 have been disrupted. The additional stability, the added benefit of vertical reduction facilitation, and the additional load-bearing fusion surface area make this the preferred technique for atlantoaxial instability cases [1].

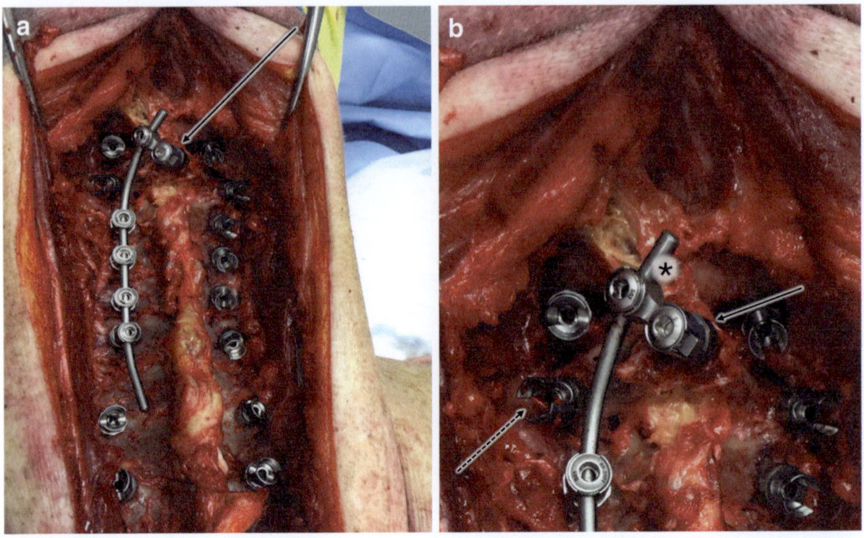

Fig. 13.2 A cadaveric image demonstrating the C2 translaminar screw and also the C2 pars screw for an illustrative example of the proximity of these screws in location. In (**a**) the instrumentation shown includes C1 lateral mass screw (top of the image) through T2 pedicle screw. The arrow in (**a**) is demonstrating a C2 translaminar screw placed into the C2 lamina on the left. In (**b**) a closer look shows the C2 pars screw (hashed arrow), the C2 translaminar screw (solid arrow), and the cross connector used to connect to the lower construct (∗)

13.4 Case Presentations

Case 1, Fig. 13.3
A 76-year-old woman who has a history of prior C4-C7 anterior and posterior spinal fusion (9 years prior) for cervical spondylotic myelopathy presented after worsening hand numbness and function. An MRI at this time revealed a pseudotumor and stenosis at C1-C2, which was felt to be a result of microinstability at the C1-C2 complex. This was treated with a decompression laminectomy at C1 and C2 and revision and extension of fusion up to C1. A transarticular screw was used on the left side because despite distraction between the C1 and C2 space, it was not possible to visualize the lateral mass given the severe and somewhat rigid hyperextended position. Under navigation following an intraoperative CT, a transarticular screw was placed on the left.

Case 2, Fig. 13.4
A 73-year-old man with a history of progressive growth of a lesion on the right side at C1-C2 consistent with an enlarging synovial cyst likely as a result of microinstability at C1-C2. A C1 lateral mass and C2 pedicle screw were placed for fixation, and a laminectomy of C1 and C2 was performed with subsequent removal of capsule and contents of the lesion that was ultimately consistent with a synovial cyst.

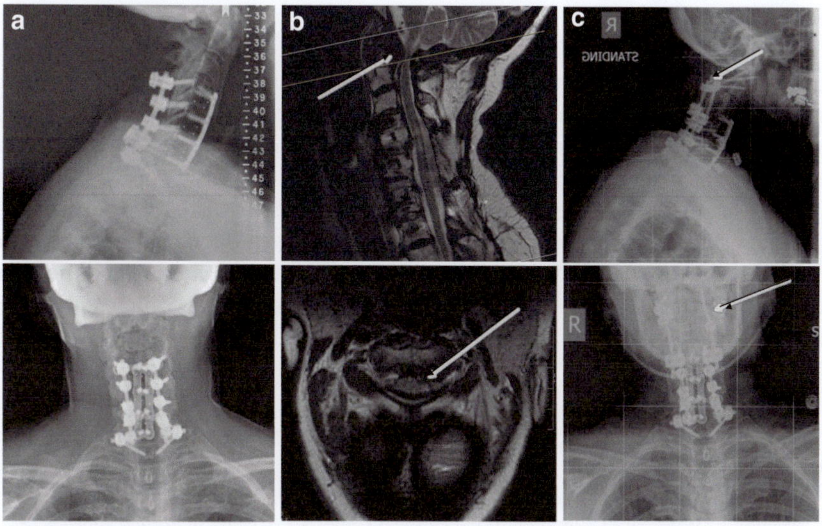

Fig. 13.3 In (**a**) the preoperative X-rays are shown (lateral and A/P) demonstrating a prior C4-T1 posterior instrumentation and C4-C7 ACDF. In (**b**) the sagittal and axial T2-weighted MRI demonstrate the panus and region of greatest central stenosis upon the spinal cord (arrow). In (**c**) the postoperative X-rays are shown (lateral and A/P) demonstrating the C2 fixation utilized with a transarticular screw, on the left (arrow)

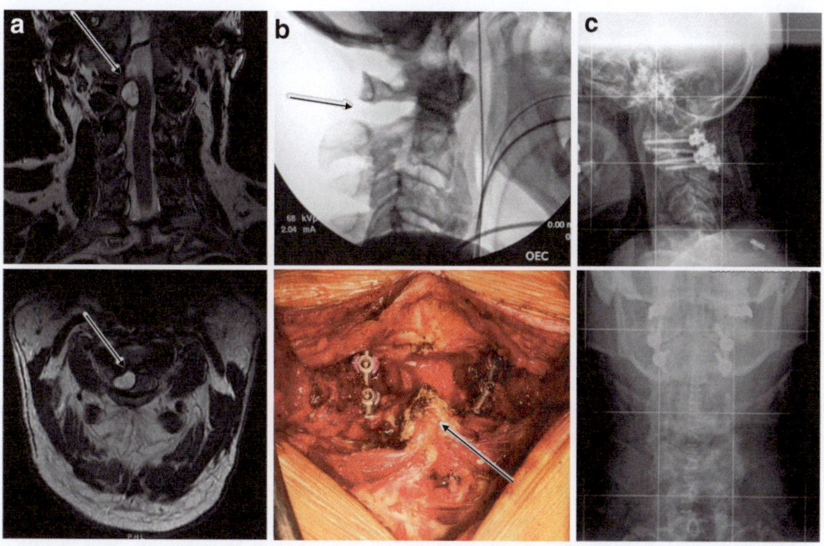

Fig. 13.4 A 73-year-old man who presented with radiculopathy who was referable to a C1/2 enlarging lesion consistent with a synovial cyst causing severe cord compression. A C1/2 instrumented fusion was performed together with decompression of the facet cyst. In (**a**) the facet cyst is shown in the T2-weighted coronal and axial image of the MRI. In (**b**) intraoperative fluoroscopy is used to confirm head position and cervical spine alignment prior to the procedure. Also in (**b**), intraoperative photographs are shown of the final construct with minimal disruption to the C2 musculature. In (**c**) the final A/P and lateral X-rays are shown of the C1 lateral mass and C2 pedicle screws

13.5 Conclusions

This chapter focuses on fixation techniques in the atlanto-axial region of the spine, which is a complex area that entails unique articular surfaces, ligaments that are specific to the region and factor into surgical management, and the vertebral artery that courses intimately within this region. The evolution of the common techniques was described, and examples were presented showing the variations that can exist in practice. Although the development of the more current operative techniques has been refined over time and often these more recent techniques are the most frequently used, there are still instances where the complex spinal column anatomy or pathology encountered require more antiquated techniques to be utilized for the best potential fixation.

References

1. Penning L, Wilmink JT. Rotation of the cervical spine. A CT study in normal subjects. Spine (Phila Pa 1976). 1987;12(8):732–8.
2. Fried LC. Atlanto-axial fracture-dislocations. Failure of posterior C.1 to C.2 fusion. J Bone Joint Surg Br. 1973;55(3):490–6.
3. Dickman CA, Sonntag VK. Surgical management of atlantoaxial nonunions. J Neurosurg. 1995;83(2):248–53.
4. Abou Madawi A, Solanki G, Casey AT, Crockard HA. Variation of the groove in the axis vertebra for the vertebral artery. Implications for instrumentation. J Bone Joint Surg Br. 1997;79(5):820–3.
5. Tokuda K, Miyasaka K, Abe H, Abe S, Takei H, Sugimoto S, et al. Anomalous atlantoaxial portions of vertebral and posterior inferior cerebellar arteries. Neuroradiology. 1985;27(5):410–3.
6. Gallie WE. Skeletal traction in the treatment of fractures and dislocations of the cervical spine. Ann Surg. 1937;106(4):770–6.
7. Brooks AL, Jenkins EB. Atlanto-axial arthrodesis by the wedge compression method. J Bone Joint Surg Am. 1978;60(3):279–84.
8. Dickman CA, Sonntag VK, Papadopoulos SM, Hadley MN. The interspinous method of posterior atlantoaxial arthrodesis. J Neurosurg. 1991;74(2):190–8.
9. Moskovich R, Crockard HA. Atlantoaxial arthrodesis using interlaminar clamps. An improved technique. Spine (Phila Pa 1976). 1992;17(3):261–7.
10. Fielding JW, Cochran G, Lawsing JF III, Hohl M. Tears of the transverse ligament of the atlas. A clinical and biomechanical study. J Bone Joint Surg Am. 1974;56(8):1683–91.
11. Harms J, Melcher RP. Posterior C1-C2 fusion with polyaxial screw and rod fixation. Spine (Phila Pa 1976). 2001;26(22):2467–71.
12. Grob D, Crisco JJ 3rd, Panjabi MM, Wang P, Dvorak J. Biomechanical evaluation of four different posterior atlantoaxial fixation techniques. Spine (Phila Pa 1976). 1992;17(5):480–90.
13. Stillerman CB, Wilson JA. Atlanto-axial stabilization with posterior transarticular screw fixation: technical description and report of 22 cases. Neurosurgery. 1993;32(6):948–54; discussion 54-5.
14. Goel A, Laheri V. Plate and screw fixation for atlanto-axial subluxation. Acta Neurochir. 1994;129(1–2):47–53.
15. Goel A, Desai KI, Muzumdar DP. Atlantoaxial fixation using plate and screw method: a report of 160 treated patients. Neurosurgery. 2002;51(6):1351–6; discussion 6-7.
16. Goel A, Pareikh S, Sharma P. Atlantoaxial joint distraction for treatment of basilar invagination secondary to rheumatoid arthritis. Neurol India. 2005;53(2):238–40.

Occipito-Cervical Fixation Techniques

14

Yann Philippe Charles

14.1 Indications

Posterior fixation techniques are usually considered in pathologies leading to instability of the occipito-cervical junction. The main indications can be grouped into four categories [1–6].

- ***Trauma:*** Occipito-cervical dislocations, fractures of the occipital condyle, unstable atlas fractures including the lateral mass, and complex C1-C2 fractures might require a posterior occipito-cervical fusion. Temporary fixation may be indicated in younger patients and instrumentation is removed after fracture consolidation in order to restore the range of motion of the atlanto-axial complex.
- ***Tumors:*** Primary tumor resections of the axis may necessitate an occipito-cervical reconstruction. Bone metastases of the cranio-cervical junction leading to spinal cord compression or osteolysis with subsequent atlanto-axial subluxation may require a posterior stabilization.
- ***Congenital malformations:*** Cranio-cervical junction abnormalities may be specific structural abnormalities or belong to general systemic disorders that affect skeletal growth. Structural abnormalities include: os odontoideum, Klippel-Feil syndrome, Chiari malformation, basilar invagination, atlas hypoplasia, or congenital fusion between atlas and occiput. Systemic disorders that affect skeletal development and involve the cranio-cervical junction include: achondroplasia, Down syndrome, Morquio syndrome, or osteogenesis imperfecta, which can cause atlanto-axial subluxation or dislocation.

Y. P. Charles (✉)
Service de Chirurgie du Rachis, Hôpitaux Universitaires de Strasbourg,
Strasbourg Cedex, France
e-mail: YannPhilippe.CHARLES@chru-strasbourg.fr

E. Tessitore et al. (eds.), *Surgery of the Cranio-Vertebral Junction*,
https://doi.org/10.1007/978-3-030-18700-2_14

- ***Inflammatory diseases:*** Rheumatoid polyarthritis can cause an inflammatory pannus, osteolysis of the dens axis, and ligamentous insufficiency, which can lead to anterior-posterior or vertical atlanto-axial instability and basilar impression. A resection of the dens or posterior decompression and occipito-cervical fusion might be indicated in these cases.

14.2 Historical Techniques

Historically, in situ bone fusion, wiring techniques, and rod-loop constructs using Harthsill rectangles have been described [7]. Removing its posterior rim with a Kerrison rongeur enlarged the foramen magnum and a series of holes were drilled in the occipital bone on either side of the midline. Wires or cables were passed epidurally from the drill holes to the foramen magnum. The ligamentum flavum was detached from instrumented vertebrae and wires were passed under the laminae of C2, C3, and the posterior arch of C1 on the right and the left side. A contoured rod or frame with a sagittal angle of less than 110° was inserted and the wires were tightened on the rod. An on lay auto graft was placed over the posterior aspect of the decorticated occiput, atlas, and axis. These techniques were safe with little proximity to vital structures and easy to perform. However, the three-dimensional stabilization was poor compared to rigid contemporary techniques using occipital fixation plates connected to cervical rod-screw constructs.

14.3 Patient Positioning

The operation is performed with the patient prone in a slight reverse Trendelenburg position in order to reduce intraocular pressure [8]. The use of as Jackson spine table with a Mayfield clamp is helpful as the patient is positioned on his chest and iliac wings, thus avoiding abdominal compression and subsequent venous obstruction. The radiographic access to the occiput and to the cervical spine is checked at this stage, which facilitates 2D or 3D fluoroscopic control during the procedure. If intraoperative computed tomography (CT) is used, the gantry is entered from cranial and the patient is placed on a carbon table. Accurate positioning of the head and sagittal setting of cervical alignment is achieved using a Mayfield clamp attached to the table via an articulated system (Fig. 14.1). A fluoroscopic image is mandatory before surgery to verify the occipito-cervical alignment (Fig. 14.2). An adequate alignment is crucial in order to provide a horizontal gaze postoperatively. Furthermore, the occiput-C2 alignment influences the lordosis of the subaxial spine, which plays a role for the functional outcome and the avoidance of postoperative dysphagia [9–11]. The McGregor line represents a reproducible radiographic marker that is drawn between the hard palate and the caudal aspect of the occiput. Its normal slope measures −4° on average and ranges between −20 and 9° [10]. The McGregor slope might be used as a simple parameter of skull alignment allowing an estimation of horizontal gaze. The posterior occipito-cervical angle (POCA) represents a second reliable radiographic parameter estimating intraoperative alignment.

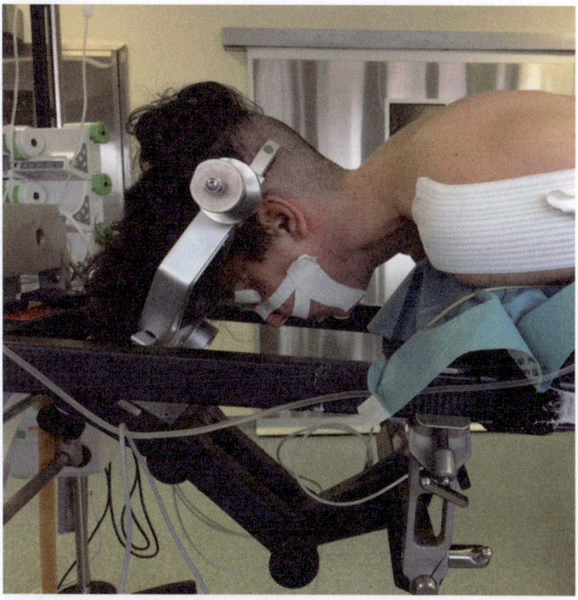

Fig. 14.1 Patient positioning and setting of sagittal occipito-cervical alignment on a Jackson table using a Mayfield clamp

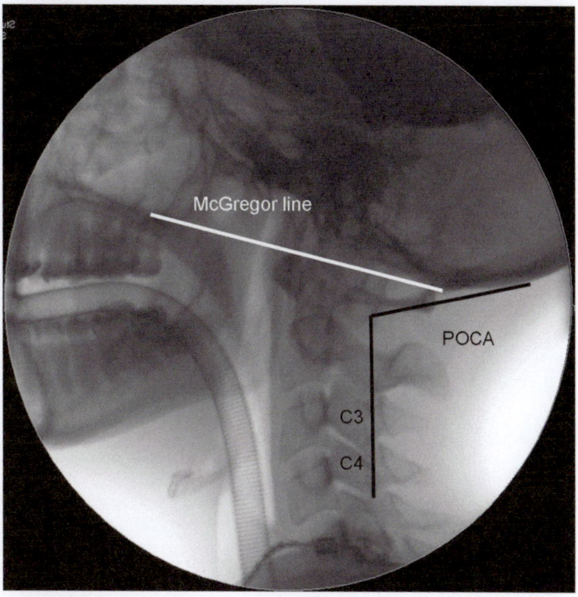

Fig. 14.2 Lateral intraoperative fluoroscopy for setting of sagittal occipito-cervical alignment based on the slope of the McGregor line and the posterior occipito-cervical angle (POCA)

It is defined as the angle formed by the intersection of a line drawn tangential to the flat posterior aspect of the occiput between the foramen magnum and occipital protuberance and the line determined by the posterior aspect of the third and fourth cervical facets. The average POCA is at 109° and the majority of measurements range between 101 and 119° [12, 13].

14.4 Surgical Approach

Extensive shaving of the posterior head and neck is required. The area from the cranio-cervical junction to the cervicothoracic junction and the skin over the iliac crest are prepared and draped in a sterile fashion. The posterior approach is made from the external occipital protuberance to C4-C5 (Fig. 14.3). The caudal extent of the incision depends on the distal instrumentation level and the patient's local anatomy. After splitting the subcutis, self-retaining retractors are applied and the nuchal ligament is approached at the level of the spinous processes C2 and C3, or further if necessary. Subperiosteal dissection is performed using a small Cobb elevator and a diathermy knife. Cranially, the nuchal ligament is divided in the midline and the occipital bone is easily identified. The part of the occipital squama that lies caudal to the external protuberance is exposed and the median part of the trapezius and semispinalis capitis muscle insertions is detached in a reversed T-shape fashion. The spinous process of C2 and its musculo-ligamentous attachment are usually very

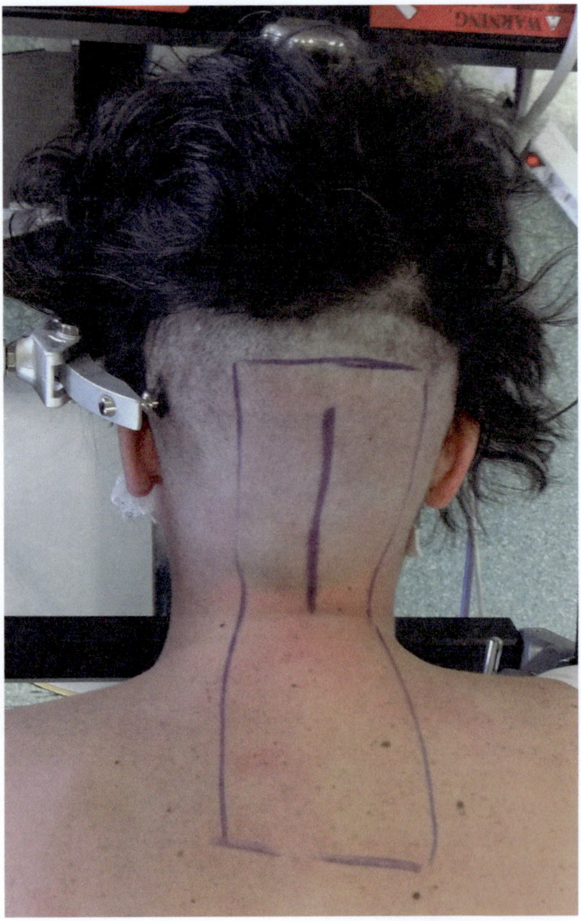

Fig. 14.3 Posterior view of the patient demonstrating the prepared area for sterile draping from the cranio-cervical junction to the cervicothoracic junction and incision line from the external occipital protuberance to the mid-cervical spine

prominent. Beginning at the second spinous process and proceeding caudally, the short rotator and multifidus muscles are dissected from the spinous processes, the laminae and the lateral masses. Once the occiput and the posterior aspect of C2 are exposed, the posterior tubercle of C1 is easily palpated and the posterior arch of the atlas can be dissected while the tip of the electrocautery and the periosteal elevator maintain constant bone contact to avoid vertebral artery injury cranially and laterally. Care should further be taken not to extend too far laterally at the level of C1 and C2 in order to avoid venous plexus bleeding. Hemostasis may be achieved by insertion of hemostatic gauze, gelfoam, and eventually thrombin. Because this segment is very unstable, periosteal elevators should be applied with care. Too much pressure exerted on posterior bony elements can cause motion at subluxated levels in trauma, tumor, or inflammatory diseases.

14.5 Occipital Fixation

For occipital fixation, the plate is fitted to the occipital bone and screws are inserted into a drilled pilot hole. The bone is thickest in the midline and the ideal zone of screw placement is up to 2 cm lateral to the external occipital protuberance along the superior nuchal line. The drilling depth can be measured preoperatively on CT and optimal occipital screw lengths can be predetermined. Occipital screw lengths usually range between 8 mm and 12 mm. Bicortical screws may increase the pullout strength (Fig. 14.4). Nevertheless, intracranial injuries to venous sinuses have been reported. As there is no universal position for safe insertion of occipital screws that is applicable to all individuals, preoperative angio-CT studies have been recommended [14, 15]. In biomechanical studies, unicortical screw fixation at the midline

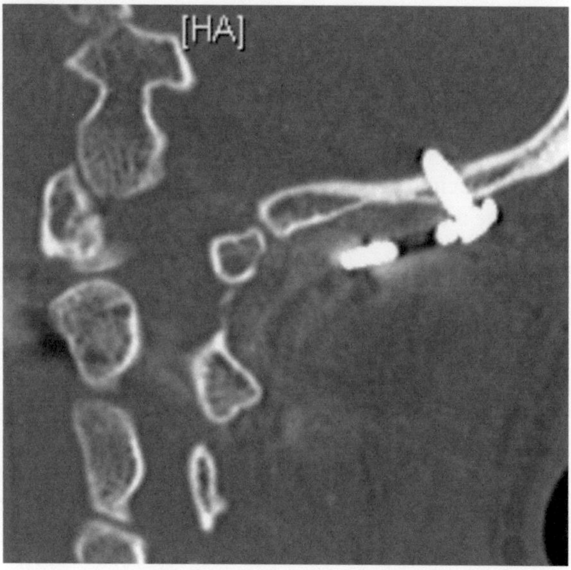

Fig. 14.4 Postoperative sagittal CT showing a bicortical occipital screw fixation

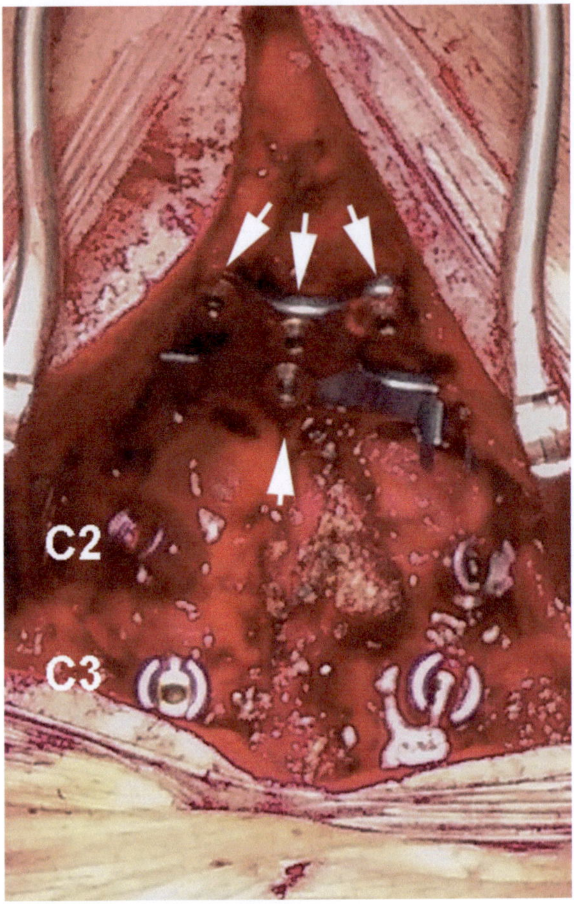

Fig. 14.5 Intraoperative view of occipital plate fixation using 4 screws (arrows) along the midline and the superior nuchal line, C2 isthmus, and C3 lateral mass screws

ridge approached the pullout strength of bicortical fixation at other sites of the occiput [16]. This fixation method can be improved by using screws that have a large thread, similar to cancellous bone screws, which enhances the unicortical purchase in occipital bone. A stable plate fixation is usually achieved with 3 or 4 screws along the midline and the superior nuchal line (Fig. 14.5).

14.6 Cervical Fixation

Distal cervical fixation is usually achieved at C2, C3, and C4. Lateral mass screws are rarely used at C1 as the occipital plate is very close, which makes the rod insertion difficult at its angulated part. At C2, pedicle or isthmus screws can be used depending on the local anatomy of the vertebral artery, which should be studied on a preoperative CT-angiogram. The ideal screw length can also be premeasured on CT in order to avoid any vascular injury (Fig. 14.6). Intraoperative CT or 3D

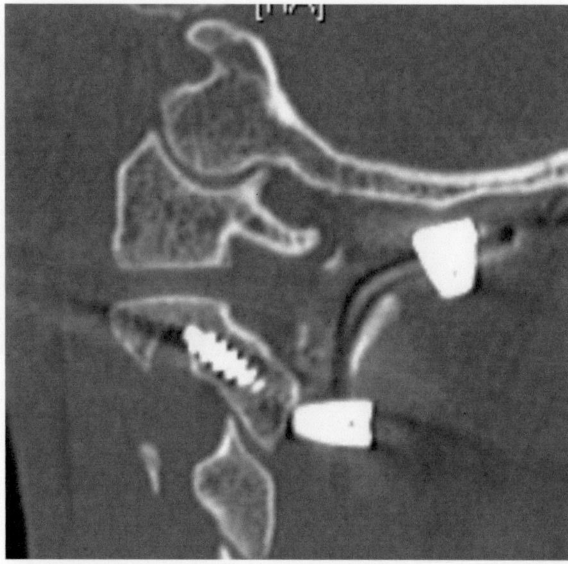

Fig. 14.6 Postoperative sagittal CT showing a C2 isthmus screw with its tip posterior to the vertebral artery

fluoroscopy navigated screw insertion might be an additional tool that increases accuracy and safety [17]. The entry point for the drill is opened using an awl in the cranial-medial quadrant of the C2 lateral mass. The C2 pedicle can be palpated inside the canal, which is helpful when determining the drilling direction, which is around 15° toward the midline and 35° cranially. If standard lateral fluoroscopic guidance is used, drilling can be monitored in the sagittal plane. Shorter isthmus screws appear to be a safe option, which reduced the risk of a vertebral artery injury. If the local anatomy allows positioning of long pedicle screws, this trans-isthmic fixation offers a higher pullout strength [18]. At subaxial levels, lateral mass screws are additionally used at C3 and eventually C4, depending on pathologic findings and the stability of the construct. The two most popular techniques for lateral mass screws are the Roy-Camille and the Magerl technique, offering similar biomechanical pullout strength [19]. The entry point is at the middle of the lateral mass. The drilling direction is straightforward in the sagittal plane and 10° lateral according to Roy-Camille, whereas the orientation is 30° cranially and 30° laterally according to Magerl.

A clamp construct using a supra-laminar hook at C3 and a sub-laminar hook at C4 represents a valuable alternative (Fig. 14.7). This technique is less common compared to screw fixation techniques. It is safe and easy to perform, and it allows a stable construct that might be superior in the case of osteoporosis or rheumatoid polyarthritis as the claw is fixed on dense cortical laminae [20, 21]. The flavum ligament and the caudal-lateral portion of the C2 lamina are resected using a Kerrison rongeur, which allows sliding a hook under the C3 lamina from cranial, as lateral as possible, at the junction with the lateral mass. The hook at C4 is placed under the lamina from caudal, which does not require any ligamentous resection. A stable construct is achieved by tightening the claw under compression once the rods are in place.

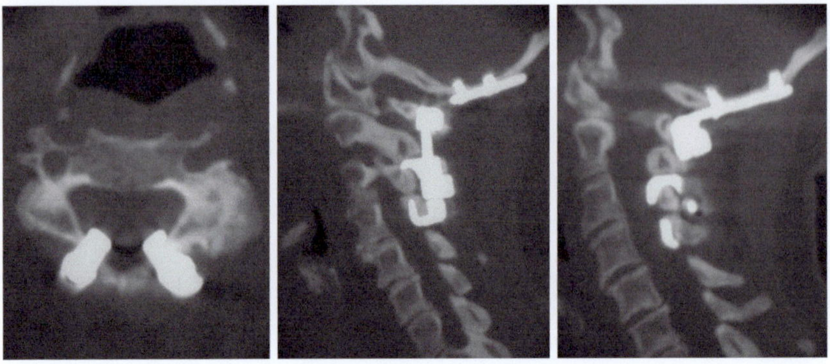

Fig. 14.7 Postoperative axial and sagittal CT demonstrating a C3-C4 claw construct which gets stable after bilateral compression and fixation on rods

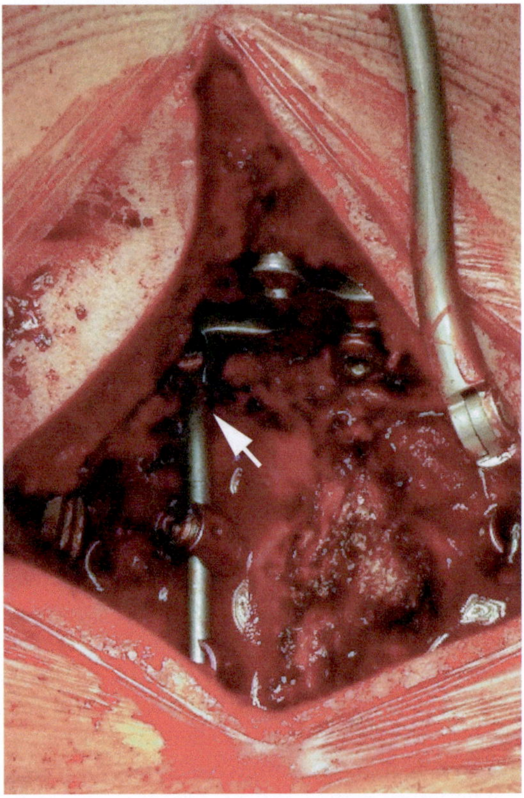

Fig. 14.8 Intraoperative view of the occipital plate, rod and screw connection where the POCA is set by previous rod bending at its angulated part (arrow)

The rod is contoured according to the sagittal posterior occipito-cervical angle (POCA) around 110° and fixed to the occipital plate and cervical implants (Figs. 14.8, 14.9 and 14.10). There are different kinds of occipito-cervical rod-plate fixation systems. Some of them offer an integrated smaller plate at the end of the rod, which necessitates an occipital fixation lateral to the midline ridge.

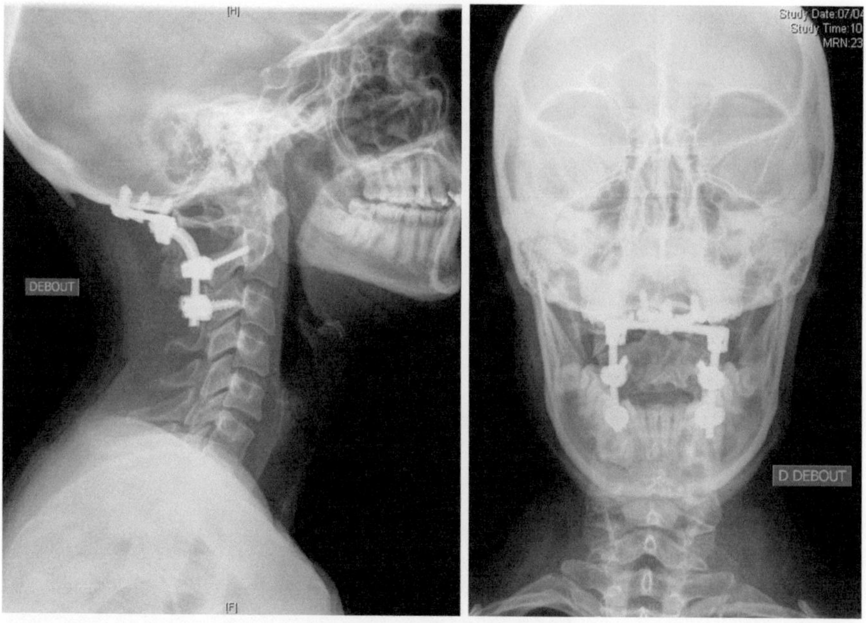

Fig. 14.9 Postoperative lateral and anterior-posterior radiographs showing an occipito-cervical instrumentation using C2 isthmus and C3 lateral mass screws

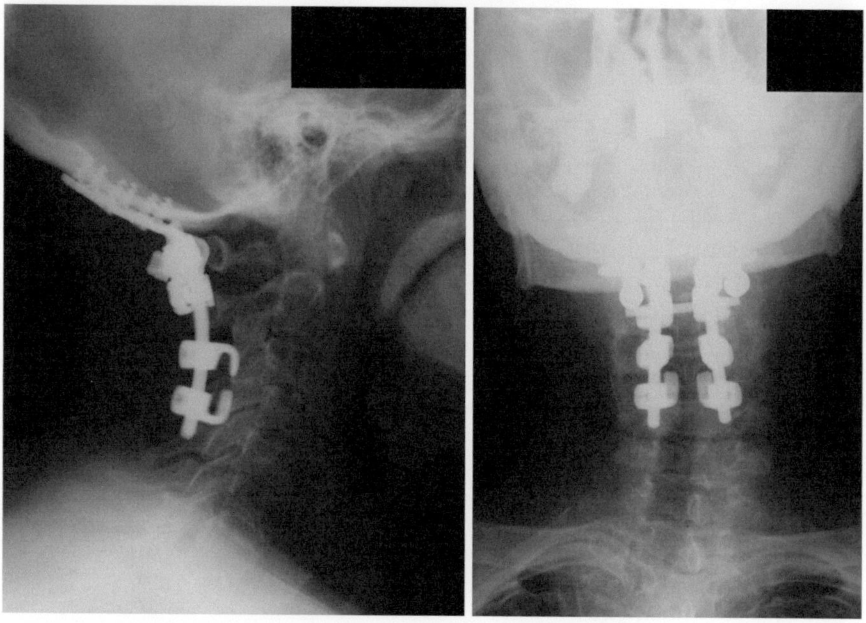

Fig. 14.10 Postoperative lateral and anterior-posterior radiographs showing an occipito-cervical instrumentation using a C3-C4 claw construct

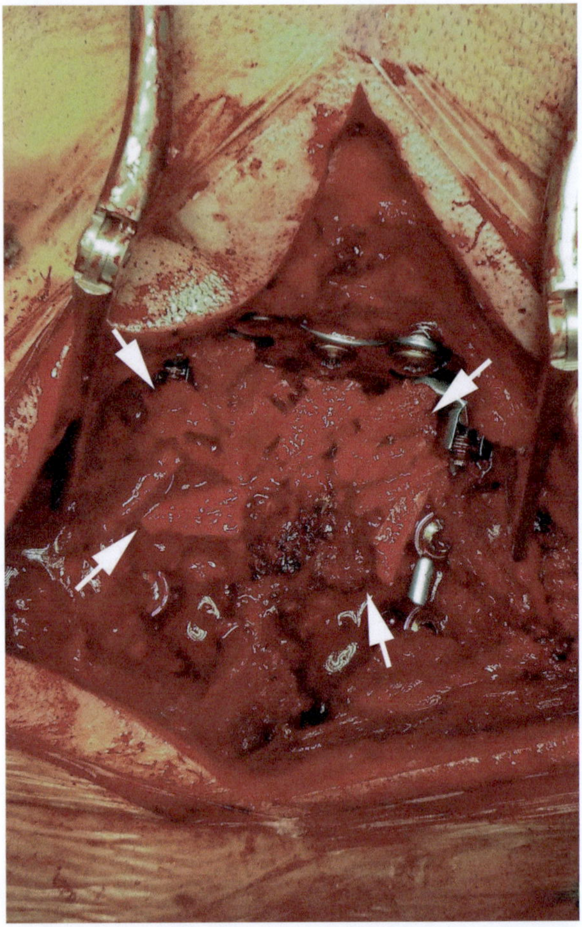

Fig. 14.11 Intraoperative view of posterior bone grafting with cortical and cancellous bone from the iliac crest (arrows)

14.7 Fusion Techniques

Occipito-cervical fusion is best achieved by cancellous bone from the iliac crest. Local bone harvested from spinous processes combined with bone substitutes may be used as an alternative, such as allograft in form of cortical/cancellous chips. The off-label use of bone morphogenetic protein (BMP) has been described anecdotally [22], but this application might not be necessary in general. The occipital bone, the posterior arch of C1 and the laminae of instrumented vertebrae C2-C4 are decorticated using a drill or a Kerrison rongeur. This will enhance the fusion potential of cancellous bone, which is locally applied to the decorticated area (Fig. 14.11).

Conflict of Interest None.

References

1. Zhao D, Wang S, Passias PG, et al. Craniocervical instability in the setting of os odontoideum: assessment of cause, presentation, and surgical outcomes in a series of 279 cases. Neurosurgery. 2015;76(5):514–21.
2. Landi A, Marotta N, Morselli C, et al. Pannus regression after posterior decompression and occipito-cervical fixation in occipito-atlanto-axial instability due to rheumatoid arthritis: case report and literature review. Clin Neurol Neurosurg. 2013;115(2):111–6.
3. Schnake KJ, Pingel A, Scholz M, et al. Temporary occipito-cervical stabilization of a unilateral occipital condyle fracture. Eur Spine J. 2012;21(11):2198–202.
4. Cappuccio M, De Iure F, Amendola L, et al. Occipito-cervical fusion in post-traumatic instability of the upper cervical spine and cranio-cervical junction. Eur Spine J. 2013;22(Suppl 6):S900–4.
5. Ehlinger M, Charles YP, Adam P, et al. Survivor of a traumatic atlanto-occipital dislocation. Orthop Traumatol Surg Res. 2011;97(3):335–40.
6. Zimmermann M, Wolff R, Raabe A, et al. Palliative occipito-cervical stabilization in patients with malignant tumors of the occipito-cervical junction and the upper cervical spine. Acta Neurochir. 2002;144(8):783–90.
7. MacKenzie AI, Uttley D, Marsh HT, Bell BA. Craniocervical stabilization using Luque/Hartshill rectangles. Neurosurgery. 1990;26(1):32–6.
8. Carey TW, Shaw KA, Weber ML, DeVine JG. Effect of the degree of reverse Trendelenburg position on intraocular pressure during prone spine surgery: a randomized controlled trial. Spine J. 2014;14(9):2118–26.
9. Inada T, Furuya T, Kamiya K, et al. Postoperative increase in occiput-C2 angle negatively impacts subaxial lordosis after occipito-upper cervical posterior fusion surgery. Asian Spine J. 2016;10(4):744–7.
10. Matsubayashi Y, Shimizu T, Chikuda H, et al. Correlations of cervical sagittal alignment before and after occipitocervical fusion. Global Spine J. 2016;6(4):362–9.
11. Tian W, Yu J. The role of C2-C7 and O-C2 angle in the development of dysphagia after cervical spine surgery. Dysphagia. 2013;28(2):131–8.
12. Riel RU, Lee MC, Kirkpatrick JS. Measurement of a posterior occipitocervical fusion angle. J Spinal Disord Tech. 2010;23(1):27–9.
13. Kunakornsawat S, Pluemvitayaporn T, Pruttikul P, et al. A new method for measurement of occipitocervical angle by occiput-C3 angle. Eur J Orthop Surg Traumatol. 2016;27:1051. https://doi.org/10.1007/s00590-016-1881-9.
14. Lee DH, Hong JT, Sung JH, et al. Morphologic analysis of occipital sinuses for occipital screw fixation using digital subtraction angiography. World Neurosurg. 2016;91:279–84.
15. Izeki M, Neo M, Fujibayashi S, et al. Utility of the analysis of intracranial venous sinuses using preoperative computed tomography venography for safe occipital screw insertion. Spine (Phila Pa 1976). 2013;38(18):E1149–55.
16. Hasher TR, Yeung AW, Caruso SA, et al. Occipital screw pullout strength. A biomechanical investigation of occipital morphology. Spine (Phila Pa 1976). 1992;24(1):5–9.
17. Smith JD, Jack MM, Harn NR, et al. Screw placement accuracy and outcomes following O-arm-navigated atlantoaxial fusion: a feasibility study. Global Spine J. 2016;6(4):344–9.
18. Lucas F, Mitton D, Frechede B, Barrey C. Short isthmic versus long trans-isthmic C2 screw: anatomical and biomechanical evaluation. Eur J Orthop Surg Traumatol. 2016;26(7):785–91.
19. Barrey C, Mertens P, Jund J, et al. Quantitative anatomic evaluation of cervical lateral mass fixation with a comparison of the Roy-Camille and the Magerl screw techniques. Spine (Phila Pa 1976). 2005;30(6):E140–7.
20. Espinoza-Larios A, Ames CP, Chamberlain RH, et al. Biomechanical comparison of two-level cervical locking posterior screw/rod and hook/rod techniques. Spine J. 2007;7(2):194–204.
21. Motosuneya T, Hirabayashi S, Yamada H, Sakai H. Occipitocervical fusion using a hook and rod system between cervical levels C2 and C3. J Clin Neurosci. 2009;16(7):909–13.
22. Molinari RW, Molinari C. The use of bone morphogenetic protein in pediatric cervical spine fusion surgery: case reports and review of the literature. Global Spine J. 2016;6(1):e41–6.

Far Lateral Transcondylar Transtubercular Approach

15

Naveed Kamal, Renuka K. Reddy, Takanori Fukushima, and James K. Liu

15.1 Indications

The far lateral transcondylar approach (commonly referred to as the "far lateral approach") provides excellent exposure and a lateral viewing trajectory for accessing intradural and extradural lesions located at the craniovertebral junction (consisting of the lower one-third of the clivus, the foramen magnum, and the C1 and C2 vertebrae), thereby reducing the need for brain retraction [1, 2]. The approach typically involves a lateral suboccipital craniectomy behind the sigmoid sinus, a C1 hemilaminectomy, partial resection of the posteromedial one-third of the occipital condyle, and partial resection of the jugular tubercle. The degree of bone removal varies based on the patient, depending on the location and pathology of the lesion. The approach is useful for several tumors, which arise in the craniovertebral

N. Kamal
Department of Neurological Surgery, Rutgers University-New Jersey Medical School, Center for Skull Base and Pituitary Surgery, Rutgers Neurological Institute of New Jersey, Newark, NJ, USA

R. K. Reddy
Department of Otolaryngology-Head and Neck Surgery, Rutgers University-New Jersey Medical School, Newark, NJ, USA

T. Fukushima
Department of Neurosurgery, Duke University, Durham, NC, USA

Carolina Neuroscience Institute, Raleigh, NC, USA

J. K. Liu (✉)
Department of Neurological Surgery, Rutgers University-New Jersey Medical School, Center for Skull Base and Pituitary Surgery, Rutgers Neurological Institute of New Jersey, Newark, NJ, USA

Department of Otolaryngology-Head and Neck Surgery, Rutgers University-New Jersey Medical School, Newark, NJ, USA
e-mail: james.liu.md@rutgers.edu

E. Tessitore et al. (eds.), *Surgery of the Cranio-Vertebral Junction*,
https://doi.org/10.1007/978-3-030-18700-2_15

junction, including foramen magnum meningiomas, schwannomas, chordomas, chondrosarcomas, and neurenteric cysts [3–6]. The far lateral approach can also be used to access vascular lesions, such as vertebral artery-posterior inferior cerebellar artery (VA-PICA) junction aneurysms, vertebrobasilar junction aneurysms, and ventrolaterally located brainstem cavernous malformations. Unlike the anterior transoral approaches or endoscopic endonasal approaches, the far lateral approach has no risk of contamination with oral flora or nasal cavity, respectively. When compared to a midline posterior approach, the far lateral approach offers better visualization of the vertebral arteries and its branches. Some limitations of the far lateral approach are the risk of lower cranial nerve deficits and potential difficulty for dural closure.

15.2 Anatomy

15.2.1 Muscle Layers

An understanding of the upper cervical muscles and the suboccipital triangle is important in performing the far lateral approach safely. There are three layers of muscle identified during the dissection. The most superficial layer includes the sternocleidomastoid muscle and the trapezius. The middle layer consists of four muscles: the splenius capitis, splenius cervicis, longissimus capitis, and semispinalis capitis. The deepest layer consists of the muscles comprise the suboccipital triangle, which is bound medially by the rectus capitis posterior major, inferiorly by the inferior oblique, and superolaterally by the superior oblique muscle. The rectus capitis major muscle inserts into the inferior nuchal line superiorly and to the spinous process of C2 inferiorly. The inferior oblique inserts to the transverse process of C1 superiorly and to the spinous process of C2 inferiorly. The superior oblique inserts at the temporo-occipital suture superiorly and on the transverse process of C1 inferiorly. The suboccipital triangle harbors the vertebral artery (V3 segment), situated in the vertebral sulcus on the arch of C1. The artery is typically covered by a dense venous plexus.

15.2.2 Bony Anatomy

The key bony structures involved in the far lateral approach include the occipital condyle, the hypoglossal canal, and the jugular tubercle. The occipital condyles are found in the anterolateral border of the foramen and extend inferiorly. It is an oval shaped structure, which articulates with the superior facet of C1. The hypoglossal canal is found directly superior to the middle of the occipital condyle. It faces anterolaterally at a 45-degree angle from the sagittal plane and its intracranial opening is approximately 5 mm above the posterior and middle third of the occipital condyle. Superior to the hypoglossal canal is the jugular tubercle, which is the second protuberance of the occipital bone. The jugular tubercle projects medially from the occipital bone and is found rostral and anterior to the occipital condyle. Cranial nerves IX, X, and XI wrap around the posterior aspect of the jugular tubercle along their course into the jugular foramen. Knowledge of the anatomic relationships between cranial nerves and bony protuberances is crucial to safe and effective drilling of the occipital condyle and jugular foramen during the far lateral approach. The hypoglossal canal separates the jugular tubercle from the occipital condyle and serves as a useful landmark in guiding the drilling of the occipital condyle and jugular tubercle.

15.2.3 Vertebral Artery

One of the keys of the extradural stage of the far lateral approach is determining the location and course of the vertebral artery. Anatomic variants of the vertebral artery can lead to vascular complications such as arterial injury if they are not recognized. As the vertebral artery ascends from the foramen transversarium of C2 and C1, it is ventral to the ventral ramus of the C2 nerve root, which is found between the laminae of C1 and C2, and can be traced laterally until it crosses the vertical segment of the vertebral artery [7, 8]. As the vertebral artery exits the foramen transversarium of C1, it is encased in a venous plexus, sometimes referred to as the suboccipital cavernous sinus, and courses posteriorly behind the lateral mass of C1 in the J-shaped vertebral groove ("J-groove"), or vertebral sulcus. It then turns medially as it pierces the atlanto-occipital membrane and the dura mater [9]. The posterior meningeal artery and several small branches arise from the horizontal segment of the extradural vertebral artery; these branches can be safely coagulated. In rare cases, the posterior inferior cerebellar artery may arise from the extradural segment of the vertebral artery [10, 11]. Inadvertent injury to this vascular variant can potentially result in a postoperative brainstem stroke.

15.3 Surgical Technique

15.3.1 Preoperative Considerations

The far lateral approach is performed on the side of the lateral extension of the lesion. If the lesion is midline, the anatomy of the vertebral artery, the sigmoid sinus, and the jugular bulbs is considered to decide the side of the approach. In these cases, the side of the nondominant vertebral artery or nondominant jugular bulb is preferred [7]. Preoperative imaging, including MRI, CT angiography, magnetic resonance angiography, magnetic resonance venography, or conventional angiography should be studied carefully to evaluate the features of the lesion, its neighboring vasculature, and the bony anatomy of the foramen magnum, occipital condyles, jugular tubercles, and the atlantoaxial complex. If the tumor encases the vertebral artery, a balloon test occlusion should be performed to determine if the artery can be safely sacrificed during surgery, if needed. This information can determine whether revascularization with a bypass may be needed if vessel occlusion is not tolerated. Otherwise, the vertebral artery must be preserved with residual adherent tumor. Intraoperative monitoring includes somatosensory evoked potentials, motor evoked potentials, brainstem auditory evoked responses, and monitoring of cranial nerves VII, X, XI, and XII. An electromyographic endotracheal tube may be used to monitor cranial nerve X. Meanwhile, electrodes placed directly into the sternocleidomastoid muscle and the tongue may be used to monitor cranial nerves XI and XII, respectively.

15.3.2 Positioning and Skin Incision

The patient is placed in a modified lateral park bench position (Fig. 15.1). The body is initially positioned laterally with the head secured in three-point pin fixation. The neck is slightly flexed, the vertex is angled slightly downward, and the face is rotated slightly ventrally, so that the mastoid body is at the highest point. This positioning allows for improved exposure and inferior-to-superior viewing angle to the ventral craniovertebral junction. An axillary roll is placed on the dependent side with care not to compress the axilla, and the contralateral arm rests on a Krauss armrest. The

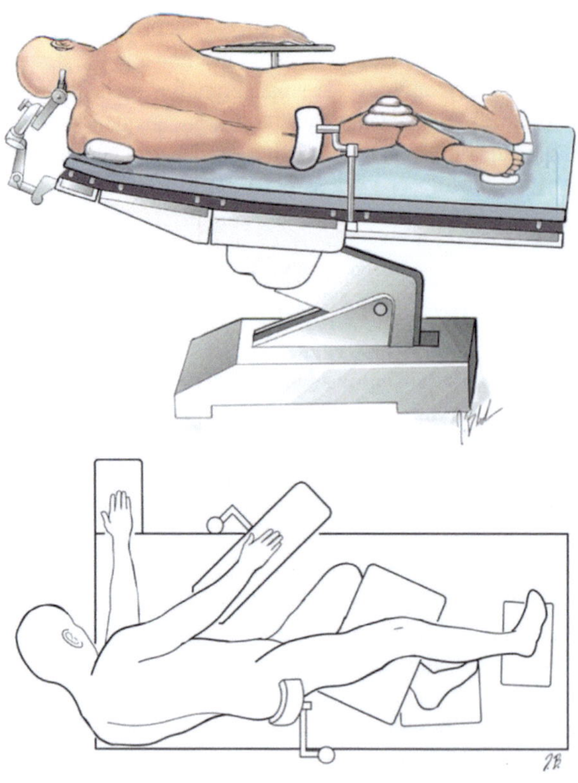

Fig. 15.1 Modified lateral park bench positioning. The top shoulder is rotated slightly anteriorly and the top arm rests on an arm rest at 45°. An axillary roll is placed beneath the dependent arm. All pressure points are adequately padded. The head is fixed in Mayfield head holder, and rotated so that the nose is pointing toward the floor (vertex down), slight flexion of the neck, and bending of the of the head away from the top shoulder to open up the space between the mastoid and the shoulder. This positioning allows for improved exposure and inferior-to-superior viewing angle to the ventral craniovertebral junction. (Reproduced with permission from Fukushima T. Manual of skull base dissection. AF NeuroVideo, Inc.; 1996)

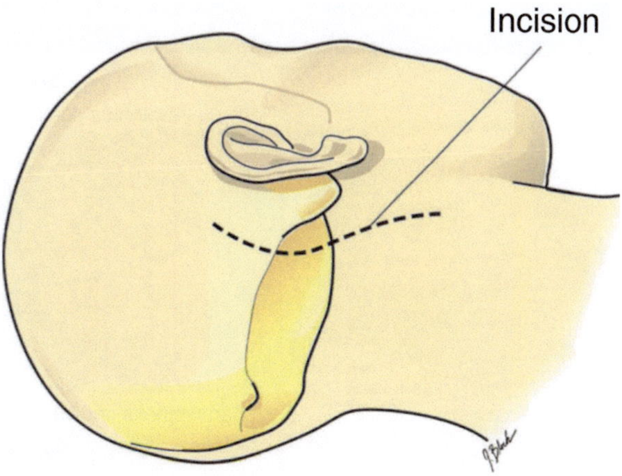

Fig. 15.2 Right retroauricular c-shaped incision. (Reproduced with permission from Fukushima T. Manual of skull base dissection, AF NeuroVideo, Inc.; 1996)

elevated shoulder is rotated anteriorly and the arm is placed inferiorly toward the foot approximately at 45-degrees of the table in order to provide more room for the surgeon working above the shoulder. All pressure points are carefully padded with foam or gel pads, and the patient is secured to the operating table with adhesive tape to allow safe rotation of the table during the operation to improve the surgeon's line of sight. At the time of skin incision, intravenous glucocorticoids and antibiotics are administered.

Although a variety of skin incisions can be used for the far lateral approach, we typically use a retroauricular C-shaped incision that is roughly three finger breadths behind the pinna of the ear and continues inferiorly in a curvilinear fashion into the neck over the posterior border of the sternocleidomastoid muscle to the level of C3 or C4 (Fig. 15.2). The skin is incised with a no. 10 blade. The upper part of the C-shaped incision is raised as a myocutaneous flap (includes the posterior aspect of the temporalis muscle and the occipital belly of the occipitofrontalis muscle) to expose the mastoid body and the upper suboccipital region. The attachment of the sternocleidomastoid muscle and splenius capitis muscle at the superior nuchal line are preserved. The inferior limb of the skin incision is raised as a galeocutaneous flap, leaving the sternocleidomastoid muscle intact. The scalp is held with fish hooks and rubber bands and reflected anteriorly.

15.3.3 Muscle Dissection and Suboccipital Triangle

For the muscle dissection, we prefer to incise the muscles as a single layer rather than dissecting each individual layer of muscles, which can create more dead space and pathways for pseudomeningocele formation (Fig. 15.3). The superficial and middle muscle layers are carefully incised and reflected with sutures or a self-retaining retractor. The arch of C1 is frequently palpated and then exposed at the medial extent near the midline. This is done with a monopolar cautery to expose the most medial aspect of the C1 arch. Dissection is then carried from a medial to lateral

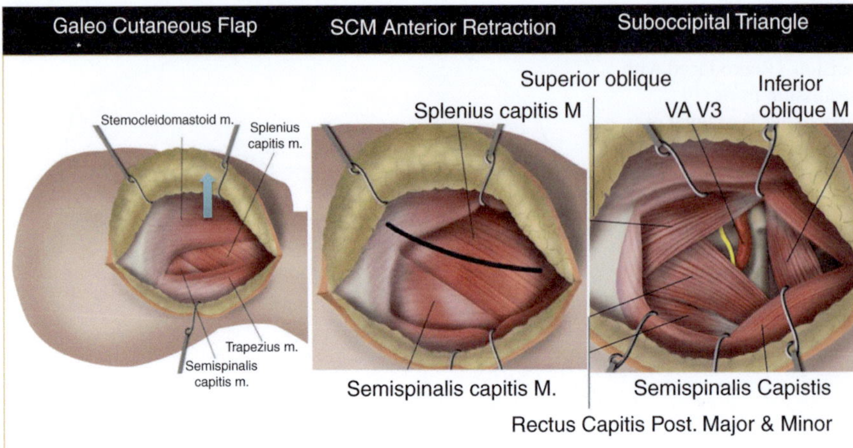

Fig. 15.3 Muscular layers of the lateral neck dissection. (Reproduced with permission from Fukushima T. Manual of Skull Base dissection, 3rd ed. AF NeuroVideo, Inc.; 2014)

direction using subperiosteal dissection with a key periosteal elevator. Care is taken to identify the J-groove to identify the V3 segment of the vertebral artery (Fig. 15.4). Once C1 is confirmed, further exposure of the laminae of C2 and C3 can be performed if more inferior exposure is needed. The foramen magnum is also carefully exposed subperiosteally from the midline keel medially, to the occipital condyle laterally.

15.3.4 Exposure of the Extradural Vertebral Artery

The extradural vertebral artery is identified at the J-groove of the C1 arch. In order to reduce bleeding from the venous plexus surrounding the vertebral artery, subperiosteal dissection from the vertebral sulcus can be performed to maintain integrity of the venous plexus around the artery to minimize venous bleeding [12]. Any venous bleeding from the suboccipital and vertebral venous plexus can be controlled with gelfoam and pressure with a cottonoid pattie or alternatively, with injection of flowable gelatin and thrombin (Surgiflo, Ethicon, Somerville, New Jersey) followed by pressure with a cottonoid pattie.

15.3.5 Suboccipital Craniectomy and C1 Laminectomy

The lateral suboccipital craniectomy is initially performed with a high-speed drill and rongeurs similar to a retrosigmoid fashion (Fig. 15.5). We prefer to perform a craniectomy instead of a craniotomy to avoid the risk of dural tear or sigmoid sinus injury. The extent of the craniectomy usually extends toward the midline keel medially, to the inferior nuchal line superiorly, to the rim of the foramen magnum inferiorly, and up to the occipital condyle laterally. If further superior access is needed to

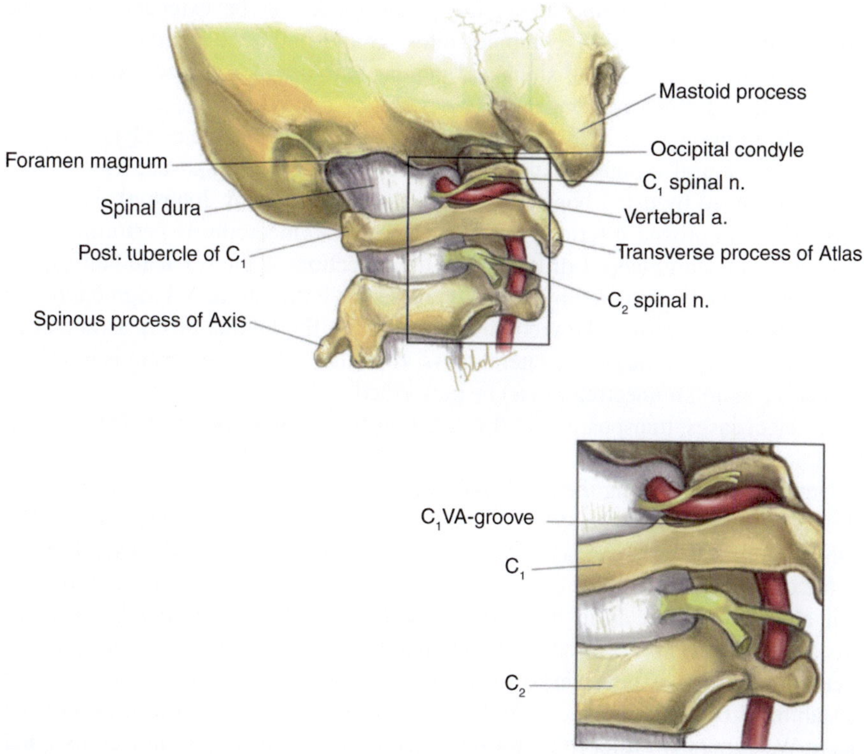

Fig. 15.4 Exposure of the foramen magnum and extradural vertebral artery. The V3 segment of the vertebral artery can be identified on the C1 arch at the vertebral sulcus ("J-groove"). The C2 nerve root crosses over the vertebral artery between C1 and C2. (Reproduced with permission from Fukushima T. Manual of skull base dissection. AF NeuroVideo, Inc.; 1996)

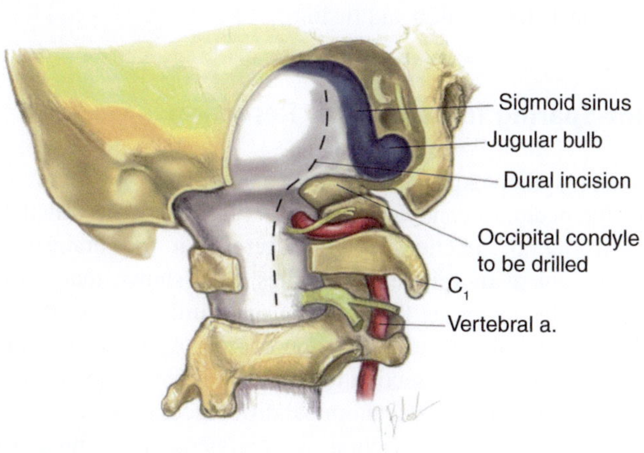

Fig. 15.5 Lateral suboccipital craniectomy and C1-hemilaminectomy. The foramen magnum is unroofed and the posterior aspect of the sigmoid sinus is exposed. Dural incision (dotted line) is made behind the sigmoid sinus and behind the entrance of the vertebral artery. (Reproduced with permission from Fukushima T. Manual of skull base dissection. AF NeuroVideo, Inc.; 1996)

access the cerebellopontine angle, the craniectomy can be extended up to the transverse-sigmoid junction (combined retrosigmoid-far lateral approach). The posterior margin of the sigmoid sinus and jugular bulb are skeletonized with a high-speed drill and Kerrison rongeurs. The posterior condylar emissary vein, which travels from the jugular bulb and exits the condylar fossa via the condylar canal to join the extradural venous plexus, is encountered during the exposure. Hemostasis can be achieved by using bone wax and Surgicel (Johnson & Johnson). The dural exposure is improved inferiorly when a C1 hemilaminectomy is performed with rongeurs and a high-speed drill. During the resection of the C1 hemilamina, the vertebral artery is protected by placing a dissector between the V3 segment of the artery and the J-groove. We recommend removing the lamina of C1 as lateral as possible to where it meets the lateral mass. If further inferior exposure is required, C2 and C3 hemilaminectomies can be performed.

In select cases, transposition of the vertebral artery can be performed by opening the foramen transversarium at C1 with a high-speed diamond drill and Kerrison rongeurs, and mobilizing the artery inferomedially from the atlanto-occipital joint. However, this is rarely needed in the vast majority of cases in our experience. The indication for this is if one needs to resect the lateral mass of C1, the lateral aspect of the occipital condyle, the odontoid process, and the inferior clivus (extreme lateral approach), such as in cases of extradural chordomas or chondrosarcomas involving the atlanto-occipital joint and odontoid process. Subsequent occipitocervical stabilization is necessary in these cases where the atlanto-occipital joint is destabilized by the tumor invasion preoperatively, or by surgical resection of the mass. We generally prefer to perform the occipitocervical stabilization at a second stage through a traditional midline posterior cervical incision in the prone position at about 24–48 h later. This allows better bilateral fixation in the anatomical position, whereas stabilization performed during the far lateral approach only allows for unilateral stabilization, which can risk fixation of the head in an awkward and suboptimal position. The patient is kept intubated and in a cervical collar prior to definitive occipitocervical stabilization and fusion.

15.3.6 Joint-Sparing Transcondylar Resection

Ventral foramen magnum exposure can be further extended by removing the posterior aspect of the occipital condyle. This allows for improved visualization of the ventral craniovertebral junction without cerebellar or brainstem retraction (Fig. 15.3). Anatomical morphometric studies have shown that partial condylar resection sequentially increases the angle of exposure as more of the condyle is resected [13–16]. Recommendations for the degree of occipital condyle removal vary widely, ranging from no resection to complete resection [8, 15, 17]. This variability is largely due to individual anatomical differences between patients and their preexisting pathology. Prior to resection, the preoperative CT images of the skull base must be evaluated because not all patients will require a condylar resection to increase the surgical corridor. In addition, condylar resection may not be necessary if the patient has small occipital condyles, a large foramen magnum, or if the tumor has eroded the condyle and displaced the brainstem medially. If greater than 50% of the condyle has been eroded by tumor or resected by the surgeon, occipitocervical stabilization should be strongly considered [18]. In our experience, removal of the posterior and medial one-third of the condyle is adequate for visualization of the ventral foramen magnum region. We generally use the proximal extradural hypoglossal canal as a surgical landmark to mark the extent of the condyle removal. The hypoglossal canal is also useful in that it separates the jugular tubercle superiorly from the occipital condyle inferiorly (Fig. 15.6). Once the hypoglossal canal is identified, further bony resection anteriorly beyond the plane of the hypoglossal canal is not necessary when addressing intradural lesions, such as foramen magnum meningiomas, brainstem cavernous malformations, and vertebrobasilar junction aneurysms. In addition, further resection inferiorly toward the atlanto-occipital joint space is also unnecessary. It is critical to preserve the "ball-socket" joint space of O-C1 to avoid the risk of occipitocervical instability (joint-sparing condylar resection).

The posteromedial aspect of the occipital condyle is removed with a high-speed diamond drill while protecting the vertebral artery. Once the cortical layer of bone is removed, the soft cancellous bone is encountered. Venous bleeding from the condylar emissary vein within the condylar canal is controlled with bone wax and

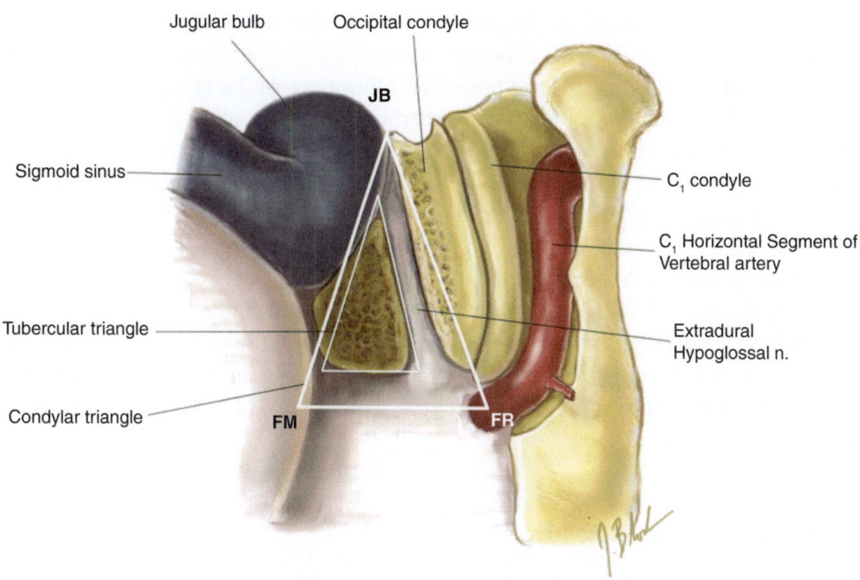

Fig. 15.6 The occipital condyle is drilled while sparing the condyle-C1 lateral mass joint. Once the extradural hypoglossal canal is exposed, the medial aspect of the jugular tubercle (situated between the jugular bulb and hypoglossal canal) can be removed to increase lateral trajectory to the craniovertebral junction. (Reproduced with permission from Fukushima T. Manual of skull base dissection. AF NeuroVideo, Inc.; 1996)

Surgicel. Further drilling exposes another cortical layer which covers the hypoglossal canal. The hypoglossal canal is situated between the occipital condyle and jugular tubercle. Within the canal, the hypoglossal nerve, a meningeal branch of the ascending pharyngeal artery, and the venous plexus of the hypoglossal canal (which allows the basilar venous plexus to communicate with the plexus surrounding the foramen magnum) are found. Identification of the medial one-third of the hypoglossal canal indicates that approximately one-third of the posterior condyle has been resected. If the lesion does not involve the hypoglossal canal, the hypoglossal canal can be left intact as the condylectomy proceeds. Because the hypoglossal canal is oriented anterolaterally at a 45° angle from the midline in the axial plane, further skeletonization of the canal to its lateral extent results in removal of the lateral aspect of approximately two-thirds of the posterior condyle. This is generally not necessary to perform when accessing intradural foramen magnum lesions. Bone removal is then directed superiorly toward the inferior margin of the jugular bulb by removing the jugular tubercle.

15.3.7 Transtubercular Resection

Located at the junction of the basilar and condylar sections of the occipital bone, the rounded prominence of the jugular tubercle obstructs the view of the basal cisterns and clivus anterior to the lower cranial nerves. Resection of this tubercle helps to maximize visualization of the intradural space around the anterior surface of the brainstem and mid-clivus. This exposure is also important when operating on vertebrobasilar junction aneurysms and posterior inferior cerebellar artery aneurysms. In performing the resection of the jugular tubercle, special attention should be paid to the superomedial portion as this is the key area of obstruction. Additionally, cranial nerves IX, X, and XI closely traverse the posterior region of the jugular tubercle prior to entering the jugular foramen. The nerves at this site are particularly sensitive to surgical manipulation, such as direct trauma, stretching of the dura mater, and heat released from the surgical drill. Damage to the nerves can be avoided by using a high-speed diamond drill to core the center of the tubercle, leaving an eggshell-thin layer that can be delicately manipulated with a microdissector. Copious irrigation is used during drilling to avoid thermal injury to the lower cranial nerves. The bottom of the inferior point of the jugular bulb should be free of any bone prior to opening the dura.

15.3.8 Intradural Exposure

For intradural lesions, such as meningiomas, schwannomas, vascular malformations, and aneurysms, a curvilinear incision is made several millimeters posterior to the sigmoid sinus, extending inferiorly toward the top of the C2 lamina (or further inferiorly if exposure was extended) and staying posteriorly to the vertebral artery where it pierces the dura mater (Figs. 15.7, 15.8, 15.9, 15.10, and 15.11). Increased

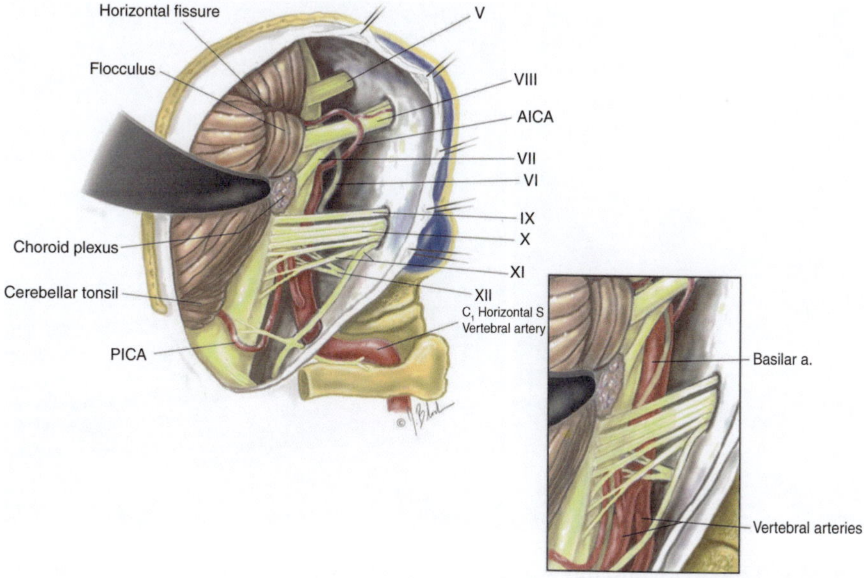

Fig. 15.7 Intradural exposure of the lower cerebellopontine angle and craniovertebral junction. (Reproduced with permission from Fukushima T. Manual of skull base dissection. AF NeuroVideo, Inc.; 1996)

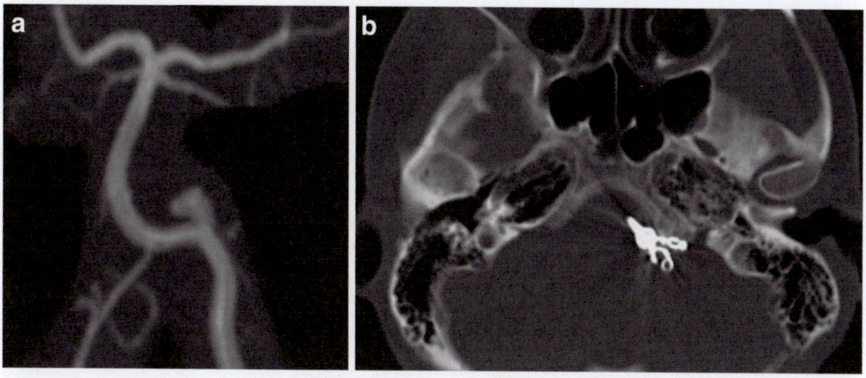

Fig. 15.8 (**a**) MR angiogram showing a left posterior inferior cerebellar artery aneurysm microsurgically clipped via a left far lateral approach. (**b**) Postoperative CT scan showing clip placement

exposure anteriorly can be achieved by incising the dura laterally above the entrance to the vertebral artery, leaving a dural cuff around the artery. Further exposure of the tentorium and upper cerebellopontine angle can be obtained by extending the incision superiorly up to the junction of the transverse-sigmoid sinus. The anterior leaflet of the dura mater is reflected laterally and retracted with tacking sutures. Adequate resection of the occipital condyle and jugular tubercle generally provides

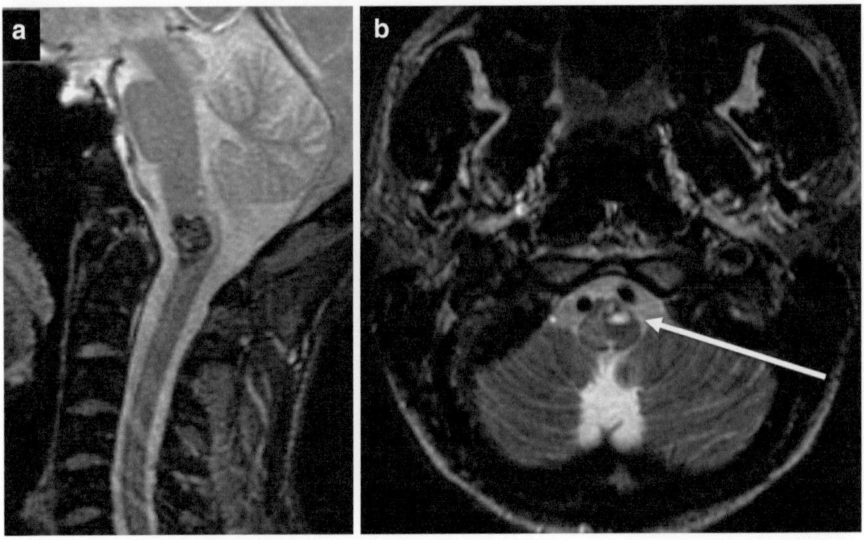

Fig. 15.9 T2-weighted MRI ((**a**): sagittal view; (**b**): axial view) demonstrating a brainstem cavernous malformation presenting to the ventrolateral medulla that was resected via a left far lateral approach

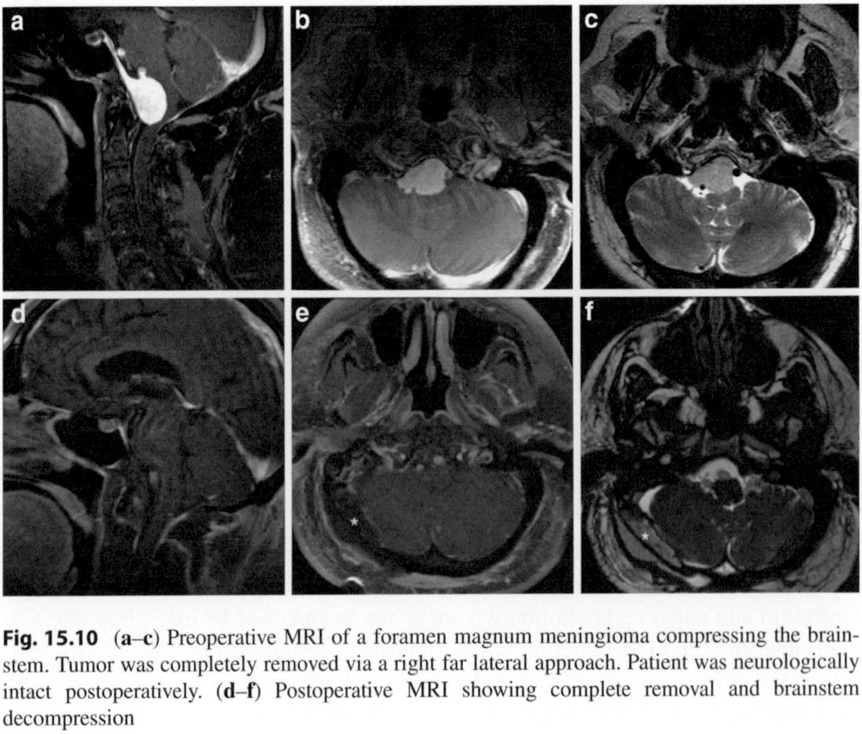

Fig. 15.10 (**a**–**c**) Preoperative MRI of a foramen magnum meningioma compressing the brainstem. Tumor was completely removed via a right far lateral approach. Patient was neurologically intact postoperatively. (**d**–**f**) Postoperative MRI showing complete removal and brainstem decompression

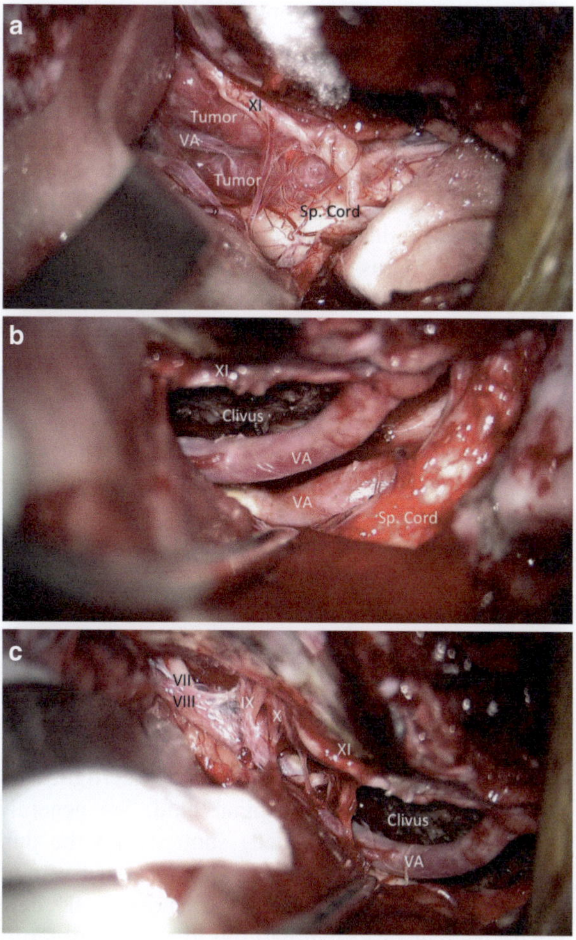

Fig. 15.11 (**a**) Intraoperative view of right far lateral approach for resection of foramen magnum meningioma shown in Fig. 15.9. The tumor was compressing the brainstem and spinal cord (Sp. Cord) and partially encasing the vertebral artery (VA). Cranial nerve XI is visualized. (**b** and **c**) Intraoperative view of the resection cavity after tumor was completely removed. The vertebral arteries and cranial nerves are visualized. The dural attachment at the clivus was cauterized (Simpson Grade II resection)

a straight surgical trajectory to the craniovertebral junction parallel to the intracranial course of the vertebral artery. Sharp arachnoid dissection is performed to expose deeper structures, including cranial nerves V through XII, the basilar artery, the vertebral artery, the vertebrobasilar junction, the posterior inferior cerebellar artery, and the anteroinferior cerebellar artery. Division of the dentate ligament and the C1 and C2 nerve roots can provide more ventral access to the upper cervical spinal cord, if needed. Definitive treatment of the underlying pathology is performed with standard microsurgical techniques depending on the lesion.

For posterior inferior cerebellar artery (PICA) aneurysms (Fig. 15.8), it is important to obtain proximal control at the ipsilateral vertebral artery as it enters the dura. Alternatively, proximal control can be established at the V3 extradural segment as well. Clip reconstruction should be performed in such a way that avoids injury to the lower cranial nerves. Generally, the clip configuration is below the level of cranial nerves 9–11.

For cavernous malformations (Fig. 15.9) that present themselves to the ventrolateral cervicomedullary junction, the far lateral exposure allows direct access to the point of entry to the malformation. In some instances, the cavernous malformation may have an exophytic component that has a typical mulberry appearance, or there may be only a hint of hemosiderin stained tissue on the surface of the pia. Removal should be performed with minimal manipulation of the neural tissue.

For foramen magnum meningiomas (Figs. 15.10 and 15.11), the dentate ligaments should be sharply divided and the vertebral artery should be dissected from the proximal fibrous ring toward the vertebrobasilar junction. This is particularly important in tumors that may have partial or complete encasement of the artery. Internal tumor debulking is performed with an ultrasonic aspirator. Extracapsular dissection can then be performed to dissect the tumor away from critical neurovascular structures. In general, these tumors will elevate the lower cranial nerves (9–11 complex) and dissection is carried out in an inferior-to-superior working corridor. The tumor attachment is then carefully devascularized with bipolar cautery and detached from the ventral clivus attachment. Care must be taken to identify the hypoglossal nerve complex, which can be ventral or inferior to the tumor. If there is any tumor that is strictly adherent to nerves or important vasculature, a small remnant is left on the critical structures to avoid neurovascular complications.

15.3.9 Wound Closure

Proper wound closure entails primary watertight closure of the dura in order to prevent leakage of cerebrospinal fluid. We generally use an acellular dermal allograft (AlloDerm, LifeCell) sutured into the dural defect as a patch graft (Fig. 15.12). Any small areas of CSF leakage are reinforced with primary sutures or with a small muscle or fat graft anchored to the defect with a figure of 8 suture. A Valsalva maneuver can be used to confirm watertight closure of the dura. The exposed mastoid air cells are sealed with bone wax. We then place an autologous fat graft in the craniectomy dead space and the dead space over the spinal cord dura. The fat graft is placed over the suture line. Care is taken not to overpack the dead space so as to avoid compression of the cervicomedullary junction. A cranioplasty is performed with a titanium mesh plate embedded within two sheets of porous polyethylene (Medpor Titan, Stryker, Kalamazoo, Michigan). The Medpor Titan is cut to the appropriate size with heavy scissors and plated to the skull to bolster the fat graft. This applies pressure on the fat graft to the suture line to prevent any postoperative CSF fistulas and pseudomeningoceles. Postoperative lumbar drainage is generally not necessary unless there is concern for suboptimal watertight dural closure. Meticulous multi-layered closure of the neck muscles, fascia, galea, and skin are performed. A headwrap or mastoid dressing is placed for three days to prevent pseudomeningocele formation.

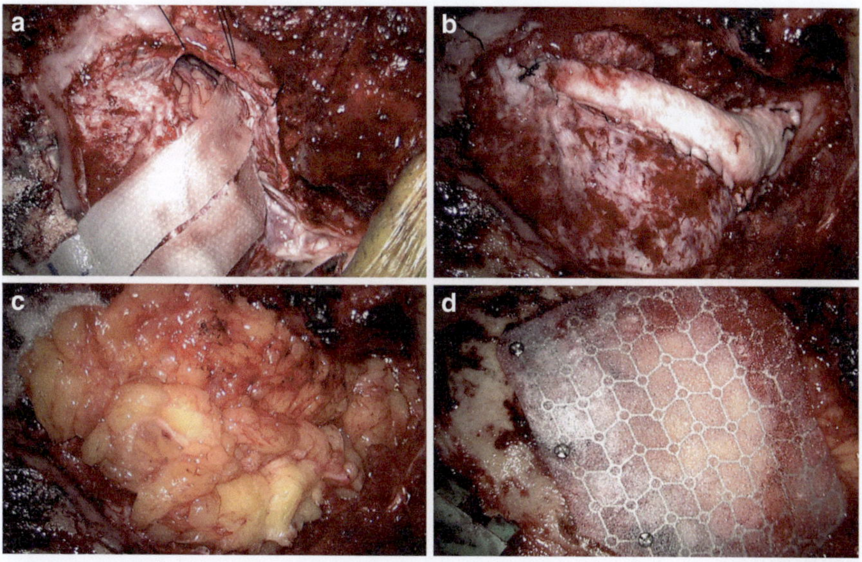

Fig. 15.12 Closure technique for far lateral approach to prevent CSF leakage. (**a**) Dural opening of right far lateral approach. (**b**) An Alloderm dural patch graft is sewn into the defect. (**c**) Autologous fat graft is placed over dural closure in the craniectomy defect. (**d**) A Medpor Titan implant is secured to the skull to buttress the fat graft against the suture line

15.3.10 Occipitocervical Stabilization

There is a risk of destabilization of the craniovertebral junction when performing a far lateral exposure. The craniovertebral junction is stabilized by the occipital condyle, the C1 lateral mass, and the ligamentous attachments at the craniovertebral junction. If these structures are damaged, either by resection or by the tumor itself, an occipito-cervical fusion becomes necessary. A biomechanical study conducted by Vishteh et al. demonstrated significant hypermobility at the atlanto-occipital joint when greater than 50% of the occipital condyle was resected [18]. Further resection of the condyle produced increased hypermobility at C1-C2, especially after 75% resection. However, an anatomical study by Kshettry et al. demonstrated that 50% condylar resection did not lead to significantly increased motion in the cardinal directions [19]. They did find that 75% and 100% resection led to significantly increase the range of motion in the cardinal directions, which indicates that larger resections may necessitate fusion. Another cadaveric study by Mazur et al. showed that changes in the biomechanics of the atlanto-occipital joint may be observed when as little as one-third of the occipital condyle is resected [20]. We generally monitor the patients with interval postoperative CT scans and flexion and extension cervical spine radiographs to detect for any early or delayed occipitocervical instability. We have not experienced any instability when resection of the occipital condyle and jugular tubercle was limited to the posterior one-third, or limited to the proximal hypoglossal canal. However, occipitocervical fusion should be considered when 50% or more of the occipital condyle is resected.

15.4 Conclusion

The far lateral transcondylar transtubercular approach provides excellent exposure with minimal brainstem retraction for the treatment of intradural and extradural lesions found in the craniovertebral junction, inferior clivus, ventral foramen magnum, and the ventral and ventrolateral brainstem. Reduction of the occipital condyle and jugular tubercle is the key maneuver in increasing the lateral viewing angle past the mid-clivus. It is important to keep in mind that the removal of these structures should be tailored to the individual patient and the pathology so that bone is not removed in excess. Removal of more than 50% of the occipital condyle can result in occipitocervical instability, requiring occipitocervical fusion.

References

1. Bertalanffy H, Seeger W. The dorsolateral, suboccipital, transcondylar approach to the lower clivus and anterior portion of the craniocervical junction. Neurosurgery. 1991;29:815–21.
2. Seeger W. Atlas of topographical anatomy of the brain and surrounding structures for neurosurgeons, Neuroradiologists, and Neuropathologists. Wien, New York: Springer-Verlag; 1978.
3. Fukushima T. Manual of skull base dissection. Pittsburgh, PA: AF NeuroVideo, Inc; 1996.
4. Fukushima T. Fukushima manual of skull base dissection. Raleigh, NC: AF NeuroVideo, Inc; 2014.
5. Liu JK, Couldwell WT. Far-lateral transcondylar approach: surgical technique and its application in neurenteric cysts of the cervicomedullary junction. Report of two cases. Neurosurg Focus. 2005;19:E9.
6. Patel SK, Liu JK. Staged bilateral far-lateral approach for bilateral cervicomedullary junction neurenteric cysts in a 10-year-old girl. J Neurosurg Pediatr. 2013;12:274–80.
7. al-Mefty O, Borba LA, Aoki N, Angtuaco E, Pait TG. The transcondylar approach to extradural nonneoplastic lesions of the craniovertebral junction. J Neurosurg. 1996;84:1–6.
8. Nanda A, Vincent DA, Vannemreddy PS, Baskaya MK, Chanda A. Far-lateral approach to intradural lesions of the foramen magnum without resection of the occipital condyle. J Neurosurg. 2002;96:302–9.
9. Arnautovic KI, al-Mefty O, Pait TG, Krisht AF, Husain MM. The suboccipital cavernous sinus. J Neurosurg. 1997;86:252–62.
10. Rhoton JAL. The far-lateral approach and its transcondylar, supracondylar, and paracondylar extensions. Neurosurgery. 2000;47:S195–209.
11. Wen HT, Rhoton JAL, Katsuta T, de Oliveira E. Microsurgical anatomy of the transcondylar, supracondylar, and paracondylar extensions of the far-lateral approach. J Neurosurg. 1997;87:555–85.
12. Kawashima M, Tanriover N, Rhoton JAL, Ulm AJ, Matsushima T. Comparison of the far lateral and extreme lateral variants of the atlanto-occipital transarticular approach to anterior extradural lesions of the craniovertebral junction. Neurosurgery. 2003;53:662–75.
13. Dowd GC, Zeiller S, Awasthi D. Far lateral transcondylar approach: dimensional anatomy. Neurosurgery. 1999;45:95–100.

14. Patel AJ, Gressot LV, Cherian J, Desai SK, Jea A. Far lateral paracondylar versus transcondylar approach in the pediatric age group: CT morphometric analysis. J Clin Neurosci. 2014;21:2194–200.
15. Spektor S, Anderson GJ, McMenomey SO, Horgan MA, Kellogg JX, Delashaw JJB. Quantitative description of the far-lateral transcondylar transtubercular approach to the foramen magnum and clivus. J Neurosurg. 2000;92:824–31.
16. Wanebo JE, Chicoine MR. Quantitative analysis of the transcondylar approach to the foramen magnum. Neurosurgery. 2001;49:934–43.
17. Sen C. The transcondylar approach to the lower clivus, foramen magnum and C1-C2. Clin Neurosurg. 1996;43:113–26.
18. Vishteh AG, Crawford NR, Melton MS, Spetzler RF, Sonntag VK, Dickman CA. Stability of the craniovertebral junction after unilateral occipital condyle resection: a biomechanical study. J Neurosurg. 1999;90:91–8.
19. Kshettry VR, Healy AT, Colbrunn R, Beckler DT, Benzel EC, Recinos PF. Biomechanical evaluation of the craniovertebral junction after unilateral joint-sparing condylectomy: implications for the far lateral approach revisited. J Neurosurg. 2016;127:829–36.
20. Mazur MD, Couldwell WT, Cutler A, Shah LM, Brodke DS, Bachus K, Dailey AT. Occipitocervical instability after far-lateral transcondylar surgery: a biomechanical analysis. Neurosurgery. 2017;80:140–5.

16 Anterolateral and Extreme Lateral Approaches

Kentaro Watanabe, Moujahed Labidi, Shunya Hanakita, Bernard George, and Sébastien Froelich

16.1 Introduction

Lesions of the cranio-vertebral junction (CVJ) are complex lesions to treat because of their deep location and complex surrounding anatomy composed of muscles, ligaments, joints, bony structures, cranial nerves, and critical vessels. They also frequently have an intricate morphology, involve the para-pharyngeal space, extend rostrocaudally, and from one side to the other. CVJ tumors can also extend both in the intradural and extradural compartments, often making closure and reconstruction challenging.

To help choose the optimal surgical route, many anatomically based classification schemes have been proposed for CVJ lesions. One such classification system is based on the location of the lesion in relation to the dura mater and divides CVJ lesions in three categories:

K. Watanabe · S. Hanakita · B. George · S. Froelich (✉)
Department of Neurosurgery, Hôpital Lariboisière, Assistance Pubique—Hôpitaux de Paris, Paris, France

Paris Diderot University, Paris, France
e-mail: Sebastien.froelich@aphp.fr, sebastien.froelich@lrb.aphp.fr

M. Labidi
Department of Neurosurgery, Hôpital Lariboisière, Assistance Pubique—Hôpitaux de Paris, Paris, France

Paris Diderot University, Paris, France

Division of Neurosurgery, Centre Hospitalier de l'Université de Montréal, Montréal, QC, Canada

E. Tessitore et al. (eds.), *Surgery of the Cranio-Vertebral Junction*,
https://doi.org/10.1007/978-3-030-18700-2_16

- *Intradural lesions*, such as lower clivus, foramen magnum, and C1-C2 meningiomas and schwannomas. Posterior circulation aneurysms can also be included in this category.
- *Extradural lesions*, which most often are tumors of bony origin from C1-C2, the occipital condyle, and lower clivus. Prototypical lesions are chordomas and chondrosarcomas, but also include plasmocytoma, lymphoma, secondary tumors, etc.
- *Mixed extra- and intradural lesions* of the CVJ, which are also most frequently chordomas and chondrosarcomas but also include glomus tumors and dumbbell tumors of the jugular and hypoglossal foramina.

The precise location of the tumor in the antero-posterior and lateral axes must also be taken into account in the surgical strategy: (1) anterior arch/clivus, (2) lateral mass of C1-C2/occipital condyle, and (3) posterior arch and occipital bone. In fact, many surgical approaches have been developed to reach these different anatomical regions and the surgeon must carefully select which is the most suitable route to be able to reach all tumor extensions. Among these surgical approaches, the retrocondylar and transcondylar posterolateral "far lateral," the extreme lateral transcondylar and the extreme lateral infrajugular transcondylar exposure (ELITE), with its anterolateral ELITE, and dorsolateral ELITE variations [1–15]. Each of these surgical approaches has specific indications, operative nuances, and limitations. In and around the foramen magnum, the surgeon must also be able to gain exposure and control of the jugular foramen, the vertebral artery, the occipital condyle, the dens, and the lower cranial nerves in the neck (Fig. 16.1).

In 1995, Bernard George et al. described the anterolateral approach (ALA) to access extradural and mixed intra- and extradural lesions of the anterior aspect of

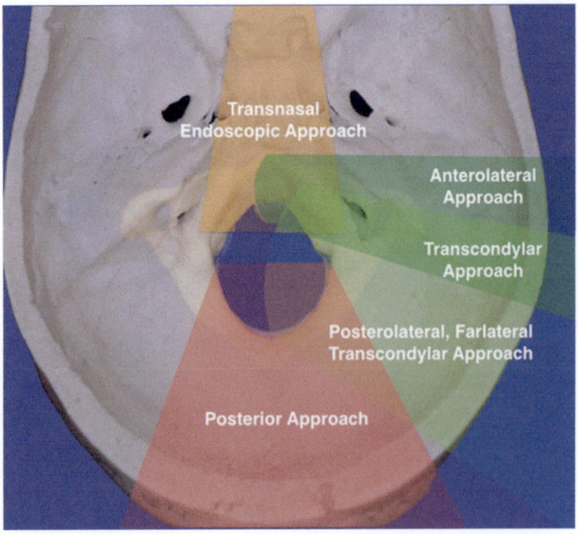

Fig. 16.1 Surgical corridors to the craniovertebral junction

the lower clivus and C1-C2 [3]. He also championed the general principles of vertebral artery management. In comparison to other lateral approaches to the CVJ, the ALA provides a very unique trajectory that is more "down-up" and from the high cervical to intracranial compartment. Conversely, the ELITE approaches have a trajectory that traverses the intracranial compartment first, before reaching the high cervical region [13, 16].

In this chapter, we summarize these different "lateral approaches" and focus particularly on the anterolateral approach. In addition, we describe extensions of the ALA, including classic skull base techniques such as vertebral artery transposition, but also endoscopic assistance. In fact, endoscopic visualization through transcervical exposures provides a wide range of possibilities in the CVJ, which we will discuss in detail in this chapter.

Through cadaveric dissections, we will first review the surgical anatomy relevant to the ALA and describe, step-by-step, the surgical technique to expose the CVJ through an ALA. Finally, clinical cases are presented in order to illustrate potential indications for the ALA and its different variations.

16.2 Anterolateral Approach

The anterolateral approach (ALA) was developed by Bernard George et al. as a novel surgical route for the anterior and lateral aspects of the CVJ. In fact, this region is difficult to reach though a posterior route without manipulation of neurological structures. Although it can be adequate in some cases, an anterior route to the lower CVJ, such as the submandibular approach, is usually limited by the mandibular bone and the salivary glands. The surgical trajectory of the ALA to the cranio-vertebral junction is from inferior to superior and from posterior to anterior. In addition to the cervical vertebrae, that are seen from a lateral perspective, the ALA allows exposure of the lower clivus and jugular foramen from below.

However, the first, second, and third segments of the vertebral artery (VA), located in the foramen transversarium of C1 to C6 vertebrae, is located in the center of the surgical field in an ALA. Therefore, careful management of the VA is an important issue in this area and has preoperative, operative, and postoperative consequences.

16.3 Differential Diagnosis of CVJ Lesions and Indications for ALA (cf. Table 16.1)

ALA is mainly indicated for lesions involving the occipital condyle, C0-C1 joint, lateral mass, and anterior arch of C1, odontoid process, lateral mass, and body of C2.

Table 16.2 summarizes the key characteristics of the different surgical approaches that can be discussed along with the ALA to treat lesions at the CVJ.

Table 161 The history of surgery of the lateral craniocervical junction and differences of the name of approach, a position, a skin incision, exposures of cervical area, vertebral translocation, and a target lesion, between the surgeons

Author (year)	Name of approach	Target lesion	Position	Skin incision	w/o high cervical exposure	w/o VA transposition	w/o mastoidectomy	Main corridor
Heros [4]	Far lateral	VA, VA-BA junction, proximal BA trunk, AVM of the inferolateral cerebellum	Park-bench	Vertical paramedian	–	–	–	Extreme lateral removal of the rim of the foramen magnum, C1 laminectomy
Yamamoto (1990) [17]	Unilateral suboccipital transcondylar	Intradural, anterior to lower brainstem, upper cervical cord, VA, basilar trunk	Sitting	Paramedian	+	–	–	Medial third, C1 laminectomy
Bertalanffy and Seeger (1991) [18]	Dorsolateral suboccipital transcondylar	Condyle, hypoglossal canal	Sitting	Vertical paramedian, straight, trans muscular		+	–	Condyle
George and Lot [3]	Anterolateral	VA, O-C condyle, anterior arch of C1, C2, C3 corpus body	Supine head rotation 30–45	Post-auricular linear incision, mastoid to cervical	+	+/–	–	C0, C1 condyle, C1 lateral mass
George (1997) [19]	Posterolateral	Posterior arch of C1, intradural CC junction	3/4 lateral position	Hockey stick	–	–	–	Retrosigmoid + C1, C2 posterior lamina
Fukushima (1996) [20]	Antero lateral ELITE[a]	Jugular foramen, mid-lower clivus, dumbbell-type schwannoma, Glomus meningioma	Supine head lateral	Post-auricular question mark	+	–	+	Infralabyrinthine transjugular approach with high cervical exposure, C1 laminectomy

Fukushima (1996) [20]	Dorsolateral ELITE[b]	Lower clivus, foramen magnum, VA_PICA complex aneurysm, V-B junction	Lateral	Lazy S	–	+/–	–	Infrajugular transcondylar transjugular tubercle
Sen and Sekhar [11]	Extreme lateral transcondylar	Foramen magnum, C1-C2 meningioma, ventral of brainstem	Modified Park-bench lateral	Lazy S	–	+	–/+	Retrosigmoid
Babu and Sekhar (1994) [21]	Extreme lateral transcondylar	Extradural tumor, intradural tumor	Modified Park-bench lateral	U shaped or C shaped	–	+	–/+	Intradural lesion; one-third to one half condyle resection, extradural lesion; transfacetal
Canalis et al. (1993) [22]	Lateral	Extradural tumor, intradural tumor	Supine and head rotated	Post-auricular to hyoid bone at midline	+	+	Partial	C1 laminectomy
Al-Mefty [1]	Transcondylar	Odontoid, extradural	Half-lateral decubitus	C shaped	+/–	+/–	Partial	OC-C1 condyle, odontoid
Matsushima (2010) [7]	Transcondylar fossa approach	Intradural lower clivus, foramen magnum lesion	Lateral	U shaped	–	+/–	–	Condyle fossa (C0 foramen magnum), infracondyle, transjugular tubercle

(continued)

Table 16.1 (continued)

Author (year)	Name of approach	Target lesion	Position	Skin incision	w/o high cervical exposure	w/o VA transposition	w/o mastoidectomy	Main corridor
Vallée (1993) [23]	Juxta-trans condylar approach	Tumor and aneurysm of the anterior or anterior-lateral of the foramen magnum	Lateral	Hockey stick	–	–	+	Condyle, suboccipital
S. Froelich	Endoscope assisted minimum, transcondylar	Medial jugular, clivus, anterior arch of C1, odontoid, contralateral condyle	Lateral	Small C shaped	–	+/–	–	Infrajugular bulb, transcondyle
S. Froelich	Endoscope assisted transmastoid	Medial jugular clivus, suprajugular foramen, mid-clivus, petrous apex, foramen lacerum, contralateral jugular foramen	Lateral	Small C shaped	+/–	–	+	Infralabyrinthine, suprajugular

AVM arteriovenous malformation, *BA* basilar artery, *PICA* posterior inferior cerebellar artery, *VA* vertebral artery
[a]Extreme lateral infralabyrinthine transjugular exposure with high cervical exposure
[b]Extreme lateral infrajugular transcondylar transtubercle exposure

Table 16.2 Surgical indications of the ALA, PLA

	Indications	Pathology
Anterolateral approach (ALA)	Extradural lesions Bone lesion C1-C2 Midline/lateral	– Chordomas – Myeloma – Metastasis – Tuberculosis – Primary bone tumors (chondroid tumor, sarcoma, fibrous dysplasia, osteoid osteoma)
Posterolateral approach	Intradural lesions Lower clivus/C2	– Meningiomas (foramen magnum, lower clivus) – Hemangioblastomas – Schwannomas (vestibular schwannoma, jugular foramen schwannoma, hypoglossal schwannoma) – Neurofibromas – Glomus tumors – Vascular pathology (VA, PICA, BA)
Extended endoscopic endonasal approach	Extra- and intradural lesions Midline Above C2 Soft tumors	– Chordomas – Primary bone tumors (chondroid tumor, sarcoma, myeloma) – Rheumatoid arthritis – Congenital bony abnormalities

ALA Anterolateral Approach, *BA* basilar artery, *PICA* posterior inferior cerebellar artery, *PLA* Posterior lateral approach, *VA* vertebral artery

16.4 Preoperative Considerations

A detailed study of the preoperative images should be done by an experienced multidisciplinary skull base team. An angio-CT of the vessels of the neck with bony reconstructions is mandatory. The head and cervical spine CT scan should be examined in detail to identify all areas of bony destruction of infiltration that need to be resected and/or reconstructed. All cases should also have an MRI of the head and cervical spine preoperatively, including contrast-enhanced sequences. In tumor cases, all extensions of the lesion to be resected should be delineated and recorded. Careful attention should also be given to extensions causing neurological compression, those that will not be accessible to adjuvant radiation therapy (i.e., close to the brainstem, bone infiltration, or near metallic implants, etc.).

The relationship of the lesion with the lower cranial nerves, namely the 9th, 10th, and 11th at the level of the jugular foramen and the 12th cranial nerve in its hypoglossal canal is another critical element to establish preoperatively. Their function should be assessed and documented, and in cases of severe preoperative dysfunction, a precautionary tracheostomy should be discussed in order to protect the airways during the postoperative period. When the lower cranial nerves function is impaired on one side and the contralateral nerves are involved or at risk during surgery, care should be taken to avoid catastrophic bilateral deficits and such a risk should be discussed frankly and in details with the patient and his/her family.

Preoperative assessment of CVJ instability with dynamic studies may be required in some tumor cases. Extent of condylar osteolysis, the presence of "dynamic" cervical pain and/or a hypoglossal palsy may be useful as clinical and radiological indicators of potential CVJ instability.

16.4.1 Vertebral Artery

Envisioning the precise localization of the VA is imperative at all times during an ALA. The VA is divided into four segments: (1) V1, or the “ostial” segment, is located between the subclavian artery and the *foramen transversarium* of C6, (2) V2, the “transversary segment” runs from C6 to C2 in the *foramen transversarium*, (3) V3 or the “suboccipital” segment extends from the *foramen transversarium* of C2 to the point of entry of the VA in the intradural compartment, and (4) V4 is the “intradural” segment [14]. The V3 segment can be further divided into a vertical segment between the transverse foramen of C2 and the transverse foramen of C1 and a horizontal segment along the posterior arch of C1.

The VA is surrounded by a dense venous plexus, which should be kept intact and not be disrupted when manipulating the VA, in order to avoid profuse venous bleeding.

Moreover, anatomic variations of the VA are frequent, including loops and anomalous locations. Elderly patients are particularly prone to vascular ectopia, atherosclerosis, and calcifications. Bone anatomical variations such as arcuate foramen, occipitalization of the atlas, and defect of the posterior arch of C1, defect of the transverse foramen of C1 can also occur leading to surgeon disorientation and VA injury [24–26].

One should also be aware that with the head rotation that is needed for ALA, the vertical segment of the V3 becomes horizontal and can be identified immediately below the posterior arch of C1 (Fig. 16.2).

In other cases, there can be an extradural origin of the posterior inferior cerebellar artery (PICA) [24, 27]. It is thus critical that anatomical variations be recognized preoperatively on a CTA.

When the tumor involves the vertebral artery, it is important to clarify if and how the VA can be sacrificed. In some pathology, resection of an invaded VA may be required for oncological control of the tumor while in other tumors, adjuvant therapy is sufficient to ensure long-term control of residual tumor. Ideally, this should be discussed in multidisciplinary tumor boards. In cases where VA ligature/resection is considered, a balloon test occlusion (BTO) should be performed preoperatively. If the patient fails the BTO, a revascularization procedure may be required before the actual resection can take place safely.

16.5 Surgical Anatomy and Technique

16.5.1 Positioning

The patient is placed supine and the head rotated laterally, approximately 30–45° to the contralateral side (Fig. 16.2a–d). Placing the head in slight extension is

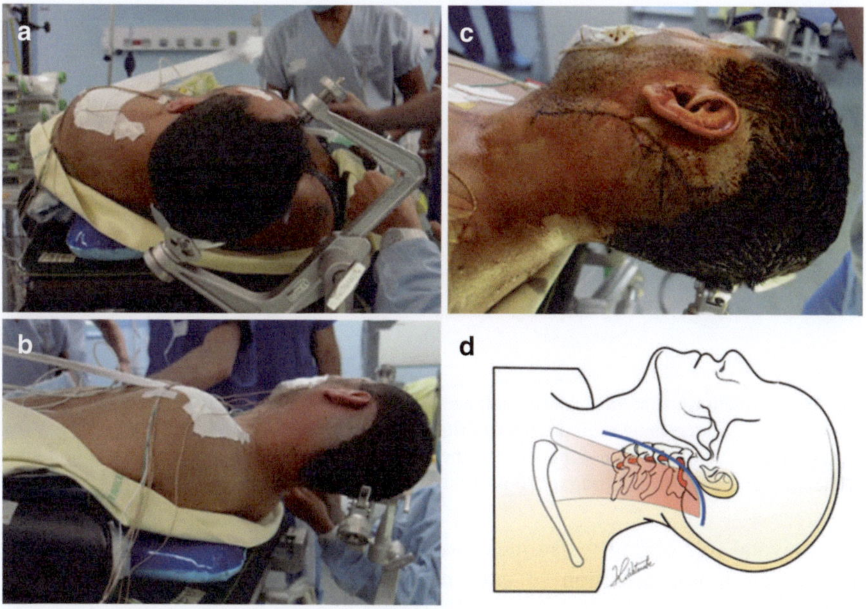

Fig. 16.2 Surgical positioning in an anterolateral approach. (**a**) The patient is placed supine and the head is rotated laterally, approximately 30–45° to the contralateral side. A Mayfield head holder can be used in most cases (as shown in the figure), but a "horseshoe" headrest can allow neutral repositioning of the head during cases when fixation or vertebral reconstruction are planned. (**b**) A wide area around the planned skin incision should be prepped to have a large working space. The head should not be rotated too much. (**c**) Skin incision in an anterolateral approach. It is made along the upper third of the anterior border of the sternocleidomastoid muscle and is curved at the level of the mastoid process (skin markings) and the occipital crest

important to disengage the angle of the mandible. A horseshoe headrest is preferred since it allows modification of the position of the head if necessary. More importantly, if the need for osteosynthesis or vertebral reconstruction arises during the case, the head can then be placed in a neutral position to do so.

The shoulders should be as flat as possible and should not impede the surgeon. Rotation of the head can be adjusted depending on the location of the lesion and its extensions; with increasing rotation, the anterior arch of C1 becomes progressively hidden by the transverse process of C1 and the vertebral artery (Fig. 16.3).

16.5.2 Neurophysiological Monitoring and Surgical Adjuncts

Electromyographic (EMG) monitoring of the 7th, 9th, 10th, 11th, and 12th nerves, motor and sensory evoked potentials are done in all cases of ALA. Direct stimulation with an EMG probe can be useful in cranial nerve identification and preservation (especially 11th cranial nerve). Neurophysiological monitoring with somatosensory evoked potentials (SSEPs) and motor evoked potentials (MEPs) also

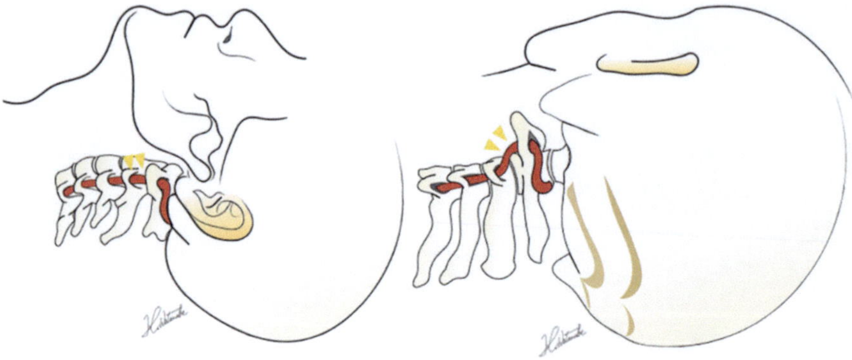

Fig. 16.3 Rotation of the head can be adjusted depending on the location of the lesion and its extensions; With increasing rotation, the anterior arch of C1 becomes progressively hidden by the transverse process of C1. More importantly, the vertebral artery's trajectory is altered by rotation of the head as the vertical portion of V3 is "horizontalized"

has a pivotal role during the surgical positioning of unstable high cervical lesions and during tumor resection in case of brainstem or high cervical medullary compression.

Neuronavigation is not used routinely since its precision in the CVJ, especially through an ALA, is usually inadequate. Electromagnetic neuronavigation and intra-operative imaging might be used in select cases. We routinely use the micro-Doppler probe in all ALA cases.

16.5.3 Skin Incision

The skin incision is made along the upper third of the anterior border of the sterno-cleidomastoid (SCM) muscle and is curved at the level of the mastoid process and the occipital crest (Fig. 16.3). The anterior border of the SCM can be approximated by a line connecting the manubrium and the mastoid tip. The height of the incision can be adapted to the surgical goals and strategy. For instance, when a mastoidec-tomy is planned, the incision needs to reach the level of the transverse sinus. The inferior border of the incision also depends on the pathology at hand, but 5–6 cm below from the mastoid tip on the anterior border of the sternocleidomastoid muscle is usually adequate for CVJ exposures.

16.5.4 High Cervical Dissection and Exposure of the Vertebral Artery

16.5.4.1 Dissection Between the SCM and Internal Jugular Vein

After the skin and hypodermis are incised, the first layer that is encountered is the platysma, which is dissected and incised parallel to the skin incision. The SCM is then exposed and its medial border followed. The great auricular nerve can be dissected on the surface of the SCM (Fig. 16.4a). This nerve can be used for nerve reconstruction in case of cranial nerve injury or sutured back at the end of the procedure. The cervical fascia is then opened along the medial aspect of the SCM muscle and the internal jugular vein (IJV) is identified (Fig. 16.4b, c). The facial vein is usually encountered and can be ligated safely. The mastoid insertion of the SCM is then cut and the insertion of the splenius capitis muscle and longissimus muscle are detached from the mastoid process and occipital bone. These muscles are translocated posteriorly (Fig. 16.4d, e).

16.5.4.2 Identification of the Posterior Edge of the Digastric Muscle

The IJV is dissected and followed distally up to the posterior border of the digastric muscle. The digastric muscle is found under the SCM, and can be easily identified and traced anteriorly starting from its groove posterior to the mastoid tip. During this dissection, the occipital artery (OA) can be found coming from under the digastric muscle. The OA can be ligated or preserved to serve as a donor vessel if the need for revascularization arises.

16.5.4.3 Detachment and Mobilization of the Digastric Muscle

In order to further expose the jugular foramen and lower cranial nerve that exit from the foramen, it is necessary to detach the digastric muscle from the digastric groove of the mastoid process and to mobilize it inferiorly (Fig. 16.4f). The facial nerve exits from the stylomastoid foramen and runs medially to the deep fascia of the digastric muscle toward the inferior aspect of the parotid gland. In this segment, the facial nerve gives off a branch to the digastric muscle, about 1 cm below the mastoid tip. Although the facial nerve branch is usually covered with fat tissue, manipulation, partial resection, and/or retraction of the digastric muscle should be done carefully so as not to injure the facial nerve. Thus, when the digastric muscle is sectioned, the anterior aponeurosis of the muscle should be preserved to protect the facial nerve.

A common mechanism of injury of the facial nerve is prolonged and overly aggressive retraction with autostatic retractors that are positioned too high immediately below the tip of the mastoid.

16.5.4.4 Identification of the Accessory Nerve and Dissection of the Fat Pad (Fig. 16.4d, e)

The C1 lateral process, which can be easily identified by palpation, is found approximately 1 cm below the tip of the mastoid. The C1 lateral process is a very important landmark for the vertebral artery (VA) and the accessory nerve (XIth). In most patients, the XIth can be found 0.5–1 cm below the transverse process of C1. From there, the nerve runs more or less obliquely superomedially to infero-laterally in direction of the medial border of the SCM muscle at the C3–C4 level. The carotid fat pad, located in the triangle formed by the posterior edge of the digastric muscle, the splenius muscle, and internal jugular vein encloses the XIth. The XIth is

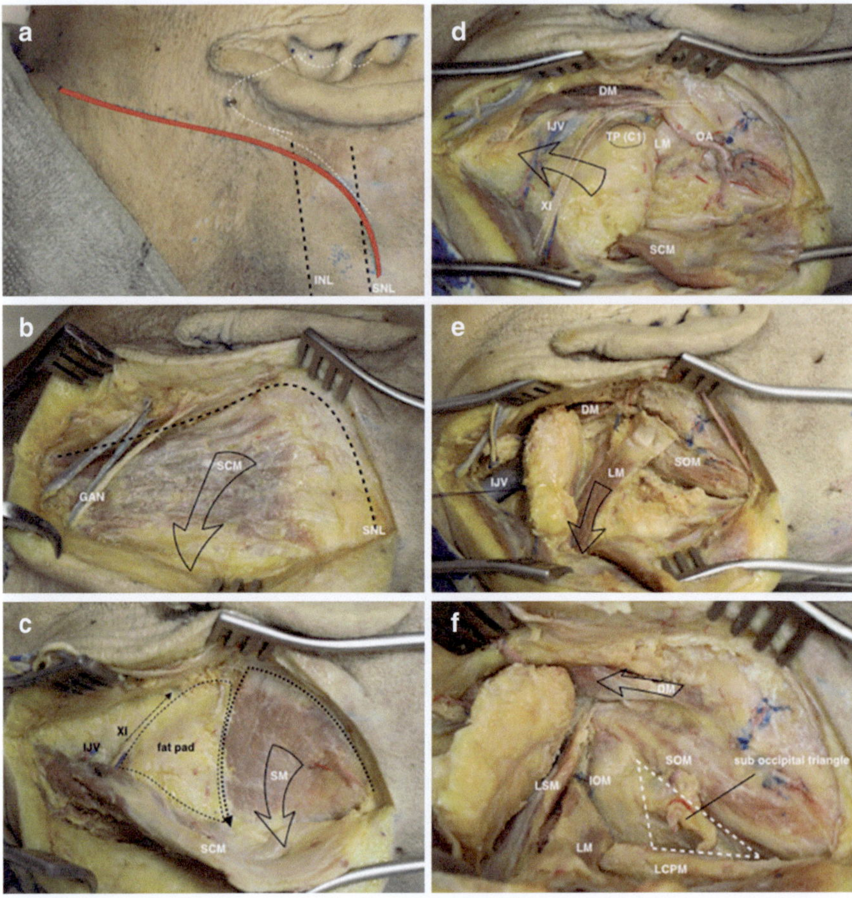

Fig. 16.4 (**a**) The skin incision is made along the upper third of the anterior border of the sternocleidomastoid (SCM) muscle and is curved at the level of the mastoid process and the occipital crest. (**b**) The Greater auricular nerve can be seen running above the SCM. The SCM is detached from the mastoid and transposed inferiorly. *GAN* greater auricular nerve, *SCM* sternocleidomastoid muscle. (**c**) Under the SCM, the splenius muscle and a fat pad are exposed. The accessory nerve can be identified in the fat pad inferiorly. *IJV* internal jugular vein, *XI* accessory nerve. (**d**) After transposition of the splenius muscle posteriorly, the fat pad can also be detached from the surrounding tissues and can be transposed inferiorly and kept as a protective layer for the accessory nerve. *DM* digastric muscle, *IJV* internal jugular vein, *OA* occipital artery, *LM* longissimus muscle, *TP* transvers process, *XI* accessory nerve. (**e**) Under the fat pad, the longissimus muscle can be exposed and detached from the mastoid inferiorly. The superior oblique muscle is exposed. *DM* digastric muscle, *IJV* internal jugular vein, *LM* longissimus muscle, *SOM* superior oblique muscle. (**f**) The suboccipital triangle, defined by the superior oblique muscle, the inferior oblique muscle, and the rectus capitis posterior major muscle. *DM* digastric muscle, *IOM* superior oblique muscle, *LM* longissimus muscle, *LSM* Levator scapulae muscle, *SOM* superior oblique muscle

superficial in this fat pad and can be readily detected with electric stimulation. Once the XIth nerve is identified, the fat pad can then be detached superiorly and mobilized downward from the digastric, splenius muscles and from the dense fibro-fatty tissue covering the suboccipital triangle. It is then used as a natural protection for the retraction of the XIth nerve inferiorly [28].

16.5.4.5 Identification of the Suboccipital Triangle (Fig. 16.4f)

In addition to the transverse process, the suboccipital triangle is also an important landmark for identification of the VA. This triangle is defined by the superior oblique muscle, the inferior oblique muscle, and the rectus capitis posterior major and is covered by a layer of dense fibro-fatty tissue. It is located beneath the semispinalis capitis.

At the level of the C1 posterior lamina, the vertebral artery as well as the vertebral venous plexus and C1 nerve root can be found in the center of this triangle. Muscular branches often arise from the horizontal segment of the VA in this area. Rarely, a PICA with an extradural origin may originate from the V3 segment on its horizontal portion, just outside the dura or further laterally above the transverse foramen of C1. The incidence of an extradural origin of the PICA is between 5 and 20% (George). In this configuration, the PICA courses parallel to the VA and the C1 nerve root extradurally.

16.5.4.6 Exposure of the Transverse Process (TP) of C1

To fully expose the transverse process of C1 and easily identify the foramen transversarium at this level; the muscles inserted on the TP of C1 are detached. Five muscles insert on the TP of C1: the rectus capitis lateralis, the superior oblique, the inferior oblique, the splenius cervicalis, and the levator scapulae muscles (Fig. 16.5a, b). The muscle insertion on the TP of C1 are progressively coagulated and sectioned until the posterior aspect of the TP of C1 is identified and further exposed using subperiosteal dissection. The opening of the transverse foramen is identified with a dissector along the superior and inferior aspect of the TP of C1, in this area, large venous plexuses are found in the retrocondylar fossa, around the vertebral artery and between the TP of C1 and the lateral mass of C2. These venous plexuses should be left intact as much as possible to avoid profuse bleeding. Coagulation is often ineffective while injectable hemostatic agents are usually sufficient in controlling such venous bleeding (Fig. 16.5d–f).

16.5.4.7 VA Exposure

Safe tumor removal and adequate access requires mobilization, translocation, or at least identification of the VA above and below the transverse foramen of C1 (V2 and V3 segments) (Fig. 16.5c). The superior surface of the posterior arch of C1 has an osseous groove in which the VA is located, the *sulcus arteriosus*. The safest way to identify the VA is to follow laterally the posterior arch of C1 from the midline. The sulcus arteriosus, along the superior surface of the posterior arch of C1, is exposed subperiostally, from medial to lateral until the superior opening of the transverse foramen of C1 is identified. It is imperative that this dissection be done

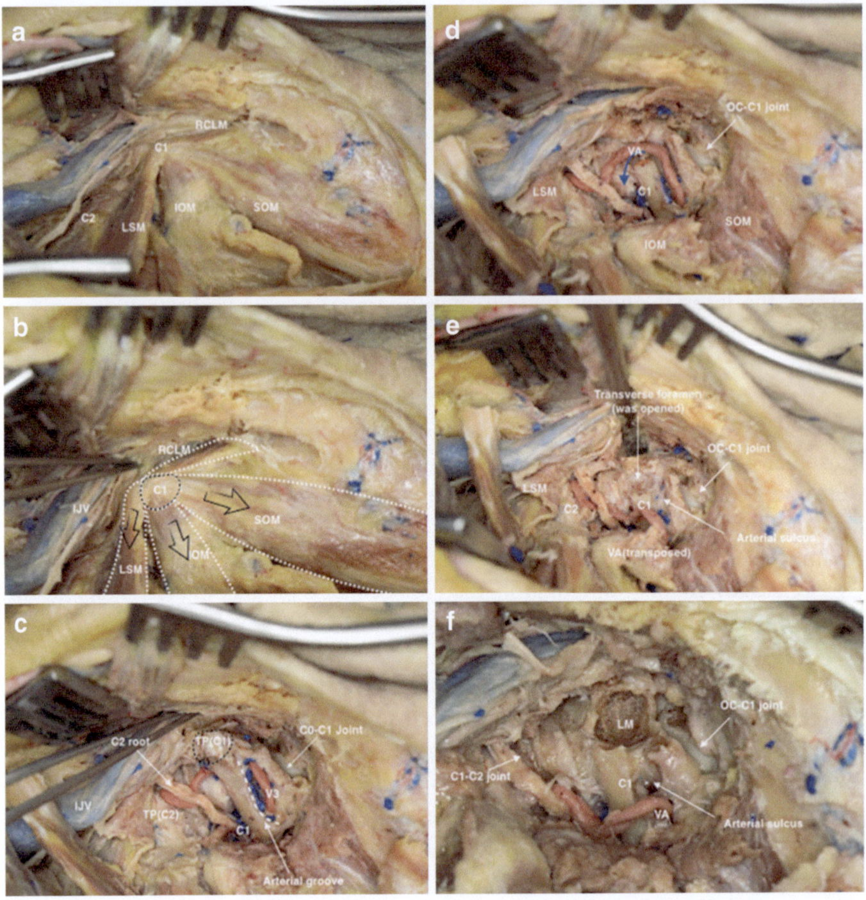

Fig. 16.5 (**a**) C1 transverse process is exposed and the rectus capitis lateralis muscle is exposed below the mastoid. *IOM* superior oblique muscle, *LM* longissimus muscle, *LSM* Levator scapulae muscle, *SOM* superior oblique muscle. (**b**) The muscles which are attached to the C1 transverse process can be coagulated and detached. *IOM* superior oblique muscle, *LM* longissimus muscle, *LSM* levator scapulae muscle, *SOM* superior oblique muscle, *RCLM* rectus capitis lateralis muscle. (**c**) After transposition of the cervical muscles and the transvers process of C1 has been denuded, the vertebral artery (V3) can be seen in the C1 arterial groove and between the C1 and C2. *TP* transverse process, *IJV* internal jugular vein. (**d**) The transverse foramen is opened, uncovering this whole 3^d^ segment of the vertebral artery. *IOM* superior oblique muscle, *LM* longissimus muscle, *LSM* levator scapulae muscle, *SOM* superior oblique muscle, *VA* vertebral artery. (**e**) The vertebral artery is transposed posteriorly and medially from the transverse foramen. *LSM* levator scapulae muscle, *VA* vertebral artery. (**f**) The transverse process is drilled and lateral mass is exposed. *LM* lateral mass, *VA* vertebral artery

subperiosteally. In fact, the periosteum acts as a protective layer for the venous plexus around the VA. Then, the TP of C1 is removed (Fig. 16.5c, d). The tip can be first removed with a rongeur. Once the cancellous bone of the TP is exposed, we favor the use of a high-speed diamond drill in order to progressively unroof the transverse foramen of C1. The last shell of cortical bone that form the posterior margin of the foramen is then removed with a kerrison rongeur. Once the transverse foramen of C1 is completely open, the third segment of the VA can be separated from the foramen and fully mobilized. The vertebral artery can also be followed downward toward the transverse foramen of C2. At this level, the C2 nerve root is identified. Once the transverse foramen of C2 is identified, the foramen can be opened, and the TP of C2 removed to allow further mobilization of the VA (Fig. 16.5e, f).

16.5.4.8 Rectus Capitis Lateralis Muscle (RCLM) (Fig. 16.5a, b)

The rectus capitis lateralis muscle (RCLM) is one of the key muscles to access the anterior aspect of the cranio-vertebral junction. The RCLM is a short muscle attached to the upper surface of the TP of C1 and to the jugular process located between the mastoid process and the occipital condyle. To access the cranio-vertebral segment of the IX, X, XI, XII nerves and the IJV or the anterior part of C1, the odontoid process, and the lower clivus, both the TP of C1 and the RCLM should be removed. If a tumor extends to the high cervical region, in the case of a dumbbell-type jugular foramen lesion or a lower clivus and cervical chordoma, removing the RCLM is usually required to gain enough space to access the anterior aspect of the CVJ and benefit from the look up view to the jugular foramen and clivus that the ALA can provide.

16.5.5 Variations and Extensions

16.5.5.1 Transposition of the VA

If the VA is not already occluded by the tumor and when the condyle, the lateral mass of C1, odontoid process or the clivus is invaded by tumor, transposition of the VA is often necessary to fully expose the lesion. In case of a soft chordoma, full transposition may be avoided. After identifying the horizontal segment of the vertebral artery along the sulcus arteriosus, the TP of C1 is removed and the transverse foramen of C1 is opened. The V3 segment is then displaced posteriorly and out of the transverse foramen of C1, freeing a corridor to the lateral mass of C1 and beyond. The periosteal sheath and vertebral plexus around the VA should be kept intact to protect the VA, reduce venous bleeding, and minimize the risk of dissection. When additional mobility is needed, the transverse foramen of C2 can also be opened, liberating completely the suboccipital segment of the VA.

After translocation of the VA and exposure of the lateral mass of C1, the anterior arch of C1 is followed in direction of the midline and even to the contralateral side of the anterior arch (Fig. 16.6a). Subsequent resection of the tumor infiltrating the lateral mass of C1, the odontoid process and surrounding ligaments (alar, transverse and apical) and the contralateral mass of C1 can be performed (Fig. 16.6b, c). Care must be taken to preserve the contralateral vertebral artery, especially if the ipsilateral vertebral artery is occluded by the tumor or has been already been sacrificed during the surgery. The use of a Doppler probe is mandatory to identify the contralateral VA.

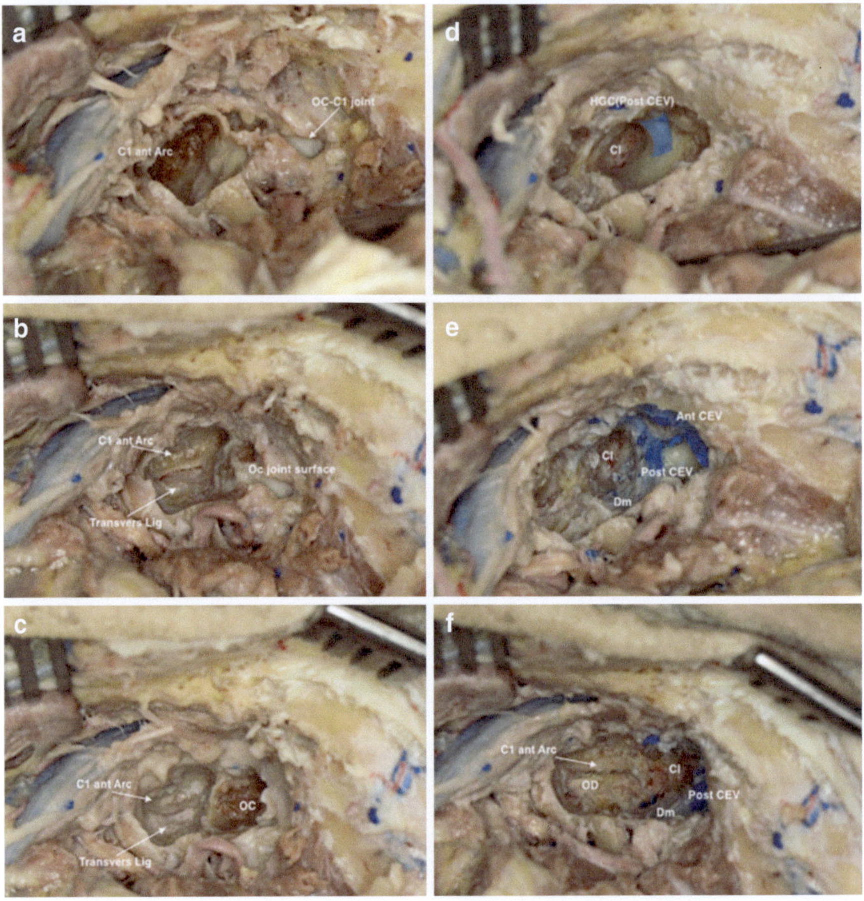

Fig. 16.6 (**a**) After drilling of the C1 lateral mass, the anterior arch of C1 can be accessed. *C1 ant Arc* C1 anterior arch. (**b**) The C1 anterior arch is drilled until the midline, the transverse ligament of the odontoid process is exposed. *Transverse lig* transverse ligament. (**c**) The occipital condyle can be also drilled to gain an upper view to the lower clivus. *C1 ant Arc* C1 anterior arch, *OC* occipital condyle, *Transvers lig* transverse ligament. (**d**) The hypoglossal canal with the posterior condyle emissary vein can be seen in the condyle. Anterior to the hypoglossal canal, an area of cancellous bone is found. This finding indicates entry into the lower aspect of the clivus. *Cl* clivus, *HGC* hypoglossal canal, *Post CEV* posterior condyle emissary vein. (**e**) The anterior condyle emissary vein and the posterior condyle emissary vein can be skeletonized during condylar drilling. These veins connect to the occipital venous plexus. *Cl* clivus, *HGC* hypoglossal canal, *Ant CEV* anterior condyle emissary vein, *Post CEV* posterior condyle emissary vein. (**f**) The view obtained after drilling the anterior arch of C1 and condyle. The odontoid process and dura mater of the spine are exposed. *C1 ant Arc* C1 anterior arch, *Cl* clivus, *HGC* hypoglossal canal, *Dm* dura mater, *OD* odontoid process, *Post CEV* posterior condyle emissary vein

16.5.5.2 Condylar Resection

In case of a tumor extending in the condyle and the lower clivus, such as chordomas, chondroid tumors, myeloma, hypoglossal schwannoma, etc. a resection of the condyle may become necessary. To gain adequate exposure of these lesions, the inferior part of the sigmoid sinus and the jugular bulb is skeletonized. The retrocondylar fossa is exposed and the posterior condylar emissary vein are identified. After partial condylectomy, the anterior condylar emissary vein can also be seen (Fig. 16.6d, e). It runs with the hypoglossal nerve in the hypoglossal canal and is exposed with the inferior aspect of the sigmoid sinus and jugular bulb (Fig. 16.6e, f). This is the combination of an anterolateral approach and a far lateral transcondylar approach.

It is important to limit bony resection if it is not necessary for surgical exposure or from an oncological standpoint. However, oftentimes the tumor has already compromised the structural integrity of the C0-C1 joint. When involvement of the condyle is superior to 75%, occipitocervical fusion is usually necessary, although some reconstruction strategies can obviate the need for rigid fixation. Limiting the drilling to the posterolateral third of the condyle also reduces the risk of injury to the hypoglossal canal and nerve, which is located in the anteromedial aspect of the condyle.

To access the anterior arch of C1 or the odontoid process, opening of the C0-C1 joint with condylar and lateral mass removal provide an adequate trajectory. Slight downward mobilization of the horizontal segment of the V3 segment of the VA is needed to expose the lateral mass of C1. Rather than a complete translocation of the VA and resection of the rectus capitis lateralis muscle, this can be an alternative strategy to reach the anterior aspect of the CVJ.

16.5.5.3 Inferior Extension to the C2-4 Vertebrae

When the target lesion extends inferiorly to C2-C3, exposure of the V2 segment of the VA is necessary [14]. The C2 lateral process and the longus colli and longus capitis muscles can be exposed and removed to expose the VA and gain access to the body of C2 and the lower cervical vertebrae. In this situation, care must be taken to avoid injuring the sympathetic chain and the superior cervical ganglion, which run under the prevertebral fascia over the longus coli muscle. The vagus nerve gives off the superior and recurrent laryngeal nerves. These nerves run medially to the carotid-jugular sheath and, contrarily to an anterior approach, are not at risk of injury. However, care must be taken not to compress the vagal nerve in order to avoid laryngeal nerve dysfunction.

16.5.5.4 Intradural Extension, Combined Extradural, and Intradural Approach

In cases when the tumor originates intradurally, the far lateral transcondylar approach is usually preferred as a larger surface of posterior fossa dura can be exposed and better neurovascular control can be insured than through an ALA. When there is extradural extension of a mostly intradural tumor, for example a meningioma invading the clival bone, these extensions can often be reached transdurally though the intradural exposure provided by the far lateral transcondylar or posterolateral approach. Similarly, and as it is often the case for chordomas, intradural tumor extensions of mostly extradural tumors can usually be resected through the ALA extradural exposure, after tumor resection has provided the space and corridor to do so.

16.5.5.5 Endoscope Assistance Through an ALA

In addition to classic skull base techniques such as mastoidectomy, unroofing the hypoglossal canal, or transposition of the vertebral artery, the use of endoscopic assistance has also proven to be an invaluable tool to increase the exposure provided by the ALA. The endoscope increases both illumination and visualization in these deep locations. It should be used as a tool to navigate and operate in the depths of the triangles defined by the lower cranial nerves and vertebral artery. When using the endoscope through these "deep keyholes," further tumor resection can be accomplished in the lower clivus more anteriorly in the prevertebral retropharyngeal space, medially and inferiorly in the periodontoid region and, controlaterally in the opposite lateral mass of C1, in and around the odontoid process and around the contralateral occipital condyle.

Through the condylar corridor, and with careful protection of the hypoglossal nerve, endoscopic assistance can provide visualization of tumor extensions higher up into the middle and superior third of the clivus, toward the petrous apex and sphenoid sinus. With the cervical muscles retracted inferiorly and the high cervical dissection already providing the look up trajectory, exposure can indeed reach the level of the sphenoid sinus. When the tumor is soft and easily aspirated, the resection cavity becomes an additional corridor to deepen the exposure.

16.6 Complication Avoidance and Management

The most frequent complications encountered during and after and ALA are cranial nerve palsy, vertebral artery injury, and cervical hematoma. As in all cervical surgery, careful hemostasis is mandatory and can prevent the occurrence of a potentially life-threatening hematoma. The "coagulate and cut" technique helps providing a dry surgical field and probably reduces the occurrence of a postoperative hematoma. The use of a subcutaneous drain can also be considered depending on the situation.

In case of intraoperative injury to the VA, and when a BTO has not been obtained before the surgery or has been failed, the objective should be to preserve flow and avoid emboli. A primary repair of the VA can be attempted when the arterial wall defect is small. When the risk of intraoperative rupture is high, i.e., after radiation therapy or when there is tumor encasement, the arm can be draped to be prepared for radial artery graft harvest. The radial artery is an ideal donor in terms of size match with the VA and long-term patency. Otherwise, the occipital artery can serve as a donor vessel when it is of adequate size and has been preserved while performing the approach [29].

16.7 Clinical Cases

Case Illustration 1 (Figs. 16.8 and 16.9)
A 72-year-old male was referred to our clinic after multiple previous operations for a cervical chordoma. The patient initially presented an acute tetraparesis secondary to a C2-C3 lesion. The patient underwent in another center emergency laminectomy but this posterior approach did not allow exposure of the tumor and a subsequent anterior surgery for tumor biopsy was done.

The patient improved neurologically after the first surgery but presented unrelenting cervical pain that required constant immobilization with a Minerva orthosis. On the MRI, a lesion centered on the vertebral body of C3 with an extradural extension behind the inferior half of the body of C2 was found. Its characteristics on T1 and T2-weighted images were concordant with chordoma (Fig. 16.7a–f).

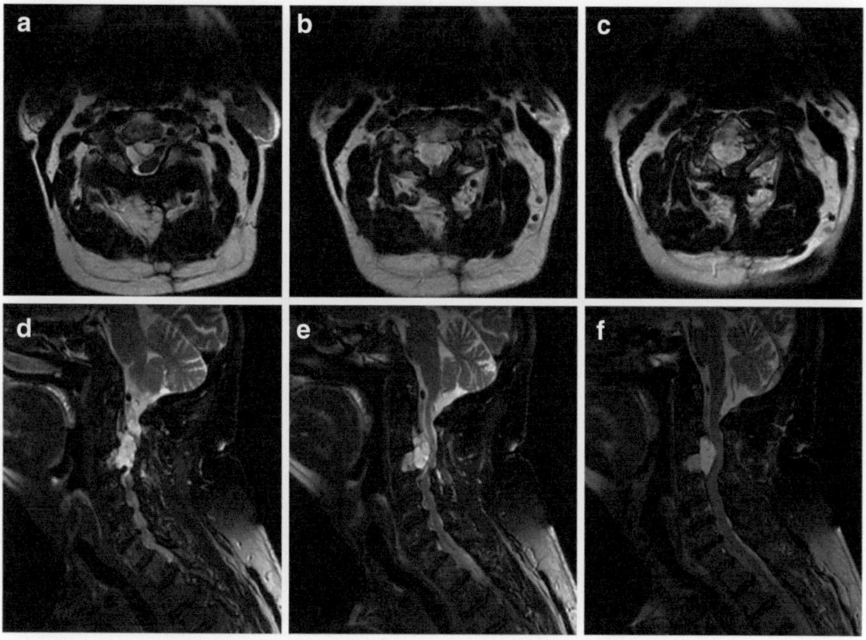

Fig. 16.7 T2-weighted MR images (**a**–**c**; axial and **d**–**f**; sagittal) showing a lesion at the posterior aspect of the C2-C3 vertebral bodies and causing compression on the spinal cord

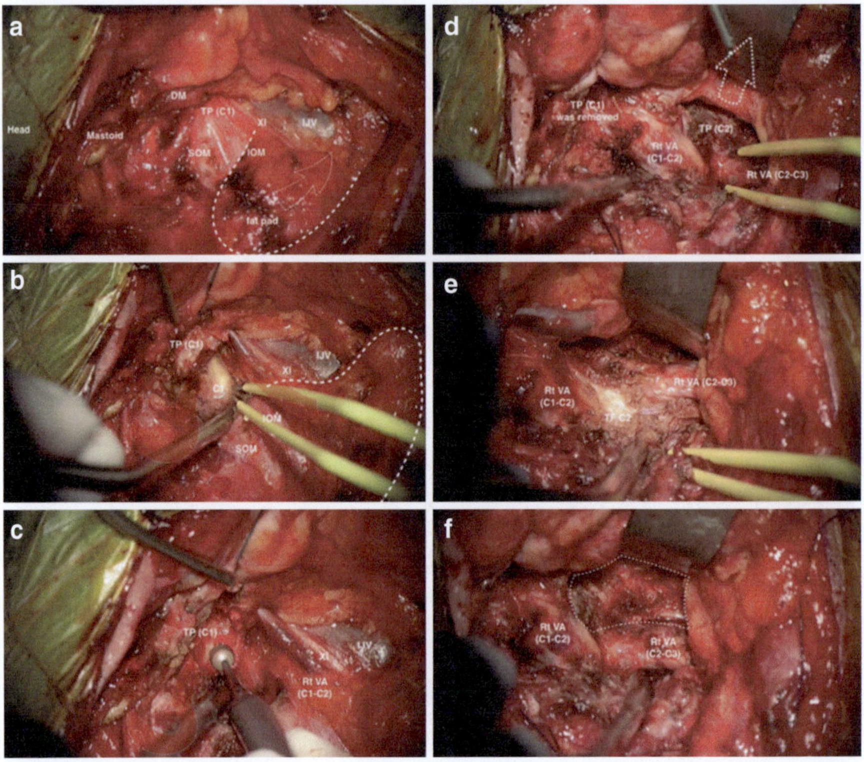

Fig. 16.8 (**a**) The fat pad, and the accessary nerve, inferior jugular vein, transverse process are exposed. The accessory nerve is protected with the fat pad. *DM* digastric muscle, *IOM* inferior oblique muscle, *IJV* internal jugular vein, *SOM* superior oblique muscle, *TP* transverse process, *XI* accessory nerve. (**b**) The fat pad is translocated inferiorly with protection of the accessory nerve. The C1 posterior arch is exposed by detaching the superior oblique and inferior oblique muscles from the C1 transverse process. *IOM* inferior oblique muscle, *IJV* internal jugular vein, *SOM* superior oblique muscle, *TP* transverse process, *XI* accessory nerve. (**c**) The C1 transverse process is drilled and the transverse foramen opened, thus uncovering V3. *IJV* internal jugular vein, *Rt. VA* right vertebral artery, *XI* accessory nerve. (**d**) C2 transverse process is also removed, allowing mobilization of the segment of the vertebral artery between its exit from C3 transverse foramen to its intradural entry. The internal jugular vein is retracted anteriorly, opening a corridor to the anterior aspect of the C2-C3 vertebral bodies. *Rt. VA* right vertebral artery, *TP* transverse process, (**e**) The transverse foramen of C2 is opened, exposing the vertebral artery from C1 to C3. *TF* transverse foramen. (**f**) The surgical corridor to the anterior aspect of the C2-C3 vertebral bodies. *Rt. VA* right vertebral artery

Gross total resection of the lesion was accomplished through an anterolateral approach. Considering that the vertebral bodies of C2 and C3 were only partially resected (Figs. 16.8 and 16.9), neither vertebral body reconstruction nor posterior cervical fixation was required. Clinically, the cervical pain remitted and the patient did not present any neurological deficit. He underwent adjuvant proton beam therapy.

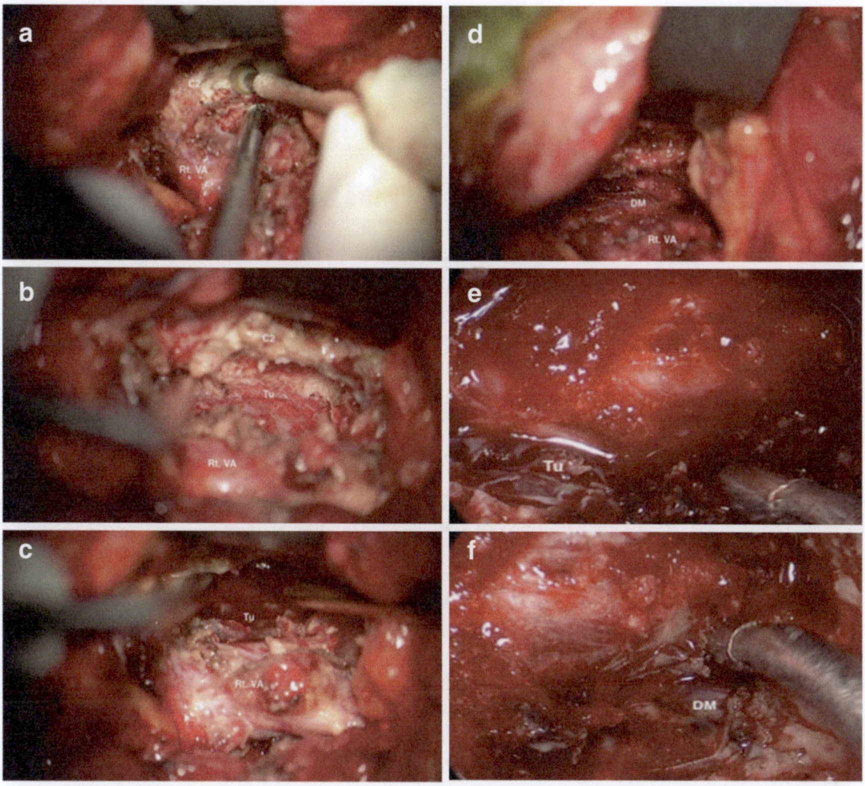

Fig. 16.9 (**a**) The posterior past of the vertebral body of C2 is drilled to expose the tumor. *Rt. VA* right vertebral artery. (**b**) The tumor is seen between the C2 vertebral body and the vertebral artery. *Rt. VA* right vertebral artery, *Tu* tumor. (**c**) An area of soft tumor can be seen in the vertebral body. *Rt. VA* right vertebral artery, *Tu* tumor. (**d**) After resection of the tumor, the dura mater of the cervical spine is seen. *DM* dura mater. (**e**) Endoscopic view in the anterolateral corridor. The border between the tumor and normal structures can be inspected precisely. *Tu* tumor. (**f**) After removing the tumor and fibrous tissue, the clean dura mater can be seen. *DM* dura mater

Case Illustration 2 (Figs. 16.10 and 16.11)
A 41-year-old man initially presented with headaches. On imaging, a tumor was found in the left petrous apex. The patient underwent surgical resection through a left anterior petrosectomy and was diagnosed with chondrosarcoma. Four years later, he was referred to us with hoarseness, dysphagia, and partial deviation of the tongue. The tumor was found to have grown and was causing mass effect on the jugular foramen. It was extending to level of C2 inferiorly and to the sphenoid sinus superiorly. We performed anterolateral and posterolateral transmastoid combined approach with endoscopic-assisted resection of this large lesion. Care was taken to preserve a barrier between the extradural and intradural compartment of the lesion. Two corridors were used to access the tumor (multiportal surgery): (1) the high cervical anterolateral approach, to benefit from the look up view to the lower clivus and medial aspect of

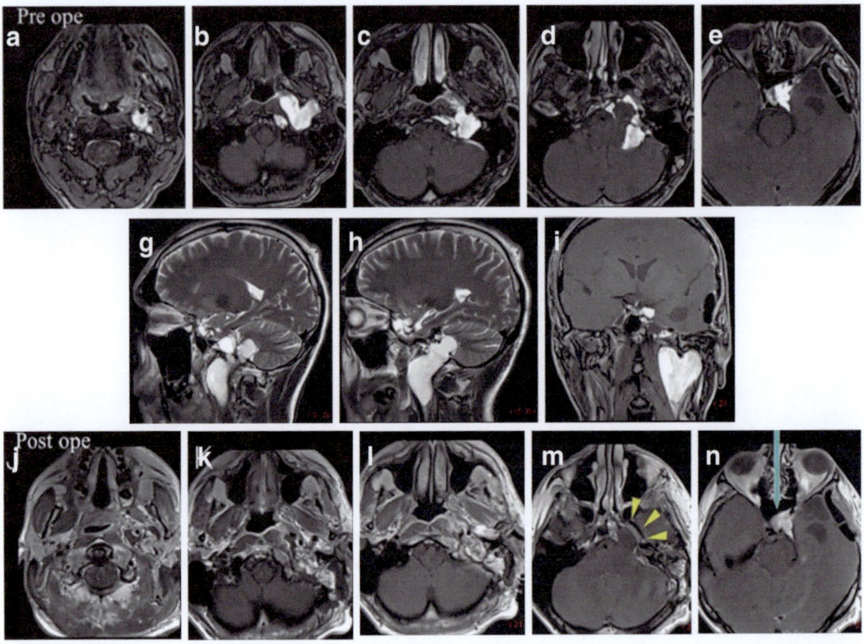

Fig. 16.10 The MRI shows a lesion in the area of the jugular foramen and extending from C2 to the sphenoid sinus. The tumor engulfs the internal carotid artery and extends into the intracranial compartment through the jugular foramen. (**a**–**e**) Preoperative gadolinium enhanced T1weighted axial images show the tumor engulf the carotid artery and jugular foramen. (**g**–**i**) Preoperative MRI T2 weighted sagital images show the tumor located from the C2 level to the sphenoid sinus. (**j**–**n**) Postoperative MRI Gadolinium enhanced T1 image show the tumor was removed except the sphenoid sinus lesion. The part of the tumor that was located in the mastoid area was partly resected during the previous surgery. Postoperative MRI image shows a small residual tumor in the sphenoid sinus

the jugular foramen, and (2) transmastoid presigmoid, suprajugular bulb look down view on the medial jugular foramen. The transmastoid corridor also allowed better visualization of the lesions extending toward the petrous apex. A small residual tumor that was left in the sphenoid was subsequently resected though an endoscopic endonasal approach. Clinically, the patient did not present any new neurological deficit.

16.8 Summary

The anterolateral approach grants a unique surgical trajectory to the cranio-vertebral junction that is in an inferior to superior and posterior to anterior direction. In addition to the cervical vertebrae, including C1 and C2 that are seen from a lateral perspective, the ALA allows exposure of the lower clivus and jugular foramen from below. Detailed knowledge of the 3D surgical anatomy, especially of the vertebral artery, is paramount for safe dissection and exposure through an ALA. In our practice, it is most often used to resect chordomas and other bony lesions of the CVJ. Endoscopic assistance as a surgical tool is an important adjunction that can enhance the exposure provided by the ALA in order to reach deep tumor extensions.

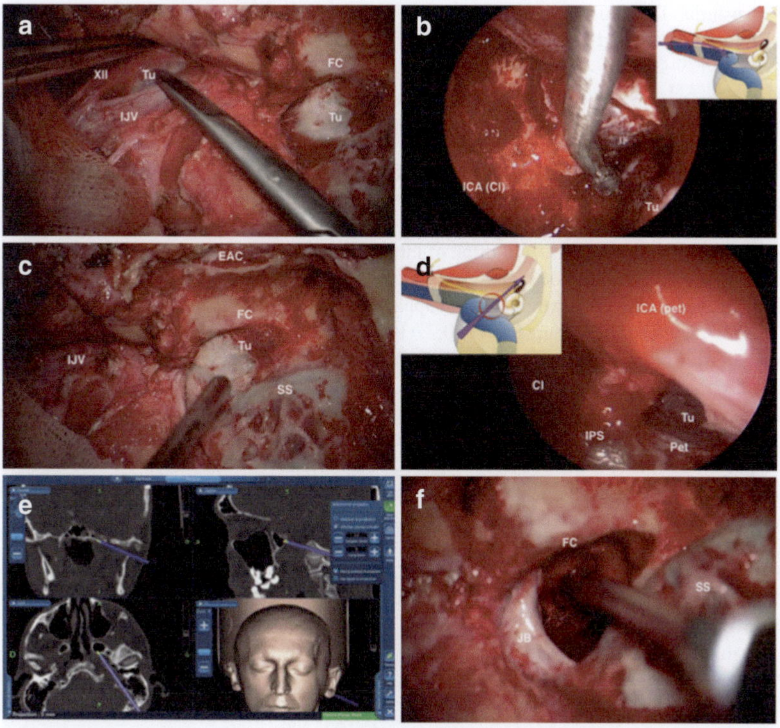

Fig. 16.11 (**a**) After an anterolateral approach and dissection, the internal jugular vein and hypoglossal nerve are seen. The tumor is exposed between the internal jugular vein and hypoglossal nerve. (**b**) Endoscopic assisted tumor removal is performed through the high cervical corridor, in the space between the internal jugular vein and hypoglossal nerve. The endoscope improved visualization of the tumor, which was located medial to the jugular foramen. (**c**) The fallopian canal and sigmoid sinus are exposed after mastoidectomy. The tumor can be seen between the fallopian canal and sigmoid sinus. (**d**) Endoscopic-assisted tumor removal is performed through the retrofacial presigmoid, suprajugular corridor. The inferior petrosal sinus is seen between the petrous bone and clivus. Through this corridor, the petrous segment of the internal carotid artery is identified. (**e, f**) The neuronavigation indicates the area of the petrous apex, confirming that the tumor was totally removed in this location

References

1. Al-Mefty O, Borba LA, Aoki N, Angtuaco E, Pait TG. The transcondylar approach to extradural nonneoplastic lesions of the craniovertebral junction. J Neurosurg. 1996;84:1–6.
2. Dehdashti AR. The suboccipital midline approach to foramen magnum meningiomas; feasible, but is it optimal? Acta Neurochir (Wien). 2015;157:875.
3. George B, Lot G. Anterolateral and posterolateral approaches to the foramen magnum: technical description and experience from 97 cases. Skull Base Surg. 1995;5:9–19.
4. Heros RC. Lateral suboccipital approach for vertebral and vertebrobasilar artery lesions. J Neurosurg. 1986;64:559–62.
5. Lanzino G, Paolini S, Spetzler RF. Far-lateral approach to the cranio-vertebral junction. Neurosurgery. 2005;57:367–71; discussion 367–71.
6. Li D, Wu Z, Ren C, Hao SY, Wang L, Xiao XR, Tang J, Wang YG, Meng GL, Zhang LW, Zhang JT. Foramen magnum meningiomas: surgical results and risks predicting poor outcomes based on a modified classification. J Neurosurg. 2017;126:661–76.

7. Matsushima T, Fukui M. [Lateral approaches to the foramen magnum: with special reference to the transcondylar fossa approach and the transcondylar approach]. No Shinkei Geka. 1996;24:119–24.
8. Menezes AH. Surgical approaches: postoperative care and complications "posterolateral-far lateral transcondylar approach to the ventral foramen magnum and upper cervical spinal canal". Childs Nerv Syst. 2008;24:1203–7.
9. Patel AJ, Gressot LV, Cherian J, Desai SK, Jea A. Far lateral paracondylar versus transcondylar approach in the pediatric age group: CT morphometric analysis. J Clin Neurosci. 2014;21:2194–200.
10. Sekhar LN, Ramanathan D. Evolution of far lateral and extreme lateral approaches to the skull base. World Neurosurg. 2012;77:617–8.
11. Sen CN, Sekhar LN. An extreme lateral approach to intradural lesions of the cervical spine and foramen magnum. Neurosurgery. 1990;27:197–204.
12. Velat GJ, Spetzler RF. The far-lateral approach and its variations. World Neurosurg. 2012;77:619–20.
13. Wanibuchi M, Fukushima T, Zenga F, Friedman AH. Simple identification of the third segment of the extracranial vertebral artery by extreme lateral inferior transcondylar-transtubercular exposure (ELITE). Acta Neurochir (Wien). 2009;151:1499–503.
14. Bruneau M, George B. Foramen magnum meningiomas: detailed surgical approaches and technical aspects at Lariboisiere Hospital and review of the literature. Neurosurg Rev. 2008;31:19–32; discussion 32–3.
15. Bulsara KR, Sameshima T, Friedman AH, Fukushima T. Microsurgical management of 53 jugular foramen schwannomas: lessons learned incorporated into a modified grading system. J Neurosurg. 109(5):794–803.
16. Fukushima T. Fukushima ELITE approach. Manual of skull base dissection. Raleigh: AF Neuro Video; 2004.
17. Yamamoto S, Sunada I, Matsuoka Y, Hakuba A, Nishimura S. Persistent primitive hypoglossal artery aneurysms. Neurol Med Chir. 1991;31(4):199–202.
18. Bertalanffy H, Seeger W. The dorsolateral, suboccipital, transcondylar approach to the lower clivus and anterior portion of the craniocervical junction. Neurosurgery. 29(6):815–21.
19. George B, Lot G, Boissonnet H. Meningioma of the foramen magnum: a series of 40 cases. Surg Neurol. 1997;47(4):371–9.
20. Fukushima T, Maroon JC, Bailes JE, Kennerdell JS, Chen DA, Celin S, Arriage MA. *Manual of skull base dissection*. United States, A F Neurovideo Inc; Lslf edition, 1996.
21. Babu RP, Sekhar LN, Wright DC. Extreme lateral transcondylar approach: technical improvements and lessons learned. J Neurosurg. 81(1):49–59.
22. Canalis RF, Martin N, Black K, Ammirati M, Cheatham M, Bloch J, Becker DP. Lateral approach to tumors of the craniovertebral junction. Laryngoscope. 103(3):343–9.
23. Vallée B, Besson G, Houidi K, Person H, Dam Hieu P, Rodriguez V, Mériot P, Sénécail B. Juxta- or trans-condylar lateral extension of the posterior suboccipital approach. Anatomical study, surgical aspects. Neurochirurgie. 1993;39(6):348–59.
24. Bodon G, Glasz T, Olerud C. Anatomical changes in occipitalization: is there an increased risk during the standard posterior approach? Eur Spine J. 2013;22(Suppl 3):S512–6.
25. Kim MS. Anatomical variant of atlas: arcuate foramen, occpitalization of atlas, and defect of posterior arch of atlas. J Korean Neurosurg Soc. 2015;58:528–33.
26. Senoglu M, Safavi-Abbasi S, Theodore N, Bambakidis NC, Crawford NR, Sonntag VK. The frequency and clinical significance of congenital defects of the posterior and anterior arch of the atlas. J Neurosurg Spine. 2007;7:399–402.
27. Lister JR, Rhoton AL Jr, Matsushima T, Peace DA. Microsurgical anatomy of the posterior inferior cerebellar artery. Neurosurgery. 1982;10:170–99.
28. Yasuda M, Bresson D, Cornelius JF, George B. Anterolateral approach without fixation for resection of an intradural schwannoma of the cervical spinal canal: technical note. Neurosurgery. 2009;65:1178–81; discussion 1181.
29. Kubota H, Tanikawa R, Katsuno M, Izumi N, Noda K, Ota N, Ishishita Y, Miyazaki T, Okabe S, Endo S, Niemela M, Hashimoto M. Vertebral artery-to-vertebral artery bypass with interposed radial artery or occipital artery grafts: surgical technique and report of three cases. World Neurosurg. 2014;81:202.e1–8.

Minimally Invasive Techniques Applied to the Cranio-Vertebral Junction

17

Ken Hsuan-kan Chang, John Paul G. Kolcun, and Michael Y. Wang

17.1 Introduction

Minimally invasive surgery (MIS) has gained popularity among spine surgeons in recent decades. MIS techniques involve less blood loss and tissue damage, reducing the physical stress of surgery and potentially shortening recovery time and hospital stay [1, 2]. These procedures are therefore safer in elderly or otherwise frail patients, a segment of the population projected to increase dramatically in coming decades [3, 4]. MIS procedures have also been associated with significant cost reductions following their adoption [5, 6].

While the early applications of MIS to the spine were in lumbar surgery, significant advances have been made across the spectrum of spinal pathology. In this chapter, we will describe a variety of MIS fixation techniques at the craniovertebral junction (CVJ), including their indications, technique, perioperative considerations, and common complications.

K. H.-k. Chang · J. P. G. Kolcun
Department of Neurological Surgery and Rehabilitation Medicine, University of Miami Miller School of Medicine, Miami, FL, USA

M. Y. Wang (✉)
Department of Neurological Surgery and Rehabilitation Medicine, University of Miami Miller School of Medicine, Miami, FL, USA

Lois Pope Life Center, Miami, FL, USA
e-mail: mwang2@med.miami.edu

E. Tessitore et al. (eds.), *Surgery of the Cranio-Vertebral Junction*,
https://doi.org/10.1007/978-3-030-18700-2_17

17.2 Anterior Odontoid Screw Fixation

17.2.1 Indications

Odontoid screw fixation attempts to restore bony integrity from odontoid fracture through internal fixation. Nearly 50% of axial rotation of the CVJ is provided by the C1-2 structure. Odontoid screws avoid compromising the physiological function of the C2 odontoid bone by fusing the C1-2 complex, thereby maintaining the rotatory motion of atlantoaxial joint. Open odontoid screw fixation has been performed for decades since its first introduction in the 1980s [7]. Recently, several publications have advocated a minimally invasive (MIS) approach for anterior odontoid screw placement.

The indications for MIS odontoid screw fixation are very similar to the open surgery. The best indication for odontoid screw is type II and some rostral type III odontoid fracture, according to Anderson and D'Alonzo's classification. The odontoid fracture must be reducible. This technique is contraindicated with a displaced odontoid fracture unless anatomical reduction can be achieved with skull traction. Other contraindications include a disrupted C1-2 transverse ligament, C2 vertebral body fracture, pathologic fracture, etc. The fusion rate of chronic fracture or nonunion using odontoid screw fixation is low. In cases of chronic nonunion >6 months, C1-2 arthrodesis carries a greater chance for bone fusion.

17.2.2 Preoperative Planning

Complete X-ray (XR) examination of the cervical spine, including open-mouth view, is mandatory to evaluate the fracture type and the stability of atlantoaxial joint. MRI is recommended to evaluate the integrity of the transverse ligament. CT scan with coronal and sagittal reconstruction is helpful in clarifying the integrity of the entire bone structure and verifying the fracture type.

It may be difficult to obtain an ideal angle for screw insertion for patients with obesity, short neck, barrel chest, or cervical kyphotic deformity. Preoperative CT and MRI can be useful for planning the proper angle of screw insertion and thereby previse any obstacles.

Nasotracheal intubation is preferred. Radiolucent mouth bite is used to facilitate intraoperative fluoroscopic imaging of the open-mouth view. The patient's skull must be secured with either a head-fixation device or the Gardner-Wells tongs traction system. After positioning, anteroposterior (AP) open-mouth view and lateral XR should be obtained before surgery to assure the visualization of the C1 lateral mass, C2 body, and odontoid process.

17.2.3 Surgical Technique

After the patient is positioned supine and the head is secured, a 5 mm–1 cm incision is made at approximately the level of C4-5 and slightly medial to the sternocleidomastoid (SCM) muscle. The platysma muscle is then divided. The medial border of the SCM muscle was dissected sharply. With blunt dissection, the anterior surface of the cervical spine is approached from the natural tissue plane between the carotid sheath and the esophagus/trachea. *Hashizume* et al. also published an alternative technique for anterior approach with endoscopic assistance [8]. A guide tube is then placed. The tip of the tube is pointed at the anterior and inferior tip of the C2 body under lateral XR guidance. Under AP XR imaging, the guide tube should be docked on the midline of the C2 body as the entry point. A power drill is used to create a proper tract across the fracture line to the tip of the odontoid process under fluoroscopic guidance. The drill is exchanged for a guidewire, which is inserted into the tract created by the power drill. The guide tube is replaced with a working channel. The screw tract is then tapped via the working channel. The screw length can be measured with a depth-gauge. Finally, a 4-mm cannulated screw is inserted into the C2 body. The screw is advanced under XR guidance to reach the superior tip of the odontoid process (Fig. 17.1).

As an alternative, the screw entry point can be placed under the inferior endplate of C2 and pass through the anterior C2-3 disc space. This may allow the surgeon to obtain a more adequate trajectory and conceal the screw head in the disc space by

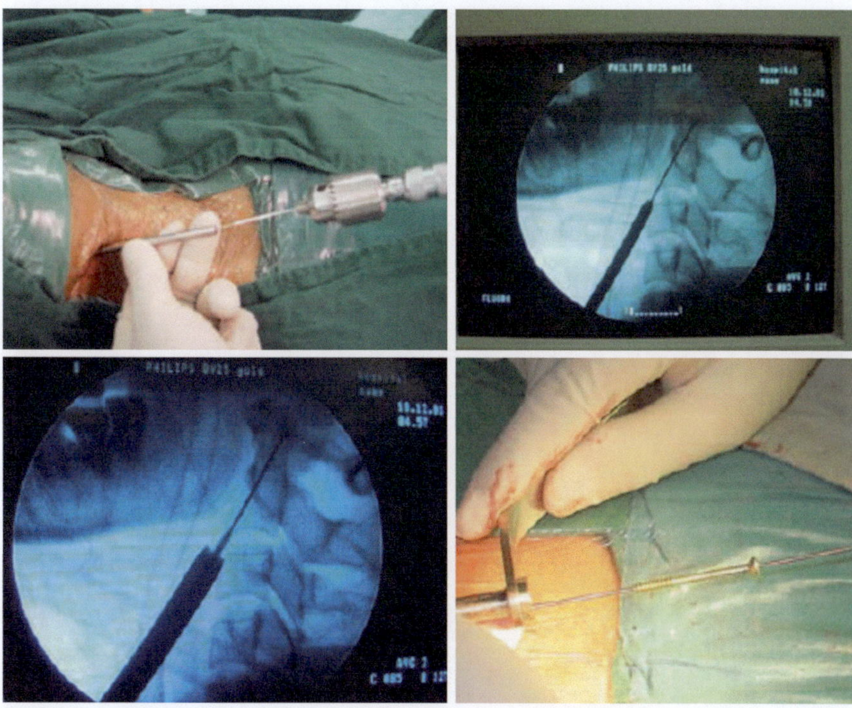

Fig. 17.1 Percutaneous anterior odontoid screw. *Upper figures:* A power drill was used to create a proper tract across the fracture line to the tip of odontoid process under fluoroscopic guidance. *Lower figures:* a 4-mm cannulated screw was inserted into the C2 body and aimed toward the superior tip of odontoid process under the monitor of X-ray image. (Adapted from *Chi YL, Wang XY, Xu HZ, et al. Management of odontoid fractures with percutaneous anterior odontoid screw fixation. Eur Spine J. 2007;16(8):1157–1164*)

removing a small portion of C2-3 disc. This technique does involve the disruption of an intact C2-3 disc, and may therefore accelerate disc degeneration at this level.

In the open technique, two odontoid screws can be inserted to prevent odontoid rotation around a single screw. However, inserting two screws is technically challenging under MIS setting and has not been reported in the literature.

Robotic arm-assisted placement of odontoid screws has been reported in literature [9]. The robotic arm can move spontaneously, providing a preoperatively planned trajectory to serve as a drill guide. A Kirschner wire can be inserted after drilling. The screw is then placed manually.

17.2.4 Postoperative Care

On postoperative day one, follow-up XR (AP, lateral, and open-mouth view) should be obtained to check screw position. A cervical collar is prescribed to immobilize the cervical spine for 3 months. In severe osteoporotic cases, a halo brace may be considered to enhance fusion.

Current studies regarding MIS odontoid screw fixation are scarce. The reported radiographic fusion rate was approximate 90% after an average of 15 months follow-up in a small clinical series. There was no procedure-related complication. No screw loosening or breakage was seen in that series [10]. Wang et al. compared a percutaneous technique to open surgery and demonstrated equivalent fusion rates in both group. There was no procedure- or implant-related complication for patients who underwent MIS surgery [11]. In summary, the literature regarding MIS odontoid screw fixation remains limited. The outcome and safety of MIS odontoid screw fixation require further validation (Fig. 17.2).

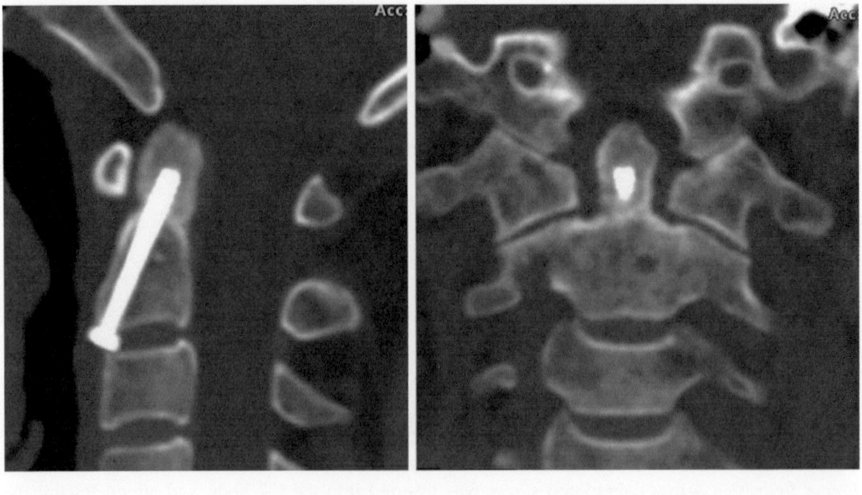

Fig. 17.2 CT confirmation of percutaneous anterior odontoid screw. (Adapted from *Wu AM, Wang XY, Xia DD, Luo P, Xu HZ, Chi YL. A novel technique of two-hole guide tube for percutaneous anterior odontoid screw fixation. Spine J. 2015;15(5):1141–1145*)

17.2.5 Complications

Complications of this surgery are associated with the technique, the implant, and the bone fusion. The most common presentation of nonunion is persistent high neck pain beyond the normal fusion period (approximately 3–6 months). Myelopathy can develop if a nonunion dens fragment causes compression of the spinal cord. Soft tissue growth around a dens fragment may also cause spinal cord compression. Implant-related complications include screw breakage, loosening, and pullout. Screw malposition may occur if the surgeon lacks experience with the MIS approach. MIS techniques can potentially cause any of the complications seen with open surgery, including postoperative hematomas, dysphagia, and hoarseness. Serious morbidities, such as esophageal perforation, carotid artery laceration, neurologic deterioration, and airway obstruction are also possible.

17.3 Anterior Transarticular Screw Fixation

17.3.1 Indications

Atlantoaxial instability can result from C1-2 dislocation with transverse atlantal ligament incompetence (rheumatoid arthritis, trauma, local infection, Down syndrome, etc.), chronic nonunion after odontoid fracture, or os odontoideum. The most common surgical treatment for atlantoaxial instability is posterior transarticular screw fixation or C1-C2 fixation. Anterior transarticular screw fixation has been advocated to treat atlantoaxial instability, as it avoids the excessive muscle damage and bleeding associated with the posterior cervical approach. Anterior transarticular screws achieve similar biomechanical stability when compared to posterior screw fixation [12].

Additional indications for anterior transarticular screw fixation include odontoid fracture with displacement and odontoid process invasion by tumor. Generally, anterior transarticular screw fixation can be useful when C1-2 fusion is indicated. MIS methods of anterior transarticular screw fixation have been described in several studies in the literature. A minimally invasive approach may further reduce the tissue damage and bleeding from surgery.

Patients with irreducible atlantoaxial dislocation may prove poor candidates for anterior transarticular fixation. Irreducible dislocation requires more extensive release and intraoperative reduction, which may be more appropriately treated with C1-C2 screw fixation. In open surgery, previous cervical spine operation is usually not a contraindication for anterior transarticular screw fixation. However, previous operation may increase the risk of vital structure injury (i.e., artery, vein, and esophagus) during the approach. It is certainly not recommended to perform percutaneous procedure under such circumstances.

17.3.2 Preoperative Planning

The preoperative planning, anesthetic considerations, and patient positioning are similar to MIS odontoid screw fixation. Preoperative MRI, CT, and full set of XR images (AP, lateral, and open-mouth view) should be carefully examined. CT angiography is of paramount importance to investigate the course of vertebral artery (VA) at the C1-2 region, as VA anomalies are not uncommon. Patient characteristics such as obesity, short neck, barrel chest, and kyphotic cervical spine are taken into consideration to planning for proper screw angle.

Nasotracheal intubation and radiolucent mouth bite are recommended to facilitate the quality of intraoperative fluoroscopy. AP, lateral, and open-mouth fluoroscopic views are checked after patient's head is secured with a Mayfield skull clamp or Gardner-Wells tongs traction system.

17.3.3 Surgical Technique

The percutaneous approach is similar to MIS odontoid screw placement. The patient is positioned supine with the head secured. A 5–10 mm incision is made at approximately the level of the C4-5 disc space, medial to the sternocleidomastoid (SCM) muscle. The platysma muscle is then divided. The anterior border of the cervical spine is approached with blunt dissection via the natural tissue plane between the carotid sheaths and the esophagus/trachea. A guide tube is placed at the inferior border of the C2 vertebral body. The entry point should be 5–10 mm from the midline on AP imaging. A sharp-tip K-wire is used to drill a tract from the C2 body to the center of the C1 lateral mass with a power drill. Xu et al. proposed that the direction of the drill should aim toward the C1 lateral mass at an angle of 20–30° from midline on the AP view and 20–28° from the vertical line on the lateral view (Fig. 17.3) [13].

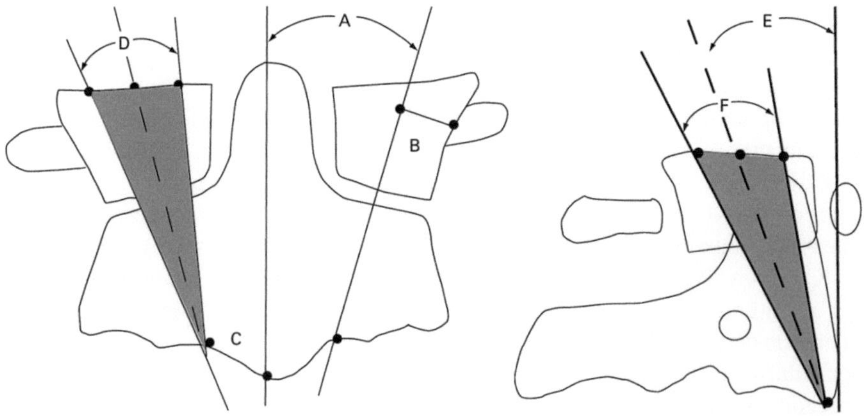

Fig. 17.3 The trajectory of drill aims toward the C1 lateral mass at an angle of 20–30° from midline on the AP view and 20–28° from the vertical line on the lateral view. The gray area represents the safety zone. (Adapted from *Li WL, Chi YL, Xu HZ, et al. Percutaneous anterior transarticular screw fixation for atlantoaxial instability: a case series. J Bone Joint Surg Br. 2010;92(4):545–549*)

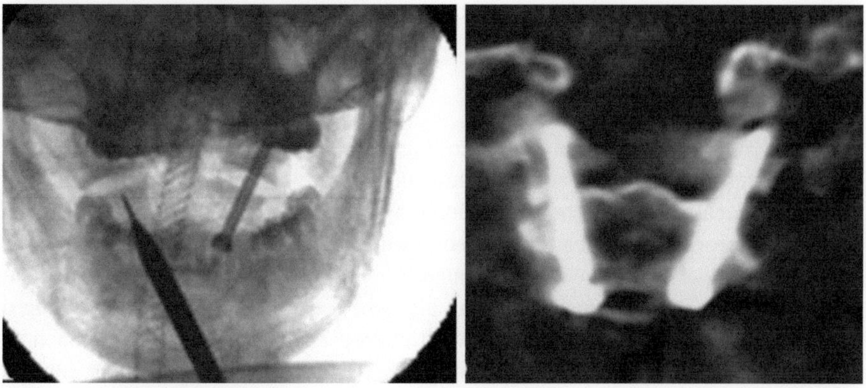

Fig. 17.4 *Left:* Intraoperative fluoroscopic image of percutaneous anterior transarticular screw placement. *Right:* The postoperative CT confirmation, coronal view. (Adapted from *Wang J, Zhou Y, Zhang Z, Li C, Zheng W, Zhang Y. Minimally invasive anterior transarticular screw fixation and microendoscopic bone graft for atlantoaxial instability. Eur Spine J. 2012;21(8):1568–1574*)

They concluded this to be a safe trajectory as it avoided VA injury in a series of patients, which was confirmed with three-dimensional (3D) CT [14]. A protective sleeve is then inserted along the guide tube. After the guide tube is removed, a 3.5 mm partially-threaded self-tapping cannulated screw is then placed along the K-wire, inside the protective sleeve. The screw is advanced to the tip of the C1 lateral mass (Fig. 17.4). The K-wire is then removed. The anterior C1-2 articular process is then exposed on both sides and grafted with autologous or heterologous bone grafts through the protective sleeve.

17.3.4 Postoperative Care

After surgery, patients are braced with a cervical collar for 3 months until bone fusion is achieved. Periodic follow-up XR to assess implants is recommended.

Radiological and clinical outcomes with percutaneous anterior transarticular screws demonstrate favorable results in the current literature [13, 15]. Solid fusion can be achieved without serious screw misplacement and surgical complication. However, there are few reports on the efficacy of anterior transarticular screws for atlantoaxial instability. More study is required to confirm its safety and feasibility.

17.3.5 Complications

Potential serious complications involve VA and nerve injury, which are often caused by misplacement of the instruments and implants. Cautious examination of neurovascular and bony anatomy as well as planning of screw trajectory are imperative to avoid devastating neurovascular complications. Careful monitoring of intraoperative fluoroscopy while drilling and instrumenting may help to reduce these complications. Other possible complications are esophageal or vascular injury during the percutaneous approach. Previous neck surgery is considered a contraindication in a MIS setting.

17.4 Posterior Atlantoaxial Fixation

17.4.1 Indications

In general, atlantoaxial instability due to fracture is the most common indication for fusion. Other common indications include degenerative changes, spondylosis, and rheumatic disease. Less frequently, fusion may be indicated for mal-union, stenosis, congenital deformity, dislocation, or neoplasm [16].

MIS techniques are generally indicated in elderly or frail patients with medical co-morbidities. The MIS approach may also prove useful in revisions, avoiding a larger dissection through scar tissue with altered anatomy. An MIS approach to atlantoaxial fusion spares the posterior tension band, the deep extensor muscle attachment to C2, and the multifidus and semispinalis cervicis muscles [17]. The preservation of these structures may help reduce postoperative loss of cervical lordosis.

17.4.2 Preoperative Planning

Preoperative CT scanning should be performed to note the dimensions of the C1 lateral mass, the C2 pedicles, and the vertebral artery, and to plan the ideal screw trajectory. The patient is positioned prone on chest rolls or a Jackson frame, with the head secured with skull clamp fixation device. Neuromonitoring is performed with somatosensory evoked potentials (SSEPs) and motor evoked potentials (MEPs). Cervical alignment should be carefully maintained and verified fluoroscopically. The surgical area is prepped and draped in the usual fashion.

17.4.3 Surgical Technique

Small vertical paramedian incisions are made 2–4 cm from midline on either side. The first dilator is docked at superior aspect of the C2 facet, after standard blunt tissue dissection. Following sequential dilation, the MIS tubular retractor is docked in the superior aspect of the C2 lateral mass under fluoroscopy. Electrocautery and dissectors can be used to remove any soft tissue overlying the C2 lateral mass and pars in order to visualize the C2 nerve root, the articulating facet of the C1 lateral mass, the C1-2 joint, and the C2 pars. The C2 nerve root may be sacrificed and divided by electrocautery if necessary. Alternately, the inferior oblique muscle can be transected by electrocautery to visualize the C1 posterior arch, the posterior atlantoaxial membrane, and the C2 pars. The posterior atlantoaxial membrane is then divided by sharp dissection.

Further dissection for the venous plexus between the C1 and C2 lateral mass can be performed with bipolar and unipolar electrocautery, in order to visualize entry points for C1 lateral mass and C2 pedicle screws. Bleeding from the venous plexus is often massive and can usually be controlled with bipolar cautery, tissue sealant, and hemostatic agents. A C1-2 joint spacer is then introduced. The joint space can be distracted manually with a Penfield dissector. Following endplate preparation, a graft can be placed into the joint space. The C1 lateral mass screws, C2 pedicle screws, and connecting rods are then be introduced by standard methods. Of note, the angle of the tubular retractor may require adjustment during screw insertion (Fig. 17.5) [18, 19].

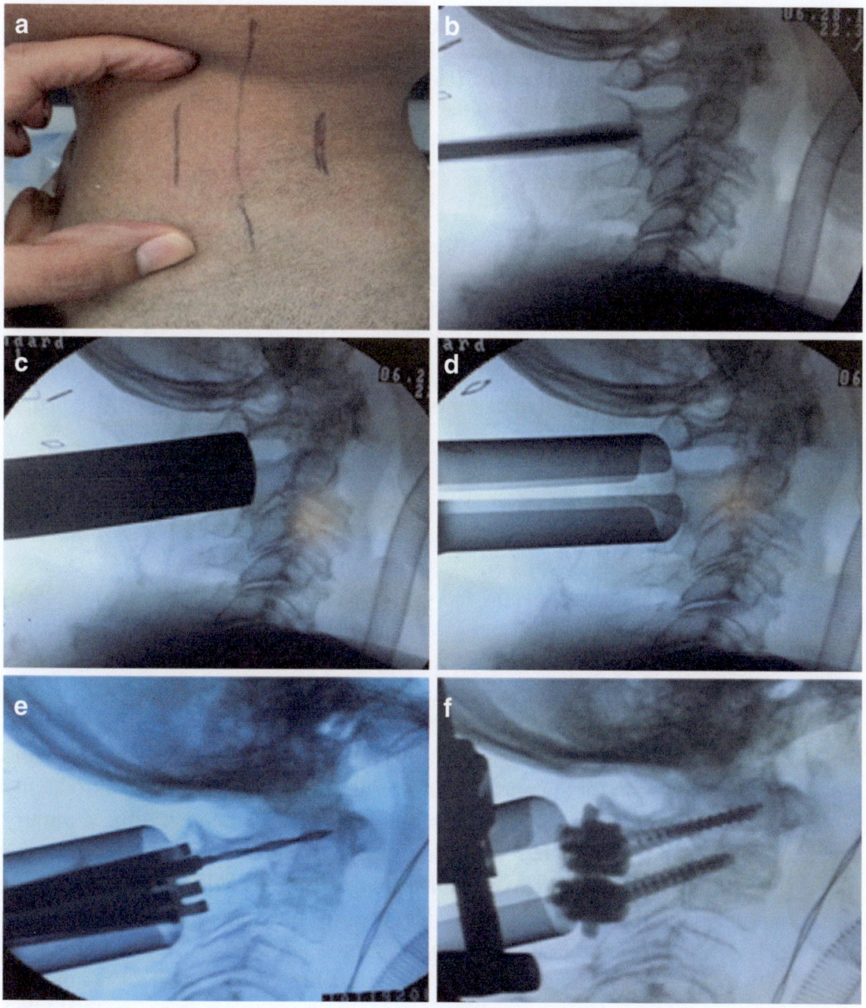

Fig. 17.5 (**a**) Image showing the skin marking and stretch ability of the skin in the cervical region, allowing for a smaller incision. (**b–e**) Intraoperative fluoroscopy images showing initial docking over the C-2 facet (**b**), after sequential dilation (**c**), placement of an expandable retractor (**d**), the C-1 lateral mass drill hole being prepared (**e**), and the final construct (**f**). (Adapted from *Srikantha U, Khanapure KS, Jagannatha AT, Joshi KC, Varma RG, Hegde AS. Minimally invasive atlantoaxial fusion: cadaveric study and report of 5 clinical cases. J Neurosurg Spine. 2016;25(6):675–680*)

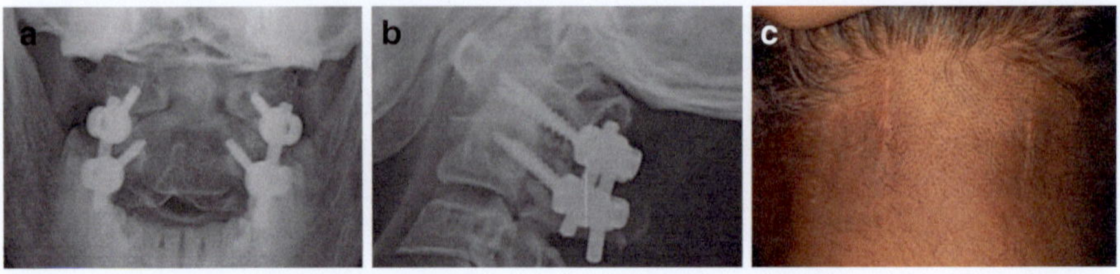

Fig. 17.6 (**a**, **b**) Postoperative anteroposterior (**a**) and lateral (**b**) radiographs showing the position of the screws. (**c**) Appearance of the wound at follow-up. (Adapted from *Srikantha U, Khanapure KS, Jagannatha AT, Joshi KC, Varma RG, Hegde AS. Minimally invasive atlantoaxial fusion: cadaveric study and report of 5 clinical cases. J Neurosurg Spine. 2016;25(6):675–680*)

17.4.4 Postoperative Care

Postoperative CT imaging can be used to confirm screw placement. The cervical spine should be immobilized postoperatively. A halo brace is mandatory for 3–4 months in patients with rheumatoid arthritis or osteopenia. In patients without these co-morbidities who undergo rigid fusion with screws, and hard collar is acceptable. Although there are as yet no large-scale investigations of MIS atlanto-axial fusion, a recent study in five patients reported an average postoperative hospital stay of 7.4 days (Fig. 17.6) [19].

17.4.5 Complications

As in conventional atlantoaxial fusion, the vertebral artery (VA) is at risk during placement of the C1 lateral mass screw and C2 pedicle screw. Patients with a "ponticulus posticus" at C1 are at higher risk for injury. Ponticulus posticus is known as the abnormal bony formation at the posterior arch of C1. A complete ponticulus posticus can easily be recognized as a thickened posterior arch and therefore be mistaken as an incorrect entry site for C1 screws (Fig. 17.7). This risk is mitigated by (1) reviewing the preoperative CT scan for the presence of a posterior ponticulus and (2) introducing 10–15° of medial angulation during C1 lateral mass screw placement [20]. VA injury can also occur during C2 pedicle screw insertion due to a small or absent pedicle, or a major vertebral artery anomaly. Preoperative images such as MRI and CT angiography should be scrutinized in detail before surgery. We recommend thin cut CT angiography (1–2 mm) as a routine study. This allows spine surgeons to evaluate imperative anatomical features, such as the pedicle diameter, the course of the VA, and the patency of bilateral vessels. If the pedicle is narrower than 4 mm, it is very likely that the screw diameter will be larger than the pedicle size. This may result in screw breach or pedicle fracture. One must be cautious in patients with unilateral vertebral artery obstruction or hypoplasia. Damage to the contralateral patent VA can have serious consequences, such as cerebrovascular stroke due to a complete obstruction of arterial flow to the brain stem. Dural tear, dysphagia, and dystonia occur infrequently. As with any instrumented fusion, nonunion, screw loosening, and rod breakage are possible.

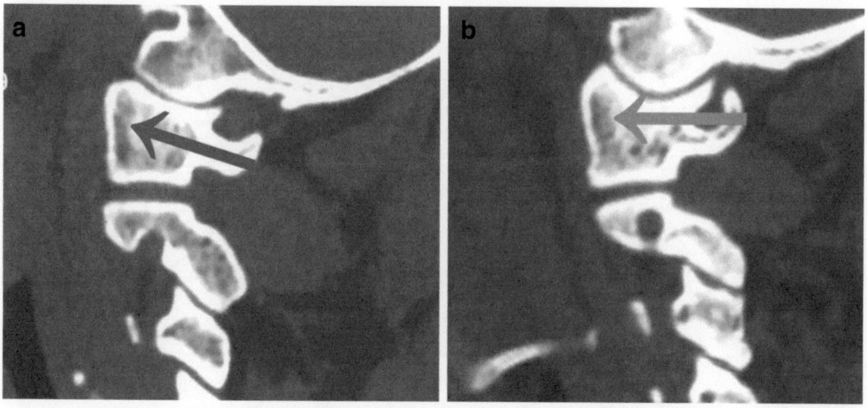

Fig. 17.7 (**a**) C1 lateral mass screw in a normal posterior arch of atlas; (**b**) A misplaced screw trajectory when a "ponticulus posticus" is mistaken as a thicken posterior arch of atlas. (Adapted from *Zhang XL, Huang DG, Wang XD, et al. The feasibility of inserting a C1 pedicle screw in patients with ponticulus posticus: a retrospective analysis of eleven patients. Eur Spine J. 2017;26(4):1058–1063*)

There is typically a steep learning-curve associated with the new adoption of MIS techniques. Thorough training in a laboratory setting is therefore recommended to familiarize the surgeon with the restricted view of the relevant anatomy, as well as the operation and nuances of the MIS equipment.

17.5 Anterior Occipito-Cervical Fixation

Occipito-cervical (OC) fusion is commonly performed from a posterior approach with screws, rods, and plate fixation. Solid fusion can be achieved for atlanto-occipital instability with open posterior OC fixation. However, there is a substantial lack of literature applying the MIS techniques to OC fusion.

Dvorak et al. have described a technique of anterior occiput-to-axis fixation in an open setting [21]. Subsequent biomechanical investigation demonstrated comparable stability to posterior plate and screw fixation in axial rotation and lateral bending, but inferiority in extension and flexion [22]. A Chinese group published a clinical series of MIS anterior occiput-to-axis screw fixation [23]. With a mini-open approach, a guide tube is placed at the antero-inferior border of the C2 body, 5–10 mm from the midline. Under C-arm control, a power drill and K-wire oriented approximately 10–20° laterally and 15–36° posteriorly across the C1 lateral mass is aimed toward the posterolateral third of the occipital condyle (Fig. 17.8). Self-tapping cannulated screws are then inserted inside a protective channel on both sides. Iliac cancellous bone is grafted at the occiput-C1 and C1-C2 articular surfaces through the protective channel. In this study, anterior surgery was indicated in patients with anatomic restraints precluding posterior fixation or with previous suboccipital decompressive craniectomy. Five of six patients in their series achieved solid fusion after an average 20 months of follow-up.

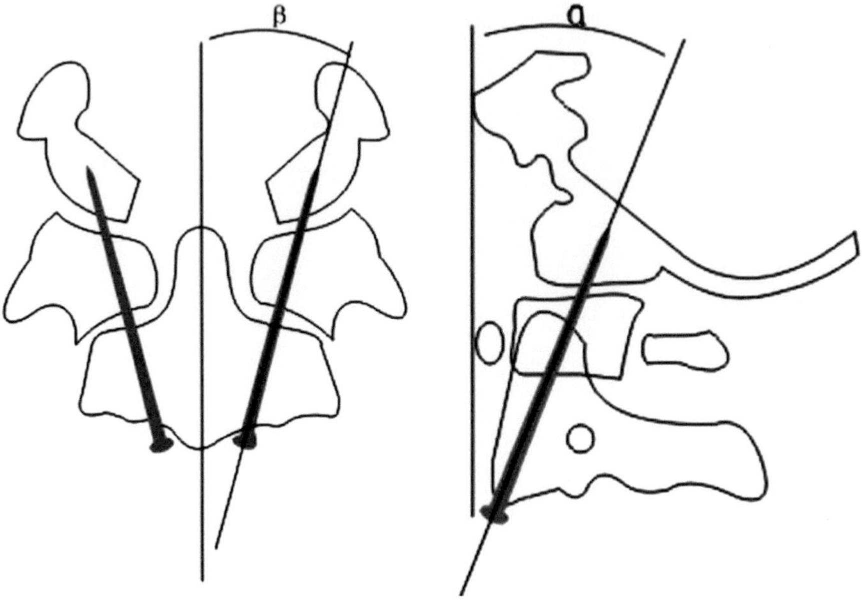

Fig. 17.8 The trajectory of percutaneous anterior occiput-to-axis screw. (Adapted from *Wu AM, Chi YL, Weng W, Xu HZ, Wang XY, Ni WF. Percutaneous anterior occiput-to-axis screw fixation: technique aspects and case series. Spine J. 2013;13(11):1538–1543*)

17.6 Conclusion

Minimally invasive surgery at the craniovertebral junction remains an evolving field in spine surgery. Although percutaneous screw fixation has been implemented with some success, the majority of procedures at the craniovertebral junction are still performed with open techniques. Minimally invasive odontoid screws and anterior/posterior transarticular screw fixation may yield promising outcomes with further study. For now, while minimally invasive surgery of the thoracolumbar and subaxial cervical spine is a thriving field in modern spine surgery, much progress remains in developing these techniques at the craniovertebral junction.

References

1. Fan S, Hu Z, Zhao F, Zhao X, Huang Y, Fang X. Multifidus muscle changes and clinical effects of one-level posterior lumbar interbody fusion: minimally invasive procedure versus conventional open approach. Eur Spine J. 2010;19(2):316–24.
2. Kim CW. Scientific basis of minimally invasive spine surgery: prevention of multifidus muscle injury during posterior lumbar surgery. Spine (Phila Pa 1976). 2010;35(26 Suppl):S281–6.
3. Colby SL, Ortman JM. Projections of the Size and Composition of the U.S. Population: 2014 to 2060. U.S. Census Bureau, U.S. Department of Commerce, March, 2015.

4. Shamji MF, Goldstein CL, Wang M, Uribe JS, Fehlings MG. Minimally invasive spinal surgery in the elderly: does it make sense? Neurosurgery. 2015;77(Suppl 4):S108–15.
5. McGirt MJ, Parker SL, Lerner J, Engelhart L, Knight T, Wang MY. Comparative analysis of perioperative surgical site infection after minimally invasive versus open posterior/transforaminal lumbar interbody fusion: analysis of hospital billing and discharge data from 5170 patients. J Neurosurg Spine. 2011;14(6):771–8.
6. Vertuani S, Nilsson J, Borgman B, et al. A cost-effectiveness analysis of minimally invasive versus open surgery techniques for lumbar spinal fusion in Italy and the United Kingdom. Value Health. 2015;18(6):810–6.
7. Bohler J. Anterior stabilization for acute fractures and non-unions of the dens. J Bone Joint Surg Am. 1982;64(1):18–27.
8. Hashizume H, Kawakami M, Kawai M, Tamaki T. A clinical case of endoscopically assisted anterior screw fixation for the type II odontoid fracture. Spine (Phila Pa 1976). 2003;28(5):E102–5.
9. Tian W, Wang H, Liu YJ. Robot-assisted anterior odontoid screw fixation: a case report. Orthop Surg. 2016;8(3):400–4.
10. Chi YL, Wang XY, Xu HZ, et al. Management of odontoid fractures with percutaneous anterior odontoid screw fixation. Eur Spine J. 2007;16(8):1157–64.
11. Wang J, Zhou Y, Zhang ZF, Li CQ, Zheng WJ, Liu J. Comparison of percutaneous and open anterior screw fixation in the treatment of type II and rostral type III odontoid fractures. Spine (Phila Pa 1976). 2011;36(18):1459–63.
12. Lapsiwala SB, Anderson PA, Oza A, Resnick DK. Biomechanical comparison of four C1 to C2 rigid fixative techniques: anterior transarticular, posterior transarticular, C1 to C2 pedicle, and C1 to C2 intralaminar screws. Neurosurgery. 2006;58(3):516–21; discussion 516–21.
13. Li WL, Chi YL, Xu HZ, et al. Percutaneous anterior transarticular screw fixation for atlantoaxial instability: a case series. J Bone Joint Surg Br. 2010;92(4):545–9.
14. Xu H, Chi YL, Wang XY, et al. Comparison of the anatomic risk for vertebral artery injury associated with percutaneous atlantoaxial anterior and posterior transarticular screws. Spine J. 2012;12(8):656–62.
15. Wang J, Zhou Y, Zhang Z, Li C, Zheng W, Zhang Y. Minimally invasive anterior transarticular screw fixation and microendoscopic bone graft for atlantoaxial instability. Eur Spine J. 2012;21(8):1568–74.
16. Derman PB, Lampe LP, Lyman S, et al. Atlantoaxial fusion: sixteen years of epidemiology, indications, and complications in New York state. Spine (Phila Pa 1976). 2016;41(20):1586–92.
17. Bodon G, Patonay L, Baksa G, Olerud C. Applied anatomy of a minimally invasive muscle-splitting approach to posterior C1-C2 fusion: an anatomical feasibility study. Surg Radiol Anat. 2014;36(10):1063–9.
18. Taghva A, Attenello FJ, Zada G, Khalessi AA, Hsieh PC. Minimally invasive posterior atlantoaxial fusion: a cadaveric and clinical feasibility study. World Neurosurg. 2013;80(3–4):414–21.
19. Srikantha U, Khanapure KS, Jagannatha AT, Joshi KC, Varma RG, Hegde AS. Minimally invasive atlantoaxial fusion: cadaveric study and report of 5 clinical cases. J Neurosurg Spine. 2016;25(6):675–80.
20. Lall R, Patel NJ, Resnick DK. A review of complications associated with craniocervical fusion surgery. Neurosurgery. 2010;67(5):1396–402; discussion 1402–393.
21. Dvorak MF, Fisher C, Boyd M, Johnson M, Greenhow R, Oxland TR. Anterior occiput-to-axis screw fixation: part I: a case report, description of a new technique, and anatomical feasibility analysis. Spine (Phila Pa 1976). 2003;28(3):E54–60.
22. Dvorak MF, Sekeramayi F, Zhu Q, et al. Anterior occiput to axis screw fixation: part II: a biomechanical comparison with posterior fixation techniques. Spine (Phila Pa 1976). 2003;28(3):239–45.
23. Wu AM, Chi YL, Weng W, Xu HZ, Wang XY, Ni WF. Percutaneous anterior occiput-to-axis screw fixation: technique aspects and case series. Spine J. 2013;13(11):1538–43.

Endovascular Approaches: Indications and Techniques

18

Elias Atallah, Nohra Chalouhi, and Pascal Jabbour

18.1 Part 1: Craniovertebral Junction Aneurysms

18.1.1 Vertebral Artery Aneurysms

One of the major blood supplying vessels to the central nervous system, the vertebral artery (VA) branches from the postero-superior aspect of the first part of the subclavian artery, travels in the neck and enters intracranially *piercing the dura* at the level of the first cervical vertebrae. It can be divided into four consequent anatomical segments: the extra-osseous segment (V1) originating from the subclavian artery toward the C6 transverse foramina, the foraminal segment (V2) traveling from C6 to C1 within the transverse foramina, the sub-occipital segment as the VA emerges from the transverse foramina of C1 where it describes a siphon-like tortuosity before entering the skull through the foramen magnum and wanders intradurally (V4) along the medulla toward the basilar artery (BA). Whether single or dually aberrant or anomalous, VAs are predominantly damaged via dissection of the arterial wall [24]. VA aneurysms (VAA) are not encountered repeatedly but are increasingly recognized as dissecting in nature. Although the majority of dissecting VAAs are subsequent to significant blunt or penetrating injury, several spontaneous VAAs ensue after a trivial trauma involving a certain degree of cervical distortion. Rare associations between VAA and neurofibromatosis type I, fibromuscular dysplasia, autosomal dominant polycystic kidney disease and Ehler-Danlos disease have been reported.

E. Atallah · N. Chalouhi · P. Jabbour (✉)
Division of Neurovascular Surgery and Endovascular Neurosurgery, Department of Neurological Surgery, Thomas Jefferson University Hospital, Philadelphia, PA, USA
e-mail: elias.atallah@jefferson.edu; nohra.chalouhi@jefferson.edu; pascal.jabbour@jefferson.edu

E. Tessitore et al. (eds.), *Surgery of the Cranio-Vertebral Junction*,
https://doi.org/10.1007/978-3-030-18700-2_18

Vertebral artery dissection (VAD) is often an underdiagnosed entity because of the repeatedly vague nature and insidious early symptoms: although not always obvious, patients would experience an initially severe occipital headache with a posterior nuchal pain following a head or neck injury and manifest with focal neurologic signs attributable to the ischemia of the brainstem or the cerebellum. The variable presentation attributed to VAD is vindicated by the reckoned anatomic variability of the collaterals connecting the different arteries of the circle of Willis—completely intact in only about 20% of individuals. This is why sacrificing one VA, while treating VAD, can be tolerated while the contralateral supposedly intact VA suffuses adequately the BA. Several reports have identified mortality rates, as high as 46%, with untreated VAAs. Patients presenting with bleeding or ruptured VAAs have a pronounced 71% prospect of rebleeding especially within the first 24 h following hemorrhage, and within the first week if left untreated. However, relatively benign natural histories have been reported in cases presenting with ischemic symptoms and the indications or timings for treatment of non-SAH cases remain controversial.

Patients presenting with symptomatic or ruptured VAA have been mainly treated with a deconstructive procedure of the vertebral artery or a reconstructive procedure with flow diversion keeping in mind the challenge of starting patients with SAH on dual anti-platelet therapy. Those dissecting aneurysms are rarely coiled due to their nature and the fact that they are considered more as pseudoaneurysms as compared to real aneurysms. On the other hand, unruptured asymptomatic VAA tend to follow a relatively benign clinical course, and because the prognosis tends to be agreeable, conservative treatment has been proposed.

Endovascular management of dissecting VAAs is a safe procedure. It warrants a remarkable low recurrence rate of aneurysm refilling-bleeding in those initially presenting with a SAH, whether proximal or distal to the PICA, treatment options of VAAs are clearly elucidated and accessible; but those involving the PICA have been renowned endovascularly challenging. In such cases, neurointerventionists tend to use the [balloon transitory occlusion (BTO)] Transient Balloon Occlusion technique (TBO) in order to evaluate the likelihood of the neurological damage subsequent to sacrificing the PICA with or without VA revascularization. Currently, the treatment of PC aneurysms has somewhat shifted away from microsurgical clipping to endovascular techniques. Pipeline embolization device (PED) has been exceedingly deployed in the treatment of anterior circulation aneurysms, nonetheless, it has not been quietly implicated in the treatment of posterior circulation (PC) aneurysms. Few centers have successfully installed the PED across the VAA's neck in order to divert the blood flow and consequently prompt its occlusion [5, 13]. Parent vessel occlusion, trapping, coiling, stent-assisted coiling, or stent monotherapy are also used to treat these aneurysms. Parent artery occlusion is a reliable technique for obliteration of the aneurysm, but it may not be feasible for cases with dominant artery or major branch (PICA or anterior spinal artery) involvement without collateral flow. In these cases, flow diversion with the cylindrical meshwork

PED may be the preferred treatment modality. One of the major advantages of the PED in this setting is to maintain patency of branching vessels or perforators arising from the parent artery.

18.1.2 Posterior Inferior Cerebellar Artery Aneurysms

PICA, the largest branch of the VA, usually arises from the intradural segment (V4) of the VA near the inferior olives and passes posteriorly around the medulla. At the lateral margin of the medulla, it passes between the rootlets of the hypoglossal nerve, and courses rostral to the fila of the glossopharyngeal, vagus, and accessory nerves, then, it courses in a tortuous manner toward the fourth ventricle. PICA aneurysms (PICAA) are relatively uncommon (0.5–3%) among intracranial aneurysms (IA) but they count for roughly 18% of infratentorial aneurysms, making it the second in frequency following the basilar apex aneurysms.

PICAA can sprout at the PICA origin (saccular) or—not infrequently—at a distal location along p2 to p5 segments of the artery. These aneurysms are usually "atypical" with an increased incidence of fusiform or dolichoectatic morphology, lobulated and distally located beyond the arterial origin. This is mostly due to the rebellious turns in the course of the PICA, and excessive sheer stress forces contributing to the elastic lamina injury and subsequent aneurysm formation. As with all other IA, patients are often diagnosed subsequently to subarachnoid hemorrhage (SAH) or to symptoms involving the medulla or cranial nerves IX-XI [23]. Natural history studies have demonstrated that PC aneurysms have a higher risk of rupture and a higher associated mortality than their anterior circulation counterparts. Selecting the best treatment protocol for PICAA is vital because of their somewhat elevated risk of recurrence and its overwhelming risk of fatality.

Blood vessel reconstruction via open surgery has been the optimal choice for treating PICAA for decades. Nevertheless, surgeons nowadays tend to prefer minimally invasive endovascular procedures as first-line treatment for several but not all PICAAs. It is challenging to elucidate the gold standard treatment of these aneurysms now that flow diversion techniques are easily accessible and flow diversion stents straightforwardly deployable across the aneurysms neck. Xu F. et al. 2017 [23] discussed this latter postulation, and pondered the challenging technique and the potential neurological damage accompanying open surgery—due to its proximity to the brainstem—, and compared it to the more "luxurious" endovascular therapy that offers a less invasive alternative. They confirmed, in a series of 42 PICAA, the effectiveness of the endovascular treatment in achieving long-term stability and preventing rebleeding. It can be technically performed either by occluding the aneurysm with endosaccular coiling or an assisted bypass with parent artery preservation—with a decreased risk of ischemic complications—or by inducing reversed blood flow by occluding parent artery, forming an assisted bypass or diverting the blood flow with the PED that would preserve and reconstruct the main vessel and induce a progressive aneurysm occlusion [2]. The morbi-mortality rate associated with endovascular embolization of PICAA—related to the small and tortuous anatomy of the main artery sometimes preventing catheterization—has ranged between 8.6 and 12.7% [2, 3, 10, 20]. Still, the risk of brainstem ischemia seems to be relatively low, because of commonly seen sufficient collateral vascularization impending from the contralateral PICA or from the ipsilateral anterior cerebellar artery and/or the superior cerebellar artery.

The primary complications encountered with the endovascular PICAA treatment are aneurysm recurrence (5.4%), rebleeding phenomenon (3.2%) and thrombosis of the main artery, and the utmost portrayed complication of the surgical approach is the injury affecting the lower set of cranial nerves IX-XII (18.5%). For this reason, the microsurgical anatomy has been portrayed as a series of triangular corridors for limiting nerve injury while approaching such aneurysms with an open surgical procedure. While treating a series of 113 PICAA (65 microsurgically and 37 endovascularly) Bohnstedt et al. 2015 [2] reported a higher significant tendency to use shunts (31% vs 23%) in patients treated microsurgically compared to endovascular treatment. Around 41% of ruptured and unruptured aneurysms undergoing surgical treatment, experience postoperative deficits compared to only 16% of the endovascularly managed ruptured aneurysms. Despite statistically significant differences in complications between endovascularly or microsurgically treated patients, these same differences were not observed in final patient outcomes at 1 year follow-up [2].

Decisions to treat PICAA with a microsurgical far-lateral approach or endovascularly are selected on a case-by-case basis according to aneurysm location, morphology—broad neck aneurysm or ruptured state—, presenting neurologic condition, medical comorbidities, preferences of the treatment team and of the patient. Comparing both approaches in variable settings remains essential in order to define the primary treatment of care for every PICAA (Figs. 18.1, 18.2, and 18.3).

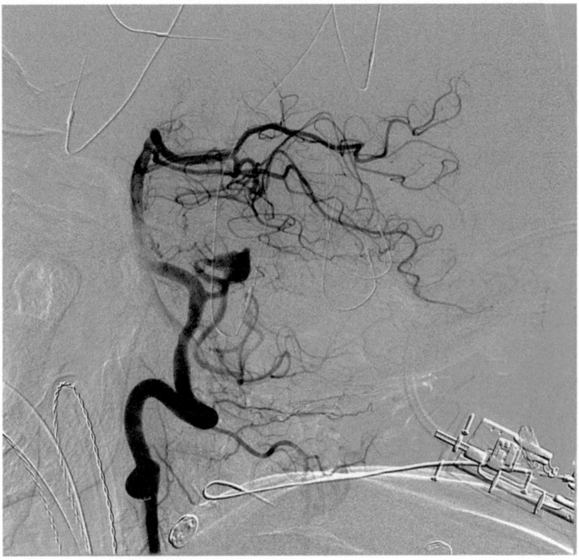

Fig. 18.1 Angiogram showing a Left vertebral artery (Lvert) catheterization with contrast injection. Wide necked saccular aneurysm at the lateral medullary segment (P2) of the left poterior inferior cerebellar artery (PICA)

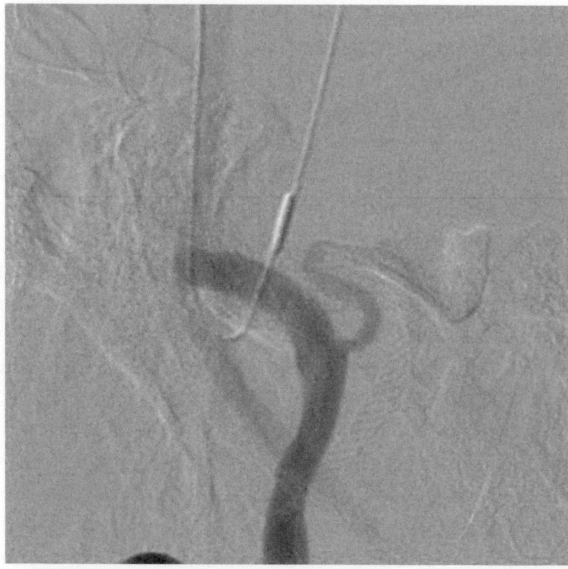

Fig. 18.2 Flow diversion pipeline embolization device (PED) deployment, at the lateral medullary segment of the left poterior inferior cerebellar artery (PICA), across the neck of the aneurysm

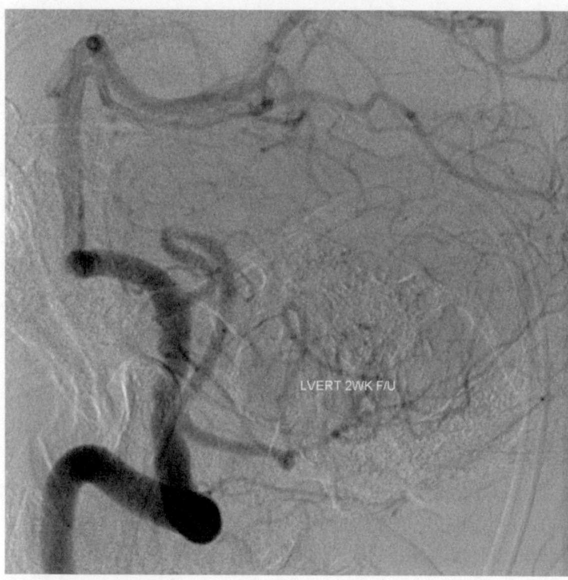

Fig. 18.3 One-year follow-up digital subtraction angiography (DSA) with left vertebral artery (Lvert) catheterization and contrast injection. Complete resolution of the saccular aneurysm, at the left poterior inferior cerebellar artery (PICA), after treatment with the pipeline embolization device (PED)

18.1.3 Vertebro-Basilar Aneurysms

Vertebro-basilar junction (VBJ) is an intracranial midline union of the intradural segments of the right and left VAs. It gives rise to the BA which is divided into junctional, trunk and tip segments and branches into the anterior inferior cerebellar artery (proximal BA trunk) and the superior cerebellar artery (proximal to BA tip). Aneurysms of the VBJ (VBJA) are often large, giant in size and mostly of non-saccular geometry, dissecting in nature characterized by elongation, dilation, and/or tortuosity of the vessel. This has been related in almost 70% of VBJAs to defects of embryogenesis manifesting as fenestration of the intracranial vasculature arising from the incomplete fusion of primitive neural arteries. The main underlying pathologic mechanism behind the aneurysms at this site has been linked to the delicate arterial wall media defects rendering it susceptible to wall shear stress and altered hemodynamics. VBJAs are relatively rare, with an incidence of almost 0.5%. Asymptomatic patients tend to precipitate ischemic disease rather than IA rupture and SAH. Most symptomatic patients present with a SAH. Mizutani et al. suggested, in 1999, a benign progression of the disease of the dolichoectatic VBJAs. In opposition to this proposition, Nasr et al. 2016 [17] deliberated, in their analysis on the imaging characteristics associated with growing and ruptured non-saccular and dolichoectatic aneurysms of the VB tree, the likelihood of dolichoectatic aneurysm to grow (8%) during the follow-up period similarly but less frequently than transitional and fusiform aneurysms. These results are analogous to those displayed by Passero and Rossi [19] who found that approximately 5% of dolichoectactic aneurysms progressed (defined as either increasing tortuosity and/or enlargement) over a 5-year follow-up period.

Surgical access to the VBJ is challenging, local anatomy is complex due to the existence of perforators to the brainstem and lower cranial nerves. In addition, the complicated geometry of the fenestration makes clipping of the aneurysms difficult. With the results of the subarachnoid aneurysm Trial, the endovascular treatment of VBJAs has been widely acknowledged and has become the first-line treatment of these lesions ranging from coiling, balloon remodeling techniques, stenting, parent vessel occlusion, and trapping [25]. The rate of technical success of endovascular interventions has been reported close to 95.5% with only 10% risk of per-procedural complications [25]. Meckel et al. [14] demonstrated the safety and the efficacy of single pipeline or pipeline/coiling combined treatment of complex VBJAs. Nevertheless, they have debated the persisting risk of recurrent SAH, late intra-PED thrombosis, progressive mass effect and delayed intracranial hemorrhage, coupled to the endovascular approach. Consequently, the use of PED in the treatment of VBJAs should be pondered and reserved for those cases in which alternative approaches either are deemed unsafe or are likely to be ineffective.

18.2 Part 2: Arteriovenous Malformations and Tumors Encasing the Vertebral Artery—Temporary Balloon Occlusion and Tumor Embolization

18.2.1 Arteriovenous Malformations and Fistulas of the Vertebral Artery

Spinal arteriovenous malformations and fistulas (AVM/F) are uncommon lesions in adults (4%) and rarer still in children. These vascular lesions may cause serious neurologic morbidities, are regularly categorized based on nidus anatomical location and its corresponding angioarchitecture, four groups have been described: dural AVF, glomus AVM, juvenile metameric AVM, and pial AVF. The dural type is the most frequent lesion (70%) of all spinal AVMs. One AVM could be supplied by multiple feeders arising from anterior/posterior or VAs. Previous reports have assembled a heterogeneous collection of VA arteriovenous lesions, including arterial contributions from the upper and lower VAs draining into a variety of spinal and paraspinal collectors.

Embryologically, the CVJ represents a transition point from a spinal intersegmental arterial organization to a carotid-based system. In the first few weeks of embryogenesis, while the temporary connections between the first six cervical segments and the dorsal aorta go on to regress, the VAs originate as the C7 intersegmental branches. With regression of the other cervical intersegmental branches, the longitudinal axis of the definitive VAs within the *foramen transversarium* results from the coalescence of the first six cervical intersegmental arteries. In contrast, at the CVJ, development is instead organized along the carotid-vertebral anastomoses. These temporary connections between the carotid arteries and the plexiform longitudinal neural arteries go on to regress, and the longitudinal neural arteries unite to form the definitive basilar artery. Thus, for arteriovenous lesions affecting the upper vertebral artery, distinct embryological pathways of coalescence and regression between the cervical intersegmental and the longitudinal neural arteries may be related to developmental anatomic variants. However, the mid and lower cervical longitudinal axis of the VA represents purely intersegmental development, and is thus thought less likely to be a congenital lesion originating from anatomic variants.

Based on the latter embryological inscription, several authors suggested that upper VAs angio-malformations tend to be spontaneous lesions whereas those affecting the mid and lower segments of the VA are mostly subsequent to various traumatic aggressions and dissections. It was Rodesch and Lasjaunias who proposed, in a classification of vertebral-vertebral AVF (VVAVF), the likelihood of having lower vertebral AVF as typically low flow with large paraspinal collecting venous pouches. Nevertheless, this is not always the case [1]. Clinical manifestations of these lesions has been correlated to the anatomic location of the malformation and regrouped a few or many of the following signs and symptoms: objective bruit, pain, paresthesia, congestive myelopathy-related to retrograde intradural venous drainage-, paresis, paralysis, subarachnoid, epidural, or intramedullary hemorrhage, high-output cardiac failure, and VB insufficiency secondary to arterial steal.

Many authors have labeled the microsurgical approach as a primordial treatment for AVMs. Surgical treatment of VVAVFs include radical fistula resection/trapping, clip ligation of the fistulous point, VA sacrifice, and surgical decompression. Given the potential blood loss and the morbidity of such a delicate surgical technic, a fairly large number of these vascular malformations are difficult to treat with primary microsurgical occlusion. Endovascular management of these vascular "*nests*" has gained significant popularity and has become common practice with the recent escalation of catheter and guidewire technology and novel embolic materials. Detachable latex balloons and coils have the longest historical track record for this purpose, although more recently liquid embolic agents have also been used for the spinal AVF treatment. However, unlike coils which can be retrieved before detachment—only if the pattern of deployment appears unfavorable—, liquid embolic agents are not retrievable after injection and pose the potential risk of distal embolization through the epidural plexus or proximal embolization through the VA. Although modern endovascular approach for treating AVM/Fs is becoming increasingly effective, it still lags behind surgical success rates which approach 100% [12]. The outcome of both treatment options is similar if complete obliteration of AVM/F is obtained and depends mainly on the severity of neurological dysfunction before treatment (Figs. 18.4, 18.5, and 18.6).

18.2.2 Tumors Encasing the Vertebral Artery

Mass occupying lesions are commonly encountered in this anatomical location. Several neoplastic lesions can occupy the CVJ: chordomas, osteoblastomas, meningiomas, hemangioblastoma, ependymoma, metastatic tumors, etc. The surgical management of these tumors, particularly with associated neurovascular compromise, is challenging in terms of achieving proper resection, spinal stabilization and guaranteeing minimal probability of recurrence. Whenever the tumor is at proximity or encircling the VA, additional investigations with digital subtraction angiography or magnetic resonance angiogram is desirable with possible embolization or

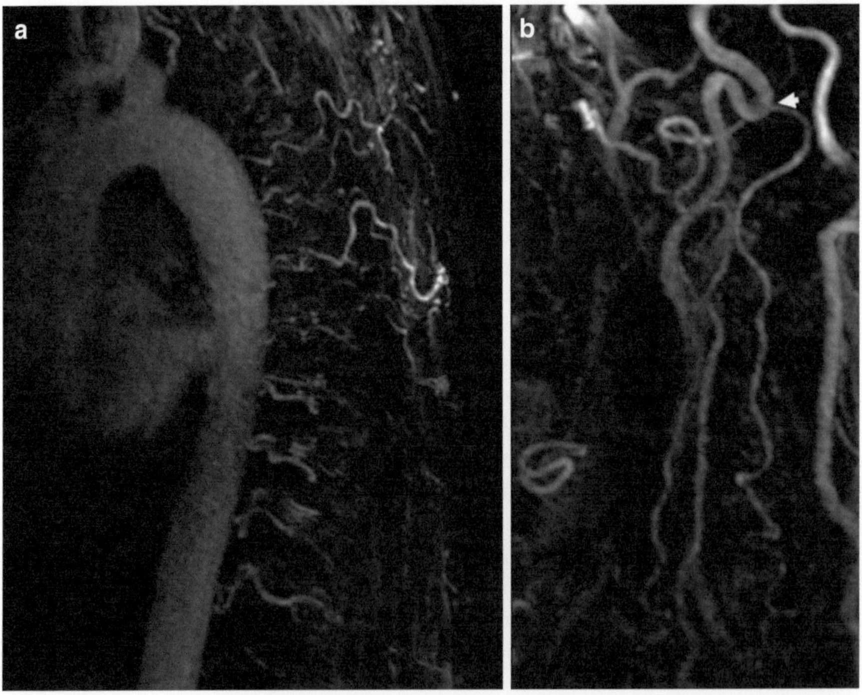

Fig. 18.4 Sagittal T_2-weighted short-tau inversion recovery (STIR) images of the thoracic (**a**) and cervical (**b**) spine. Dilated dorsal perimedullary veins are seen throughout the imaged spinal canal, but significant cord signal change is seen only from T8 to the conus medullaris

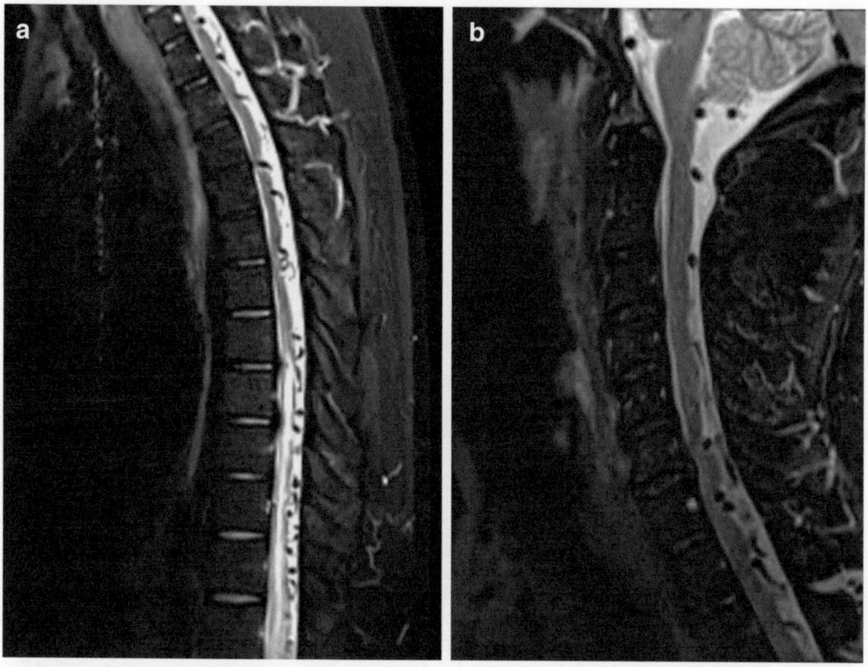

Fig. 18.5 Thoracic (**a**) and cervical (**b**) time-resolved MR angiogram (TR-MRA) using TRICKS protocol (General Electric Inc., Chicago, USA). There is no evidence of fistulous lesion seen on thoracic TR-MRA, but is clearly seen in the cervical images (arrow) at the level of the craniovertebral junction

temporary balloon occlusion. Preoperative VA angiograms or highly specific CT angiograms should be routinely completed to demonstrate the relation between VAs, the cervical spine and the tumor. This step is primordial in the planning of the right surgical technique.

18.2.2.1 Tumor Embolization

VA angiograms are usually gold standard in the preoperative visualization of the vascular anatomy and serves as a tactical approach to perform adjuvant endovascular tumor embolization (TE), only if feeders happen to be accessible.

Embolic agents may be permanent or of temporary use. Choosing the best agent relies on the tumor infiltration, on the vascular anatomy and on the interventionist's expertise in manipulating liquid embolic agents or particles that can penetrate into the smallest vessels but withhold a relatively considerable risk of damage to the normal adjacent tissues. Superselective micro-catheterization is often necessary for complete evaluation of individual distal vessels and to assess for intratumoral shunting. Close attention should be paid to the presence of anastomoses between extra and intracranial circulation or anastomoses to critical structures such as the eye or *vaso nervosum* supplying various cranial nerves [11].

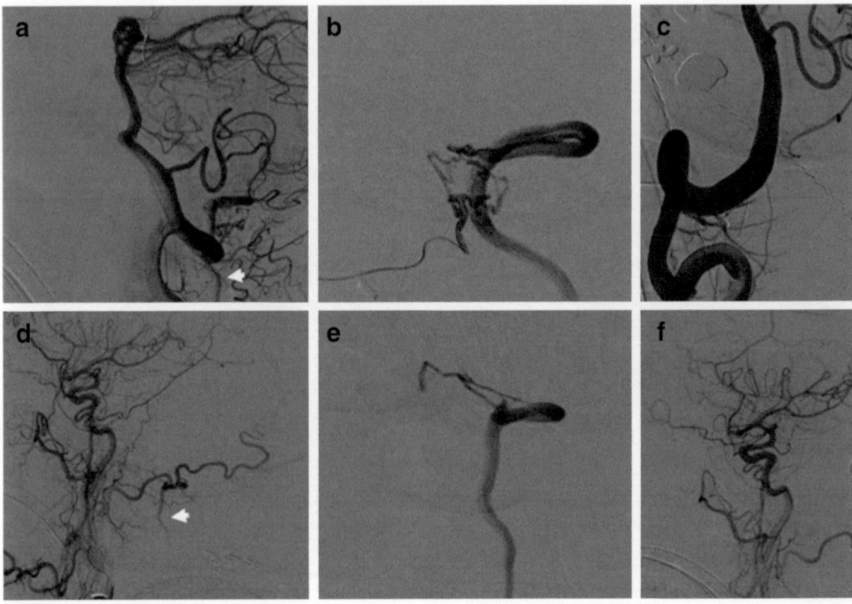

Fig. 18.6 Digital subtraction angiography (DSA) of the right vertebral artery (VA) (**a**–**c**) and common carotid artery (CCA) (**d**–**f**) systems. Evidence of a large early-draining vein is seen at the level of the craniovertebral junction on both VA and CCA injections (**a**, **d**, arrows). Superselective catheterization shows filling of the fistula through branches of the posterior meningeal artery and ascending pharyngeal artery (**b**, **e**). Control runs after superselective embolization of the dural arteriovenous Fistula show complete occlusion of the fistula (**c**, **f**)

The procedure is considered technically successful once the surgeon is capable of occluding the designated vessels. Clinical success is attained if minute blood is lost during surgery, if it has participated in limiting surgical morbidity by allowing better visualization of the surgical field, shortening of the operative procedure time, increased the chances of complete surgical resection and limited the damage to adjacent normal tissue.

18.2.2.2 Vertebral Artery Deconstruction: The Role of Temporary Balloon Occlusion

The safety and the efficacy of preoperative endovascular deconstruction of the encircled VA has been shown to facilitate safe CVJT resection. Chalouhi et al. [4] described a new technique in 2013 for carotid and VA deconstruction using a combination of Onyx and coils, and assessed its feasibility, safety, and efficacy. Nevertheless, the use of trans-arterial detachable coils has been described as time-consuming and costly expensive since it frequently requires several coils deployment to achieve flow interruption. Ogungbemi et al. 2015 re-evaluated the safety and the efficacy of the primal endovascular detachable balloons, performed without prior TBO in the preoperative management of these tumors. The only absolute contraindication to occlusion was absent or severely hypoplastic intradural segment of the contralateral VA considered angiographically inadequate to support the posterior circulation. Temporary VA balloon test conventionally precedes complete perprocedural VA sacrificing with CVJT resection in order to establish the integrity of the circle of Willis and identify patients prone to ischemic complications [8]. In opposition to several statements, VA TBO is not always deemed necessary as its veracity in predicting subsequent ischemia has not been, so far, clearly elucidated [9, 22, 26]. In fact, TBO is one of many preoperative indicators-like regional cerebral blood flow evaluation with computed tomography and magnetic resonance imaging, measurement of arterial stump pressure, transcranial Doppler ultrasound, deemed significant in order to predict inadequate perfusion. Although it seems logical that cerebral blood flow evaluation and/or other adjunctive tests performed during TBO should help to reveal marginal areas of perfusion that might lead to neurologic deficits after permanent arterial occlusion, this has not been convincingly shown.

Published data suggested that clinically evident ischemic complication is relatively infrequent following unilateral VA occlusion. Dominance of the affected VA is not considered to be a contraindication to vessel deconstruction. Dual VA inflow to BA and multiple potential collateral inputs to the distal VA from cervical and external carotid arteries as well as retrograde flow from the circle of Willis are protective against ischemic complications. Although the use of detachable balloons carries several risks of potential disastrous distal embolization as well as balloon deflation and delayed vessel recanalization if used inappropriately, in experienced hands, they may offer further advantages including accuracy of placement, cost effective flow arrest with lower consequent radiation dose knowing that those balloons were removed from the US market.

18.3 Part 3: Mechanical Thrombectomy in the Management of Vertebro-Basilar Artery Strokes

Posterior ischemic stroke (PIS) represents approximately 20% of all ischemic strokes. Small lesions can cause significant deficits as compared to anterior circulation strokes, due to the close proximity of major afferent and efferent tracts and cranial nerve nuclei in Brainstem [18]. A PIS is defined by an infarction occurring within the vascular territory supplied by the VB arterial system [18]. Although the posterior circulation (PC) is branded with a highly interconnected vasculature, around 70% of VB infarcts are clinically manifest due to the concomitant anatomical variability of the PC vasculature: unilateral VA hypoplasia and BA curvature.

Multiple stroke registries have been analyzed to determine the most characteristics and common etiologies of PIS. Large vessel and small vessel stroke ensuing from causal atherosclerotic disease have been responsible for 35% and 13% of PIS, respectively. The most common location of VA atherosclerosis and consequently thrombus formation are V1 and V4 segments. It is noteworthy to consider VA dissection whenever stenosis involves the V2 and V3 segments. Similar to ICA atherothrombotic accidents, lesion irregularity and plaque morphology correlate with the severity of the ischemic presentation in the PC. De facto, ischemia due to intracranial disease may result from tissue hypoperfusion, in situ-thrombosis or artery to artery thromboembolis (20% in PIS disease). The failure of compensatory mechanisms—typically witnessed in “Tandem” extra-intracranial VA lesions—can be responsible for a wide range of severe neurologic damage, which has been labeled as the “misery perfusion phenomenon.”

Chemical and mechanical revascularization options have been considered lately as primary modalities in the management of PISs. The use of mechanical thrombectomy (MT) in the management of acute ischemic stroke (AIS) has become increasingly popular throughout the past decade. It provides an option for flow restoration in those who are arbitrated non-eligible for receiving chemical intravenous thrombolysis with the classical fibrinolytic agents (IV-rtPA). It augments the chances of completely reversing the patients’ symptoms by offering to extend the treatment window from 4.5 h with the IV-rtPA to 8 h from the initial time of their early symptoms manifestation. It is worthy to mention that although to a much less extent, some patients still benefit from the use of MT after 8-h mark [6].

Multiple factors affect the clinical outcome and the complication rates in patients with AIS treated with mechanical flow restoration devices. The first device was the Merci Retriever (Concentric Medical, Kalamazoo, Michigan), which was approved by the US Food and Drug Administration (FDA) in 2004, and the second mechanical thrombectomy device was the Penumbra, which was approved in 2007. In 2012, a newer generation of MT devices, the Solitaire flow restoration (FR) revascularization device (ev3/Covidien Vascular Therapies, Irvine, California) and the Trevo stent retriever devices (Stryker, Kalamazoo, Michigan), were approved by the FDA. Better clinical outcomes, recanalization rates, and significantly less complications have been recently quantified with the Solitaire® device.

Current MT interventionists prefer the use of stentrievers over its predecessors [6, 21]. The use of such devices has been associated with high rates of recanalization with a low probability of complications and a consequent improved functional outcome in patients with AIS involving the PC [7]. The rate of good clinical outcome was higher in young patients <80 years (67%) [6]. Nevertheless, a discrepancy has been described between a high thrombolysis in cerebral infarction (TICI) perfusion scale grade and clinical outcome. Not all patients with good recanalization grade go on to having favorable outcomes, especially patients with internal carotid or BA occlusion, elderly and those with higher NIHSS score at admission. In a retrospective study conducted by Daou et al. [6], 89 patients presenting with AIS symptoms underwent MT. Although eight of nine patients with a VB thrombus had substantial revascularization, the only statistically significant predictors of increased mortality after Solitaire® thrombectomy were thrombus location in the PC with a mortality rate of 33%, and a high NIHSS score. An occlusion of the VB circulation is often associated with higher odds of morbidity and mortality. A comparable result has been reported by Mordasini et al. [15] where all the included patients had successful revascularization however, the mortality rate was 35.7%. Mourand et al. 2014 [16] included 31 patients in their designed prospective single center study and were diagnosed with acute BA occlusion; they underwent MT and reported an analogous mortality rate of 32% also. Nonetheless, neurointerventionists should tend to include MT in the urgent management of PISs, for it is regarded as a life-saver, an indispensable procedure and remains capable of improving the clinical outcome of approximately 70% of the PIS patients.

18.4 Conclusion

The craniovertebral junction is an anatomical region where a multitude of pathologies can occur. Endovascular techniques play a major role in either treating or as an adjunct to the final surgical treatment of those lesions, knowing the indications and limitations of those techniques is key to screen patients and reduce complications.

References

1. Ashour R, Orbach DB. Lower vertebral-epidural spinal arteriovenous fistulas: a unique subtype of vertebrovertebral arteriovenous fistula, treatable with coil and Penumbra Occlusion Device embolization. J Neurointerv Surg. 2016;8:643–7.
2. Bohnstedt BN, Ziemba-Davis M, Edwards G, Brom J, Payner TD, Leipzig TJ, et al. Treatment and outcomes among 102 posterior inferior cerebellar artery aneurysms: a comparison of endovascular and microsurgical clip ligation. World Neurosurg. 2015;83:784–93.
3. Chalouhi N, Jabbour P, Starke RM, Tjoumakaris SI, Gonzalez LF, Witte S, et al. Endovascular treatment of proximal and distal posterior inferior cerebellar artery aneurysms. J Neurosurg. 2013;118:991–9.
4. Chalouhi N, Starke RM, Tjoumakaris SI, Jabbour PM, Gonzalez LF, Hasan D, et al. Carotid and vertebral artery sacrifice with a combination of Onyx and coils: technical note and case series. Neuroradiology. 2013;55:993–8.
5. Chalouhi N, Tjoumakaris S, Dumont AS, Gonzalez LF, Randazzo C, Starke RM, et al. Treatment of posterior circulation aneurysms with the pipeline embolization device. Neurosurgery. 2013;72:883–9.
6. Daou B, Chalouhi N, Starke RM, Dalyai R, Hentschel K, Jabbour P, et al. Predictors of outcome, complications, and recanalization of the solitaire device: a study of 89 cases. Neurosurgery. 2015;77:355–60; discussion 360–51.
7. Du S, Mao G, Li D, Qiu M, Nie Q, Zhu H, et al. Mechanical thrombectomy with the Solitaire AB stent for treatment of acute basilar artery occlusion: a single-center experience. J Clin Neurosci. 2016;32:67–71.
8. Gonzalez CF, Moret J. Balloon occlusion of the carotid artery prior to surgery for neck tumors. AJNR Am J Neuroradiol. 1990;11:649–52.
9. Graves VB, Perl J 2nd, Strother CM, Wallace RC, Kesava PP, Masaryk TJ. Endovascular occlusion of the carotid or vertebral artery with temporary proximal flow arrest and microcoils: clinical results. AJNR Am J Neuroradiol. 1997;18:1201–6.
10. Isokangas JM, Siniluoto T, Tikkakoski T, Kumpulainen T. Endovascular treatment of peripheral aneurysms of the posterior inferior cerebellar artery. AJNR Am J Neuroradiol. 2008;29:1783–8.
11. Lazzaro MA, Badruddin A, Zaidat OO, Darkhabani Z, Pandya DJ, Lynch JR. Endovascular embolization of head and neck tumors. Front Neurol. 2011;2:64.
12. Maimon S, Luckman Y, Strauss I. Spinal dural arteriovenous fistula: a review. Adv Tech Stand Neurosurg. 2016; 43:111–37.

13. Mazur MD, Kilburg C, Wang V, Taussky P. Pipeline embolization device for the treatment of vertebral artery aneurysms: the fate of covered branch vessels. J Neurointerv Surg. 2016;8:1041–7.
14. Meckel S, McAuliffe W, Fiorella D, Taschner CA, Phatouros C, Phillips TJ, et al. Endovascular treatment of complex aneurysms at the vertebrobasilar junction with flow-diverting stents: initial experience. Neurosurgery. 2013;73:386–94.
15. Mordasini P, Brekenfeld C, Byrne JV, Fischer U, Arnold M, Heldner MR, et al. Technical feasibility and application of mechanical thrombectomy with the Solitaire FR Revascularization Device in acute basilar artery occlusion. AJNR Am J Neuroradiol. 2013;34:159–63.
16. Mourand I, Machi P, Milhaud D, Picot MC, Lobotesis K, Arquizan C, et al. Mechanical thrombectomy with the Solitaire device in acute basilar artery occlusion. J Neurointerv Surg. 2014;6:200–4.
17. Nasr DM, Brinjikji W, Rouchaud A, Kadirvel R, Flemming KD, Kallmes DF. Imaging characteristics of growing and ruptured vertebrobasilar non-saccular and dolichoectatic aneurysms. Stroke. 2016;47:106–12.
18. Nouh A, Remke J, Ruland S. Ischemic posterior circulation stroke: a review of anatomy, clinical presentations, diagnosis, and current management. Front Neurol. 2014;5:30.
19. Passero SG, Rossi S. Natural history of vertebrobasilar dolichoectasia. Neurology. 2008;70:66–72.
20. Peluso JP, van Rooij WJ, Sluzewski M, Beute GN, Majoie CB. Posterior inferior cerebellar artery aneurysms: incidence, clinical presentation, and outcome of endovascular treatment. AJNR Am J Neuroradiol. 2008;29:86–90.
21. Saver JL, Jahan R, Levy EI, Jovin TG, Baxter B, Nogueira RG, et al. Solitaire flow restoration device versus the Merci Retriever in patients with acute ischaemic stroke (SWIFT): a randomised, parallel-group, non-inferiority trial. Lancet. 2012;380:1241–9.
22. Sorteberg A, Bakke SJ, Boysen M, Sorteberg W. Angiographic balloon test occlusion and therapeutic sacrifice of major arteries to the brain. Neurosurgery. 2008;63:651–60; discussion 660–51.
23. Xu F, Hong Y, Zheng Y, Xu Q, Leng B. Endovascular treatment of posterior inferior cerebellar artery aneurysms: a 7-year single-center experience. J Neurointerv Surg. 2017;9(1):45–51.
24. Yuan SM. Aberrant origin of vertebral artery and its clinical implications. Braz J Cardiovasc Surg. 2016;31:52–9.
25. Zhu DY, Fang YB, Wu YN, Li Q, Duan GL, Liu JM, et al. Treatment of fenestrated vertebrobasilar junction-related aneurysms with endovascular techniques. J Clin Neurosci. 2016;28:112–6.
26. Zoarski GH, Seth R. Safety of unilateral endovascular occlusion of the cervical segment of the vertebral artery without antecedent balloon test occlusion. AJNR Am J Neuroradiol. 2014;35:856–61.

Part IV

Management of Cranio-Vertebral Junction Lesions

Craniovertebral Junction Instability and Mechanisms of Injury

19

Cédric Barrey, Mehdi Afathi, Théo Broussolle,
Corentin Dauleac, and Philippe Bancel

19.1 Introduction

The most important challenge in managing craniovertebral junction (CVJ) traumas mainly lies in recognizing and differentiating stable and unstable lesions which may result into severe neurological complication(s). With this objective, one must understand the normal anatomy and biomechanics of the CVJ [5, 25–28, 34, 37], and also the mechanisms of the injury, in order to diagnose the unstable post-traumatic lesions which may lead to a surgical indication.

Biomechanically, the cranio-cervical junction supports the weight of the head and represents one of the most mobile segment of the spine [6, 29, 35, 36, 37]. Physiological range of motion must be understood with approximately 25–30° of flexion-extension at C0-C1 and C1-C2, and around 35–40° of rotation at C1-C2. The stability is ensured by both soft tissues including joint capsules, membranes and ligaments, and sub-occipital muscles with the key-role played by the transverse ligament and bony structures. According to the mechanisms of injury (compression, distraction, rotation, and translation), it is possible to categorize specific injury patterns that is helpful to assess the stability of the injury and may influence the treatment option.

This book chapter is mainly focused on the biomechanics of the injured CVJ to help the clinician for treatment decision-making.

C. Barrey (✉) · M. Afathi · T. Broussolle · C. Dauleac
Spine and Spinal Cord Surgery Department, Pierre Wertheimer University Hospital,
Hospices Civils de Lyon, Claude Bernard University of Lyon 1, Lyon, France
e-mail: cedric.barrey@chu-lyon.fr

P. Bancel
Orthopaedic Surgery Department, Cochin Hospital, Assistance Publique des Hôpitaux
de Paris, Paris, France

E. Tessitore et al. (eds.), *Surgery of the Cranio-Vertebral Junction*,
https://doi.org/10.1007/978-3-030-18700-2_19

19.2 Biomechanics of the Injured Spine

Different mechanisms of injury, which will be detailed further, may result into excessive range of motion and therefore overtake the physiological resistance of ligaments, capsules, and/or bony structures. Damage of the bony structures and/or soft tissues elements may lead to severe CVJ instability with compromise of the integrity of the neurological structures [9, 10, 19, 38]. The objective of this part III is to analyze what are the biomechanical consequences according to which structure is injured.

19.2.1 Ligamentous Injuries

Ligaments represent uniaxial structures that can resist to direct traction forces. Some ligaments may resist to forces from a range of directions because of the multidirectional orientation of their fibers. In fact, ligaments are the most resistant when they are stressed along the direction of their predominant fibers. Otherwise, not only the amount of load but also the rate of load application may affect the nature of injury produced, as reported by Goel and al [20, 21].

Also, severe ligamentous injuries are incapable to heal spontaneously. Ligamentous lesions thus result into permanent and definitive instability and surgical stabilization has to be considered in most cases.

19.2.1.1 Rupture of the Transverse Ligament

The transverse ligament (TL) is the thickest and strongest ligament of the entire spine. Another mechanical particularity of the transverse ligament is represented by its poor elasticity [14]. During CJV injury, the thick and inelastic transverse ligament resists and suddenly disrupts. It tears suddenly as an "all-or-nothing" mechanism and does not fail partially or gradually, potentially leading to horizontal C1-C2 instability with C1 anterior subluxation (up to 12 mm), Fig. 19.1.

The transverse ligament represents the main stabilizing structure of C1-C2 constraining C1 around the dens. When torn, TL is incapable to repair and surgical C1-C2 fusion has strongly to be considered.

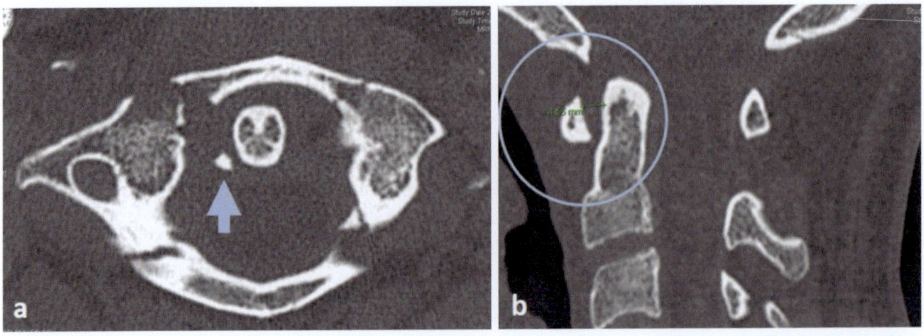

Fig. 19.1 (**a**, **b**). Avulsion of transverse ligament (blue arrow) resulting into C1-C2 horizontal instability with increase of ADI (atlanto-dens interval, which normally should be less than 3 mm) (from personal series)

19.2.1.2 Rupture of the Joint Capsules

Capsular C1-C2 ligaments are relatively loose and provide a small of C1-C2 stability. In the presence of intact transverse and alar ligaments, unilateral rupture of C1-C2 capsules result to augmented ROM into contralateral rotation. Isolated injury of C1-C2 capsular ligaments injury is considered not sufficient to induce C1-C2 instability [7].

19.2.1.3 Rupture of the Alar Ligament

It has been reported that isolated and unilateral rupture of alar ligaments on one side will cause increased contralateral axial rotation by approximately 30% [11].

Both alar and capsular ligaments compromise, without rupture of the transverse ligament, are unlikely to induce significant risk for C1-C2 translation, as demonstrated by Puttlitz et al. [30].

19.2.2 Bony Injuries

Not only ligamentar elements play a role for stability of CVJ but also bony structures [5]. Among them, the dens represents a major pivot element for stability of C0-C1-C2 complex. The dens and the intact transverse ligament are considered as the elements providing the major stability at the C1-C2 articulation. As an example, trans-oral or trans-nasal odontoidectomy, which is performed to decompress the upper spinal cord or the brain stem, may significantly jeopardize the CVJ stability (Fig. 19.2). This phenomenon is easy to understand seeing the crucial role of the

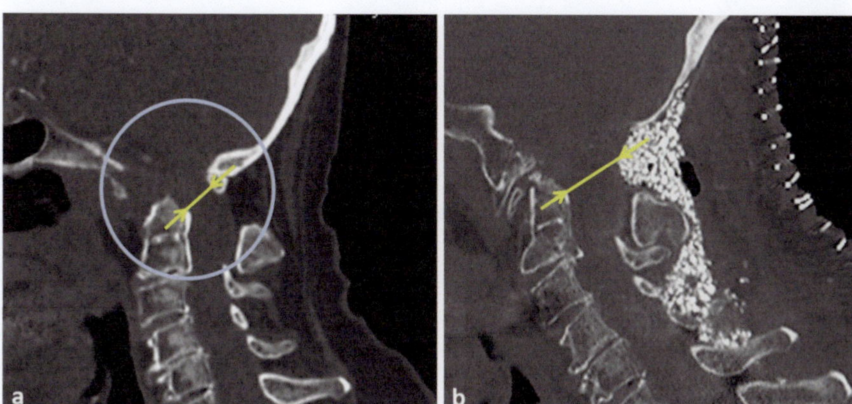

Fig. 19.2 (**a**, **b**) Illustrative case. Eighty-year-old woman who underwent a trans-sphenoidal odontoid process resection for a compressive rheumatoid pannus developed a severe CVJ instability. The neurological symptoms progressively relapsed, and the CT-scan showed a severe mixed vertical and horizontal CVJ instability with anterior translation of the C0-C1 complex regarding C2 vertebra (**a**) and associated with basilar invagination. The patient had to go through a revision surgery in order to decompress the spinal cord, reduce the displacement and the deformity and perform a posterior instrumented stabilization from C0 to T1 with bone grafting (**b**). The case illustrates the importance of the dens integrity to ensure the stability of the CVJ (from personal series)

dens which is the pivot around which C1 vertebra and the transverse ligament articulate. The laxity of C1 (translational movements) was proven to significantly increase after a trans-oral odontoidectomy, principally into the antero-posterior direction [9, 30]. C0-C2 posterior instrumented stabilization should systematically be discussed after partial/complete resection of the dens.

Otherwise, in contrast to ligamentous injuries, bony injuries have the potential of healing and orthoses may play a role for treatment until the consolidation of the bone occurs.

19.3 Mechanisms of Injury

In the context of normal biomechanics, understanding the mechanism of injury permits to fully appreciate the potential instability of the injured CVJ. In fact, CVJ injury is the result from the application of moments (with a certain magnitude of force, a certain length of lever arm, and a certain angle of application) to a particular site of the craniovertebral junction. The summary of theses torques are called major injuring vector (MIV). The mechanism of injury depends on the MIV, which conditions the damage of one or multiple anatomical element. By analyzing the type of injury force vectors, post-traumatic cervical lesions can be categorized into specific injury patterns. Also, according to the mechanism of injury, one must pay attention to the expected specific lesions associated with that mechanism.

Even if this organizational approach based on the predominant force vector is a kind of simplification, it is helpful to understand more precisely the potential instability consecutive to a trauma.

19.3.1 Pure Compression

The structures that bear the compressive forces at the CVJ are mainly the bony structures (and the discs into the sub-axial cervical spine) and are represented by the occipital condyles, the lateral masses of C1 and C2, and the vertebral body of C2. In fact, pure compression is rarely observed and most often compression is associated with flexion (flexion-compression vector) or rotation (rotation-compression vector).

19.3.1.1 Fracture of the Occipital Condyle

Fracture of the occipital condyle may result from different primary force vectors including: axial compression, axial traction, rotation-compression, asymmetrical compression, asymmetrical traction, and translation (Fig. 19.3). In fact, pure compression is very rare and most often more complex mechanism is the cause of the injury [31]. Most widely used classification is the one reported by Anderson and Montesano [2] into three types: compression fracture (type I), skull base fracture extended to occipital condyle (type II), and avulsion fracture of the alar ligament (type III).

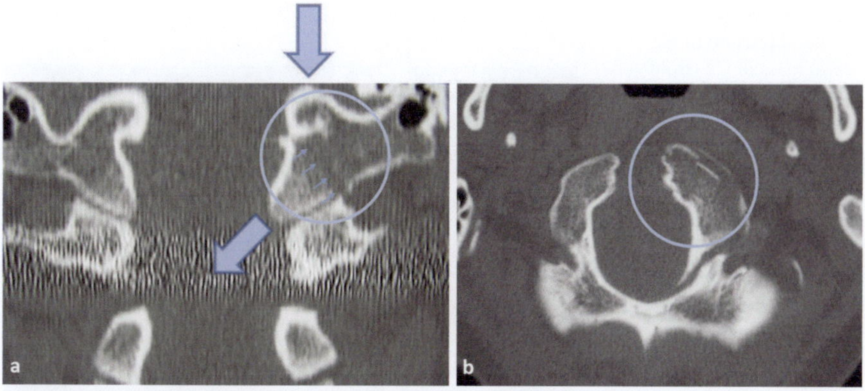

Fig. 19.3 (**a**, **b**) Fracture of the occipital condyle (left side). Type I injury according to Anderson and Montesano grading (from personal series)

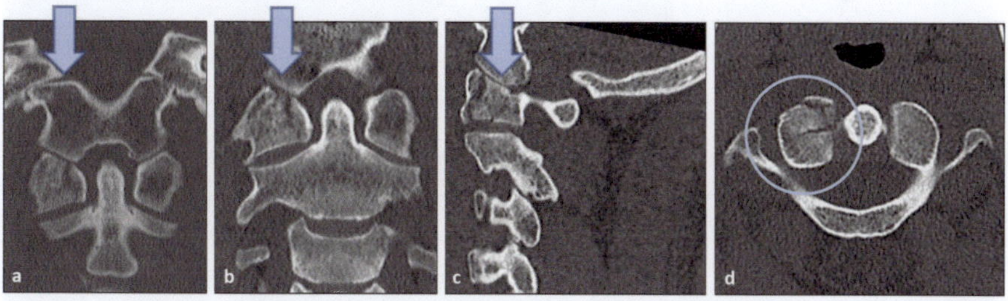

Fig. 19.4 (**a**–**d**) Unilateral lateral mass fracture of C1 consecutive to a pure compression mechanism. Type IV injury according to Gehweiler grading (from personal series)

19.3.1.2 Fracture of the Lateral Mass of C1

Atlas injuries represent the second most frequent type of bony lesions in the CVJ after odontoid fractures and are essentially caused by axial compression [32]. They are rarely isolated and are associated with C2 fracture in approximately 1 case over 2. The most relevant classification is the one reported by Gehweiler et al. [16] dividing theses fractures into five types: isolated fracture of the anterior arch (type I), isolated fracture of the posterior arch (type II), fracture of both anterior and posterior arch (type III), fracture of the lateral mass (type IV), and fracture of the transverse process (type V), Fig. 19.4.

19.3.1.3 Fracture of the Lateral Mass of C2

Isolated lateral mass fracture of C2 is rare (Fig. 19.5) and most often associated with a more complex vertebral body fracture of C2.

19.3.1.4 Fractures of C2 Vertebral Body

C2 vertebral body fractures are uncommon (7.2% among a series of 417 C1-C2 traumas as reported by Barrey and Charles [3]) and were classified into three main types by Benzel et al. [4, 17] according to the predominant direction of the fracture: coronally oriented (type I), sagittally oriented (type II), and transversally

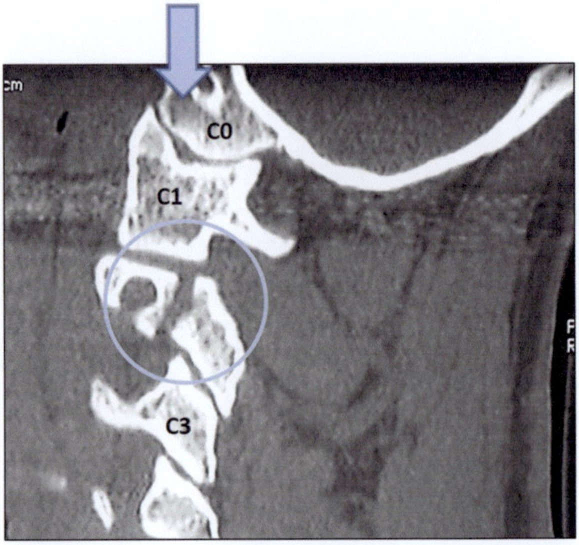

Fig. 19.5 Isolated unilateral fracture of the lateral mass of C2 (from personal series)

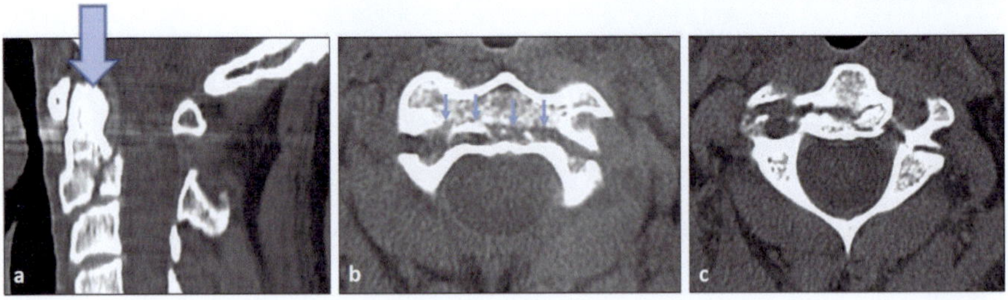

Fig. 19.6 (**a–c**) Fracture of C2 vertebral body, coronally oriented (i.e., Benzel type I), and consecutive to a predominant axial compression vector (from personal series)

oriented (type III), Fig. 19.6. In fact, Benzel type III is equivalent to type III odontoid fracture according to Anderson and D'Alonzo classification for odontoid fractures.

Type I (coronal) and type II (sagittal) are consecutive to axial compression mechanisms when type III is caused by hyperflexion or hyperextension mechanisms.

19.3.2 Distraction (Hyperflexion or Hyperextension)

Distraction injuries are typically consecutive to rapid acceleration or deceleration of the spine with the trunk staying in place and the head keeping to move. They are divided into hyperflexion and hyperextension mechanisms. According to the location of the center of rotation, hyperflexion injuries can result into pure flexion-distraction or flexion-compression injury patterns. Hyperextension will result into excessive stresses on the posterior elements and particularly on the posterior arches of C1 and C2, which are compressed between the occiput and the bony structures below.

19.3.2.1 Occipital Cervical Dislocation

Occipital-cervical dislocation (OCD) is also called cranio-cervical dislocation or dissociation [22, 23]. OCD is consecutive to application of enormous distraction energy pulling the head vertically (Fig. 19.7). This devastating injury is generally fatal. Traynelis et al. [33] categorized OCD into three types according to the main force vector: anterior (type I), vertical (type II), and posterior (type III).

19.3.2.2 Jefferson Fracture

Jefferson fracture was first reported in 1920, consists of both anterior and posterior arch fracture of C1 (Fig. 19.8) and corresponds to type 3 according to the classification system by Gehweiler [16]. Combination of hyperflexion and hyperextension is now considered as the main mechanism injury for Jefferson fracture with the posterior arch of C1 compressed between the occiput and the posterior of C2 during hyperextension and the anterior arch of C1 compressed between the basion and the body of C2 during hyperflexion [32].

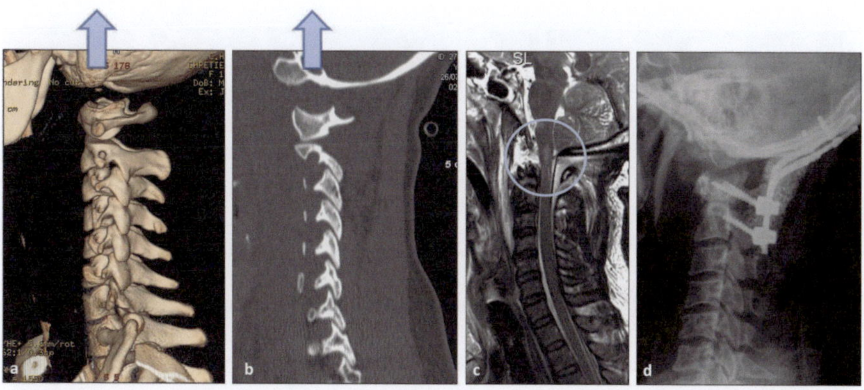

Fig. 19.7 (**a**–**d**) Complete C0-C1 dislocation secondary to a pure vertical distraction mechanism (**a**, **b**). Note the injury of the spinal cord (**c**). The treatment consisted of C0-C2 posterior stabilization (**d**) (from personal series)

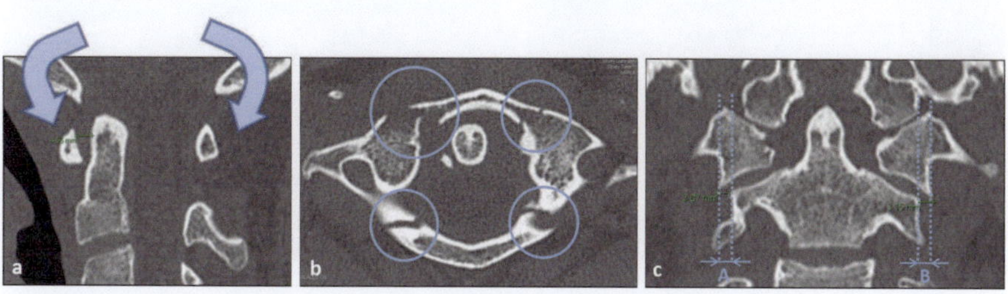

Fig. 19.8 (**a**–**c**) Jefferson fracture with fracture of both the anterior and posterior arches of C1 (**a**, **b**). According to the "rule of Spence," if the sum of A + B is more than 7 mm, instability should be considered (**c**) (from personal series)

19.3.2.3 Atlantoaxial Dislocation

In the case of atlantoaxial dislocation (Fig. 19.9), enormous energy is necessary to separate C1 from C2. The vertical portion of crucial ligament is sectioned whereas the horizontal part (i.e., the transverse ligament) is still intact. If the section occurs below the transverse ligament, atlantoaxial dislocation is observed, if the section is above, occipito-atlantal dislocation will occur.

19.3.2.4 Type II Odontoid Fracture

Type II odontoid fractures represent the most common type of bony lesion in the upper cervical spine [24]. They may result into atlantoaxial instability, antero-posterior translation and, therefore, compromise of the neurological structures [1]. Type II odontoid fractures generally result from hyperflexion or hyperextension, with the main injury mechanism determining the direction of the displacement (Fig. 19.10). When the main force vector is hyperflexion, typically, an anterior displacement of the dens will be observed. On the contrary, hyperextension will result into a posterior translation of the dens. The most common classification used

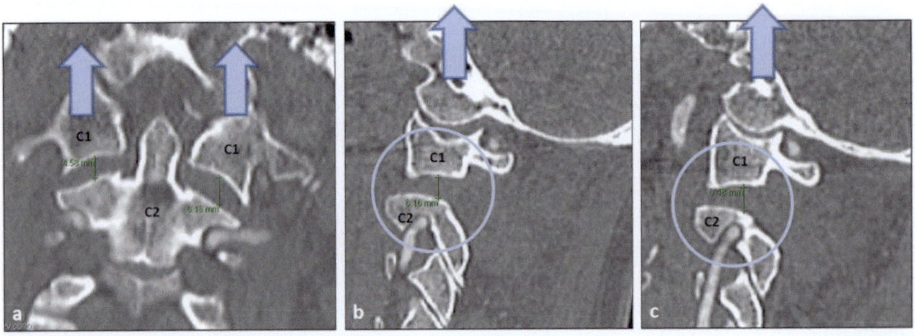

Fig. 19.9 (**a–c**) Atlantoaxial dislocation due to high-energy distraction mechanism (from personal series)

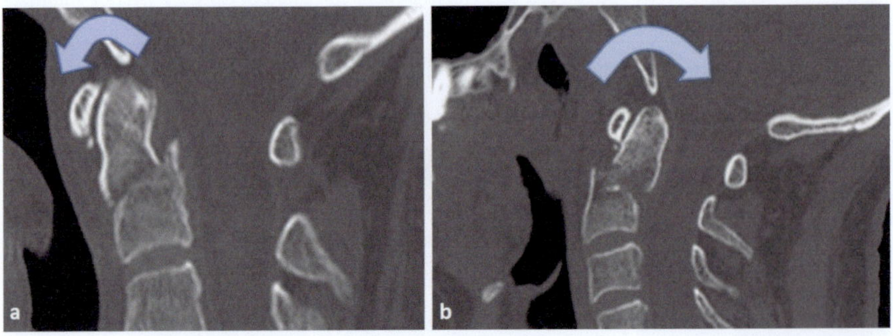

Fig. 19.10 (**a**, **b**) Type II odontoid fracture with antero-inferior direction of the fracture and anterior displacement of the dens by hyperflexion mechanism (**a**); and type II with posterior displacement by hyperextension mechanism (**b**) (from personal series)

nowadays is the one reported by Anderson and Alonzo who distinguish: fracture of the tip of odontoid process (type I), fracture of the base (type II), and fracture passing through C2 vertebral body (type III).

19.3.2.5 Hangman's Fracture

Hangman's fracture is also referred as the bilateral isthmic fracture of C2 or post-traumatic cervical spondylolisthesis of C2. Hyperextension, generally associated with axial compression forces, will result to shear stresses on the isthmus of C2, which may lead to bilateral C2 pars fracture, also referred as the Hangman's fracture (Fig. 19.11). Effendi et al. [13] divided the lesions into three main types: non-displaced fracture with no kyphotic deformity (type I), fracture associated with translation more than 3.5 mm and/or angulation more than 11° (type II), and fracture associated with unilateral or bilateral complete C2-C3 facet dislocation (type III).

19.3.3 Translation

19.3.3.1 Occipito-Cervical Dislocation

Occipito-cervical dislocation can result from a pure vertical distraction force vector (see Fig. 19.7) but also from an anterior or posterior translation vector, corresponding respectively to Traynelis type I and III.

19.3.3.2 Rupture of the Transverse Ligament

In normal conditions, the transverse ligament (TL) serves as the restraint to anterior translation of C1 and represents the strongest ligamentous structure of the cranio-cervical junction [14]. In case of rupture of TL, this allows the anterior translation of C1 (up to 12 mm) with the risk of compromise of neurological structures, Fig. 19.12.

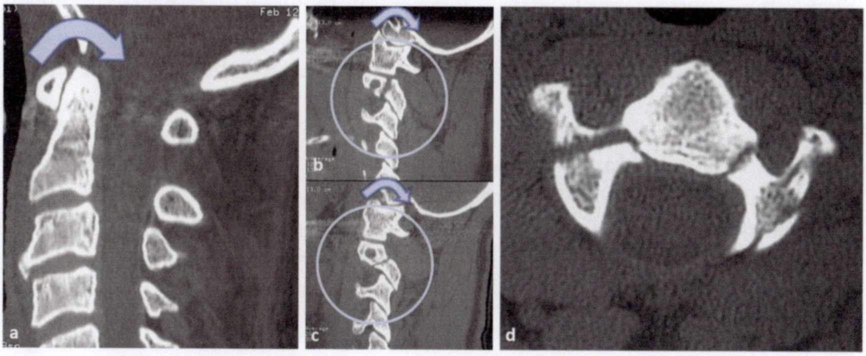

Fig. 19.11 (**a–d**) Bi-isthmic fracture of C2, Effendi type I, consecutive to a hyperextension mechanism (from personal series)

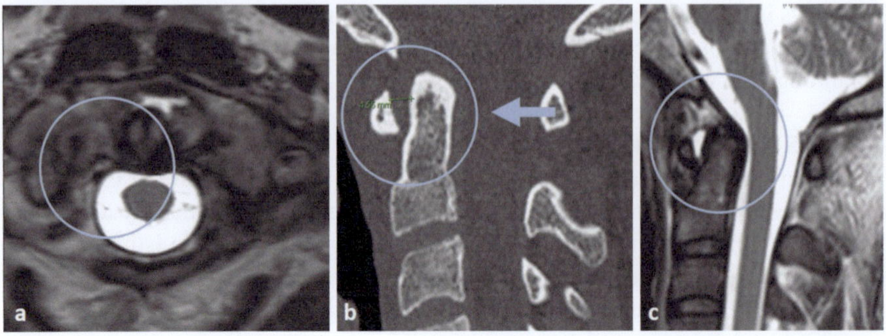

Fig. 19.12 (**a**–**c**) Rupture of the transverse ligament associated with anterior translation of C1 (abnormal increase of the ADI). In normal conditions, the TL permits to restraint the anterior arch of C1 (from personal series)

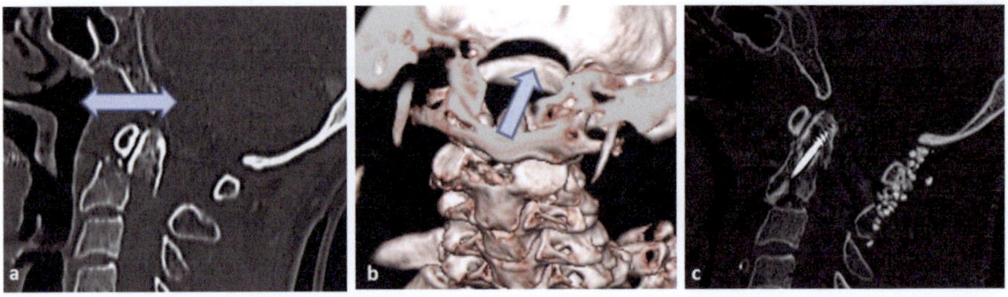

Fig. 19.13 (**a**–**c**) Type II odontoid fracture with severe antero-posterior translation (**a**, **b**). The fracture necessitated a combined surgery with anterior screw and posterior C1-C2 fixation to control the post-traumatic C1-C2 instability (from personal series)

Imaging modalities (CT-scan and MRI) permit to differentiate type I and II injuries according to Dickman's classification [8] for atlantal-transverse ligaments lesions. Type I corresponds to an intra-ligamentous rupture with respect to the attach zone of the TL at the inner aspect of lateral mass of C1. Type II is characterized by the bony avulsion of the transverse ligament from the medial border of the lateral mass of C1.

19.3.3.3 Type II Odontoid Fracture

Most odontoid fractures result from complex force vectors including distraction, lateral bending, axial compression, and translation forces. Importance of fracture-displacement indicates the severity of the instability (not the only parameter), Fig. 19.13.

19.3.4 Rotation

The rotation at the CVJ is neutralized by the alar ligaments at first line, with contribution from the tectorial membrane, joint capsules, and transverse ligament. In case of excessive rotatory force vector, these structures may be ruptured and lead to rotatory subluxation or dislocation. Also, asymmetrical injuries, including asymmetrical fracture or ligamentar rupture, suggest a part of rotational force vector.

19.3.4.1 Rupture of C1-C2 Capsular Ligaments

Capsular C1-C2 ligaments function predominantly into control axial rotation. Isolated injury of C1-C2 capsular ligaments injury is considered not sufficient to induce C1-C2 instability.

19.3.4.2 Atlantoaxial Rotatory Subluxation

The first case of atlantoaxial rotatory subluxation was reported by Charles Bell in 1930. In the case of C1-C2 rotatory subluxation, it is important to determine if the subluxation is partial/complete and reducible/irreducible [12, 18]. Fielding and Hawkins [15] proposed a classification into four types: rotatory subluxation of C1-C2 with no anterior displacement of C1 (type I), rotatory subluxation of C1-C2 with anterior displacement of C1 by 3–5 mm (type II), rotatory subluxation of C1-C2 with anterior displacement >5 mm (type III), and rotatory subluxation of C1-C2 with posterior displacement of C1 (type IV) in Fig. 19.14.

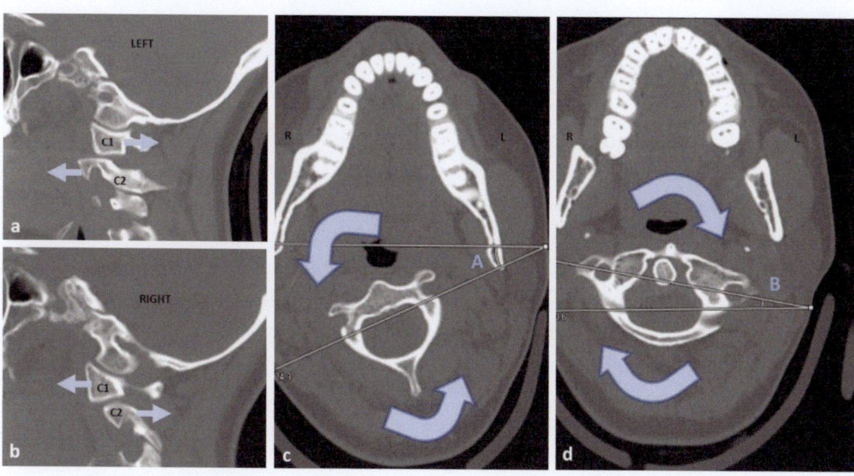

Fig. 19.14 (**a–d**) Incomplete rotatory subluxation of C1-C2. The lateral masses of C1 and C2 are still in contact (**a**, **b**). If the sum of angle A + B is more than 45°, significant instability should be suspected (**c**, **d**) (from personal series)

Key-Messages from the Mechanism Injury

- Main injury vectors are compression, distraction, translation, rotation, and a combination of all of them.
- Most post-traumatic lesions can be categorized into specific injury patterns even if they result most often from a combination of primary forces.
- Compression injuries affect predominantly bony structures.
- Distraction and rotation affect predominantly ligamentar elements.
- Asymmetrical injuries suggest a part of rotational force vector.
- The main injury mechanisms dictate the nature of post-traumatic lesions observed and the direction of the displacement.
- Mechanisms of injury for type II odontoid fracture, which represent the most common injury in the upper cervical spine, are often complex and multidirectional.

19.4 Recognize the Unstable Lesions

The stability of the injury is the determining factor for decision-making in term of surgical indication. Determining instability in the case of ligament injury can be particularly challenging. Indeed, ligamentous instability will not heal by itself and generally requires a surgical fusion. Radiological analysis is fundamental in that it shows indirect or direct signs of instability.

19.4.1 Indirect Signs

Unstable lesions can lead to abnormal displacements or diastasis between the occipital bone and the cervical spine, or between C1 and C2. In contrast to bony injuries, ligament injuries are much more difficult to diagnose and assess. Some radiological measurements were described (see below) that must lead to the suspicion of unstable lesions and call for the realization of an MRI imaging. Abnormal displacements indirectly reflect the injury of soft tissues and are typically observed on multiaxial CT-scan and/or dynamic X-rays.

Indirect signs suggesting instability:

- axial rotation between C0 and C1 superior to 8°
- axial rotation between C1 and C2 superior to 45°
- translation superior to 1 mm between the dens and the basion (caudal extremity of the clivus) between flexion and extension
- more than 2.5 mm between the occipital condyle and the lateral mass of C1 (this is suggestive of atlanto-cervical dislocation)
- lateral translation between lateral masses of C1 and lateral masses of C2 more than 7 mm (suggesting rupture of transverse ligament)

- atlanto-dens interval (ADI) superior to 3 mm in adults and superior to 5 mm in children
- space available for the cord (SAC) between the posterior cortex of the dens and the posterior arch of C1 inferior to 13 mm
- distance from the lateral mass of C1 to the lateral mass of C2 should not exceed 2.6 mm on coronal CT-scan

19.4.2 Direct Signs

The most specific test to diagnose unstable lesions that require surgical fusion in the CVJ is the MRI (Fig. 19.15). T2 STIR sequence allows the direct visualization of capsules and/or ligaments ruptures that represent unstable lesions. Abnormal signal and/or Intra-capsular hematoma with the presence of fluid observed on MRI (T2 sequence) is suggestive of capsules injury (Fig. 19.16). MRI in now considered safer and far more sensitive and specific than dynamic X-rays to evaluate the ligamentar structures.

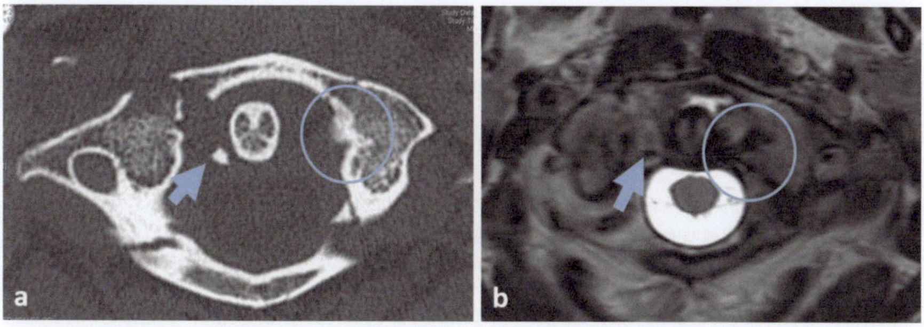

Fig. 19.15 (**a**, **b**) Rupture of transverse ligament (TL) was suspected on CT-scan with the presence of bony fragment avulsion on the inner aspect of right lateral mass of C1 (blue arrow). Axial MRI could confirm the rupture of transverse ligament. TL was still intact on the left side (blue circle) (from personal series)

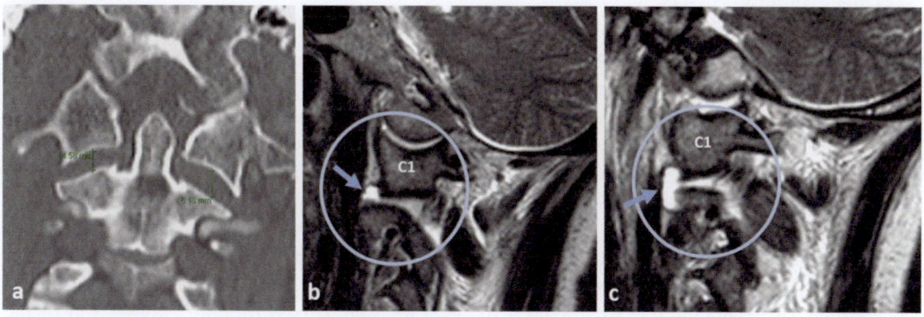

Fig. 19.16 (**a**–**c**) Atlantoaxial dislocation with the presence of intra-capsular fluid between C1-C2 on both sides on MRI (T2 sequence) (from personal series)

19.5 Conclusions

The comprehension of the normal anatomy, normal biomechanics, and normal physiological range of motion is essential to recognize the unstable lesions of the CVJ. The post-traumatic unstable injuries result from specific force vectors which may induce failure of bony and/or ligamentar stabilizing structures. Most lesions result from a combination of basic primary force vectors including compression, distraction, translation, and rotation. Bony injuries are detected on multiplanar CT-scan (thin slices). Ligament injuries can be suspected on CT-scan in the presence of abnormal displacements; however, they can be observed directly on MRI (T2-STIR sequence). These two modalities are therefore complementary to fully explore post-traumatic injuries of the CVJ.

References

1. Anderson PA, D'Alonzo RT. Fractures of the odontoid process of the axis. J Bone Joint Surg Am. 1974;56:1663–74.
2. Anderson PA, Montesano PX. Morphology and treatment of occipital condyles fractures. Spine. 1988;13:731–6.
3. Barrey C, Charles YP, French Spine Surgery Society (SFCR). Symposium on C1-C2, based on 417 C1-C2 post-traumatic injuries. Presented at SFCR Annual Meeting. Lyon; 2016.
4. Benzel EC, Hart BL, Ball PA, Baldwin NG, Orrison WW, Espinosa M. Fractures of the C2 vertebral body. J Neurosurg. 1994;81:206–12.
5. Bleys RL. Chapter 1: Anatomy of the cervical spine. In: Vialle LR, editor. Cervical spine trauma, AOspine Masters Series, vol. 5: Thieme Medical Publishers; 2015. p. 1–16.
6. Bogduk N, Mercer S. Biomechanics of the cervical spine I: normal kinematics. Clin Biomech. 2000;15:633–48.
7. Crisco JJ, Oda T, Panjabi MM, Bueff HU, Dvorak J, Grob D. Transections of the C1-C2 joint capsular ligaments in the cadaveric spine. Spine. 1991;16:S474–9.
8. Dickman CA, Greene KA, Sonntag VK. Injuries involving the transvers atlantal ligament: classification and treatment guidelines based upon experience with 39 injuries. Neurosurgery. 1996;38:44–50.
9. Dickman CA, Crawford NR. Chapter 3: Biomechanics of the craniovertebral junction. In: Dickman CA, Spetzler RF, Sonntag VK, editors. Surgery of the craniovertebral junction: Thieme Publisher; 1998. p. 59–80.
10. Dickman CA, Greene KA, Sonntag VK. Chapter 8: Traumatic injuries of the craniovertebral junction. In: Dickman CA, Spetzler RF, Sonntag VK, editors. Surgery of the craniovertebral junction: Thieme Publisher; 1998. p. 175–96.
11. Dvorak J, Panjabi MM. Functional anatomy of the alar ligaments. Spine. 1987;12:183–9.
12. Dvorak J. CT-functional diagnostics of the rotatory instability of upper cervical spine—part 1. An experimental study on cadavers. Spine. 1987;12:197–205.
13. Effendi B, Roy D, Cornish B, Dussault RG, Laurin CA. Fractures of the ring of the axis. A classification based on the analysis of 131 cases. J Bone Joint Surg Br. 1981;63-B:319–27.
14. Fielding JW, Cochran G, Lawsing J, Hohl M. Tears of the transverse ligament of the atlas. A clinical and biomechanical study. J Bone Joint Surg Am. 1974;56:1683–91.
15. Fielding JW, Hawkins RJ. Atlantoaxial rotatory fixation. (Fixed rotatory subluxation of the atlanto-axial joint). J Bone Joint Surg Am. 1977;59:37–44.
16. Gehweiler JA, Osborne RL, Becker RF. The radiology of vertebral trauma. Philadelphia: WB Saunders; 1980.

17. German JW, Hart BL, Benzel EC. Nonoperative management of vertical C2 body fractures. Neurosurgery. 2005;56:516–21.
18. Gire JD, Roberto RF, Bobinski M, Klineberg EO, Durbin-Johnson B. The utility and accuracy of computed tomography in the diagnosis of occipitocervical dissociation. Spine J. 2013;13:510–9.
19. Ghori A, Leonard D, Cha T. Chapter 2: Biomechanics of the cervical spine: from the normal state to the injury state. In: Vialle LR, editor. Cervical spine trauma, AOspine Masters Series, vol. 5: Thieme Medical Publishers; 2015.
20. Goel VK, Clark CR. Moment-relationships of the ligamentous occipito-atlanto-axial complex. J Biomech. 1988;21:673–80.
21. Goel VK. Chapter 6: Biomechanics of the unstable craniovertebral junction. In: Goel A, Cacciola F, editors. The craniovertebral junction: Thieme Publishers; 2011. p. 39–47.
22. Gonzalez LF, Fiorella D, Crawford NR. Vertical atlanto-axial distraction injuries: radiological criteria and clinical implications. J Neurosurg Spine. 2004;1(3):273–80.
23. Gonzalez LF, Webb KM, Crawford NR, Sonntag VK. Chapter 32: Trauma to the craniovertebral junction. In: Goel A, Cacciola F, editors. The craniovertebral junction: Thieme Publishers; 2011. p. 338–56.
24. Jackson RS, Banit DM, Rhyne AL, Darden BV. Upper cervical spine injuries. J Am Acad Orthop Surg. 2002;10(4):271–80.
25. Louis R. Chirurgie du rachis (anatomie chirurgicale et voies d'abord), french. 2e édition. Springer; 1993.
26. Panjabi MM, et al. Three dimensional movements of the upper cervical spine. Spine. 1988;13:726–30.
27. Panjabi MM, Oxland TR, Parks EH. Quantitative anatomy of cervical spine ligaments. Part I. Upper cervical spine. J Spinal Disord. 1991;4(3):270–6.
28. Panjabi MM. Posture affects motion coupling patterns of the upper cervical spine. J Orthop Res. 1993;11:525–36.
29. Penning L. Normal movements of the cervical spine. AJR Am J Roentgenol. 1978;130:317–26.
30. Puttlitz CM, Goel VK, Clark CR, traynelis VC, Scifert JL, grosland NM. Biomechanical rationale for the pathology of rheumatoid arthritis in the craniovertebral junction. Spine. 2000;25(13):1607–16.
31. Schleicher P, Scholz M, Kandziora F. Chapter 5: Occipital condyle fractures and occipitocervical dissociation. In: Vialle LR, editor. Cervical spine trauma, AOspine Masters Series, vol. 5: Thieme Medical Publishers; 2015. p. 49–60.
32. Scholz M, Schleicher P, Kandziora F. Chapter 6: Atlas injuries. In: Vialle LR, editor. Cervical spine trauma, AOspine Masters Series, vol. 5: Thieme Medical Publishers; 2015. p. 61–72.
33. Traynelis VC, Marano GD, Dunker RO, Kaufman HH. Traumatic atlanto-occipital dislocation. Case report. J Neurosurg. 1986;65:863–70.
34. Watier B. Étude expérimentale du rachis cervical: comportement mécanique in vitro et cinématique in vivo [thèse]. Paris: Ensam; 1997. p. 1–184.
35. Watier B. Mechanical behavior of cervical spine: literature update. ITBM-RBM. 2006;27:92–106.
36. Wen N. Contribution à l'étude expérimentale du comportement mécanique in vitro du rachis cervical [thèse]. Paris: Ensam; 1993. p. 1–234.
37. White AA. Clinical biomechanics of the spine. 2nd ed. Philadelphia: Lippincott; 1990.
38. Wolfla CE, Yoganandan N. Chapter 5: Biomechanics of the craniovertebral junction. In: Goel A, Cacciola F, editors. The craniovertebral junction: Thieme Publishers; 2011. p. 33–8.

Classification and Radiological Assessment of CVJ Trauma

20

Juan Barges-Coll and John M. Duff

20.1 Introduction

Trauma to the craniovertebral junction (CVJ) require complex clinical diagnosis and management in survivors reaching a hospital setting. Several classification systems are currently available that which combine clinical and radiological data to obtain a treatment algorithm. Recently, the role of ligaments as primary stabilizers at the CVJ has been recognized. Comprehensive assessment of soft tissue component of the injury requires MR imaging, making classifications even more complex to assess post-traumatic stability of the CVJ [1].

Although the overall incidence of CVJ fractures is not fully elucidated, these may represent 2–6% of all spine trauma and 20% of cervical trauma. While conventional radiographs or CT scans can reveal detailed bone anatomy and have a high sensitivity for fractures, MR imaging plays a very important role in evaluating the presence or likelihood of instability caused by ligamentous injury at the CVJ [2].

Approximately 10–20% of all spinal trauma results in spinal cord injury and associated morbidity and mortality, particularly among young people. Clinical examination of upper cervical spine trauma may be limited, particularly where the patient has an associated head injury with altered level of consciousness [3].

The craniovertebral junction (CVJ) has specific injury patterns on CT and MRI. High-resolution axial T2 MR images from CVJ should be obtained to fully assess the stabilizing ligaments and surrounding soft tissues. MRI techniques, including volumetric sequences, high resolution can be attained, allowing for detailed analysis of the ligaments, particularly in trauma patients [4].

J. Barges-Coll
Spine Unit, Department of Clinical Neurosciences, CHUV, Lausanne, Switzerland

J. M. Duff (✉)
Spine Center, Clinique de Genolier, Genolier, Switzerland

E. Tessitore et al. (eds.), *Surgery of the Cranio-Vertebral Junction*,
https://doi.org/10.1007/978-3-030-18700-2_20

This chapter will focus on classification of CVJ trauma and the complementary role of different radiologic modalities in the diagnosis of patients with traumatic CVJ injuries.

The role of imaging CVJ trauma classifications will be addressed. The importance of MR imaging in the assessment of soft tissue injury and the increasing role of advanced imaging techniques such as dynamic MRI, or 3D printed models, for prognostication of the traumatic spine could play a role in the near future [5].

20.2 Atlanto-Occipital Dislocation (AOD)

Craniocervical ligamentous injuries without dislocation of the occipito-atlantal or atlantoaxial motion segments have been described rarely. The most important soft tissue structures that are usually involved are the alar ligaments, the occipito-atlantal joint capsules, the tectorial membrane, the rectus capitis muscles, and the suboccipital muscles [6].

The distractive forces necessary for AOD are extremely high. This is often a lethal injury with many if not most victims succumbing in the field, likely due to acute cardiopulmonary insufficiency or arrest. The number of survivors is increasing due to more efficient and faster interventions in the field followed by transfer to acute medical centers. This lesion is often missed on the initial trauma evaluation, and must be considered in any high energy impact.

Due to extensive ligamentous disruption, there can be significant mobility in all axes between the skull base and C1. In surviving cases, the diagnosis may be obvious due to significant C0-C1 joint dislocation. In more subtle screening radiological findings, any suspicion of this injury mandates appropriate immobilization followed by rapid MR imaging for ligamentous assessment. Placement and maintaining a cervical collar may be hazardous. Halo vest placement with gentle compression may be placed in the emergency room, followed by imaging and subsequent surgical management. MRI procedures performed at 3-T may be particularly problematic for patients with external orthosis because of the higher field strength and frequency causing excessive heating, and artifacts. Ceramic-tipped pins and compression-molded, glass composite halos are the only ones that can be used with 3 T MRIs [7–9].

AODs are classified by Traynelis in anterior, vertical, and posterior according to where the condyles are projected compared to the atlas lateral masses.

20.2.1 Occipital Condyle Fractures (OCF)

Patients with an OCF often have head injuries that may be difficult for the clinical and neurologic examination. Patients which are neurologically intact may present only with pain and tenderness in the posterior cervical region, whereas others may have significant neurologic deficits with lower cranial nerve palsies can occur in nearly 20% of patients with an OCF and sometimes even a lesion to the brainstem can be evident [10, 11].

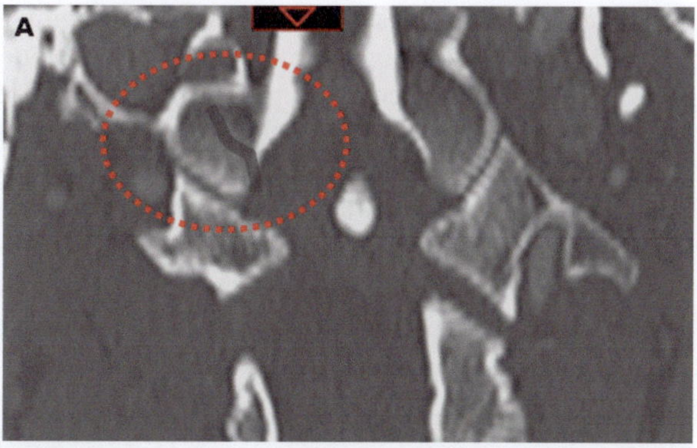

Fig. 20.1 (**a**) CT scan (coronal) shows right Type 1 Fracture (Red dotted circle). The need of MRI in this particular case is irrelevant because it does not change treatment algorithm

Classification of the OCF incorporates the mechanisms of injury and addresses the potential for instability and was introduced by Anderson and Montesano in 1988 [12] (Table below) (Fig. 20.1a).

Table	Type 1	Type 2	Type 3
Description	Small fracture of the occipital condyle secondary to axial forces with no displacement of fragments into the foramen magnum	Fracture into the base of the occipital condyle. The condyle is still at least partially attached to the base of the skull base	Excessive rotation and/or lateral bending can result in condylar avulsion and the fracture extending into the skull base
Ligament injury	Alar ligament	Alar ligament/tectorial membrane	Alar ligament/tectorial, apical (may be bilateral)
Unstable	No	No	Yes
CT	Yes	Yes	Yes
MRI	No	No	Recommended/but may not change treatment

Current cervical spine guidelines recommend CT scan but there is no recommendation for the need of MRI in OCF. It is important to note that the increased sensitivity of MRI may result in surgeons overinterpreting any abnormal signal as pathological, so caution is advised. MRI can, according to some authors, identify additional injuries in 23.6% of patients despite a normal CT scan [13].

20.2.2 C1 Fractures

Atlas fractures account for 2–10% of acute injuries of the cervical spine and 1–2% of all spinal injuries [14]. C1 fractures occur due to a traumatic axial loading and are commonly associated with other lesions in the upper cervical spine. Atlas fractures can involve lateral mass and/or the lamina. Single fractures involving the ring are rare, and a ring disruption with a fracture at two sites is common [1]. Numerous developmental anomalies also occur which can mimic trauma this is why a complete clinical and radiological evaluation should be done. Identifying fractures is even more difficult in pediatric patients, because C1 cannot be visualized radiographically until patients reach 1 year of age and the fusion of the C1 ring does not occur until the age of 5 years.

Geoffrey Jefferson was the first to report a detailed analysis on C1 fractures in 1919 to describe the action of axial loading on the traumatic mechanisms producing vertebral damage. Nearly 100 years later, this classification for C1 fractures is still in daily clinical use (Table below) (Fig. 20.2). Multiple modification had been made

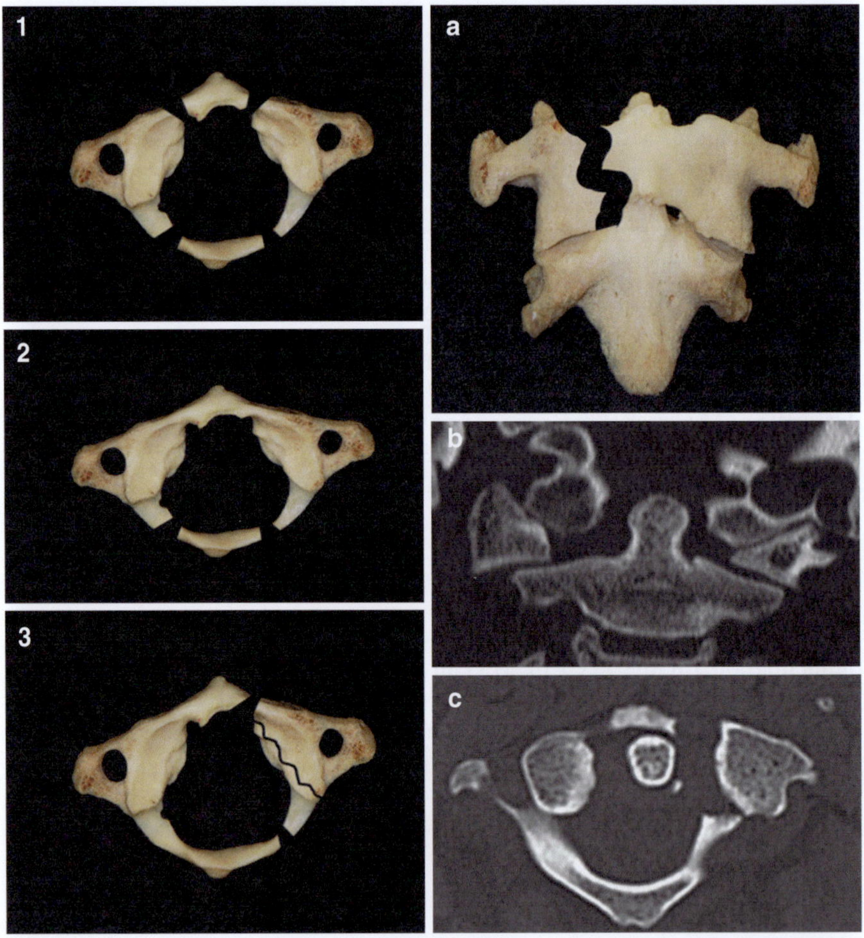

Fig. 20.2 (1) Anatomic C1 vertebrae showing an anterior and posterior C1 arch fracture (2) Anatomic C1 vertebrae showing a posterior C1 arch fracture. (3) (**a**) Anatomic fracture of lateral mass and arch of C1. Axial and coronal view. (**b**, **c**) CT scan showing a Type 3 C1 Fracture

to the original Jefferson classification but still today there is no uniformly accepted classification system for C1 fractures [1, 15, 16].

Table	Type 1 Fig. 20.2(1)	Type 2 Fig. 20.2(2)	Type 3 Fig. 20.2(2 and 3a–c)	Atlanto-occipital dislocation
Description	Isolated fracture of the anterior or posterior arch of C1	Bilateral fractures of anterior or posterior C1 arch	Lateral mass fracture	Disruption of ligament skull base and lateral mass
Ligament injury	No	No	Possible	Yes
Unstable	No	No	Possible	Yes
CT	Yes	Yes	Yes	Yes
MRI	No	No	Yes	Recommended

When deciding whether a patient requires surgical stabilization, surgeons will look at the integrity of the transverse atlantal ligament (TAL). The TAL maintains the odontoid process of C-2 in close proximity to the C-1 ring, allowing rotational movement around the long axis of the odontoid process. Other ligaments, including the capsular ligaments, alar ligaments, apical ligament, anterior longitudinal ligament, and tectorial membrane, assist the TL in providing cervical stability. TL injury has been classified by Dickman and co-workers and there are four types (Fig. 20.2a–c) [16, 17]. Transoral X ray has limited value nowadays but the MRI can provide a good view of the alar and transverse ligaments (Fig. 20.3a–d).

20.2.2.1 Shear Fracture of the Anterior Arch of C1

This is an additional rare fracture due to hyperextension at the craniovertebral junction. There are usually bilateral vertical fractures of the anterior arch of C1 with anterior displacement of the fragment which remains in articulation with the odontoid process. It is considered stable, and usually CT scan is the radiological method of choice [18].

20.2.3 C2 Fractures

The C2 vertebra consists of a body, paired pedicles, lateral masses (superior articulating facets), odontoid, pars interarticularis, inferior articulating facets, lamina, and bifid spinous process [4].

Due to the complexity of this vertebrae and the challenge that it represents for treatment algorithms we will discuss into separate entities the fractures that involve the odontoid process, the fractures that involve the body of C2, and the ones that involve the pedicles or a combination of the last two [19].

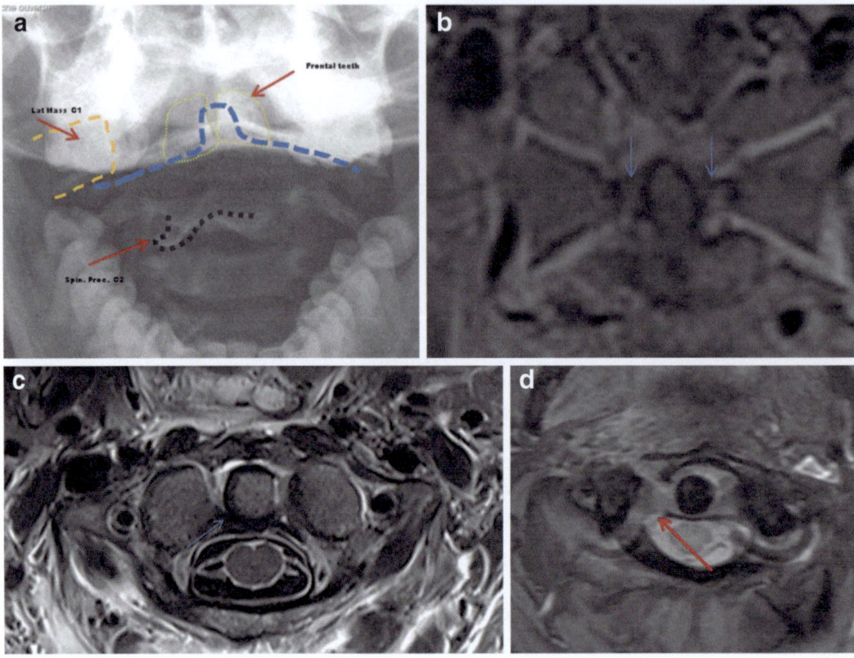

Fig. 20.3 (**a**) X Rays Transoral showing lateral mass fracture with augmentation of the Spencer rule on the right lateral mass. (**b**) MRI Coronal view showing alar ligaments (Blue arrows) (**c**) Axial MRI showing a complete transverse ligament (Blue arrow). (**d**) MRI Axial view showing a disruption of the transverse ligament 8 (red arrow)

20.2.3.1 Odontoid Fractures

Fractures of the cervical spine are relatively common odontoid process fractures account for approximately 10% of cervical spine fractures and seem to have a not well-understood behavior. In the literature, there is no clear consensus on the proper treatment and the natural history of symptomatic and asymptomatic pseudarthrosis [20].

Classification of odontoid fractures is related to the need of immobilization due to the instability that may cause a neurological deficit. Help from modern radiological techniques has evolved to better define traumatic lesions and the need for immobilization [21].

At least five classifications exist to assess the odontoid fractures [22, 19] (Table below). The best known classification is that described by Anderson–D'Alonzo in the early 1970s [23] dating from the pre-CT era. It consists of three basic types (Fig. 20.4(1–3 and a–c)) [19, 24].

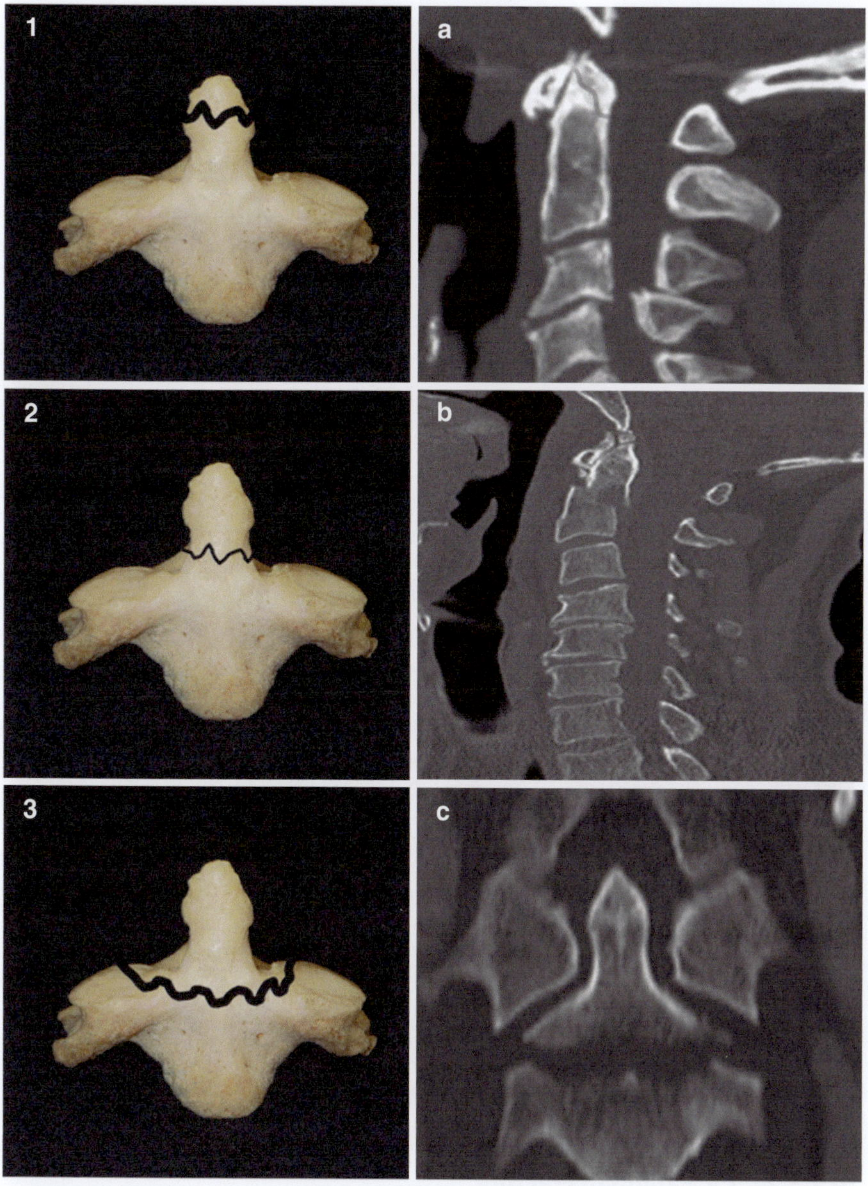

Fig. 20.4 (1–3) Anatomic representation of Type 1, 2, and 3 odontoid fractures. (**a–c**) CT Scan showing Type 1, 2, and 3 fractures of the odontoid

Table	Schatzker	Anderson–D'Alonzo	Althoff	Korres
Description	Two types (a) Tip of the odontoid (b) Base of the odontoid	Three types 1. Tip of the odontoid 2. Neck of the odontoid 3. Base of the odontoid	Four types (a) Tip of the odontoid (b) Neck of the odontoid (c) Incomplete base of the odontoid (d) Complete transverse fracture at the base	Four types (a) Avulsion fractures at the points of insertion of the alar or apical ligaments (b) Most common fracture at the level of the base of the odontoid (c) Fracture projects into the body of C2 (d) Neutral zone
Ligament injury	In type B	Type 1 Alar or apical or both. 2) Transverse 3) Non	Possible type B	B and C
Surgical treatment recommended	Type B	Type 2	Type B and possible C	B most unfavorable for conservative management.
CT	Yes	Yes	Yes	Yes
MRI	Not necessary but recommended in case of ligament injury needs to be assessed	Not necessary but recommended in case of ligament injury needs to be assessed	Not necessary but recommended in case of ligament injury needs to be assessed	Not necessary but recommended in case of ligament injury needs to be assessed

Korres classification is based on the anatomical and biomechanical properties of the odontoid process and may be the most useful for determining the need or not of surgical treatment. In the more recent classifications, CT scan is recommended. Thus far there is no consensus about using MRI systematically in patients with odontoid fractures [22].

20.2.3.2 C2 Hangman Fracture

A hangman or "hangman-like" fracture of C2 represents about 12–20% of all the fractures that involve the CVJ [19]. This may be due to one of two mechanisms, namely hyperextension and axial load that results in fractures of the pars interarticularis or the pedicle, or due to flexion/distraction mechanism results in disruption of the C2–3 disk and posterior longitudinal ligament besides de pars fracture. Multiple classification systems have been proposed [25] but the classification by Effendi published in 1981 is the one most commonly used in clinical practice [26].

Table	Type 1	Type 1A	Type 2	Type 3 Fig. 20.5(1 and 2) (a and b)
Description	Bilateral pars fractures with translation <3 mm and no angulation. C2-C3 disc remains intact.	Type IA. There is minimal translation and little or no angulation	The C2–3 disk and posterior longitudinal ligament are disrupted, resulting in translation >3 mm and marked angulation	Combination of pars fracture with dislocation of the C2–3 facet joint
Unstable	No	No	Possible	Yes
CT	Yes	Yes	Yes	Yes
MRI	No	No	Recommended for assessing disc disruption	Recommended for assessing disc disruption

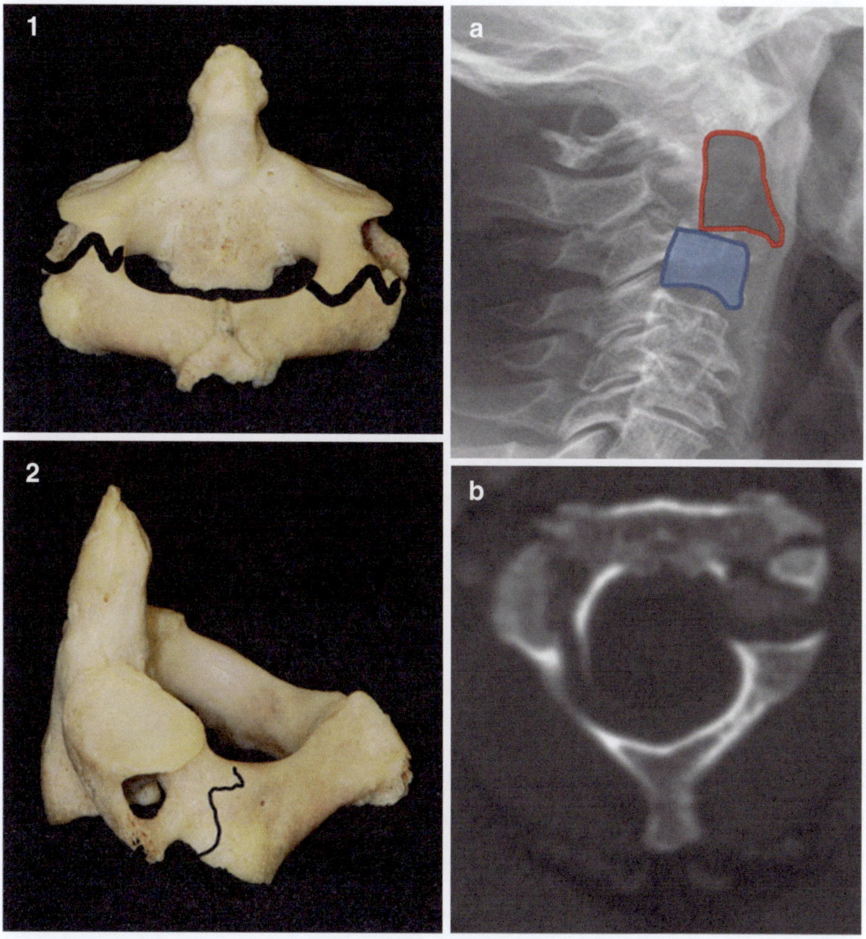

Fig. 20.5 (1and 2) Schematic anatomical specimen showing a hangman fracture. (**a**, **b**) X-ray and CT scan showing a combined hangman and burst fracture

20.2.3.3 C2 Body Fractures

Axis body fractures include fractures of the body, and may have extension into the pedicle, lateral mass, or transverse foramen. C2 body factures are classified into three types, according to the orientation of the fracture, along with subtypes in each group.

Table	Type 1	Type 2	Type 3
Description	Vertical fracture	Vertical and horizontal fractures	Horizontal fracture (Type 3 Alonzo odontoid)
Unstable	No	No	No
CT	Yes	Yes	Yes
X-rays	Yes (Transoral)	Yes (Transoral)	Yes (Transoral)
MRI	No	No	No

20.3 Radiological Assessment of CVJ Trauma

Current practice for the management of cervical spine trauma recommend CT scan in patients in whom there is a suspicion of cervical spine trauma (level 1 evidence) and the use of MRI (level 3 evidence). The ultimate decision to use MRI for a patient with a CVJ trauma relies on the judgment and bias of the treating physician [27]. Recent reviews about this topic have been published and there is a tendency in favor of using MRI since CT scan alone may underestimate the extent of the injury [17, 28].

CT is a very sensitive method for evaluating craniovertebral osseous relations and is the gold standard method for evaluating injuries in the CVJ. It also allows 3D visualization of fractures using good quality reconstruction algorithms.

MRI is occasionally useful to assess patients with neurological deficit or any suspicion of ligamentous injury (especially the transverse ligament) (Fig. 20.3).

Using X-ray alone for diagnostic purposes nowadays has limited value. Open-mouth radiographs allow visualization of the atlas, odontoid process, and lateral masses of the axis. They are useful for assessing the integrity of the odontoid process and the lateral masses. Supervised flexion and extension lateral radiographs may be helpful in recognizing instability at both occiput-C1 and C1-C2 (see traumatic C2 spondylolisthesis Type 1 or 2) (Fig. 20.5).

20.4 Conclusions

Established classification systems for CVJ injuries currently widely used in clinical practice are based primarily on bone injuries. However, CVJ stability is largely dependent on ligamentous integrity. In recent years, there has been a shift from screening high energy trauma victims with X-rays to screening with trauma protocol CT scanning of the spine. Findings of a traumatic lesion at the CVJ following high energy trauma should prompt careful examination for a second concomitant lesion lower down in the spine. Expert interpretation of the CT scan may obviate the need for MRI. However, such expert interpretation has not yet been directly compared with MRI and may not be available to all providers, so in select cases MRI can be used to rule out injury to ligaments or disc disruption so there should be a high index of suspicion for an "unseen" ligamentous injury, and a low threshold to proceed to MR imaging. Advances in more sophisticated imaging techniques may help in the future to in provide more information which will enable improved therapeutic decision making for a given traumatic CVJ lesion.

References

1. Mead LB 2nd, Millhouse PW, Krystal J, Vaccaro AR. C1 fractures: a review of diagnoses, management options, and outcomes. Curr Rev Musculoskelet Med. 2016;9(3):255–62.
2. Roy AK, Miller BA, Holland CM, Fountain AJ Jr, Pradilla G, Ahmad FU. Magnetic resonance imaging of traumatic injury to the craniovertebral junction: a case-based review. Neurosurg Focus. 2015;38(4):E3.
3. Zhang Y, Cheng K, Dong J, Li Q, Tremp M, Zhu L. Incidence and features of vertebral fractures after scalp avulsion injuries. J Craniofac Surg. 2015;26(7):2217–20.
4. Nidecker AE, Shen PY. Magnetic resonance imaging of the craniovertebral junction ligaments: normal anatomy and traumatic injury. J Neurol Surg B Skull Base. 2016;77(5):388–95.
5. Xiong C, Daubs MD, Scott TP, Phan KH, Suzuki A, Ruangchainikom M, et al. Dynamic evaluation of the cervical spine and the spinal cord of symptomatic patients using a kinetic magnetic resonance imaging technique. Clin Spine Surg. 2017;30(8):E1149–55.
6. Adams VI. Neck injuries: III. Ligamentous injuries of the craniocervical articulation without occipito-atlantal or atlanto-axial facet dislocation. A pathologic study of 21 traffic fatalities. J Forensic Sci. 1993;38(5):1097–104.
7. Riascos R, Bonfante E, Cotes C, Guirguis M, Hakimelahi R, West C. Imaging of atlanto-occipital and atlantoaxial traumatic injuries: what the radiologist needs to know. Radiographics. 2015;35(7):2121–34.
8. Yamada H, Yamanaka T. [Atlanto-axial and occipito-atlantal dislocation in Down's syndrome]. No To Hattatsu. 1987;19(4):309–14.
9. Diaz FL, Tweardy L, Shellock FG. Cervical external immobilization devices: evaluation of magnetic resonance imaging issues at 3.0 Tesla. Spine (Phila Pa 1976). 2010;35(4):411–5.
10. Aulino JM, Tutt LK, Kaye JJ, Smith PW, Morris JA Jr. Occipital condyle fractures: clinical presentation and imaging findings in 76 patients. Emerg Radiol. 2005;11(6):342–7.
11. Ueda S, Sasaki N, Fukuda M, Hoshimaru M. Surgical treatment for occipital condyle fracture, C1 dislocation, and cerebellar contusion with hemorrhage after blunt head trauma. Case Rep Orthop. 2016;2016:8634831.
12. Anderson PA, Montesano PX. Morphology and treatment of occipital condyle fractures. Spine (Phila Pa 1976). 1988;13(7):731–6.
13. Maung AA, Johnson DC, Barre K, Peponis T, Mesar T, Velmahos GC, et al. Cervical spine MRI in patients with negative CT: a prospective, multicenter study of the Research Consortium of New England Centers for Trauma (ReCONECT). J Trauma Acute Care Surg. 2017;82(2):263–9.
14. Sonntag VK, Hadley MN, Dickman CA, Browner CM. Atlas fractures: treatment and long-term results. Acta Neurochir Suppl (Wien). 1988;43:63–8.
15. Joaquim AF, Ghizoni E, Tedeschi H, Lawrence B, Brodke DS, Vaccaro AR, et al. Upper cervical injuries—a rational approach to guide surgical management. J Spinal Cord Med. 2014;37(2):139–51.
16. Findlay JM. Injuries involving the transverse atlantal ligament: classification and treatment guidelines based upon experience with 39 injuries. Neurosurgery. 1996;39(1):210.

17. Dickman CA, Greene KA, Sonntag VK. Injuries involving the transverse atlantal ligament: classification and treatment guidelines based upon experience with 39 injuries. Neurosurgery. 1996;38(1):44–50.
18. Ivancic PC. Plough fracture of the anterior arch of the atlas: a biomechanical investigation. Eur Spine J. 2014;23(11):2314–20.
19. Robinson AL, Moller A, Robinson Y, Olerud C. C2 Fracture subtypes, incidence, and treatment allocation change with age: a retrospective cohort study of 233 consecutive cases. Biomed Res Int. 2017;2017:8321680.
20. Falavigna A, Righesso O, da Silva PG, Siri CR, Daniel JW, Esteves Veiga JC, et al. Management of type II odontoid fractures: experience from Latin American Spine Centers. World Neurosurg. 2017;98:673–81.
21. Shammassian B, Wright CH, Wright J, Onwuzulike, Tomei KL. Successful delayed non-operative management of C2 neurosynchondrosis fractures in a pediatric patient: a case report and review of management strategies and considerations for treatment. Childs Nerv Syst. 2016;32(1):163–8.
22. Korres DS, Chytas DG, Markatos KN, Efstathopoulos NE, Nikolaou VS. The "challenging" fractures of the odontoid process: a review of the classification schemes. Eur J Orthop Surg Traumatol. 2017;27(4):469–75.
23. Anderson LD, D'Alonzo RT. Fractures of the odontoid process of the axis. J Bone Joint Surg Am. 1974;56(8):1663–74.
24. Sayama CM, Fassett DR, Apfelbaum RI. The utility of MRI in the evaluation of odontoid fractures. J Spinal Disord Tech. 2008;21(7):524–6.
25. Hakalo J, Wronski J. Operative treatment of hangman's fractures of C2. Posterior direct pars screw repair or anterior plate-cage stabilization? Neurol Neurochir Pol. 2008;42(1):28–36.
26. Koller H, Acosta F, Forstner R, Zenner J, Resch H, Tauber M, et al. C2-fractures: part II. A morphometrical analysis of computerized atlantoaxial motion, anatomical alignment and related clinical outcomes. Eur Spine J. 2009;18(8):1135–53.
27. Como JJ, Diaz JJ, Dunham CM, Chiu WC, Duane TM, Capella JM, et al. Practice management guidelines for identification of cervical spine injuries following trauma: update from the eastern association for the surgery of trauma practice management guidelines committee. J Trauma. 2009;67(3):651–9.
28. Martinez-Del-Campo E, Kalb S, Soriano-Baron H, Turner JD, Neal MT, Uschold T, et al. Computed tomography parameters for atlantooccipital dislocation in adult patients: the occipital condyle-C1 interval. J Neurosurg Spine. 2016;24(4):535–45.

Surgical Decision-Making in Cranio-Vertebral Junction Trauma: A Case Illustrated Chapter

21

Claudio Schonauer, Enrico Tessitore, Raffaele de Falco, Massimiliano Maione, Francesco Certo, and Giuseppe Barbagallo

21.1 Introduction

CVJ traumatic injuries represent a challenge for spine surgeons for several reasons. First, CVJ biomechanics is unique because of the high weight discrepancy between the head and the small vertebral bodies, making this transitional region subject to a high biomechanical stress. Second, the specific orientation of the facet joints in childhood and adolescence predisposes patients to secondary post-traumatic dislocations, especially when rotational forces are applied to the CVJ. Third, the occipital bone is almost everywhere extremely thin, making the occipital screws' purchase lower than in any part of the spine. Fourth, the steep angle existing between the occiput and cervical spine makes the stabilization challenging in terms of spinal alignment. At last, there is not enough space available for bone grafting between the occiput and C1-C2 region [3, 7, 8, 14].

In light of the above, the first line treatment in CVJ injuries should be the conservative one. Nevertheless, in some specific clinical and radiological scenarios there is a clear indication to perform surgical stabilization. This chapter will illustrate surgical indications and strategies in CVJ injured patients.

Case 1

- *Fracture type: C2 vertebral body (miscellaneous fracture)*
- *Surgery: C2-C3 anterior fusion*

C. Schonauer (✉)
Neurosurgical Unit, ASL Napoli 2 Nord, Naples, Italy

E. Tessitore
Neurosurgical Unit, Geneva University Hospitals, Geneva, Switzerland

R. de Falco
Neurosurgical Unit, Santa Maria delle Grazie Hospital, Napoli, Italy

M. Maione · F. Certo · G. Barbagallo
Department of Neurological Surgery, Policlinico "G. Rodolico" University Hospital, Catania, Italy

E. Tessitore et al. (eds.), *Surgery of the Cranio-Vertebral Junction*,
https://doi.org/10.1007/978-3-030-18700-2_21

A 56-year-old male patient was referred to the Emergency Unit following a car accident and complaining of severe neck pain. X-ray, CT scan, and MRI demonstrated a complex vertebral body fracture at C2 (miscellaneous fracture). Neurological examination was normal, and the patient presented only with neck stiffness.

The fracture was considered unstable and surgery was recommended. The patient underwent anterior C2-C3 fusion on day 5 after admission.

A right submandibular approach was used with the head slightly rotated contralaterally and fixed on a Mayfield clamp. Ligation of the superior tiroid artery was necessary to gain access to the upper part of C2 vertebra, the hypoglossal nerve was isolated, and protected with a patty. After complete C2-C3 discectomy, an autologous bone graft harvested from the iliac crest was inserted, and a cervical plate (Orion, Medtronic Sofamor Danek, Memphis, USA) was positioned. Surgery was uneventful and the patient was recommended to wear a soft collar for 6 weeks. Clinical and radiological follow-up was satisfactory (Fig. 21.1).

Case 2

- *Fracture type: C2 Type II odontoid fracture*
- *Surgery: Odontoid screw insertion*

A 38-year-old male was found unconscious after a car accident and transferred to the emergency unit. He quickly recovered upon admission, and the neurological examination did not reveal any deficit. The radiological work-up showed a Type II Anderson–D'Alonzo [1] odontoid fracture, associated with multiple rib fractures (from fourth to ninth with fluctuant bone flap) and hemothorax drained by a chest tube. A right laminar C6 fracture was also evident (Fig. 21.2a).

The concomitant thoracic lesions and the need for a rapid functional recovery made surgery the first option. Anterior odontoid screw fixation was then favored on the posterior fixation because: (1) Favorable fracture line (O-BAR according to Roy-Camille classification) [12]; (2) Need to avoid every thoracic compression related to the prone position that could prove potentially dangerous for the thoracic bone flap.

The operation was carried out with double fluoroscopy guidance. A standard Cloward approach with skin incision at C5-C6 level was used. The anterior part of C2-C3 disc space was then identified and the entry point prepared. A single odontoid screw was then inserted along a Kirschner wire. The operation time was 60 min with 50 mL of blood loss. The postoperative course was uneventful and the patient recovered quickly from surgery. The 1-year follow-up X-ray is shown in Fig. 21.2b.

Case 3

- *Fracture type: delayed C1-C2 ligamentous instability*
- *Surgery: C1-C2 posterior fixation*

A 73-year-old male has been involved in a car accident with cervical whiplash. The radiological work-up did not show any bony lesions and the patient was discharged. One year later, the patient came to the outpatients' clinic complaining of

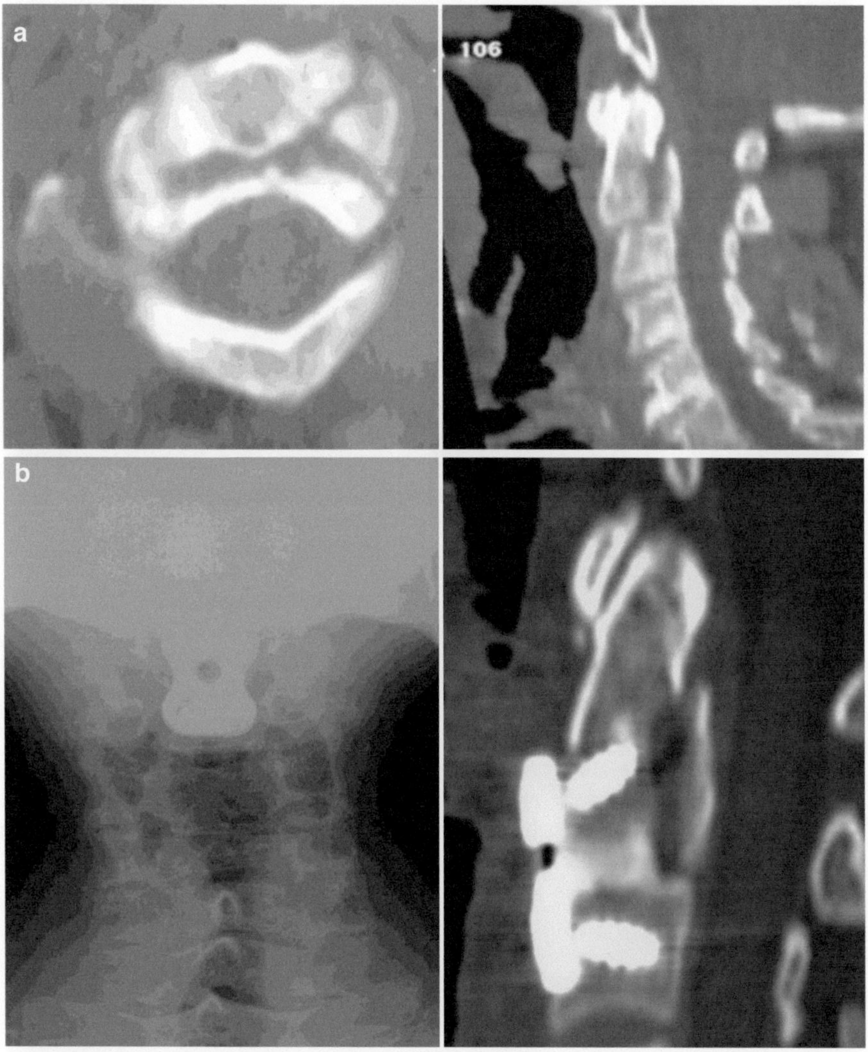

Fig. 21.1 (**a**) Case 1 Preoperative CT scan of C2 vertebral body fracture. (**b**) Case 1 Postoperative 3D CT reconstruction and X-ray after C2-C3 anterior cervical fusion

mild tetraparesis and neck pain. The MRI showed a C1-C2 myelopathy with T2-hyperintensity and associated stenosis (Fig. 21.3a).

Dynamic films revealed C1-C2 instability with increase in ADI (atlanto-dental interval) [3, 10].

The patient underwent to C1-C2 posterior fixation. Since preoperative CT angiogram showed a high riding left vertebral artery, screws were implanted in C1 lateral masses and C2 laminas to reduce the risk of VA injury (Fig. 21.3b).

The postoperative course was uneventful with prompt recovery. At 6 months follow-up the patient presented with a mild neurological improvement (Fig. 21.3c–e).

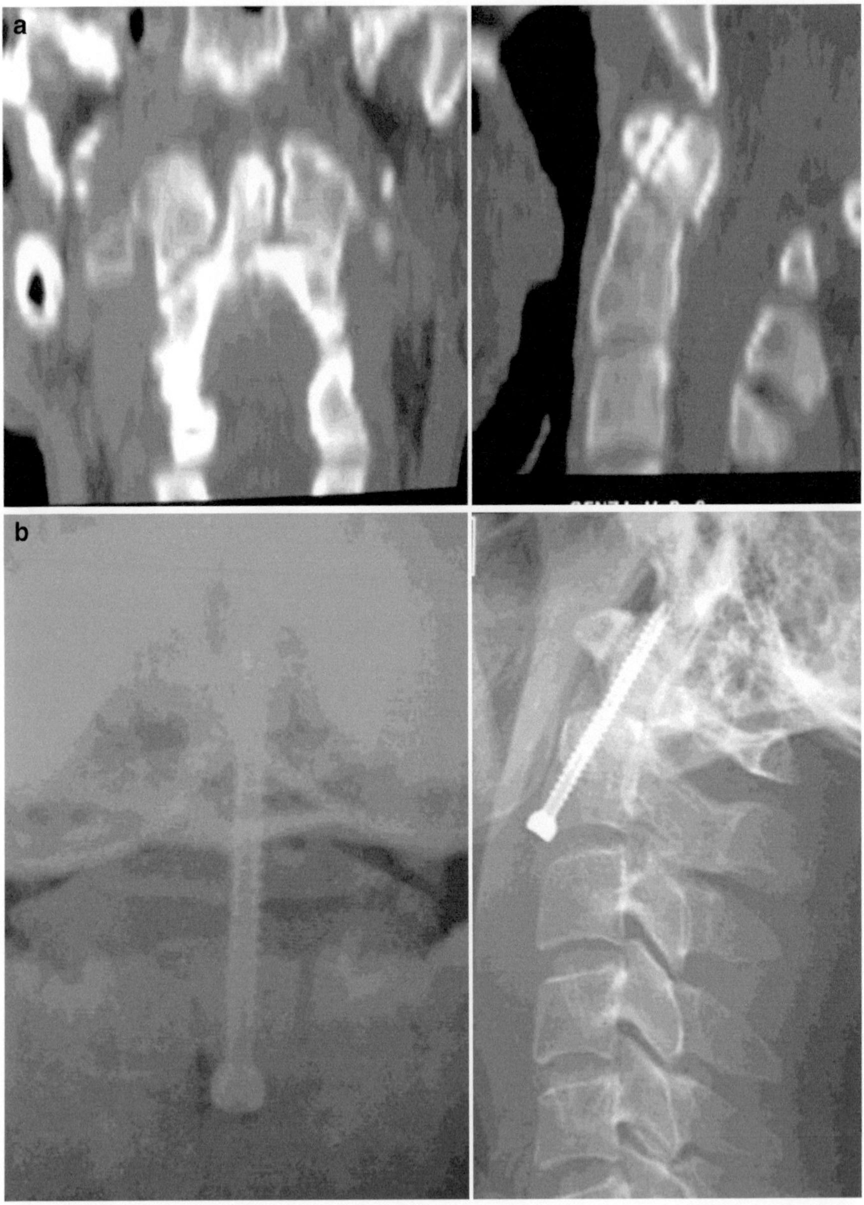

Fig. 21.2 (**a**) Preoperative CT scan showing Type II dens fracture. (**b**) Postoperative X-ray after direct dens repair

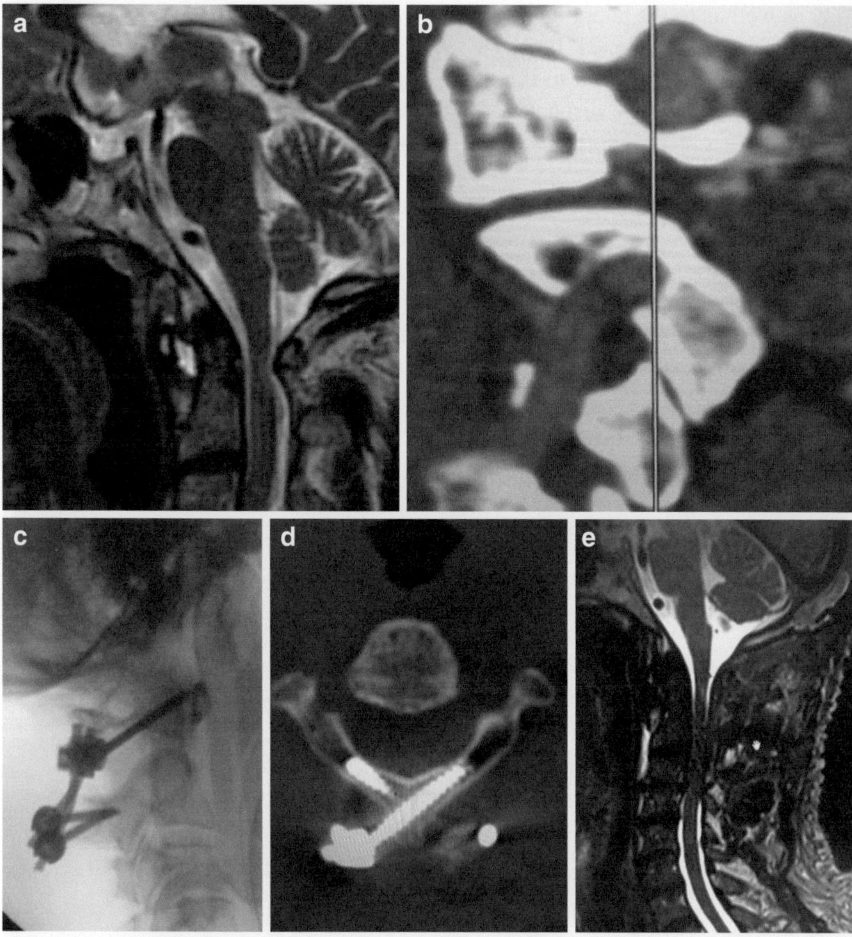

Fig. 21.3 (**a**) Preoperative T2 MRI with C1 Myelopathy. (**b**) Preoperative CT angiogram revealing a high riding vertebral artery. (**c–e**) Postoperative X-ray, CT scan, and MRI. Laminar screws were preferred to C2 isthmic/pedicle screws because of an high riding vertebral artery

Case 4

- *Fracture type: atypical type I Hangman fracture*
- *Surgery: Pars repair with Judet approach*

A 37-year-old man presented with severe neck tenderness and restricted range of motion (ROM) following a swimming injury with head hyperextension. He was admitted to the emergency department fully conscious and with no neurological impairment. Multiplanar, reconstructed, computed tomography (CT) of the cranio-vertebral junction (CVJ) showed traumatic C2 spondylolisthesis, with a fracture line crossing both C2 pedicles and extending to the posterior wall of the vertebral body as well as to the lateral masses. This fracture was classified as atypical type I hangman's fracture (Fig. 21.4a–c).

The patient was referred to the neurosurgical department. Radiological assessment included magnetic resonance (MR) of cranio-vertebral junction and cervical spine to rule out any soft tissue or ligamentous damage to the cervical spine (Fig. 21.4d).

The best treatment option for hangman's fractures is controversial [12]. Conservative management with non-rigid external fixation is considered to be effective only for resolution of type I (as well as type II) fractures without any involvement of posterior wall of C2 vertebral body [11]. Although anterior (either transoral or retropharyngeal) approach with C2-C3 intersomatic fusion, with or without plating, has been proposed as surgical option for unstable traumatic spondylolisthesis of

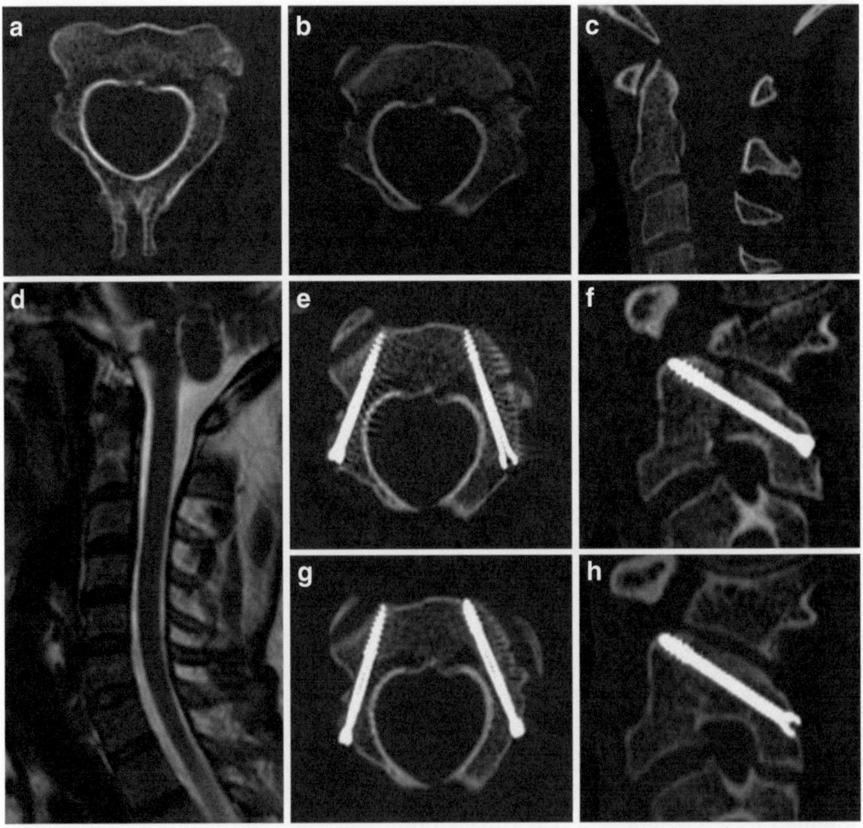

Fig. 21.4 Axial (**a**, **b**) and sagittal (**c**) CT scan showing an hairline fracture of the ring of the axis with involvement of the posterior wall of C2 vertebral body and minimal dislocation of the vertebral body (<3 mm). (**d**) Preoperative, sagittal, T2-weighted MRI showing no evidence of spinal injury. (**e**, **f**) Immediate postoperative CT scan confirming correct screws position. (**g**, **h**) Postoperative CT scan, 6 months later, demonstrating fusion across the fracture line

the axis, this technique is associated with a high rate of complications and does not always allow for preservation of the rotational motion preservation [6, 11].

The posterior approach with pars-pedicle C2 screws for "direct" fixation of hangman's type fractures was described by Judet as a motion (C1-C2) preserving technique. Lag screws facilitate the intraoperative reduction and fixation of C2 pedicle fractures, not achievable with head traction during patient positioning [9]. Vertebral artery injury, as well as neural damage, is possible and pre-operative angio-CT is mandatory to study the course of vertebral arteries in relationship to C2 pedicles [5].

Although the best indication for this surgical option seems to be the hangman's type IIa Levine-Edwards fractures [4, 5], direct transpedicular fixation of C2 using 30 mm lag screws was performed in the present case harboring an atypical type I fracture. Visualization of the medial edge of C2 pedicles assisted screw insertion maneuvers and surgery was guided by fluoroscopy. However, CT-guided technique and neuronavigation guidance for placement of C2 pars-pedicle screw according to Judet approach have also been described [2, 13].

No intra- and/or postoperative complications were observed. Postoperative CT scan showed complete reduction of the fracture lines (Fig. 21.4e, f). The patient experienced full clinical recovery, with disappearance of neck pain, as well as early mobilization and short hospitalization. Furthermore, optimal ROM was restored as documented by long-term follow-up evaluation, and a solid, long-term fusion has been achieved (Fig. 21.4g, h) (Table 21.1).

Table 21.1 CVJ injuries usually treated with surgery

Location: Occipital condyle Name of injury: Anderson and Montesano type 3 Description: Total avulsion of the condyle at the insertion of the alar ligament, worse if bilateral Operation: Occipito-cervical fusion
Location: C1 atlas Name of injury: Jefferson type III Description: Rule of Spence more than 6.9 mm in coronal CT Operation: C1-C2 posterior fusion
Location: C2 Axis Name of injury: Anderson–D'Alonzo Type 2 Description: fracture at the base of the dens at or above the junction with the vertebral body or dens displacement >6 mm Operation: Anterior odontoid screw, C1-C2 posterior fusion
Location: C2 Axis Type of injury: Levine and Edwards Type II and III Description: Traumatic spondylolisthesis of the axis with displacement over lateral plain film Operation: C2-C3 discectomy and fusion, C1-C3 posterior fusion, direct C2 pars reconstruction
Location: C1-C2 region Type of injury: Type 1 Dickman and Sonntag ligamentous injury Description: Lesion of the transverse ligament Operation: C1-C2 posterior fusion

This table links most CVJ injuries that require surgical correction

References

1. Anderson PA, Montesano PX. Morphology and treatment of occipital condyle fractures. Spine. 1988;13:731–6.
2. Arand M, Hartwig E, Kinzl L, et al. Spinal navigation in cervical fractures—a preliminary clinical study on Judet-osteosynthesis of the axis. Comput Aided Surg. 2001;6(3):170–5.
3. Dickman CA, Sonntag VK. Injuries involving the transverse atlantal ligament: classification and treatment guidelines based upon experience with 39 injuries. Neurosurgery. 1997;40:886–7.
4. Elliott MR, Kirkpatrick JS. Type IIa Hangman's fracture with pure distraction: not your typical type IIa fracture. Spine J. 2014;14(7):1360–1.
5. ElMiligui Y, Koptan W, Emran I. Transpedicular screw fixation for type II Hangman's fracture: a motion preserving procedure. Eur Spine J. 2010;19(8):1299–305.
6. Francis WR, Fielding JW, Hawkins RJ, et al. Traumatic spondylolisthesis of the axis. J Bone Joint Surg Br. 1981;63-B(3):313–8.
7. Hadley MN. Guidelines for management of acute cervical injuries. Neurosurgery. 2002;50:S1–6.
8. Joaquim AF, Patel AA. Craniocervical traumatic injuries. Global Spine J. 2011;1:37–42.
9. Judet R, Roy-Camille R, Saillant G. Actualités de chirurgie orthopédique de l'Hospital Raymond-Poin caré. VIII. Fractures du rachis cervical. Paris: Masson; 1970. p. 174–95.
10. Levine AM, Edwards CC. The management of traumatic spondylolisthesis of the axis. J Bone Joint Surg Am. 1985;67:217–26.
11. Li XF, Dai LY, Lu H, et al. A systematic review of the management of hangman's fractures. Eur Spine J. 2006;15(3):257–69.
12. Ryken TC, Hadley MN, Aarabi B, et al. Management of isolated fractures of the axis in adults. Neurosurgery. 2013;72(Suppl. 2):132–50.
13. Taller S, Suchomel P, Lukas R, et al. CT-guided internal fixation of a hangman's fracture. Eur Spine J. 2000;9:393–7.
14. Traynelis VC, Marano GD, Dunker RO, Kaufman HH. Traumatic atlanto-occipital dislocation. Case report. J Neurosurg. 1986;65:863–70.

Management of Retro-Odontoid Pseudotumor

22

Giuseppe M. V. Barbagallo, Massimiliano Maione, and Francesco Certo

22.1 Introduction

The pathologic condition firstly called retro-odontoid pseudotumor [1], but also known as pannus or phantom tumor [2], consists of a non-neoplastic, fibro-cartilaginous mass involving the odontoid process, and the surrounding structures of craniovertebral junction [3, 4].

Despite the controversies surrounding etiology and pathophysiology of retro-odontoid pseudotumor, various predisposing factors are considered to be associated with its development, including inflammatory diseases (rheumatoid arthritis [5] and psoriatic arthritis [6]) and, less frequently, noninflammatory conditions (post-traumatic dens axis pseudoarthrosis [7], unstable odontoid fractures [8], os odontoideum [9], post-laminoplasty kyphotic cervical instability [10], long-term hemodialysis [11], craniocervical junction malformations [12], and chronic atlanto-axial subluxation/instability [1, 12]).

Surgical treatment of retro-odontoid pseudotumor can be performed by direct removal of the mass, through the transnasal/transoral-transpharyngeal approach [13, 14] or the high cervical lateral approach [15] or the posterior extradural/transdural approach via laminectomy [16]. Conversely, C1 laminoplasty [2] or posterior decompression with/without atlantoaxial/occipito-cervical fixation [8, 12, 17–19] are considered to induce spontaneous pannus regression.

The aim of this chapter is to provide an overview of surgical techniques and related indications to decide which type of surgery for retro-odontoid pseudotumor should be performed. At the end of procedures' description, an illustrated case will be presented.

G. M. V. Barbagallo (✉) · M. Maione · F. Certo
Department of Neurological Surgery, Policlinico "G. Rodolico" University Hospital, Catania, Italy

E. Tessitore et al. (eds.), *Surgery of the Cranio-Vertebral Junction*,
https://doi.org/10.1007/978-3-030-18700-2_22

22.2 Surgical Techniques and Indications

Retro-odontoid pannus concentrates its action between the dens and C1 anterior arch, or the dens and transverse ligament. Its development causes spinal canal narrowing and consequent neurological symptoms. Direct spinal cord decompression is indicated when neurological deficits are present [20]. Alternatively, even if symptoms are partially silent but radiological neural structures compression is reported, posterior decompression with vertebral fixation can be performed to induce progressive pannus reabsorption [21, 22].

22.2.1 Direct Removal of Retro-Odontoid Pseudotumor

22.2.1.1 Transnasal/Transoral-Transpharyngeal Approach

An anterior approach with decompression of cervical spinal canal and odontoidectomy is needed when spinal cord compression leads to myelopathy and progressive neurologic impairment. A transoral odontoid resection is also indicated in cases of irreducible atlantoaxial kyphosis [23].

The transoral-transpharyngeal approach has been described for decades as an effective surgical technique for direct access to the anterior superior cervical spine [24], and it has been considered to be the treatment of choice to remove the retro-odontoid mass in cases without cervical instability [13, 14]. Intraoperative and postoperative complications, such as velopharyngeal incompetence, hypernasal speech, swallowing disturbance, and temporomandibular joint syndrome, are frequently reported in association with the transoral approach, regardless of whether endoscopic techniques or not are used [22].

The endoscopic transnasal transclival approach may be used as alternative to the transoral-transpharyngeal approach, achieving retro-odontoid pseudotumor removal and satisfactory decompression, in absence of surgical complications [25].

However, the anterior surgical access does not allow the surgeon to approach the posterior arch of the atlas if concomitant posterior decompression is needed [23]. Moreover, the transnasal/transoral approach is not adequate for treatment of retro-odontoid pannus associated with craniovertebral instability, and even so posterior fusion surgery would be mandatory in this case [25].

22.2.1.2 High Cervical Lateral Approach

Although the high cervical lateral approach is not routinely used for resection of retro-odontoid pannus, it may be taken into account when the retro-odontoid mass appears large and laterally extended. Removal via lateral approach alone is sufficient if cervical instability is not associated and it reveals very useful in case of rapidly progressive spinal cord symptoms, as well as via the anterior approach [15].

Preoperative evaluation of the arterial anatomy is mandatory to avoid vertebral artery injury, which represents the main risk of this approach. Despite spinal instability can occur after surgery based on the degree of bony resection, surgeon may consider this technique as an effective surgical option in selected cases, particularly if the anterior approach is undesirable (for instance, in patients presenting with dysphagia) [26].

22.2.1.3 Posterior Extradural/Transdural Approach via Laminectomy

Thanks to advances in spinal cord monitoring, posterior cervical spine procedures have become possible and considerably safe for expert spine surgeons, bypassing infective and vascular complications related to anterior (transoral) and lateral approaches.

Among posterior approaches aiming to direct removal of retro-odontoid pseudotumor, the posterior extradural resection via C1 laminectomy is the most commonly used. No vertebral fixation is usually required. Moreover, one of the advantages of this technique is that additional fusion surgery can be performed during the same approach if necessary.

Since pseudotumor is sited medially in front of the spinal cord, the posterior transdural approach—more frequently used for cervical and thoracic disk herniation—has also been described to reach more directly the retro-odontoid mass. Transdural access is encouraged by the favorable ratio of dural-to-spinal cord width at C1-C2 level. Furthermore, the transdural resection allows avoiding epidural bleeding and adhesions that could make the extradural approach hard. Careful manipulation of spinal cord and preservation of arachnoid membranes are essential cautions during this procedure [16].

22.2.2 Induced Spontaneous Regression of Retro-Odontoid Pseudotumor

22.2.2.1 C1 Laminectomy/Laminoplasty

The retro-odontoid pseudotumor is frequently observed in rheumatoid arthritis and it is associated with atlantoaxial subluxation in most cases [27]. However, retro-odontoid pannus is not necessarily related to cervical instability; indeed, subaxial fusion due to ossification of the anterior longitudinal ligament and ankylosis of adjacent segments (C0-C1, C2-C3) may occasionally induce pseudotumor development [28]. In these cases, posterior fixation would lead to the decrease of the already disturbed cervical range of motion, and thus it should be avoided [29]. Therefore, posterior decompressive procedures have been proposed as simpler, less-invasive, and relatively risk-free surgical treatment for pseudotumor without atlantoaxial instability if compared to the alternative anterior and lateral approaches.

C1 laminectomy provides satisfactory neurological improvement as result of neural structures decompression and no additional postoperative instability. Additionally, it is able to induce regression of retro-odontoid pannus in many cases, probably due to the improvement of blood flow following decompression [29].

Similar clinical and radiological outcomes are reported when C1 laminoplasty is performed in cases of cervical pannus-related myelopathy with either absent or slight atlantoaxial instability. The frequent postoperative regression of the retro-odontoid pseudotumor is attributed to posterior movement of the spinal cord and recovery of dural pulsation after C1 laminoplasty. This seems to be particularly effective if the pseudotumor is associated with synovial cysts. Moreover, laminoplasty has been suggested to limit the risk of postoperative spinal cord compression caused by scar tissue, and to prevent the postoperative kyphosis often observed after laminectomy [2].

22.2.2.2 Posterior Decompression with Atlantoaxial/Occipito-Cervical Fixation

The surgical strategies previously presented are not indicated in cases of retro-odointoid pseudotumor involving instability.

Pseudotumor associated with atlantoaxial instability—including an increased motion at the C1–C2 level as a consequence of a reduced motion of the subaxial spine secondary to spondylotic changes—are usually treated by posterior C1-C2 fixation with/without C1 laminectomy [21, 23]. Patients presenting a retro-odontoid pannus caused by spondylosis or ankylosis or ossification of the anterior longitudinal ligament could also undergo C1-C2 fixation surgery [4].

From a biomechanical point of view, the most effective strategy is represented by the C1-C2 transarticularis fixation technique; it provides both great stability and high fusion rate [17, 19, 30]. However, this procedure is associated with risk of iatrogenic vertebral artery injury [31]. Due to this reason, the C1 lateral mass-C2 pedicle/isthmus screws and rods technique has been introduced for treatment of the retro-odontoid pannus [32–34]; it presents more remarkable clinical and radiological outcomes even if compared with the transarticularis method [35]. Alternatively, bilateral crossing C2 laminar screws may be placed, allowing safer osteosynthesis in cases with high-riding vertebral artery or small C2 pedicles/isthmus [36].

Pseudotumor reduction in size significantly occurs in patients treated by posterior C1-C2 fixation, even if atlantoaxial instability is not reported [4, 8, 21].

In order to treat retro-odontoid pannus associated with either subaxial subluxation or C0-C1 fusion, an occipito-cervical fusion is needed; moreover, it may be useful in cases of poor bone quality due to extensive degenerative changes of cervical spine. This surgical strategy provides reduction of the pannus and decompression of spinal cord [21, 23].

In addition to posterior fixation procedures, C1 laminectomy is frequently performed with the purpose of achieving an early decompression of neuronal structures while safely waiting for the pannus reabsorption, which is commonly a process needing several months to take place [21].

22.3 An Illustrated Case of Retro-Odontoid Pseudotumor

A 63-year-old man presented with a 2-year history of bilateral, cervical, radicular syndrome. Neck pain and electric shock-like pain radiating down the shoulders and upper limbs to hands were rapidly worsening during the last 2 months before the admission. Neurological examination showed a severe spastic tetraparesis associated with tetrahyperreflexia; bilateral Hoffman sign was also present; grade-3 Nurick score was recorded. Moreover, urge incontinence was present.

The patient did not suffer from inflammatory diseases and no previous history of trauma or neoplastic disease was reported.

Neuroradiological examinations were performed to disclose the possible cause of this condition. Cervical X-rays with flexion-extension views and computer tomography (CT) with multiplanar reconstructions showed C1-C2 instability associated with subaxial diffuse idiopathic skeletal hyperostosis (DISH) and C5-C6 fusion. Magnetic resonance imaging (MRI) revealed cervical myelopathy secondary to a retro-odontoid mass compressing the anterior surface of the spinal cord. The retro-odontoid pseudotumor appeared hypointense on T1-weighted images, with mixed intensity on T2-weighted images (Fig. 22.1a). No gadolinium enhancement of the pseudotumor was seen.

Since neither rheumatic nor psoriatic arthritis was reported and as clear signs of cervical subaxial spondylosis with C1-C2 instability were radiologically shown, a posterior approach was chosen to treat this condition. In particular, under intraoperative fluoroscopic guidance, the patient underwent a C1-C2 Harms fixation, with

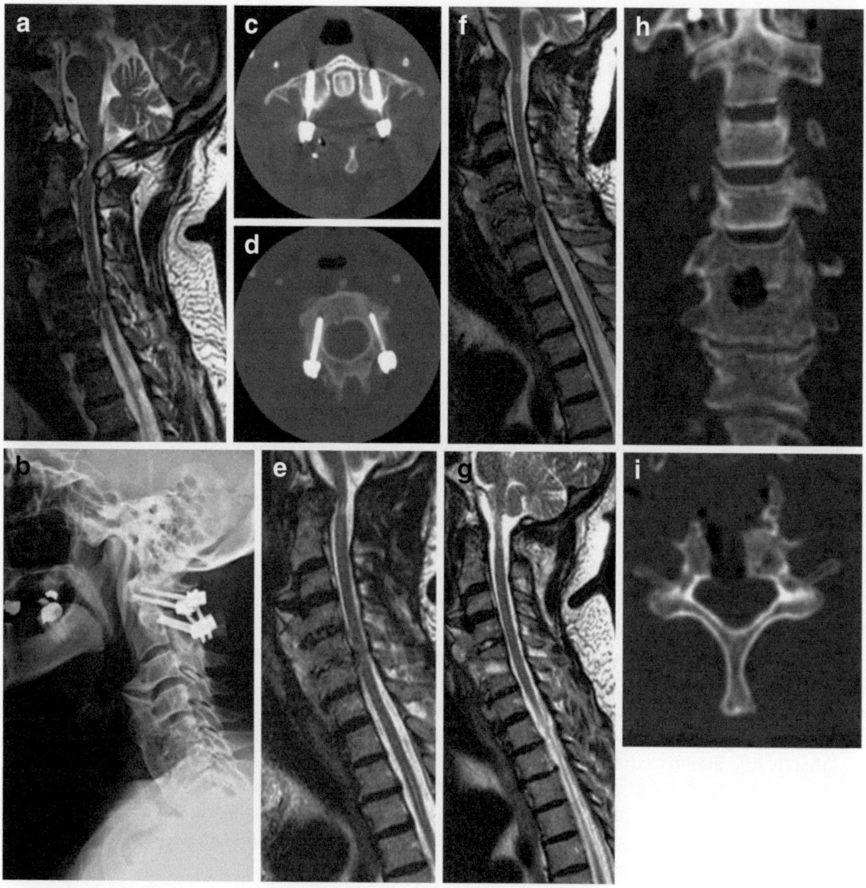

Fig. 22.1 (**a**) Sagittal, T2-weighted MRI showing severe cord compression due to a large retro-odontoid pseudotumor along with a spondylotic spinal cord compression at C5-C6 in a DISH condition. (**b**) Lateral X-ray showing C1-C2 fixation and (**c**, **d**) axial CT scan demonstrating the correct device position. Postoperative, sagittal, T2-weighted MRI confirming progressive pannus reabsorption at 5- (**e**), 8- (**f**) and 13-months (**g**) follow-up. The "key-hole" approach to remove focal compression at C5-C6 is seen on coronal (**h**) and axial (**i**) CT scan

C1 lateral mass and C2 pedicle polyaxial screw insertion and bilateral rods placement. A decompressive C1 laminectomy was also performed in order to achieve immediate spinal cord decompression. Moreover, a later focal decompression at C5-C6 level was achieved in the same patient by a "key-hole" approach. Postoperative check X-rays and CT scans showed the decompression of neural structures and correct positioning of C1 and C2 screws (Fig. 22.1b–d). Gradual neurological improvement was reported over the months following surgery. The pain completely recovered and the Nurick score improved from grade 3 to 1, allowing the patient to return to routine activities including work activities. Therefore, the patient was followed-up with serial MRI examinations showing progressive retro-odontoid pannus reabsorption to the point of its disappearance (Fig. 22.1e–g).

References

1. Sze G, Brant-Zawadzki MN, Wilson CR, et al. Pseudotumor of the craniovertebral junction associated with chronic subluxation: MR imaging studies. Radiology. 1986;161:391–4.
2. Suetsuna F, Narita H, Ono A, et al. Regression of retroodontoid pseudotumors following C1 laminoplasty. J Neurosurg Spine. 2006;5:455–60.
3. Larsson EM, Holtås S, Zygmunt S. Pre- and postoperative MR imaging of the craniocervical junction in rheumatoid arthritis. AJR Am J Roentgenol. 1989;152:561–6.
4. Tanaka S, Nakada M, Hayashi Y, et al. Retro-odontoid pseudotumor without atlantoaxial subluxation. J Clin Neurosci. 2010;17:649–52.
5. Grob D, Wursch R, Grauer W, et al. Atlantoaxial fusion and retrodental pannus in rheumatoid arthritis. Spine (Phila Pa 1976). 1997;22:1580–4.
6. Lu K, Lee TC. Spontaneous regression of periodontoid pannus mass in psoriatic atlantoaxial subluxation. Case report. Spine (Phila Pa 1976). 1999;24:578–81.
7. Yamashita Y, Takahashi M, Sakamoto Y, et al. Atlantoaxial subluxation. Radiography and magnetic resonance imaging correlated to myelopathy. Acta Radiol. 1989;30:135–40.
8. Young WF, Boyko O. Magnetic resonance imaging confirmation of resolution of periodontoid pannus formation following C1/C2 posterior transarticular screw fixation. J Clin Neurosci. 2002;9:434–6.
9. Ogata T, Kawatani Y, Morino T, et al. Resolution of intraspinal retro-odontoid cyst associated with os odontoideum after posterior fixation. J Spinal Disord Tech. 2009;22(1):58–61.
10. Matsumoto T, Takada S, Tsujimoto K, et al. Enlarging retro-odontoid pseudotumor after expanding cervical laminoplasty in the presence of kyphosis. Spine J. 2006;6(3):228–32.
11. Maruyama H, Tanizawa T, Uchiyama S, et al. Magnetic resonance imaging of pseudotumors of the craniovertebral junction in long-term hemodialysis patients. Am J Nephrol. 1999;19:541–5.
12. Lagares A, Arrese I, Pascual B, et al. Pannus resolution after occipitocervical fusion in a non-rheumatoid atlanto-axial instability. Eur Spine J. 2006;15:366–9.
13. Crockard HA, Pozo JL, Ransford AO, et al. Transoral decompression and posterior fusion for rheumatoid atlanto-axial subluxation. J Bone Joint Surg Br. 1986;68:350–6.
14. Moskovich R, Crockard H. Posttraumatic atlanto-axial subluxation and myelopathy. Efficacy of anterior decompression. Spine (Phila Pa 1976). 1990;15:442–7.
15. Oohori Y, Seichi A, Kawaguchi H, et al. Retroodontoid pseudotumor resected by a high cervical lateral approach in a rheumatoid arthritis patient: a case report. J Orthop Sci. 2004;9:90–3.
16. Fujiwara Y, Manabe H, Sumida T, et al. Microscopic posterior transdural resection of cervical retro-odontoid pseudotumors. J Spinal Disord Tech. 2015;28:363–9.
17. Cihanek M, Fuentes S, Metellus P, et al. Disappearance of retro-odontoid pseudotumor after C1-C2 transarticular fixation screw. Neurochirurgie. 2008;54(1):32–6.

18. Finn MA, Bishop FS, Dailey AT. Surgical treatment of occipitocervical instability. Neurosurgery. 2008;63(5):961–9.
19. Jun BY. Complete reduction of retro-odontoid soft tissue mass in os odontoideum following the posterior C1–C2 transarticular screw fixation. Spine (Phila Pa 1976). 1999;24:1961–4.
20. Yurube T, Sumi M, Nishida K, et al. Progression of cervical spine instabilities in rheumatoid arthritis: a prospective cohort study of outpatients over 5 years. Spine (Phila Pa 1976). 2011;36(8):647–53.
21. Barbagallo GMV, Certo F, Visocchi M, et al. Disappearance of degenerative, non-inflammatory, retro-odontoid pseudotumor following posterior C1-C2 fixation: case series and review of the literature. Eur Spine J. 2013;22(Suppl 6):S879–88.
22. Landi A, Marotta N, Morselli C, et al. Pannus regression after posterior decompression and occipito-cervical fixation in occipito-atlanto-axial instability due to rheumatoid arthritis: case report and literature review. Clin Neurol Neurosurg. 2013;115(2):111–6.
23. Kandziora F, Mittlmeier T, Kerschbaumer F. Stage-related surgery for cervical spine instability in rheumatoid arthritis. Eur Spine J. 1999;8:371–81.
24. Spetzler RF, Hadley MN, Sonntag VK. The transoral approach to the anterior superior cervical spine. A review of 29 cases. Acta Neurochir Suppl (Wien). 1988;43:69–74.
25. Wu JC, Huang WC, Cheng H, et al. Endoscopic transnasal transclival odontoidectomy: a new approach to decompression: technical case report. Neurosurgery. 2008;63(1 Suppl 1):ONSE92–4.
26. Abdullah KG, Schlenk RS, Krishnaney A, et al. Direct lateral approach to pathology at the craniocervical junction: a technical note. Neurosurgery. 2012;70(2 Suppl Operative):202–8.
27. Pettersson H, Larsson EM, Holtas S, et al. MR imaging of the cervical spine in rheumatoid arthritis. Am J Neuroradiol. 1988;9:573–7.
28. Chikuda H, Seichi A, Takeshita K, et al. Radiographic analysis of the cervical spine in patients with retro-odontoid pseudotumors. Spine (Phila Pa 1976). 2009;34:E110–4.
29. Kakutani K, Doita M, Yoshikawa M, et al. C1 laminectomy for retro-odontoid pseudotumor without atlantoaxial subluxation: review of seven consecutive cases. Eur Spine J. 2013;22(5):1119–26.
30. Magerl F, Seeman PS. Stable posterior fusion of the atlas and axis by transarticular screw fixation. In: Kehr P, Weidner A, editors. Cervical spine. Wien: Springer; 1987. p. 322–7.
31. Vergara P, Bal JS, Hickman Casey AT, et al. C1-C2 posterior fixation: are four screws better than two? Neurosurgery. 2011;71(1 Suppl Operative):86–95.
32. Goel A, Laheri V. Re: Harms J, Melcher P. Posterior C1-C2 fusion with polyaxial screw and rod fixation. (Spine. 2001;26:2467–71). Spine (Phila Pa 1976). 2002;27(14):1589–90.
33. Harms J, Melcher RP. Posterior C1-C2 fusion with polyaxial screw and rod fixation. Spine (Phila Pa 1976). 2001;26(22):2467–71.
34. Takami T, Goto T, Tsuyuguchi N, et al. Posterior C1-2 Fixation with cancellous screw and rod system for retro-odontoid pseudotumor associated with chronic atlantoaxial subluxation. Technical note. Neurol Med Chir (Tokyo). 2007;47(4):189–93; discussion 193–4.
35. Lee SH, Kim ES, Sung JK, et al. Clinical and radiological comparison of treatment of atlantoaxial instability by posterior C1-C2 transarticular screw fixation or C1 lateral mass-C2 pedicle screw fixation. J Clin Neurosci. 2010;17:886–92.
36. Wright NM. Posterior C2 fixation using bilateral, crossing C2 laminar screws: case series and technical note. J Spinal Disord Tech. 2004;17(2):158–62.

23 Classification and Radiological Assessment of CVJ Tumors

Christian F. Freyschlag and Claudius Thomé

23.1 Classification

Tumors of the craniovertebral junction (CVJ) may be classified either as primary or secondary (metastatic) disease or with respect to their localization as intradural or extradural lesions. Additionally, they are characterized as benign or malignant lesions and according to their cell of origin.

The four cell types that are involved in formation and destruction of bone are osteoblasts, osteoclasts, chondroblasts, and fibroblasts. Tumors that arise from these cells can be identified by active ossification. Involved tumors are osteoma, osteoblastoma, and osteosarcoma. Tumors arising from chondroblasts are characterized by production of cartilage; fibroblastic tumors usually exhibit production of collagen. Tumors can also originate from supporting tissues such as hemangioma, aneurysmal bone cyst and hemangiopericytoma (blood vessels) or from bone marrow (plasmocytoma, myeloma, and Ewing's sarcoma) as well as from remnants of the notochord (chordoma).

23.2 Extradural, Benign Tumors

23.2.1 Osteogenic

Both commonly diagnosed benign osteogenic tumors of the CVJ are histologically identical. Tumor size is used to differentiate between osteoid osteoma and osteoblastoma [1].

C. F. Freyschlag · C. Thomé (✉)
Department of Neurosurgery, Medical University Innsbruck, Innsbruck, Austria
e-mail: claudius.thome@tirol-kliniken.at

E. Tessitore et al. (eds.), *Surgery of the Cranio-Vertebral Junction*,
https://doi.org/10.1007/978-3-030-18700-2_23

23.2.1.1 Osteoid Osteoma

Osteoid osteoma constitutes a small, benign, and nonprogressive lesion that is smaller than 1.5 cm^2. It accounts for 11% of all primary benign bone tumors [2–4] and 25% of osteoid osteomas are located in the spine. Usually, osteoid osteomas affect male patients 5 times more frequently and occur predominately in their twenties and thirties [5]. Typically, osteoid osteoma patients present with localized pain, leading to torticollis in more severe cases. Neurological compromise is unlikely because of their small size. The pain arises from intralesional production of arachidonic acid, resulting in painful osteolysis. Traditionally, the pain is responsive to aspirin. Treatment consists of complete surgical excision of the nidus [6] with recurrence rates of up to 4.5% [5, 7].

The diagnosis of osteoid osteoma can be based on native CT scans, revealing a dense sclerotic rim and a central lucent nidus with less than 1.5 cm in diameter. Additionally, SPECT bone scans demonstrate a high tracer uptake in osteoid osteomas, whereas absence of tracer uptake has never been reported [8].

23.2.1.2 Osteoblastoma

Osteoblastomas represent 3% of all primary bone tumors. They show a predilection for the posterior spinal elements, 40% of all reported cases are located in the spinal column [9] and are located in the cervical spine in 10–40% of cases [2, 4, 10]. Unlike the histologically similar osteoid osteoma, osteoblastoma grow rather rapidly and can undergo malignant transformation. Surgical treatment of choice is en bloc excision. In CVJ osteoblastoma, however, only a piecemeal resection may be achievable [11]. Overall recurrence rates of osteoblastomas are approximately 10%, and incomplete resection leads to a high probability of recurrence [7, 12–14].

Imaging is comparable to osteoid osteomas. A hyperdense, sclerotic rim surrounds a radiolucent nidus, larger than 1.5 cm. On MR imaging, they demonstrate avid osseous and extraosseous enhancement [15].

23.2.2 Cartilageneous

These tumors are derived from remnants of cartilaginous tissue that was left behind by the epi- or apophysial growth of the endplate [16].

23.2.2.1 Osteochondroma

Osteochondroma can occur both as solitary and as multiple lesions (osteochondromatosis) [17]. The spine is involved in 6% of cases [2, 17], half of which occur in the cervical spine [4]. Multiple lesions are often familial with autosomal dominant inheritance. The lesion is typically "capped" with cartilageneous tissue that is mostly responsible for compression symptoms. Because of their very slow expansive growth, surgical decision-making has to weigh risks and benefits carefully [18, 19].

23.2.2.2 Enchondroma

Enchondroma constitutes an extremely rare disease, which is typically found in bones of hand and feet [20]. Less than 20 cases with spinal involvement have been reported. They consist of hyaline cartilage nodes that are usually surrounded by bone [21]. Surgical resection is rarely required [22]. Enchondroma can be associated with the autosomal dominant Maffucci's syndrome [22] and presents with multiple enchondromas and multiple hemangiomas.

23.2.3 Vascular

23.2.3.1 Hemangioma

With a female predominance, hemangiomas are the most common benign vertebral neoplasms [3, 20] and are frequently found on routine spine imaging. Symptoms can occur in cases with extravertebral soft-tissue extension and resulting spinal cord compression. Rarely, epidural hemorrhages may compromise neural structures. Symptoms can also occur, if the vertebral body stability is jeopardized by an extensive growth of a hemangioma [23, 24]. The indication for surgical treatment can be challenging in patients with vague pain, cases with neurologic symptoms due to compression, however, require rather straightforward treatment decisions [25].

Diagnostic procedures include MRI and CT, discovering a polka-dotted appearance on CT and T1 hyperintensity and enhancement on MR imaging.

23.2.3.2 Aneurysmal Bone Cyst

Aneurysmal bone cysts are benign expansile lesions of uncertain etiology [2] containing numerous blood-filled channels [26]. They present in patients younger than 20 years of age in 80% of cases. Aneurysmal bone cysts involve the vertebral column in 20–30% of cases (typically the posterior elements), of which approximately 40% involve the vertebral body.

They show fluid-fluid levels on MR imaging and thin peripheral/septal enhancement. These lesions may result in pain and neurologic compromise, prompting treatment [12]. Standard surgical management depends on the lesion size [27] and includes curettage, bone grafting, and internal fixation as well as en bloc or wide resection [28]. Non-surgical management by embolization or by denosumab has recently been advocated.

23.2.4 Fibrous Tissue Tumors

Non-ossifying fibromas or fibrous cortical lesions can be found commonly in the immature femur. Spinal presentation of fibrous tumors is rare but with a predilection of the upper cervical spine. The lesions are minimally expansile and mostly asymptomatic. On plain radiographs, the lesions show a well-circumscript border.

23.2.5 Fat Cell Tumors

23.2.5.1 Lipoma

Lipomas of the spinal cord account for 1% of all primary spine tumors and 40% are extradural [29] but an intradural presentation is more common [30].

The tumors show no characteristic radiological appearance and should be resected if necessary [2, 31].

23.2.5.2 Angiolipoma

Angiolipomas are composed of typical spinal lipomas with the addition of a significant vascular element. The tumors can involve the vertebral body and dorsal structures. Symptoms are usually explained by neural compression if there is a sizable epidural component.

Both fat cell tumors show the intensity of fat upon MRI and CT.

23.2.6 Miscellaneous

23.2.6.1 Eosinophilic Granuloma

Eosinophilic granulomas account for less than 4% of primary spinal tumors [2]. Spinal involvement is seen in up to 15% of cases [20, 32]. They grow locally expansile and destructive [33] although their growth pattern is often self-limited [34]. Despite their fluctuating clinical presentation [35], treatment should be conservative [12, 36].

23.2.6.2 Solitary Plasmocytoma

With only very few cases present only in bone, solitary plasmocytoma is a type of B-cell lymphocytic tumor [37]. Patients seek attention due to local pain or spinal cord compression.

Imaging shows a lytic lesion with a cystic component that can easily be identified on CT.

Treatment of choice is radiotherapy [38] but vertebroplasty may be reasonable even at the level of C1 and C2.

23.3 Malignant Tumors

23.3.1 Osteogenic

23.3.1.1 Osteosarcoma

Osteosarcomas demonstrate spinal involvement in less than 5% of cases [3]. The most common complaint caused by this invasive malignant lesion is local pain. Many patients, however, have progressed to compression of the spinal cord or nerve roots resulting in neurological deficits before they are diagnosed. Typically for its malignant behavior, osteosarcoma usually involves the anterior column of the spine

[4]. Histologically, these tumors show malignant osteoblasts in a woven bone with an extensive vascular stroma.

Imaging includes both CT and MRI, showing the destructive lesion and commonly presenting with epidural growth. CT imaging of the thorax is additionally required, as 10–20% of osteosarcomas have already metastasized to the lungs at the time of presentation.

Treatment consists of aggressive surgical resection attempting en bloc excision [39], followed by radio- and chemotherapy. If neoadjuvant treatment is considered, the pretreatment imaging has to be taken into account for surgical planning [40].

23.3.2 Cartilageneous

23.3.2.1 Chondrosarcomas

Chondrosarcomas are usually extraaxial lesions. Less than 7% affect the spine with a peak incidence in the fifth and sixth decade [41]. Half of the patients will have neurological deficits before their condition is diagnosed [42]. The radiologic appearance is consistent with the expectations of a malignant and highly vascularized tumor [3]. Preoperative CT and MR imaging is crucial for treatment planning and to delineate soft tissue and bone involvement. Typically, CT demonstrates a lytic lesion with a partly calcified soft tissue mass. In highly vascularized lesions, preoperative angiography should be considered in order to perform embolization, which could play an important role in surgical treatment [43, 44]. Even low-grade lesions have a high likelihood for recurrence [41].

Treatment consists of aggressive (en bloc) resection followed by radiotherapy [42] although these lesions were thought to be radioresistant and the use of proton beam irradiation offers additional treatment options [45]. Resection has to include bone and soft tissue, in cases where radical resection could not be obtained, repetitive debulking surgery can be helpful [46].

23.3.3 Vascular

23.3.3.1 Hemangiopericytoma

Derived from pericytes, hemangiopericytomas have a propensity for dissemination by hematogeneous routes [47]. Previously published studies found a rate of metastatic spread of 15–56% [48]. Only few of these rare malignant vascular tumors have been reported to involve the spine [47]. Plain radiographs show a soft tissue mass. When involving bone, they are predominantly lytic, and may mimic hemangiomas with a course honeycomb appearance. Angiography shows dense, well-circumscribed areas of enhancement with early draining veins and shunting. Hemangiopericytoma are described as having a pedicle formed by the arteries supplying the tumor from which vessels branch to encircle the tumor. CT depicts a density similar to muscle but with bright contrast enhancement. CTA may demonstrate large feeding vessels. MRI reveals a brightly enhancing soft tissue mass, often hyperintense on T2WI, with prominent flow voids [48]. Treatment of choice is a wide surgical resection whenever feasible [48], the 10-year survival rate is approximately 70%.

23.3.3.2 Angiosarcoma/Hemangioendothelioma

Closely related to hemangiopericytoma, angiosarcomas/hemangioendotheliomas are derived from vascular endothelium. Angiosarcoma of the spinal column is described to form lytic bony lesions with cortical destruction and extraosseous mass. Surgical resection (with or without embolization) is considered the treatment of choice [49, 50] with a 5-year survival of 25% for hemangioendothelioma, whereas patients suffering from angiosarcoma rarely survive 5 years. Radiation therapy has been advocated with the use of proton beam irradiation [51].

23.3.4 Tumors of Unknown Origin

23.3.4.1 Giant Cell Tumor (GCT)

Accounting for approximately 4% of all bone tumors, giant cell tumors are relatively uncommon [52]. They are most common in females in their second to fourth decades of life with a preference for the metaphysis of long bones [53]. However, they have been identified in the vertebral column evenly distributed in the cervical, thoracic, and lumbosacral spine. Patients present mostly with back pain that evolves over several months [54]. Radiographically, plain X-ray and CT include a narrow zone of transition, whereas a broader zone of transition is seen in more aggressive GCTs. Most of the tumors show no surrounding sclerosis (80–85%) with the overlying cortex thinned, expanded, or deficient. A periosteal reaction is seen in only 10–30% of cases with a possibility of detecting pathological fractures. MRI shows typical signal characteristics including a low to intermediate solid component and low signal periphery on T1. Solid components enhance, and help to distinguish GCT from aneurysmal bone cysts. On T2 sequences, there is a heterogeneous high signal with areas of low signal intensity due to haemosiderin or fibrosis. Their locally aggressive behavior favors early surgical resection [12, 55], offering the patients the lowest rate of recurrence. Unfortunately, many GCTs are too advanced at the time of presentation. Subtotal resections show a recurrence rate of up to 40% [55]. Recently, neoadjuvant therapy and medical management with denosumab, a receptor activator of nuclear factor κB ligand (RANKL) inhibitor, has been advocated with promising results.

23.3.4.2 Ewing's Sarcoma

Ewing's sarcoma occurs throughout the skeleton and rarely (in 3.5–15% of all cases) in the non-sacral spine [56]. These tumors typically evolve in children and adolescents between 10 and 20 years of age (95% between 4 and 25 years of age)

[57] and have a slight male predilection (M:F 1.5:1). Spinal Ewing's sarcoma often represents a metastatic lesion. They usually have an aggressive appearance on imaging [3], but are characterized by variable imaging features, including Codman triangles, spiculated (sunburst) or thick periosteal reaction and even bone expansion or cystic components. Soft tissue calcification is uncommon, seen in less than 10% of cases. MRI demonstrates a low to intermediate signal on T1, a heterogeneous but prominent enhancement on T1 with contrast and a heterogeneously high signal on T2. Treatment consists of closed needle biopsy to obtain the diagnosis of Ewing's sarcoma, followed by neoadjuvant chemotherapy and later radical (en bloc) surgical resection. Prognosis in spinal Ewing's sarcoma is still limited [58].

23.3.5 Miscellaneous

23.3.5.1 Chordoma

Chordoma is considered a histologically benign neoplasm, that is associated with a high recurrence rate and the potential for distant metastases due to local invasiveness. They are uncommon malignant tumors that account for 1% of intracranial tumors and 4% of all primary bone tumors [44]. They originate from embryonic remnants of the primitive notochord (earliest fetal axial skeleton, extending from the Rathke's pouch to the coccyx). Since chordomas arise in bone, they are usually extradural and result in local bone destruction. They are locally aggressive but uncommonly metastasize. Chordomas occur at any age but are usually seen in adults (30–70 years). Those located in the spheno-occipital region most commonly occur in patients 20–40 years of age, whereas sacrococcygeal chordomas are typically seen in a slightly older age group (peak around 50 years). They are slow growing tumors and present due to mass effect on adjacent structures (brainstem, cranial nerves, nasopharynx, spinal cord), or as a mass (e.g., sacrococcygeal chordoma). Metastatic spread of chordomas is observed in 7–14% of patients and includes nodal, pulmonary, bone, cerebral, or abdominal visceral involvement, predominantly from massive tumors. True malignant forms of chordomas occasionally have areas of typical chordoma and undifferentiated areas, most often suggestive of fibrosarcoma. Overall, the prognosis is poor.

The clival region accounts for 30–35% of cases. Typically, the mass projects in the midline posteriorly indenting the pons. This characteristic appearance has been termed the "thumb sign."

Chordomas of vertebral bodies are rare, but nonetheless the most common primary malignancy of the spine in adults [59]. They most commonly involve the cervical spine (particularly C2), followed by the lumbar spine. They often extend across the intervertebral disc space, involving more than one vertebral segment. They may extend into the epidural space, compressing the spinal cord, or along the nerve roots, enlarging the neural foramen.

MRI and CT scan have complementary roles in tumor evaluation. CT evaluation is needed to assess the degree of bone involvement or destruction and to detect patterns of calcifications within the lesion. MRI provides excellent three-dimensional analysis of the posterior fossa (especially the brainstem) [39], sella turcica, cavernous sinuses, and middle cranial fossa. MRI depicts calcifications and the precise involvement of skull base osteolysis and the cranial nerve foramina less well than CT [3].

Traditionally, surgical resection has been the first-line of treatment in feasible scenarios [60], with radiotherapy offered for recurrent cases. Ideally, en bloc resection is aimed for, but cannot be achieved in a significant portion of cases due to epidural and circumferential extension. Some advocate the combination of radiation therapy and complete or subtotal surgical resection for selected patients [3, 61]. Recurrence, including seeding along the operative tract, is common [62]. Prognosis is typically poor, due to the locally aggressive nature of these tumors with a 10-year survival of approximately 40% [63].

23.4 Secondary Tumors

Metastatic lesions to the craniovertebral junction indicate a grave progression of systemic cancer. However, the management of spinal metastasis continues to be controversial especially regarding the merits of recent advances in surgical technique and radiation oncology. All solid cancers are feasible to metastasize to the spinal column.

Imaging depends on the initial diagnosis. CT mostly discovers lytic lesions with bony destruction including the cortical surface. MRI usually shows contrast enhancement, in cases of metastatic melanoma, susceptibility weighted imaging can be used to depict the melanin rim.

Treatment consists of resection or decompression [64] (with and without stabilization) [65]. In cases without neural compression, radiation therapy can be a treatment option. Postoperative radiation is recommended. While metastatic lesions in the clivus and occiput are rare, C1 and particularly C2 are often involved in metastasis. With the region being highly mobile and representing a junctional area stability is often compromised.

23.5 Intradural Tumors

23.5.1 Neuroepithelial Tumors

Astrocytomas and ependymomas can occur in the upper cervical spinal cord. Generally, around 50% of astrocytomas are found in the cervical spinal cord [66].

As astrocytomas arise from cord parenchyma they typically have an eccentric location within the spinal cord and usually have poorly defined margins. Peritumoral edema is present in ~40%. Intratumoral cysts can be seen in ~20% and peritumoral cysts are present in ~15%. Reported signal characteristics include T1: isointense to hypointense, T2: hyperintense and T1 with contrast (Gd) depicts that the vast majority enhance, usually in a patchy fashion. Unlike ependymomas, hemorrhage is uncommon [66].

Ependymomas account for 60% of all spinal intramedullary neoplasms [67], they are predominately found in the cervical spinal cord. CT may demonstrate a nonspecific canal widening and a lesion isodense to slightly hyper-attenuating compared with normal spinal cord. The MRI is the modality of choice for evaluating suspected spinal cord tumors. Features include widened spinal cord (as ependymomas arise from ependymal cells lining the central canal, they tend to occupy the central portion of the spinal cord and cause symmetric cord expansion). Although unencapsulated, they are well-circumscribed and tumoral cysts are present in 22% of the cases [67]. Non-tumoral cysts are present in 62%. Syringohydromyelia occurs in 9–50% of cases. In contrast to intracranial ependymomas, calcification is uncommon. These lesions require microsurgical technique via a dorsal (laminectomy/laminoplasty) approach and do not pose any specific requirements if they occur at the CVJ.

23.5.2 Schwannoma

Spinal schwannomas are arising from nerve roots [68]. They represent the most common intradural extramedullary spinal tumors, representing 30% of these lesions [69]. They are most frequently seen in the cervical and lumbar regions, far more frequently than in the thoracic spine. Particularly in cases of neurofibromatosis, but also in sporadic cases they can pose a specific challenge at the CVJ due to the region's complex anatomy.

On imaging, they are usually characterized as solid and well-defined lesions with low T1 and high T2 MRI signals, and showing contrast enhancement. The signal intensity can be heterogeneous due to associated hemorrhage and fatty degeneration [70].

Schwannomas are in most instances indistinguishable from neurofibromas. In general, schwannomas appear as round lesions, which are often associated with adjacent bone remodeling. At the CVJ, these tumors often protrude out of the neural foramen, forming a dumbbell shaped mass. Although neurofibromas and schwannomas can look identical, schwannomas are frequently associated with hemorrhage, intrinsic vascular changes (thrombosis, sinusoidal dilatation), cyst formation, and fatty degeneration. These findings are rare in neurofibromas. Typical signal characteristics include: T1: 75% are isointense, 25% are hypointense, whereas on T2: more than 95% are hyper intense, often with mixed signal. T1 C+: virtually 100% enhance [69].

23.5.3 Meningioma

Meningiomas of the craniocervial junction [71] originate from the lower part of the clivus and the upper edge of the axis, laterally from the jugular tubercle to the upper aspect of the C-2 lamina [72]. Approximately 70% of all tumors in the craniocervical junction are meningiomas of benign origin [73]. Complete resection is the primary goal of surgery and is usually accomplished via a posterior neurosurgical procedure. However, it might be difficult to achieve total resection due to their close relationship to critical vascular structures, the brainstem and cranial nerves [73]. A higher risk of recurrence can be expected because a Simpson grade 1 resection is rarely achieved. The vast majority of spinal meningiomas are extramedullary in location [74].

Interestingly spinal meningiomas are also not distributed evenly along the canal: cervical spine—15%, thoracic spine—80%, lumbosacral spine—uncommon. Meningiomas are often located posterolaterally in the thoracic region and anteriorly in the cervical region. Most meningiomas are solitary lesions (98%), whereas multiple meningiomas are most often associated with NF2. CT depicts an isodense or moderately hyperdense mass. Some hyperostosis may be seen but is not as common as in intracranial meningiomas and calcification may be present [74]. On MRI, they are usually well-circumscribed and attached to the dura on a broad-base, known as a dural tail sign [74]. They share similar signal characteristics to typical intracranial meningiomas. On T1, they are isointense to slightly hypointense or may have a heterogeneous texture. On T2, they appear isointense to slightly hyperintense and T1 C+ (Gd) demonstrates moderate homogeneous enhancement. Occasionally, densely calcified meningiomas are hypointense on T1 and T2, and show only minimal contrast enhancement [74]. The ginkgo leaf sign of spinal meningiomas has been described as a useful MRI sign in distinguishing a spinal meningioma from schwannoma [75]. It is seen on axial post contrast T1 imaging, with the leaf representing the distorted spinal cord, pushed to one side of the theca by the meningioma, and the stem, seen as a non-enhancing "streak," representing the stretched dentate ligament [75] (Table 23.1).

Table 23.1 Classification of CVJ tumors

	Incidence	Imaging	Treatment	Prognosis
Extradural				
Primary benign				
Osteogenic				
Osteoid osteoma	11% of primary benign bony lesions, 25% of osteiod osteomas are located in the spine	CT: Hyperdense, sclerotic rim, surrounding a radiolucent nidus (<1.5 cm); SPECT bone scan: high tracer uptake	Excision of the nidus	Recurrence rate: 5%
Osteoblastoma	3% of all primary bone tumors, 40% of osteoblastoma are located in the spinal column	Identical to osteoid osteoma, nidus >1.5 cm	Excision of the nidus (en bloc)	Recurrence rate 10%
Cartilageneous				
Osteochondroma	Spine involved in 6% of total cases; 50% of cases occur in the cervical spine	CT: Cartilaginously capped tumor, SPECT bone scan: increased uptake	Resection in symptomatic patients	n/a
Enchondroma	Extremely rare, only around ten reported spinal cases		Resection rarely necessary	High rate of malignant transformation in patients with associated Maffucci's syndrome

(continued)

Table 23.1 (continued)

	Incidence	Imaging	Treatment	Prognosis
Vascular				
Hemangioma	Frequently	T1 and T2: hyperintense signal, fat like; vanishing on fat saturated imaging	Decompression and/or resection; consider preoperative embolisation	<5% recurrence after successful surgical resection
Aneurysmal bone cyst	20–30% of aneurysmal bone cyst cases involve the vertebral column	Fluid-fluid levels on MR imaging and thin peripheral/septal enhancement	Curettage, grafting, internal fixation, en bloc resection	
Fibrous tissue	rare	Well-circumscript border on radiographs	Watch and wait after biopsy, decompression or resection if symptomatic	n/a
Fat cell				
Lipoma	1% of all spine tumors	Show no characteristic radiological appearance	Should be resected if necessary	n/a
Angiolipoma	Rare	Both fat cell tumors show the intensity of fat upon MRI and CT		
Miscellaneous				
Eosinopholic granuloma	Less than 4% of primary spinal tumors	T1: typically low signal, T2: isointense to hyperintense, STIR: hyperintense, T1 C+ (Gd): often shows contrast enhancement	Conservative	n/a
Solitary plasmocytoma	Only few cases in spine	Lytic lesion, easily identified on CT	Radiotherapy	n/a
Malignant				
Osteogenic				
Osteosarcoma	5% of cases	Imaging consist of CT and MRI, showing the destructive lesion and commonly presenting with epidural growth	Wide resection, chemotherapy	

Cartilageneous				
Chondrosacroma	Less than 7% of spinal tumors	CT demonstrates a lytic lesion with calcified soft tissue mass. In highly vascularized lesions, preoperative angiography should be considered	Wide resection, chemotherapy	
Vascular				
Hemangiopericytoma		CT shows a density similar to muscle but with bright contrast enhancement. CTA may demonstrate large feeding vessels. MRI depicts a brightly enhancing soft tissue mass, often hyperintense on T2WI, with prominent flow voids	Surgical resection	10 years survival is approx. 70%
Angiosarcoma	Rare	Similar to Hemangiopericytoma: lytic bony lesions with cortical destruction and extraosseous mass		
Tumors of unknown origin				
Giant cell tumor	Approx. 4% of all bone tumors	MRI: low to intermediate solid component and low signal periphery on T1. Solid components enhance, and help to distinguish GCT with an aneurysmal bone cyst. On T2 sequences, the heterogeneous high signal with areas of low signal intensity due to haemosiderin or fibrosis	Wide resection	Subtotal resection shows recurrence in up to 40%
Ewing’s sarcoma	3–15% of cases	MRI shows a low to intermediate signal on T1, a heterogeneous but prominent enhancement on T1 with contrast and a heterogeneously high signal on T2	Neoadjuvant chemotherapy, followed by resection (en bloc, when feasible)	Poor

(continued)

Table 23.1 (continued)

		Incidence	Imaging	Treatment	Prognosis
Miscellaneous					
Chordoma		1% intracranial, 4% of all primary bone tumors	CT: assessment of bone involvement or destruction and to detect patterns of calcifications. MRI: precise involvement of skull base	Surgery and radiotherapy	10 years survival is approx. 40%
Secondary	*Metastasis*				
Intradural					
Neuroepithelial	Astrocytoma and ependymoma	Rare, 50% of Astrocytomas are in the cervical spine	T1: isointense to hypointense, T2: hyperintense and T1 with contrast (Gd) depicts that the vast majority enhance, usually with patchy enhancement	Resection or biopsy, radiotherapy if malignant or subtotally resected	
Schwannoma		30% of intradural, extramedullary spinal tumors	Low T1 and high T2 MRI signals, and showing contrast enhancement	Resection	n/a
Meningioma		70% of craniocervical junction tumors are meningiomas	Usually well-circumscribed and attached to the dura on a broad-base, known as a dural tail sign	Resection	

References

1. Stark RJ, Henson RA, Evans SJ. Spinal metastases. A retrospective survey from a general hospital. Brain. 1982;105:189–213.
2. Thakur NA, Daniels AH, Schiller J, Valdes MA, Czerwein JK, Schiller A, et al. Benign tumors of the spine. J Am Acad Orthop Surg. 2012;20:715–24.
3. Canete AN, Bloem HL, Kroon HM. Primary bone tumors of the spine. Radiologia. 2016;58(Suppl 1):68–80.
4. Orguc S, Arkun R. Primary tumors of the spine. Semin Musculoskelet Radiol. 2014;18:280–99.
5. Capanna R, Boriani S, Mabit C, Donati D, Savini R. [Osteoid osteoma of the spine. The experience of the rizzoli institute]. Rev Chir Orthop Reparatrice Appar Mot. 1991;77:545–50.
6. Ahmad T, Hussain MF, Hameed AA, Manzar N, Lakdawala RH. Conservative surgery for osteoid osteoma of the lumbar vertebrae. Surg Neurol Int. 2014;5:24.
7. Kadhim M, Binitie O, O'Toole P, Grigoriou E, De Mattos CB, Dormans JP. Surgical resection of osteoid osteoma and osteoblastoma of the spine. J Pediatr Orthop B. 2017;26:362–9.
8. Morley N, Omar I. Imaging evaluation of musculoskeletal tumors. Cancer Treat Res. 2014;162:9–29.
9. Redmond J 3rd, Friedl KE, Cornett P, Stone M, O'Rourke T, George CB. Clinical usefulness of an algorithm for the early diagnosis of spinal metastatic disease. J Clin Oncol. 1988;6:154–7.
10. Galgano MA, Goulart CR, Iwenofu H, Chin LS, Lavelle W, Mendel E. Osteoblastomas of the spine: a comprehensive review. Neurosurg Focus. 2016;41:E4.
11. Czigleczki G, Nagy Z, Papp Z, Padanyi C, Banczerowski P. Management strategy of osteoblastomas localized in the occipitocervical junction. World Neurosurg. 2017;97:505–12.
12. Kaloostian PE, Gokaslan ZL. Surgical management of primary tumors of the cervical spine: surgical considerations and avoidance of complications. Neurol Res. 2014;36:557–65.
13. Versteeg AL, Dea N, Boriani S, Varga PP, Luzzati A, Fehlings MG, et al. Surgical management of spinal osteoblastomas. J Neurosurg Spine. 2017;27:321–7.
14. Jiang L, Liu XG, Wang C, Yang SM, Liu C, Wei F, et al. Surgical treatment options for aggressive osteoblastoma in the mobile spine. Eur Spine J. 2015;24:1778–85.
15. Patnaik S, Jyotsnarani Y, Uppin SG, Susarla R. Imaging features of primary tumors of the spine: a pictorial essay. Indian J Radiol Imaging. 2016;26:279–89.
16. Glasser D, Cammisa F, Lane J. Benign cartilage tumors of the spine. In: Sundaresan N, editor. Tumors of the spine: diagnosis and clinical management. Philadelphia: WB Saunders; 1990. p. 146–8.
17. Albrecht S, Crutchfield JS, SeGall GK. On spinal osteochondromas. J Neurosurg. 1992;77:247–52.
18. Fukushi R, Emori M, Iesato N, Kano M, Yamashita T. Osteochondroma causing cervical spinal cord compression. Skelet Radiol. 2017;46:1125–30.
19. Hansberry DR, Gupta R, Prabhu AV, Agarwal N, Cox M, Joneja U, et al. Thoracic spinal osteochondroma: a rare presentation of spinal cord compression. Clin Imaging. 2017;45:18–21.
20. Ropper AE, Cahill KS, Hanna JW, McCarthy EF, Gokaslan ZL, Chi JH. Primary vertebral tumors: a review of epidemiologic, histological, and imaging findings, part I: benign tumors. Neurosurgery. 2011;69:1171–80.
21. Guo J, Gao JZ, Guo LJ, Yin ZX, He EX. Large enchondroma of the thoracic spine: a rare case report and review of the literature. BMC Musculoskelet Disord. 2017;18:155.
22. McCarthy CM, Blecher H, Reich S. A case of myelopathy because of enchondromas from Maffucci syndrome with successful surgical treatment. Spine J. 2015;15:e15–9.
23. Bouali S, Maatar N, Bouhoula A, Abderrahmen K, Kallel J, Jemel H. Intradural extramedullary capillary hemangioma in the upper cervical spine: first report. World Neurosurg. 2016;92:587.e581–7.
24. Nakahara M, Nishida K, Kumamoto S, Hijikata Y, Harada K. A case report of spondylectomy with circumference reconstruction for aggressive vertebral hemangioma covering the whole cervical spine (c4) with progressive spinal disorder. Eur Spine J. 2017;26:69–74.

25. Gaudino S, Martucci M, Colantonio R, Lozupone E, Visconti E, Leone A, et al. A systematic approach to vertebral hemangioma. Skelet Radiol. 2015;44:25–36.
26. Vergel De Dios AM, Bond JR, Shives TC, McLeod RA, Unni KK. Aneurysmal bone cyst. A clinicopathologic study of 238 cases. Cancer. 1992;69:2921–31.
27. Pavanello M, Melloni I, Fiaschi P, Consales A, Piatelli G, Ravegnani M, et al. A rare case of osteoblastoma associated to aneurysmal bone cyst of the spine. Case report. Br J Neurosurg. 2016;30:106–9.
28. Rajasekaran S, Aiyer SN, Shetty AP, Kanna R, Maheswaran A. Aneurysmal bone cyst of c2 treated with novel anterior reconstruction and stabilization. Eur Spine J. 2019;28(2):270–8.
29. Cavusoglu M, Ciliz DS, Duran S, Elverici E. Intramedullary lipoma of the cervico-thoracic spinal cord. JBR-BTR. 2014;97:346–8.
30. Petit D, Menei P, Fournier HD. An unusual and spectacular case of spindle cell lipoma of the posterior neck invading the spinal cervical canal and posterior cranial fossa. J Neurosurg Spine. 2011;15:502–6.
31. Tomasian A, Wallace AN, Jennings JW. Benign spine lesions: advances in techniques for minimally invasive percutaneous treatment. AJNR Am J Neuroradiol. 2017;38:852–61.
32. Song Y, Geng W, Guo T, Gao Y, Zhang Y, Li S, et al. The outcome of eosinophilic granuloma involving unilateral atlantoaxial joint: a case report and literature review. Medicine (Baltimore). 2017;96:e7197.
33. Stephens BH, Wright NM. Reconstruction of the c-1 lateral mass with a titanium expandable cage after resection of eosinophilic granuloma in an adult patient. J Neurosurg Spine. 2017;26:252–6.
34. Hu S, Hu CH, Hu XY, Wang XM, Dai H, Fang XM, et al. MRI features of spinal epidural angiolipomas. Korean J Radiol. 2013;14:810–7.
35. Turgut M. Four cases of spinal epidural angiolipoma. J Clin Neurosci. 2018;48:243–4.
36. Wang B, Yang Z, Yang J, Wang G, Xu Y, Liu P. Spinal angiolipoma: experience of twelve patients and literature. Neurol India. 2014;62:367–70.
37. Miranda AD, Rivero-Garvia M, Mayorga-Buiza MJ, Pancucci G, Valencia-Anguita J, Marquez-Rivas J. Plasmocytoma of c1 in a child. Case report. Childs Nerv Syst. 2015;31:325–8.
38. Hans FJ, Geibprassert S, Krings T, Weis J, Deckert M, Ludolph A, et al. Solitary plasmacytoma presenting as an intramedullary mass of the cervical cord. J Neurol Surg A Cent Eur Neurosurg. 2013;74(Suppl 1):e13–7.
39. D'Andrea K, Dreyer J, Fahim DK. Utility of preoperative magnetic resonance imaging coregistered with intraoperative computed tomographic scan for the resection of complex tumors of the spine. World Neurosurg. 2015;84:1804–15.
40. Clarke MJ, Price DL, Cloft HJ, Segura LG, Hill CA, Browning MB, et al. En bloc resection of a c-1 lateral mass osteosarcoma: technical note. J Neurosurg Pediatr. 2016;18:46–52.
41. Matsumoto Y, Takahashi Y, Harimaya K, Nakagawa T, Kawaguchi K, Okada S, et al. Dedifferentiated chondrosarcoma of the cervical spine: a case report. World J Surg Oncol. 2013;11:32.
42. Yang X, Wu Z, Xiao J, Feng D, Huang Q, Zheng W, et al. Chondrosarcomas of the cervical and cervicothoracic spine: surgical management and long-term clinical outcome. J Spinal Disord Tech. 2012;25:1–9.
43. Van Gompel JJ, Janus JR. Chordoma and chondrosarcoma. Otolaryngol Clin North Am. 2015;48:501–14.
44. Almefty K, Pravdenkova S, Colli BO, Al-Mefty O, Gokden M. Chordoma and chondrosarcoma: similar, but quite different, skull base tumors. Cancer. 2007;110:2457–67.
45. Stieb S, Snider JW 3rd, Placidi L, Kliebsch U, Lomax AJ, Schneider RA, et al. Long-term clinical safety of high-dose proton radiation therapy delivered with pencil beam scanning technique for extracranial chordomas and chondrosarcomas in adult patients: clinical evidence of spinal cord tolerance. Int J Radiat Oncol Biol Phys. 2018;100(1):218–25.
46. Chen B, Yang Y, Chen L, Zhou F, Yang H. Unilateral lateral mass fixation of cervical spinal low-grade chondrosarcoma with intralesional resection: a case report. Oncol Lett. 2014;7:1515–8.
47. Cole CD, Schmidt MH. Hemangiopericytomas of the spine: case report and review of the literature. Rare Tumors. 2009;1:e43.

48. Ramdasi RV, Nadkarni TD, Goel NA. Hemangiopericytoma of the cervical spine. J Craniovertebr Junction Spine. 2014;5:95–8.
49. Mattei TA, Teles AR, Mendel E. Modern surgical techniques for management of soft tissue sarcomas involving the spine: outcomes and complications. J Surg Oncol. 2015;111:580–6.
50. Nacar OA, Ulu MO, Pekmezci M, Deviren V, Ames C. Successful treatment of a very rare angiosarcoma involving the lumbar spine via en-bloc resection and radiotherapy: case report. Turk Neurosurg. 2014;24:140–5.
51. Trifiletti D, Amdur RJ, Dagan R, Indelicato DJ, Mendenhall WM, Kirwan JM, et al. Radiotherapy following gross total resection of adult soft tissue sarcoma of the head and neck. Pract Radiat Oncol. 2012;2:e121–8.
52. Dang L, Liu X, Dang G, Jiang L, Wei F, Yu M, et al. Primary tumors of the spine: a review of clinical features in 438 patients. J Neurooncol. 2015;121:513–20.
53. Zhou Z, Wang X, Wu Z, Huang W, Xiao J. Epidemiological characteristics of primary spinal osseous tumors in eastern China. World J Surg Oncol. 2017;15:73.
54. Maldonado-Romero LV, Sifuentes-Giraldo WA, Martinez-Rodrigo MA, de la Puente-Bujidos C. Giant cell tumor of the spine: a rare cause of cervical pain. Reumatol Clin. 2017;13:58–9.
55. Patil S, Shah KC, Bhojraj SY, Nene AM. Recurrent spinal giant cell tumors: a study of risk factors and recurrence patterns. Asian Spine J. 2016;10:129–35.
56. Ilaslan H, Sundaram M, Unni KK, Dekutoski MB. Primary Ewing's sarcoma of the vertebral column. Skelet Radiol. 2004;33:506–13.
57. Ozturk E, Mutlu H, Sonmez G, Vardar Aker F, Cinar Basekim C, Kizilkaya E. Spinal epidural extraskeletal Ewing sarcoma. J Neuroradiol. 2007;34:63–7.
58. Bostelmann R, Leimert M, Steiger HJ, Gierga K, Petridis AK. The importance of surgery as part of multimodal therapy in rapid progressive primary extraosseous Ewing sarcoma of the cervical intra- and epidural space. Clin Pract. 2016;6:897.
59. Awuor V, Stewart CE, Camma A, Renner J, Tongson JM. Rare case of an extraosseous cervical chordoma with both intradural and extensive extraspinal involvement. Surg Neurol Int. 2017;8:250.
60. Suchomel P, Barsa P. Single stage total endolesional c2 spondylectomy for chordoma. Eur Spine J. 2013;22:1453–6.
61. Pham M, Awad M. Outcomes following surgical management of cervical chordoma: a review of published case reports and case series. Asian J Neurosurg. 2017;12:389–97.
62. Tenny SO, Ehlers LD, Robbins JW, Gillis CC. Marginal en bloc resection of c2-c3 chordoma with bilateral vertebral artery preservation and mesh cage reconstruction with review of previously published cases. World Neurosurg. 2017;108:993.e1–7.
63. Aguiar Junior S, Andrade WP, Baiocchi G, Guimaraes GC, Cunha IW, Estrada DA, et al. Natural history and surgical treatment of chordoma: a retrospective cohort study. Sao Paulo Med J. 2014;132:297–302.
64. Park SJ, Lee CS, Chung SS. Surgical results of metastatic spinal cord compression (MSCC) from non-small cell lung cancer (NSCLC): analysis of functional outcome, survival time, and complication. Spine J. 2016;16:322–8.
65. Tang Y, Qu J, Wu J, Liu H, Chu T, Xiao J, et al. Effect of surgery on quality of life of patients with spinal metastasis from non-small-cell lung cancer. J Bone Joint Surg Am. 2016;98:396–402.
66. Koeller KK, Rosenblum RS, Morrison AL. Neoplasms of the spinal cord and filum terminale: radiologic-pathologic correlation. Radiographics. 2000;20:1721–49.
67. Smith AB, Soderlund KA, Rushing EJ, Smirniotopolous JG. Radiologic-pathologic correlation of pediatric and adolescent spinal neoplasms: part 1, intramedullary spinal neoplasms. AJR Am J Roentgenol. 2012;198:34–43.
68. Kratimenos GP, Crockard HA. The far lateral approach for ventrally placed foramen magnum and upper cervical spine tumours. Br J Neurosurg. 1993;7:129–40.
69. Cavalcanti DD, Martirosyan NL, Verma K, Safavi-Abbasi S, Porter RW, Theodore N, et al. Surgical management and outcome of schwannomas in the craniocervical region. J Neurosurg. 2011;114:1257–67.

70. Wang Z, Chen H, Huang Q, Zhang Z, Yang J, Wu H. Facial and lower cranial nerve function preservation in lateral approach for craniocervical schwannomas. Eur Arch Otorhinolaryngol. 2015;272:2207–12.
71. Arnautovic KI, Al-Mefty O, Husain M. Ventral foramen magnum meninigiomas. J Neurosurg. 2000;92:71–80.
72. Yasuoka S, Okazaki H, Daube JR, MacCarty CS. Foramen magnum tumors. Analysis of 57 cases of benign extramedullary tumors. J Neurosurg. 1978;49:828–38.
73. Duhrsen L, Emami P, Matschke J, Abboud T, Westphal M, Regelsberger J. Meninigiomas of the craniocervical junction—a distinctive subgroup of meningiomas. PLoS One. 2016;11:e0153405.
74. Hwang WL, Marciscano AE, Niemierko A, Kim DW, Stemmer-Rachamimov AO, Curry WT, et al. Imaging and extent of surgical resection predict risk of meningioma recurrence better than who histopathological grade. Neuro Oncol. 2016;18:863–72.
75. Yamaguchi S, Takeda M, Takahashi T, Yamahata H, Mitsuhara T, Niiro T, et al. Ginkgo leaf sign: a highly predictive imaging feature of spinal meningioma. J Neurosurg Spine. 2015;23(5):642–6.

Primary Osseous and Metastatic Neoplasms of the CVJ

24

Jared Fridley, Adetokunbo Oyelese, and Ziya Gokaslan

24.1 Introduction

Tumor surgery at the craniovertebral junction (CVJ) poses significant technical challenges owing to its complicated regional anatomy and unique biomechanics. Knowledge of the unique bony structure of the CVJ which includes the lower clivus, occipital condyles, atlas, and axis, as well as its surrounding neurovascular structures such as the brainstem, vertebral arteries, and lower cranial nerves, is vital prior to attempting tumor resection and spinal reconstruction in this region. In addition to considering involved anatomic structures, surgery must consider tumor pathology, as this may affect surgical strategy. Multiple types of tumors may be found at the CVJ including metastases, local extension of head and neck tumors, tumors arising from nervous system tissues, and primary osseous neoplasms. In this chapter, we will focus on the presentation, epidemiology, classification, and management of spinal metastases and primary osseous neoplasms.

24.2 Presentation

Pain is the most common presenting symptom in patients with tumors of the CVJ. It may be focal neck pain or mechanical in nature. Focal neck pain is often described as achiness or stiffness, and is often worse at night. Pain that is

J. Fridley · A. Oyelese · Z. Gokaslan (✉)
Department of Neurosurgery, The Warren Alpert Medical School of Brown University, Providence, RI, USA

Department of Neurosurgery, Rhode Island Hospital, Norman Prince Neurosciences Institute, Providence, RI, USA
e-mail: ziya_gokaslan@brown.edu, ziya.gokaslan@lifespan.org

E. Tessitore et al. (eds.), *Surgery of the Cranio-Vertebral Junction*,
https://doi.org/10.1007/978-3-030-18700-2_24

significantly relieved by aspirin is a classic characteristic of osteoid osteomas. Mechanical neck pain refers to aggravation of pain with flexion or extension of the cervical spine. In addition, rotational movement of the neck can also worsen the neck pain, which is often not seen in subaxial cervical spine tumors [1]. Occipital neuralgia due to C2 nerve root compression is often seen either due to direct tumor compression or degeneration of the atlantoaxial joint causing local inflammation or bony compression.

Symptoms and signs of myelopathy are uncommon with CVJ tumors due to the capacious spinal canal at this level. If present, either the tumor has reached a significant size, extended cranially through the foramen magnum, or eroded bony structures causing atlantoaxial subluxation and subsequent cord compression. Neurologic deficits tend to portend malignant disease and a worse overall prognosis [2]. Lower cranial nerve deficits can be seen due to either compression of the brain stem or tumor involvement of the lower cranial nerves. The spinal accessory nerve is the most common nerve root involved due to its long, looping course. This can manifest as weakness of the trapezius/sternocleidomastoid muscles, or torticollis.

24.3 Epidemiology and Classification

24.3.1 Metastases

Nearly 1.7 million people in the United States are estimated to have been diagnosed with cancer in 2016 [3]. Bone is the most common site of metastases in the body, with the spine being the most common bone structure affected. Nearly 40% of cancer patients at autopsy have pathologic evidence of spinal metastases [4]. It is estimated that 5–10% of patients with metastatic spine disease will become symptomatic and require treatment [5]. The mean age at presentation is approximately 60 years old. The thoracic spine is the most commonly affected spinal segment, followed by the lumbar spine and then cervical spine. Involvement of the CVJ accounts for only 0.5% of spinal metastases [6]. Common primary sources of metastatic spinal disease are breast carcinoma (35%), non-small cell lung carcinoma (15%), and prostate carcinoma (10%) [6].

Multiple myeloma is a hematological malignancy that frequently metastasizes to the spine. Patients typically present with neck pain, either focal or mechanical. Cervical spine metastases are often the first presentation of this disease. Myeloma lesions are lytic, and imaging usually reveals pathologic fracture on CT. At the CVJ, dens fractures are the most common, and are usually unstable, requiring external orthoses prior to definitive therapy. Multiple myeloma is radiosensitive, and radiation has been shown to be an effective treatment for pain relief even in the presence of an unstable fracture [7]. Therefore, radiation is regarded as first-line therapy, with surgery only rarely needed. Posterior occipitocervical instrumentation is an option in those patients with significant instability of the CVJ or ongoing neck pain not responsive to radiation.

24.3.2 Primary Osseous Tumors

Unlike metastatic spinal disease, primary osseous spinal tumors are rare, representing only 4.6% of all spine tumors [2]. There are nearly 3300 cases of bone cancer each year, with only approximately 10% involving the spine [3]. Multiple myeloma is the most frequently encountered primary spine tumor followed by hemangioma, eosinophilic granuloma, aneurysmal bone cyst, osteoblastoma/osteoid osteoma, chondrosarcoma, giant cell tumor, chondroma, osteosarcoma, and chordoma [8]. Like metastatic disease, the thoracic spine is most often affected, followed by the lumbar spine, sacrum, and then the cervical spine. At the CVJ chordoma is the most common primary spine tumor, followed by osteoid osteoma/osteoblastoma, osteochondroma, multiple myeloma, aneurysmal bone cyst, giant cell tumor, and Ewing's sarcoma [9]. For further details refer to Chap. 23.

24.4 Diagnostic Workup

24.4.1 Imaging

Patients in whom there is a suspicion of a CVJ neoplasm should be thoroughly imaged. Both magnetic resonance imaging (MRI) and computed tomography (CT) are helpful in tumor evaluation. MRI of the brain and spine with and without contrast in axial, sagittal, and coronal planes is helpful for defining the relationship of tumor to neural elements and adjacent soft tissue structures. CT is used to evaluate the extent of osseous disease, and whether the tumor is osteolytic or osteoblastic. Imaging of the chest, abdomen, and pelvis using CT with and without contrast is mandatory to evaluate for evidence of metastatic disease. Fluorine-18 fluorodeoxyglucose positron emission tomography (FDG-PET) and technetium-99m methylene diphosphonate (MDP) bone scintigraphy can be useful for identifying osseous metastasis originating from malignant primary spinal tumors [10].

The differential diagnosis of a primary osseous CVJ neoplasm can be narrowed based on imaging findings [11]. In the case of bone forming neoplasms such as osteoid osteoma or osteoblastoma, a nidus of immature bone surrounded by sclerotic bone, usually in the posterior elements, is characteristically seen on CT. These lesions tend to enhance on contrast enhanced MRI, and T2 sequences often reveal edema within the lamina and pedicle extending toward the vertebral body. Osteosarcoma has similar characteristics although the disease is often more extensive. Osteochondromas are common benign lesions of the CVJ, particularly at C2, and have characteristic cortical and marrow continuity with the underlying vertebra [11]. Chondroblastomas and chondrosarcomas typically show extensive bony destruction, and often soft tissue extension. Hemangiomas have a stereotypical honeycomb appearance on CT, and both T1 and T2 hyperintensity. Chordomas at the CVJ are iso- to hypointense on MRI T1 imaging, hyperintense on T2, enhance with contrast administration, and show bony erosion on CT imaging (Fig. 24.1).

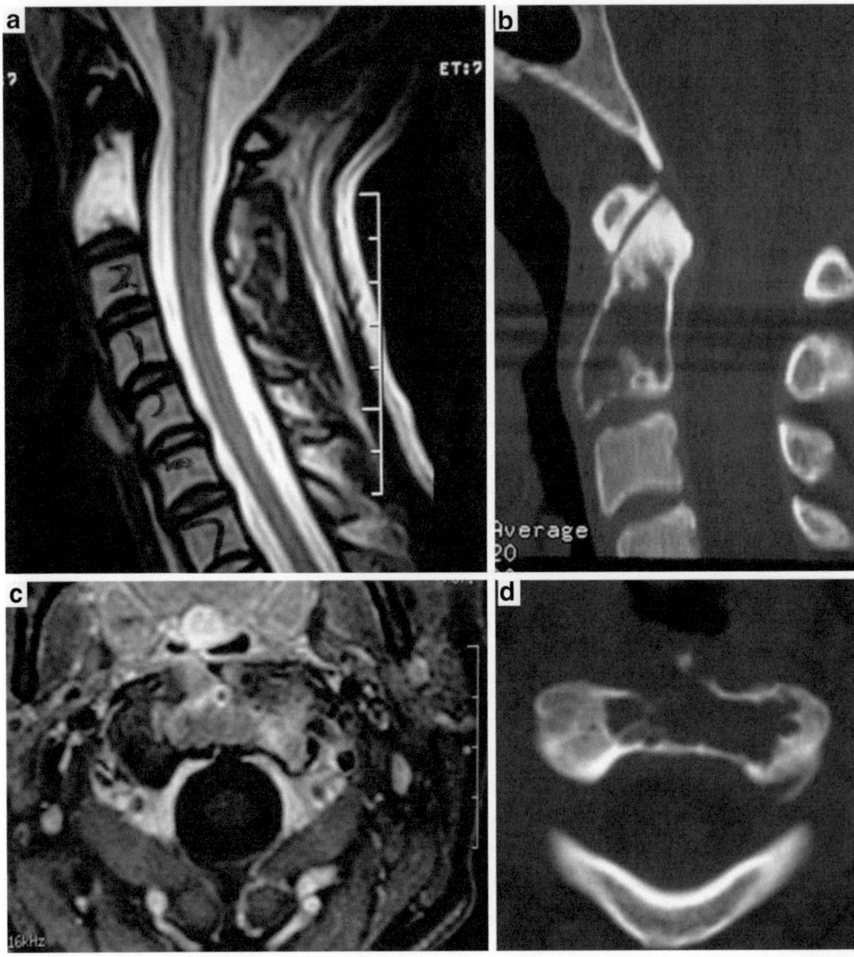

Fig. 24.1 Case illustration of a C2 chordoma on both MRI and CT imaging. (**a**) Preoperative T2-weighted MRI sagittal sequence showing a hyperintense mass within the body of C2 consistent with a chordoma. (**b**) CT sagittal reconstruction demonstrating bony erosion by the tumor. (**c**) T1-weighted with contrast axial image demonstrating an enhancing tumor within C2. (**d**) CT axial image showing a destructive tumor in the C2 body without posterior element involvement. (Reproduced with permission from the senior author Z.G.)

Due to the complex anatomy of the CVJ obtaining tumor tissue via posterior percutaneous biopsy is generally not recommended. Open incisional or excisional biopsy is generally the preferred strategy for diagnosis. In the case of a small solitary mass in the posterior elements of C1 or C2, such as with a suspected osteoid osteoma, open excisional biopsy may be the most reasonable option. An anterior transoral biopsy is contraindicated due to the risk of tumor seeding along the biopsy tract.

Vascular imaging with either CT angiography or conventional angiography is recommended to evaluate the course of the vertebral arteries and their involvement with tumor. Determining the patency and dominance of the vertebral artery is useful in surgical planning as often one of these vessels must be sacrificed. Angiographic assessment of collateral blood flow and filling of the posterior inferior cerebellar arteries is helpful to determine the risk of infarction prior to vertebral artery embolization. A balloon occlusion test of the involved vertebral artery is recommended in the case of dominant vertebral artery involvement. Tumor blush on angiography indicates hypervascularity, in which case preoperative particle or glue embolization can be useful to minimize both blood loss and operative time.

24.4.2 Laboratory Studies

In addition to imaging, laboratory studies can add information that will assist in the diagnoses of a CVJ tumor, particularly with metastatic lesions. For example, elevations in serum prostate specific antigen (PSA) or carcinoembryonic antigen (CEA) can point toward a prostate or gastrointestinal primary tumor respectively. In the case of multiple myeloma, abnormalities in hematocrit or platelet count may be seen. Additionally, serum protein electrophoresis (SPEP) or urine protein electrophoresis (UPEP) may be useful to look for a monoclonal gammopathy pointing toward multiple myeloma.

24.5 Treatment Strategy

The treatment of a CVJ neoplasm can vary significantly based on patient history/physical, suspected tumor pathology, tumor location, involvement of adjacent structures, and presence of spinal instability. The first decision-making branch point is whether the data from diagnostic workup indicates a metastasis or a primary spinal tumor. If metastatic disease is suspected, then the question becomes whether surgery or radiation should be the primary treatment. The goal with treatment of spinal metastases remains palliative and is focused on improving patient quality of life. This is unlike treatment for many primary osseous spinal tumors in which patients may live for a long time depending on the pathology. We now discuss radiation and surgery options for both metastatic and primary tumors.

24.5.1 Radiation

In patients with suspected metastatic disease that don't have evidence of either neural element compression or spinal instability, radiation is a viable first-line treatment option. External beam radiotherapy, typically 300 cGy over 10 fractions, can be an effective means of pain relief in patients with CVJ metastases. In a study of 33 patients with CVJ metastases by Bilsky et al., 23 patients without evidence of radiographic instability (defined as less than 5 mm of atlantoaxial subluxation and less than 11° of odontoid angulation) underwent initial treatment with external beam radiotherapy [12]. Over 90% of these patients had significant relief or resolution of their neck pain. Only two of the 23 patients underwent eventual surgical stabilization.

The recent advent of spinal radiosurgery (SRS) has recently been demonstrated to be efficacious in treatment of CVJ metastases, both in terms of neck pain relief and local control [13, 14]. In a small series by Azad et al., 25 patients underwent SRS for various histologies, most commonly breast and lung cancers [13]. No patient had a SINS score > 12. At a median 18-month follow-up, there was resolution or improvement in neck pain in 8 of 17 patients with preoperative pain. Sixteen out of 19 patients at last follow-up either had no change or a decrease in size of the radiated tumor. Only 2 out of 25 patients ultimately required surgery for stabilization. Given the small size of this series and inherent limitations in study design more research on SRS for CVJ metastases is needed.

In the case of primary osseous spinal tumors, the role of radiotherapy is histology specific, and its use is limited to benign aggressive and malignant primary tumors. Not only are most of these tumors radioresistant, radiation doses at the CVJ are limited due to risk of radiation toxicity to the spinal cord, brain stem, and nerve roots. This presents a problem in the treatment of these tumors as the doses required to treat them are usually rather high. For chordoma, radiation therapy has been shown to have a 5-year local control rate of only 10–40% at doses of 40–60 Gy [10]. Alternative types of radiation, such as proton-based therapy have recently been shown to be a promising treatment option for use after surgery [10]. Similar to chordoma, traditional EBRT for treatment of osteosarcoma [15] and chondrosarcoma has had poor results, but there has been ongoing research with the use of high dose proton beam or combination therapy [16]. Ewing's sarcoma is unique in that adjuvant conventional radiation has been shown to be effective following surgery or in combination with chemotherapy in cases of non-surgical candidates [17].

24.5.2 Surgery

As mentioned previously the surgical management of CVJ neoplasms is based to a large degree on underlying pathology. The goal of surgery for spinal metastases is palliative, with patient's typically succumbing to their systemic disease rather than their spinal pathology. This is contrasted with primary spinal tumor pathology in which there is usually no systemic disease, and patients can have a significantly lengthened survival with aggressive treatment [17].

24.5.2.1 Metastases

Metastatic epidural compression of the spinal cord or brain stem is uncommon at the CVJ due to size of the spinal canal at this level. In many cases, epidural disease without cord compression can be treated with radiation. However, if a patient presents with signs of myelopathy due to epidural tumor compression, surgical decompression is indicated. Dorsal decompression of the spinal cord at the CVJ involves a simple laminectomy of C1 and/or C2, followed by direct tumor resection. As with most metastatic spinal tumors, the challenge arises with ventral cord compression. While both anterior and posterior approaches to the ventral thecal sac at the CVJ are feasible, one must consider the high morbidity of approaching anteriorly such as with a transoral or high retropharyngeal procedure [18]. It must always be kept in mind that with the availability of radiosurgery and EBRT, postoperative radiation may be used to treat residual tumor, a strategy referred to as "separation surgery" [19]. In other words, if possible, a posterior or posterolateral approach to the CVJ for decompression of neural elements due to metastatic epidural disease is the preferred option. At C1 and C2, laminectomies are performed, followed by identification the C1-2 facet joints and C2 nerve roots. Sacrifice of one or both C2 nerve roots is well tolerated as it is a purse sensory root, with only rare cases of postoperative occipital neuralgia. In many cases, epidural tumor results in thecal sac displacement which creates a corridor by which tumor can be easily approached. The primary concern with a posterior approach is with vertebral artery injury. Study of the vertebral artery course on preoperative imaging is essential to minimize risk of injury. At C2 the vertebral artery courses laterally, while at C2 it turns medially and over the C1 lamina. If the vertebral artery is encased by tumor, residual disease can be reasonably be left behind with the intention to radiate this area postoperatively.

In patients with clinical or radiographic evidence of atlantoaxial instability related to either metastatic disease or from iatrogenic insult, posterior surgical stabilization is recommended. Clinical evidence of CVJ instability, while not clearly defined, may be defined as an inability of the CVJ to function under physiologic loads without pain, neurologic deficit, or spinal deformity [20]. Radiographic evidence of atlantoaxial subluxation, angulation of the dens, rotary subluxation, or destruction of the occipitoatlantal/atlantoaxial facet complexes are, in our view, indications for stabilization. In patients with mechanical neck pain but no gross radiographic evidence of instability, we generally recommend posterior instrumented stabilization. Occipitocervical instrumented fusion is preferred over atlantoaxial stabilization, even in the case of isolated C1 or C2 metastases, primarily because of the unpredictable course of metastatic disease, and the concern that involvement of adjacent areas may lead to possible construct failure and need for additional surgery (Fig. 24.2). In the series by Fourney et al., [21] occipitocervical stabilization in 19 patients with CVJ metastases resulted in a significant improvement in neck pain with minimal surgical morbidity. We perform posterolateral arthrodesis in all patients to help mitigate potential future hardware failures, though given the limited life expectancy in many metastatic disease patients it is unclear whether a more tailored approach may be beneficial.

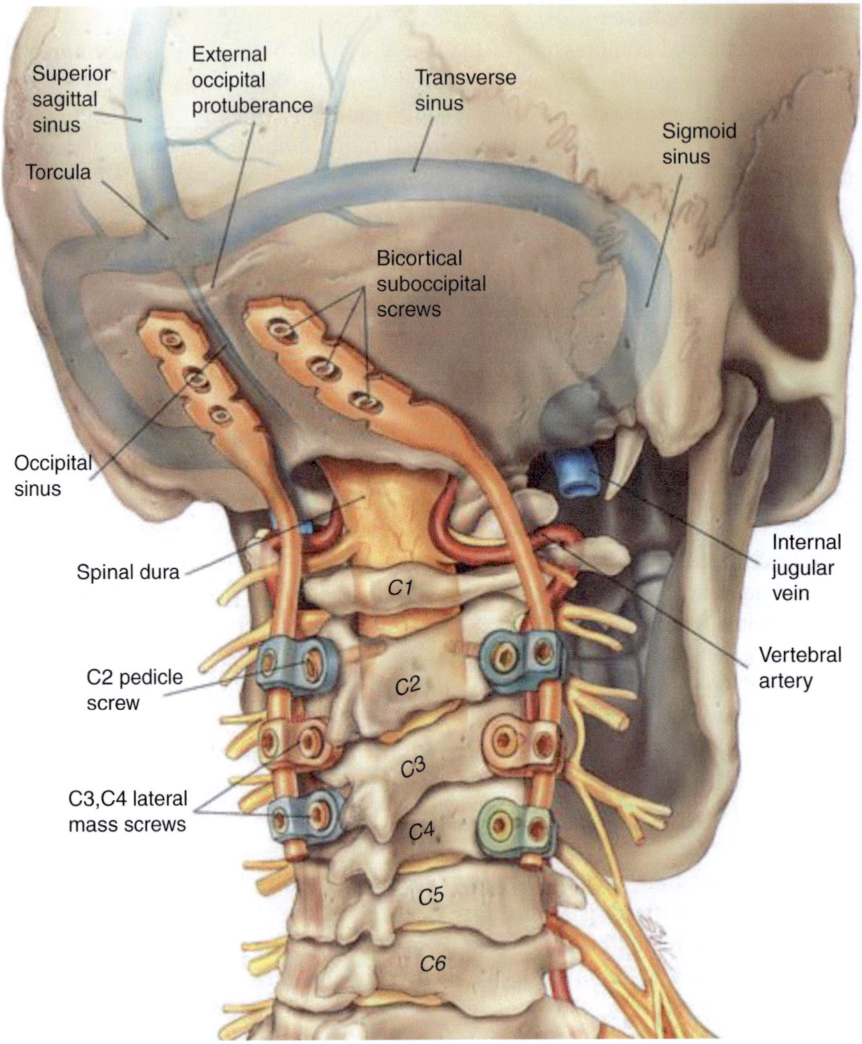

Fig. 24.2 Artist rendering of a occipitocervical fusion construct. (Illustration from Fourney DR, York JE, Cohen ZR, Suki D, Rhines LD, Gokaslan ZL. Management of atlantoaxial metastases with posterior occipitocervical stabilization. Journal of Neurosurgery: Spine. 2003 Mar;98(2):165–70)

24.5.2.2 Primary Tumors

Unlike metastatic spine disease, treatment for primary spinal tumors is performed with the goal of improving overall patient survival, with the possibility of cure in select patients. However, the unique anatomy of the CVJ makes this goal extremely challenging, and sometimes impossible, due to the risk of patient morbidity associated with injury to adjacent neurovascular structures. Tumor resection performed in en bloc fashion, defined as resection of tumor with a surrounding layer of healthy tissue, [22] has been shown to improve median survival in multiple different primary spine tumors when compared to subtotal resection [23–26].

Unlike with the thoracic, lumbar, and subaxial cervical spine, there are no CVJ specific surgical classification systems to help determine the optimal surgical approach for these tumors. However, it is helpful to adopt the principles of the Weinstein, Boriani, Biagimi staging system and the Enneking system [22]. Dividing both C1 and C2 into multiple radial zones helps to determine sites for osteotomies and the adjacent neurovascular structures that must be taken into account during tumor resection. Surgery can be divided into two stages. The first stage involves separation of the tumor from normal spine and uninvolved adjacent neural elements. C1 and C2 are ringed structures, so bony separation of tumor involves creating at least two osteotomies to disconnect the tumor from surrounding spine. Tumor in the spinal canal must then be separated from underlying neural elements. The second stage of surgery involves tumor delivery. Depending on tumor location this may involve one or more ventral and/or dorsal approaches.

Tumors within the posterior elements of C1 or C2, such as osteoid osteomas or osteochondromas are readily resected via a midline posterior cervical approach. A simple laminectomy may be all that is required for en bloc tumor resection with no need for stabilization. Involvement of facets or lateral masses requires additional surgical steps, including stabilization. Axial loading of the cervical spine occurs through the facets and lateral masses. Force is transmitted from the occipital condyles through the lateral masses of C1 and C2, and then through the subaxial cervical spine. We prefer placement of posterior instrumentation prior to tumor resection if the hardware does not obstruct the operative view during resection. The C2 nerve root must be exposed if the C1-2 facet is involved with tumor. Tumor involvement of cervical nerve roots often necessitates their sacrifice. There is little clinical consequence to sacrifice of either C1 or C2 nerve roots. Transecting the C2 nerve root will lead to occipital scalp numbness in roughly 11% of patients which typically resolves over time, but very rarely will it cause significant dysesthesias [27]. Caudal involvement of the subaxial spine nerve roots merits further consideration as sacrifice of these roots can lead to clinically significant motor weakness and disability.

Lateral mass cage reconstruction is a viable reconstruction option when CVJ facets are resected (Fig. 24.3) [28]. Reconstruction of the lateral cervical spine columns with a cage construct may help prevent pseudoarthrosis or hardware failure. It is important that the cage extend from the occipital condyle or rostral lateral mass to another lateral mass caudally, not a vertebral body, to decrease the risk of cage displacement. The cage is packed with autograft or allograft prior to placement to help achieve solid arthrodesis.

Careful consideration should be given to management of the vertebral artery if involved with tumor due to its complicated anatomic course, and devastating potential complications if sacrificed or injured. After exiting the C3 transverse foramen the vertebral artery travels rostral through the C2 foramen, then superolateral through the C1 foramen, travels posteromedial over the C1 arterial sulcus, and subsequently pierces the dura at the cervicomedullary junction after which it travels to join the contralateral vertebral artery. In about 50% of people the left vertebral

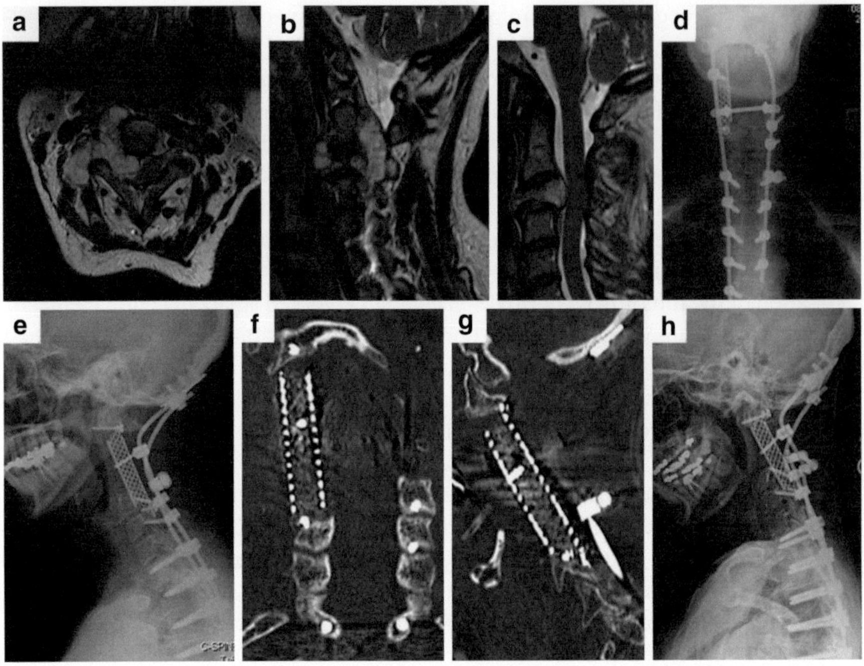

Fig. 24.3 Case illustration of cervical lateral mass reconstruction. (**a–c**) Preoperative T2-weighted MR images of biopsy-proven chondrosarcoma. (**a**) Axial image obtained at the level of the C-4 nerve root, demonstrating the tumor originating in the C-3 vertebral body with lateral extension. (**b**) Sagittal image obtained at the level of the lateral masses, demonstrating tumor extending from C-2 to C-4. (**c**) Midline sagittal image demonstrating C-3 pathological compression and canal compromise caused by the tumor. (**d–g**) Postoperative anteroposterior (**d**) and (**e**) lateral radiographs demonstrating the cage extending from the lateral masses of C1–6. Cage placement is further visualized on coronal (**f**) and sagittal (**g**) CT scans. (**h**) One year after surgery, the patient presented with neck pain and was found to have a new cervical deformity and fracture of her right posterior rod above the crossbar. (Figure from Clarke MJ, Zadnik PL, Groves ML, Sciubba DM, Witham TF, Bydon A, Gokaslan ZL, Wolinsky JP. Fusion following lateral mass reconstruction in the cervical spine. Journal of Neurosurgery: Spine. 2015 Feb;22(2):139–50)

artery is dominant, 25% of people are right artery dominant, and 25% are codominant. Determination of dominance can often be determined based on measurement of vessel caliber on preoperative imaging studies, but does not accurately predict the risk of stroke with vertebral artery sacrifice. Conventional angiography balloon test occlusion with provocative maneuvers, such as induced hypotension, can be useful to determine the clinical consequences of sacrificing a vertebral artery. If able to be sacrificed, coil embolization above and below the tumor is performed. Alternatively, intraoperative monitoring of motor and sensory evoked potentials with transient clip ligation of the vertebral artery of interest can provide similarly useful information. Prior to ligation and transection of a vertebral artery, the vessel segment rostral and caudal to the tumor must be exposed and skeletonized.

Tumors arising within the body of C2 or inferior clivus require a ventral or ventrolateral approach for either en bloc or piecemeal tumor resection. If attempting to remove these tumors en bloc a posterior approach to perform releasing osteotomies and posterior occipital cervical instrumentation is needed, after which the ventral approach is used to deliver the tumor. The transoral approach is the most direct route to the lower clivus, anterior arch of C1, vertebral body of C2, and C2-3 disc space. Supplemental splitting of the palate or mandible gives additional rostral and caudal exposure [29]. These procedures carry a substantial risk of morbidity due to entry through the oral-pharyngeal mucosa including velopharyngeal incompetence, dysphagia, odynophagia, pharyngeal wound dehiscence, cerebrospinal fluid leak, and meningitis. Another risk of a ventral approach through the pharyngeal mucosa is the potential for tumor seeding along the surgical tract, particularly with primary tumors such as chordoma.

There are alternative approaches that mitigate the risks of a transoral approach including the high transcervical approach and endoscopic-assisted approaches. The high transcervical approach allows access to ventral or ventrolateral tumors from C1 to C3 [30]. Visualization can be limited due to a narrow working corridor, and there may be difficulty seeing rostrally to the clivus. The submandibular incision can be extended to allow access further caudally to the subaxial cervical spine in the event of tumor extension inferiorly. Reconstruction of the anterior column following tumor resection is typically performed using a cage or strut graft followed by plate placement. While the high transcervical approach is generally well tolerated, there are exposure related risks including injury to the hypoglossal nerve, facial artery, facial vein, and vertebral artery.

Advances in endoscopy and image guidance using during skull base surgery and pituitary surgery have been incorporated into approaches to CVJ tumors. During a transoral approach to the CVJ the addition of endoscope assistance can improve tumor access and resection in both rostral-caudal and lateral directions. Angled endoscopes allow illumination and visualization rostral to the palate and caudal to the confines of the tongue. This can spare the need for splitting the mandible, palate, or tongue. The endoscope can also be used for a transnasal approach to the CVJ [29]. This technique uses a combination of image guidance and direct endoscopic visualization. Like a standard transnasal pituitary tumor resection, the rostrum of the sphenoid sinus is opened and the floor of the sphenoid sinus drilled flat. An endoscope is angled caudally toward the clivus and the nasopharyngeal mucosa is opened as a flap. This allows access the lower clivus, anterior C1 arch, and C2 dens. For primary tumor resection, healthy tissue margins are identified and maintained, if possible. Tumor is then resected using a combination of both straight and angled instruments. Once resection is completed the nasopharyngeal mucosa is flapped back into place. Image-guided endoscopic resection has also been described for a standard transcervical approach to the CVJ [30]. This technique takes advantage of the low morbidity of a standard transcervical exposure versus transmucosal techniques.

References

1. Daniel M, Sciubba CAM, Gokaslan ZL, Wolinsky J-P. Primary osseous and metastatic neoplasms of the craniovertebral junction. In: Bambakidis NC, editor. Surgery of the craniovertebral junction. 2nd ed. New York: Thieme; 2012. p. 560.
2. Kelley SP, Ashford RU, Rao AS, Dickson RA. Primary bone tumours of the spine: a 42-year survey from the Leeds Regional Bone Tumour Registry. Eur Spine J. 2007;16(3):405–9.
3. Society AC. Cancer facts and figures 2016. 2016. https://old.cancer.org/acs/groups/content/@research/documents/document/acspc-047079.pdf.
4. Wong DA, Fornasier VL, MacNab I. Spinal metastases: the obvious, the occult, and the impostors. Spine (Phila Pa 1976). 1990;15(1):1–4.
5. Sundaresan N, Boriani S, Rothman A, Holtzman R. Tumors of the osseous spine. J Neurooncol. 2004;69(1–3):273–90.
6. Moulding HD, Bilsky MH. Metastases to the craniovertebral junction. Neurosurgery. 2010;66(Suppl 3):A113–A8.
7. Rao G, Ha CS, Chakrabarti I, Feiz-Erfan I, Mendel E, Rhines LD. Multiple myeloma of the cervical spine: treatment strategies for pain and spinal instability. J Neurosurg Spine. 2006;5(2):140–5.
8. Chi JH, Bydon A, Hsieh P, Witham T, Wolinsky JP, Gokaslan ZL. Epidemiology and demographics for primary vertebral tumors. Neurosurg Clin N Am. 2008;19(1):1–4.
9. George B, Archilli M, Cornelius JF. Bone tumors at the cranio-cervical junction. Surgical management and results from a series of 41 cases. Acta Neurochir (Wien). 2006;148(7):741–9; discussion 9.
10. Franzius C, Sciuk J, Daldrup-Link HE, Jurgens H, Schober O. FDG-PET for detection of osseous metastases from malignant primary bone tumours: comparison with bone scintigraphy. Eur J Nucl Med. 2000;27(9):1305–11.
11. Rodallec MH, Feydy A, Larousserie F, Anract P, Campagna R, Babinet A, et al. Diagnostic imaging of solitary tumors of the spine: what to do and say. Radiographics. 2008;28(4):1019–41.
12. Bilsky MH, Shannon FJ, Sheppard S, Prabhu V, Boland PJ. Diagnosis and management of a metastatic tumor in the atlantoaxial spine. Spine (Phila Pa 1976). 2002;27(10):1062–9.
13. Azad TD, Esparza R, Chaudhary N, Chang SD. Stereotactic radiosurgery for metastasis to the craniovertebral junction preserves spine stability and offers symptomatic relief. J Neurosurg Spine. 2016;24(2):241–7.
14. Tuchman A, Yu C, Chang EL, Kim PE, Rusch MC, Apuzzo ML. Radiosurgery for metastatic disease at the craniocervical junction. World Neurosurg. 2014;82(6):1331–6.
15. Imai R, Kamada T, Tsuji H, Tsujii H, Tsuburai Y, Tatezaki S, et al. Cervical spine osteosarcoma treated with carbon-ion radiotherapy. Lancet Oncol. 2006;7(12):1034–5.
16. DeLaney TF, Liebsch NJ, Pedlow FX, Adams J, Weyman EA, Yeap BY, et al. Long-term results of Phase II study of high dose photon/proton radiotherapy in the management of spine chordomas, chondrosarcomas, and other sarcomas. J Surg Oncol. 2014;110(2):115–22.
17. Ozturk AK, Gokaslan ZL, Wolinsky JP. Surgical treatment of sarcomas of the spine. Curr Treat Options Oncol. 2014;15(3):482–92.
18. Jones DC, Hayter JP, Vaughan ED, Findlay GF. Oropharyngeal morbidity following transoral approaches to the upper cervical spine. Int J Oral Maxillofac Surg. 1998;27(4):295–8.
19. Laufer I, Iorgulescu JB, Chapman T, Lis E, Shi W, Zhang Z, et al. Local disease control for spinal metastases following "separation surgery" and adjuvant hypofractionated or high-dose single-fraction stereotactic radiosurgery: outcome analysis in 186 patients. J Neurosurg Spine. 2013;18(3):207–14.
20. White AA 3rd, Panjabi MM. The clinical biomechanics of the occipitoatlantoaxial complex. Orthop Clin North Am. 1978;9(4):867–78.
21. Fourney DR, York JE, Cohen ZR, Suki D, Rhines LD, Gokaslan ZL. Management of atlantoaxial metastases with posterior occipitocervical stabilization. J Neurosurg. 2003;98(2 Suppl):165–70.

22. Boriani S, Weinstein JN, Biagini R. Primary bone tumors of the spine. Terminology and surgical staging. Spine (Phila Pa 1976). 1997;22(9):1036–44.
23. York JE, Berk RH, Fuller GN, Rao JS, Abi-Said D, Wildrick DM, et al. Chondrosarcoma of the spine: 1954 to 1997. J Neurosurg. 1999;90(1 Suppl):73–8.
24. York JE, Kaczaraj A, Abi-Said D, Fuller GN, Skibber JM, Janjan NA, et al. Sacral chordoma: 40-year experience at a major cancer center. Neurosurgery. 1999;44(1):74–9; discussion 9–80.
25. Talac R, Yaszemski MJ, Currier BL, Fuchs B, Dekutoski MB, Kim CW, et al. Relationship between surgical margins and local recurrence in sarcomas of the spine. Clin Orthop Relat Res. 2002;397:127–32.
26. Yamazaki T, McLoughlin GS, Patel S, Rhines LD, Fourney DR. Feasibility and safety of en bloc resection for primary spine tumors: a systematic review by the Spine Oncology Study Group. Spine (Phila Pa 1976). 2009;34(22 Suppl):S31–8.
27. Elliott RE, Kang MM, Smith ML, Frempong-Boadu A. C2 nerve root sectioning in posterior atlantoaxial instrumented fusions: a structured review of literature. World Neurosurg. 2012;78(6):697–708.
28. Clarke MJ, Zadnik PL, Groves ML, Sciubba DM, Witham TF, Bydon A, et al. Fusion following lateral mass reconstruction in the cervical spine. J Neurosurg Spine. 2015;22(2):139–50.
29. Singh H, Harrop J, Schiffmacher P, Rosen M, Evans J. Ventral surgical approaches to craniovertebral junction chordomas. Neurosurgery. 2010;66(3 Suppl):96–103.
30. Hsu W, Kosztowski TA, Zaidi HA, Gokaslan ZL, Wolinsky JP. Image-guided, endoscopic, transcervical resection of cervical chordoma. J Neurosurg Spine. 2010;12(4):431–5.

Intramedullary Tumors of the Cervicomedullary Junction

25

Alessandro Landi, Giacoma M. F. Brunetto, Fabrizio Gregori, and Roberto Delfini

25.1 Introduction

Intra-axial cervicomedullary tumors (CMTs) are a heterogeneous group of tumors with a low incidence and a various range of malignancy.

These neoplasms, located at the junction of cervical spine and brainstem, were initially considered a specific subgroup of brainstem glial tumors. CMTs have been generally considered surgical inaccessible lesions, due to their perceived high risk of neurological morbidity, and associated with a poor prognosis [1].

In 1987, Epstein and Winsoff attempted to find criteria to classify brainstem gliomas; they were the first to identify five subgroups for such neoplasms: diffuse gliomas, localized gliomas, exophytic gliomas, cystic gliomas, and cervicomedullary gliomas [1]. Even if their classification was embryonal, they were pioneers in attributing a specific identity to CMTs.

Even if the first described results derived from pediatric records (brainstem gliomas have a 10% incidence in pediatric age and 2% in adult age), recent publications show a high incidence also in adult population [1]. The most represented are low grade gliomas, with a slow growth rate, considered histologically "benign" and associated with an indolent clinical presentation, with progressive and slow onset neurological symptoms.

Anatomically, cervicomedullary junction is full of eloquent structures: the areas for cardiorespiratory regulation (solitary nucleus and reticular formation), and the nuclei of the mixed motor and sensory nerves with their infranuclear portion. The corticospinal tract, spinothalamic tract, and posterior columns contribute to the anatomical complexity of this area, continuing towards the spinal cord.

Among CMTs, we can include neoplasms involving the medulla oblongata, the upper cervical region, or both with bulbo-cervical extension. According to the most

A. Landi (✉) · G. M. F. Brunetto · F. Gregori · R. Delfini
Division of Neurosurgery A, Department of Neurology and Psychiatry, Sapienza University of Rome, Rome, Italy

E. Tessitore et al. (eds.), *Surgery of the Cranio-Vertebral Junction*,
https://doi.org/10.1007/978-3-030-18700-2_25

supported hypothesis, the origin of the tumor is in the upper region of cervical spinal cord, with a secondary extension towards the medulla oblongata [2].

These tumors, mainly astrocytomas, have the capability to displace the nervous structures encountered along the growth towards the medulla oblongata, both white matter and nuclei, interrupting at the junction between pons and medulla oblongata, where white matter tracts cross [1]. This growth pattern might explain why the anatomical extension of this kind of tumors is extended in the bulbo-cervical area, without involvement of the contiguous tissue of the pons, and the growth is then "forced" dorsally into the cisterna magna or in the fourth ventricle. This hypothesis is supported by the observed histopathologic categories: is evident an overlap with purely intramedullary spinal histotypes if compared to the more aggressive and infiltrative tumors.

25.2 Epidemiology

Intramedullary tumors represent 20–30% of all the intradural tumors in the adult population, more than 50% in pediatric population.

Gliomas account for 80% of intramedullary tumors: 60–70% are astrocytomas and the remaining 30–40% are ependymomas. Astrocytomas are more represented in the pediatric age, while ependymomas are more represented in adult age [2].

The third category, accounting for 2–15%, is represented by hemangioblastomas [2]. About 2% is represented by intramedullary metastases, mainly lung or breast primary tumors, and is often encountered during autopsies [2]. Other tumors such as lipomas (1%) or tumors of other nature (mesenchymal, germ cell, dermoid, epidermoid, hematopoietic) are extremely rare in this region.

25.3 Clinical Signs and Symptoms

CMTs are, in most cases, low grade tumors, affecting mainly pediatric population. Their clinical presentation may vary, but is often encountered a clinical onset associated with a long history of clinical symptoms before the diagnosis is made.

The primary clinical manifestations can be divided into two categories: dysfunction of the lower cranial nerves and medullary impairment. Lower cranial nerves dysfunction (motor and sensory function) is characterized by deglutition and speech dysfunction. Medullary impairment can determine hemiparesis or tetraparesis and other symptoms related to a damage of the corticospinal tract (upper motor neuron). An involvement of the spinothalamic tract determines a reduction in the perception of temperature and pain. The involvement of the dorsal columns is characterized by proprioception deficit and gait disturbances (ataxia). Tumors involving the autonomous system might cause sympathetic and parasympathetic impairment. Severe spinal cord injury can determine a visceral impairment such as respiratory deficit, sphincter dysfunction, and sexual dysfunction. Paresthesia or dysesthesia can be unilateral, often encountered distally and only in a second phase they might have a proximal and a contralateral extension.

The onset of medullary symptoms is often indolent, with a slow motor impairment followed by impairment of cranial nerves after few months or years. Spinal pain is often described immediately before or just after the onset of neurological symptoms. In sporadic cases (young patients and giant CMTs), cervical pain might represent the only symptom, without neurological dysfunction. It has been postulated that pain, typically worsening in lying position and during night hours, can be derived by the distension and irritation of the dura mater.

The most frequently encountered clinical onset is characterized by lower limbs motor deficit (78.1%). Other clinical conditions include: suboccipital pain (68.8%), sensory loss (56.3%), sphincter and bowel involvement (28.1%), respiratory impairment (46.9%), vomit (46.9%) dysphagia (43.8%), nasal regurgitation (43.8%), and headache (34.4%). Cranial nerves deficits are distributed for frequency: deficit of the IX and X cranial nerve (cardiac and respiratory instability, 43.8%), XI cranial nerve (weakness and atrophy of sternocleidomastoid and trapezius muscles, 31.3%), XII cranial nerve (ipsilateral tongue palsy and atrophy, 21.9%). Symptoms related to the involvement of the posterior tracts are described in 31.3% of the patients.

Hydrocephalus is described in 1–8% of the cases of CMTs. It might be related to the obstruction of CSF flow in the subarachnoid space determined by the tumor or to an alteration in CSF reabsorption induced by an increase of the protein concentration in the CSF, produced by the tumor itself. CSF flow obstruction determined by increased proteins with xanthochromic CSF is known as Froin syndrome. CMTs often determine respiratory impairment (46.9%).

For tumors located selectively in the inferior portion of the medulla oblongata, the clinical pattern is constituted by: ipsilateral loss of tactile sensitivity of the middle and lower portion of the trunk (compression of gracile nucleus); ipsilateral loss of tactile sensitivity of the middle and upper portion of the trunk (compression of cuneate nucleus); a potential cardiac and respiratory instability (compression of solitary tract and dorsal motor nucleus of vagus) sleep apnea, known as primary alveolar hypoventilation; motor weakness of the ipsilateral hemi-tongue (compression of XII cranial nerve nucleus).

For tumors located in the ventral and lateral portion of the medulla oblongata, the clinical onset is characterized by motor weakness of the ipsilateral hemi-tongue (compression of XII cranial nerve nucleus), loss of the deglutition reflex (compression of nucleus ambiguus), loss of thermic and pain sensitivity of the contralateral half body (trunk and limbs) due to the compression of the spinothalamic tract, and loss of sensitivity in the contralateral half body (trunk and limbs) due to the compression of the medial lemniscus.

The clinical presentation of CMTs is related to their growth rate, their position, and their longitudinal extension. Other factors influencing the symptoms are: age, disc degenerative disease of the spine, dimensions of the spinal canal, the presence of other comorbidities [1, 2].

25.4 Radiological Findings

MRI represents the study of choice and is able to characterize a specific pattern on the basis of morphology, changes in signal intensity, the presence or absence of contrast enhancement, and anatomic location and extent. MRI may be helpful in differential diagnosis and to define the presence or absence of a cord–tumor interface, associated cysts, or syringomyelia. Looking at gliomas specifically (ependymomas and astrocytomas), both lesions enhance with gadolinium and demonstrate fusiform morphology over numerous vertebral segments; they both appear hypo- or isointense on T1-weighted images and hyperintense on T2-weighted images.

Ependymomas are more likely to have associated blood by-products and large satellite cysts and tend to be centrally located within the cord displaying symmetric expansion with diffuse heterogeneous enhancement. They tend to occupy the whole width of the cord and generally produce enhanced margins. Astrocytomas, in comparison, tend to be eccentrically positioned, show an exophytic component, and can be non-enhancing, heterogeneously enhancing or display only an enhancing nodule.

Hemangioblastomas are richly vascularized tumors with significant surrounding edema. They have a frequent association with syringomyelia and they are most commonly sporadic even if 30% of patients with hemangioblastomas show Von Hippel–Lindau syndrome. On MRI, they have mural nodules, which appear isointense on T1-weighted images and hyperintense on T2-weighted images with homogenous contrast enhancement.

Cavernous angiomas are lobulated masses of interwoven vessels or locules of variable size containing blood products at different stages of evolution; on CT scan, they can be negative in 30–50% of cases or they appear as well-delineated round hyperdense lesions usually <3 cm. T1-weighted sequences show different aspects depending on hemorrhage stage: the most common findings are a “popcorn ball” appearance of mixed hyper-, hypointense blood-containing locules; less frequently we can observe acute hemorrhage or reticulated “mulberry-like” lesion with a mixed signal core and complete hypointense hemosiderin rim. Cavernomas are angiographically occult vascular malformation with slow intralesional flow without artero-venous shunting.

Metastases are well-encapsulated masses and they often show cystic change or intralesional hemorrhage. Metastatic lesions are most likely eccentrically located in the cord and expand the cord parenchyma, which was historically visible on myelography and illustrated clearly on MRI. Metastases are most likely to be T1 isointense and T2 hyperintense. The amount of edema may be out of proportion to the size of the tumor, and this is evidenced by extensive T2 hyperintensity, which can be on average 3.6-fold larger than that of the enhancing portion of the lesion [2–4].

25.5 Preoperative Planning

An accurate preoperative planning is mandatory. Sometimes it might be of great importance to clearly identify the position of the vessels, including the vertebral arteries and the venous structures. The need, even if rare for intramedullary tumors, to perform a partial demolition of the occipital condyle might influence the stability of the craniovertebral junction. Therefore, it is important to perform lateral dynamic X-rays before surgery. The clinical or radiological hypothesis of a dysfunction or an involvement of the lower cranial nerves (IX, X, XI, XII) should be verified preoperatively, with a systematic examination of deglutition, phonation, and respiration. The lateral expansion of the tumor is a determining factor, but in case of a tumor extended on the midline, the anatomy of the neurovascular structures becomes more important. The dimension of the tumor combined with the direction and the extension of the tumoral growth concur to define the necessary approach, how useful it can be and if it can be helpful the combination of more approaches. The stability of the craniovertebral junction and the expected level of bony resection have to be considered before performing surgery to have a well-established plan for reconstruction, whenever needed [5].

25.6 Advanced Neuroimaging: DTI

Morphological MRI techniques provide only anatomical information while some specific sequences as diffusion-weighted imaging (DWI), diffusion tensor imaging (DTI), and fractional anisotropy (FA) are useful to described, detect, and map the extent of spinal cord lesions.

DTI and Fiber Tracking (FT) are used to describe tumors and to detect their limbs. It is also possible to envisage a histological diagnosis if you know that FA values are similar for astrocytomas, ependymomas, and metastases but are different for hemangioblastomas; in particular the lowest FA values are seen in metastases, and the highest are seen in hemangioblastomas. FT may show fibers that are destroyed or displaced by the tumor. This could be important to estimate highly infiltrative tumors and to identify their margins before surgery resection. Also neuronavigation should be used in two different ways: (1) to understand the extension of an intrinsic spinal lesion that must be removed; (2) to help in estimating tumor removal limits during surgery. The application of DTI-based fiber tracking, for diagnosis and neuronavigation, should be used in the clinical routine for the management of intramedullary high grade astrocytomas, in order to achieve a safer histological diagnosis and tumor resection [6, 7].

25.7 Treatment

25.7.1 Surgical Approaches

The most frequently used surgical approaches to perform the resection of intradural and intramedullary tumors of the craniovertebral junction are:

- Median suboccipital
- Lateral suboccipital: far lateral or postero-lateral

- Pure cervical approach with laminectomy or laminotomy (with or without a small median suboccipital craniectomy associated).

Median posterior suboccipital approach is performed with a median bilateral suboccipital craniotomy. The target lesions are located posteriorly to the dentate ligament.

The lateral or postero-lateral (far lateral) approach is performed with a suboccipital lateral craniotomy, with dissection of the muscolo-cutaneous layers with circumferential postero-lateral direction.

Postero-lateral approach is reserved to tumors located anterior to dentate ligaments. Main advantages are: the control over vertebral artery on its extradural course, the access to the anterolateral aspect of the junction without retracting brainstem or cranial nerves, and the optimal surgical control on the mixed nerves in their more lateral course. In both suboccipital approaches, for a proper rostral-caudal exposition and a better working angle, it is necessary to complete the surgical approach with the opening of foramen magnum and removal of the C1 posterior arch.

The choice of the surgical approach is determined by the anatomical location of the tumor in craniocaudal direction (suboccipital approaches for bulbar lesions, cervical approaches for cervical intramedullary lesions, and a combination of the aforementioned approaches for tumors with both bulbar and cervical extension). The approach is related also to the posterior or anterior location and median or lateral position of the tumor in the neuraxis: anterolateral and lateral tumors are reached with a postero-lateral approach (possible drilling of condylar process). For median and posterior tumors, the most considered approach is the median suboccipital with removal of C1 posterior arch and eventually associated with a posterior cervical approach.

25.7.2 Suboccipital Median Approach

The more appropriate surgical positionings for this approach are the prone position (Concorde position), the lateral-oblique and the seated position. All positions require head fixation with the Mayfield head holder for all patients older than 2 years. Neck flexion is also required, to be obtained with particular care, after excluding cervical instability and tonsil herniation through the foramen magnum.

Skin incision is performed along the posterior midline, from 1 to 2 cm above the external occipital protuberance, to end in correspondence of C4. If the tumor has a lateral location a "hockey stick" incision might be used, to allow a wider exposure and a more extended craniotomy. Skin and subcutaneous tissue are carefully dissected by the fascia on both sides of the upper half of the incision, aiming to create an adequate fascial patch for reconstruction. The dissection is then continued with autostatic retractors, aiming to spare both occipital nerves and arteries. Muscle dissection has to be performed along the midline: a deviation from midline will cause muscular bleeding during exposure of the deeper muscular layers. The next step is the Y-shaped incision of the fascia. The muscles are dissected away from the bone with the alternate use of bipolar electro-cautery and periosteum elevator. The lateral exposition is arrested as soon as the mastoid emissary vein is identified bilaterally. The muscular insertions are disinserted from the spinous processes, from C1 posterior arch and C2 laminae. Suboccipital craniotomy is performed with two burr holes, one for each side, at approximately 3 cm from the midline, just below the transverse sinus. In elderly patients, a third burr hole might be performed below the torcular herophili. The dura mater adjacent to the burr hole is detached with a Penfield dissector, and the bone flap is removed with a high speed drill or a craniotome. The transverse and sigmoid sinuses represent the upper and lateral limits for the craniotomy. Inferiorly, the craniotomy should always include the posterior margin of the foramen magnum, in order to avoid a potential cerebellar laceration touching the bony margin during retraction. A wider opening in the area of the foramen magnum reduces the potential risk of herniation due to postoperative hematomas or cerebellar swelling. The bone in correspondence of the midline is detached as last thing, because it is formed by a deep and vascularized ridge. This ridge has to be carefully detached by the surface of the dura mater, with extreme care in proximity of the median occipital sinus and of the annular sinus, near the foramen magnum. All the bony margins should be covered with bone wax to avoid air to enter into the lacunae. The dissection of C1 lamina has to be performed in craniocaudal direction, because the vertebral artery is located on the superior margin of the lamina. The removal of C1 lamina is performed with a bone rongeur or with an angled Kerrison rongeur. In some cases of cranio vertebral junction (CVJ) intramedullary tumors with caudal extension might be useful to extend laminectomy to the posterior arch of C2 and C3.

25.7.2.1 Accessory Surgical Routes to IV Ventricle

When the intramedullary tumor follows a cranial growth path towards the fourth ventricle, it is necessary to plan a second surgical step aiming to reach the superior pole of the tumor. The approaches most frequently used to reach the ventricular cavity are: the telovelar and transvermian approaches. In telovelar approach, the cerebellomedullary fissure, an arachnoid cleft located between the tonsils and the posterior surface of the medulla oblongata, is the anatomic landmark of choice to begin the dissection to reach the IV ventricle.

Telovelar incision can be divided in three parts: the first one opens the tela choroidea and begins inferiorly in proximity of the Magendie foramen, in the lowest part of IV ventricle's roof, to extend upwards until the junction of the tela with the inferior medullary velum. Once the tela choroidea is opened, the entire length of the IV ventricle's pavement is exposed. The second part of the incision consists in the opening of the inferior medullary velum, allowing to expose the entire pavement of the IV ventricle, also the ipsilateral superolateral recess (particular care has to be taken to preserve the vein of the cerebellomedullary fissure that often crosses the inferior medullary velum). The third incision performed between the tonsils and the medulla oblongata through the tela choroidea (in the portion where it forms the most caudal part of the posterior wall of the lateral recess) exposes more extensively the lateral recess and the Luschka foramen [8].

The alternative surgical corridor is the transvermian approach, performed through the splitting on the midline of the inferior portion of the vermis, in its suboccipital surface [9–11].

The entity of the resection has been scarcely described, but some authors recommend to limit as much as possible the incision on the vermis, to minimize the clinical effects related to the splitting of the cerebellar fibers [12]. Otherwise, some authors prolong the transvermian incision including also its most inferior portion and extend superiorly until the fastigium, preserving the inferior margin of the superior medullary velum [13]. Functionally, the fibers decurring from the superior cerebellar peduncles make their decussation deeply under the superior medullary velum, a subtle lamina of white matter interposed between the superior cerebellar peduncles. This first vermian incision exposes only the underlying nodule; once it has been incised together with the choroid tela and the inferior medullary velum, the access to the IV ventricle is gained. The retraction of the two inferior halves of the vermis provides a workspace of 1–2 cm between the two inferior vermis margins. Following the tonsils and vermis retraction laterally, it is possible to observe the right and left PICA in their telovelotonsillar portion. The obtained surgical corridor between the two arteries must preserve the collateral vessels. In most cases the vein of the cerebellomedullary fissure might be adequately visualized, in its horizontal course along the median vermian incision along the choroid tela and the inferior medullary velum. Many authors demonstrated that the transvermian approach does not allow to easily expose the most lateral portion of the recess, as well as the foramen of Luschka. Those structures might be reached only by performing a resection of the lateral process of the vermis and a further retraction of the tonsillar pole (foramen of Luschka) [14].

25.7.3 Far Lateral or Postero-Lateral Approach

The postero-lateral approach is also called lateral suboccipital, "basic" far lateral or retrocondylar far lateral. The far lateral approach, described for the first time by Seeger, has been an effective instrument to expose the anterior and anterolateral intradural tumors of the CVJ. The basic far lateral description does not include the occipital condyle resection, but the surgical corridor can be extended with the removal of bony components, based on the position and the extension of the tumor. The patient is in sitting position or in modified park bench position. The skin incision begins on the mastoid process, continues superiorly and then below the superior nuchal line to reach the midline until C4. The horseshoe or "hockey stick" incision allows a better exposition of the muscular layers and of the nervous and vascular structures if compared to the linear incision. A subperiosteal dissection is performed to visualize the squamous part of the occipital bone, the posterior margin of the foramen magnum, and the posterior arch of C1 and C2 by the same side of the tumor. The muscles are generally elevated in a single layer with the scalp, to expose the muscles forming the suboccipital triangle. The incision might be extended, if necessary, to expose the mastoid process and the C1 and C2 transverse processes.

Opening the triangle, the venous plexus surrounding the vertebral artery is visualized; then it passes behind the atlanto-occipital junction, above the C1 posterior arch. The C2 nerve root emerges between the posterior arch of the atlas and the lamina. Even if the suboccipital approaches do not require the anatomical dissection of every single muscular layer, the selective identification of the muscles is an important requirement to recognize early and efficiently the vascular, nervous and bony structures. Some other important anatomic landmarks include the rectus capitis lateralis, useful to identify the jugular foramen and the elevator scapulae muscle, which allows to identify the vertebral artery where it passes through the transverse foramina of C1 and C2, and the posterior belly of the digastric muscle, associated to the facial nerve. Generally the exposition is unilateral [5]. The exposition and control of the vertebral artery is mandatory to perform the surgical procedure, to ensure a vascular control, but it is not always necessary to perform also the transposition of the artery. Much care must be taken during the dissection of C1 lateral mass, in order to avoid any damage to the vertebral artery and its branches. The atlas posterior arch is removed following a subperiosteal dissection, starting from the midline towards the opposite side considering the ipsilateral foramen transversarium. The bony resection consists in a lateral suboccipital craniotomy including the margin of the foramen magnum. The remaining bone of the posterior margin can be removed with the help of a Kerrison rongeur. The bony removal from the cranial base continues towards the condylar fossa. The most useful variant of far lateral approach is the transcondylar approach [15]. Condylar resection offers a more lateral access to the inferior portion of the clivus and to the premedullary area. In the approaches performed for intramedullary tumors, the transposition of the vertebral artery, condylectomy, and the removal of the jugular tubercle do not seem to be necessary [5, 16].

25.7.4 Medulla Oblongata: Deep Tumors and Medullary Safe Entry Zones

In case of tumors located deeply in the medulla oblongata without effacement to the pial surface, the functional eloquence of the nervous tissue obliges the surgeon to plan a bulbotomy with an access as safe as possible.

25.7.4.1 Surgical Access to the Dorsal Caudal and Rostral Medulla Oblongata

The approach of choice for the access to the dorsal portion of the medulla oblongata is the median suboccipital approach. The gracile and cuneate fasciculus are considered the main anatomic landmarks for the approaches to the dorsal caudal region of the medulla oblongata. Bricolo describes three "safe entry zones" for the dorsal medulla oblongata.

They are the posterior median sulcus, below the obex; the posterior intermediate sulcus, between the gracile and cuneate fasciculus; and the posterior lateral sulcus, between the cuneate fasciculus medially and the trigeminal nucleus and trigeminal-spinal tract laterally. Tumors of the pavement of the fourth ventricle with involvement of the rostral and dorsal portion of the bulb are accessible with the pontine safe entry zones (suprafacial and infrafacial triangle) if the tumor is extended also in the pons (cavernomas). The area of the calamus scriptorius must be preserved by any surgical manipulation, to prevent dysphagia and cardiorespiratory impairment for any damage of the vagal and hypoglossal trigone. A damage of the nucleus ambiguus, located more laterally, that gives fibers to the IX, X, and XI cranial nerves, will cause a palatine velum, pharynx and larynx palsy [17–19].

25.7.4.2 Surgical Access to the Ventral Bulb

The surgical approach preferred for the access to the medulla oblongata in its ventro-lateral region is the far lateral approach. The two olivary bodies are considered the main anatomical landmarks for the ventral surface of the medulla oblongata. The two main approaches described for this region comprehend an anterolateral and a retro-olivary access. The approach is laterally limited by the corticospinal tract, laterally by the olivary bodies and in depth by the medial lemniscus. The retro-olivary approach is performed between the two olivary bodies anteriorly and by the cerebellar pedunculus inferiorly. A unilateral damage of the olivary bodies does not provide a clinically significant impairment [17–19].

25.7.5 Medulla Oblongata: Superficial and Exophytic Tumors

A different approach is demanded when the bulbar tumor, presenting with a superficial growth, is responsible for a macroscopically appreciable deformation of the bulbar surface, such as a dyschromic area or a bulky zone. In this situation, the surgeon, after a direct neurophysiological stimulation of the area and a confirmation obtained with neuronavigation or ultrasound, can perform a bulbar incision in the area of effacement/dyschromia. For the tumors with an exophytic component, the resection might be easier in the area of the cisterna magna, but will result extremely difficult in the attempt of preserving the areas of the IV ventricle pavement involved by the tumor adherence. It is frequent the decision to perform an incomplete resection, with a small tumoral residue adherent to the surface of the IV ventricle pavement, aiming to preserve the function (ependymomas are the tumors with the highest adhesion).

25.7.6 Median Posterior Cervical Approach

Surgery for rostral cervical intramedullary tumor resection is performed through a laminectomy and a subsequent posterior exploration through durotomy. Surgery is performed in general anesthesia with the patient in prone position. Usually, the incision is extended one level above and one level below the location of the tumor. The bony opening might be performed through a standard laminectomy or rarely with a laminotomy. Extensive laminectomies, performed for four or more adjacent segments, should be avoided in order to minimize the risk of kyphotic deformity (swan neck deformity). Some authors advocate the possibility of performing minimally invasive approaches to the spine, even for intramedullary tumors. Laminoplasty is an alternative solution such as the unilateral laminectomy or laminotomy. According to the experience of our department, the minimally invasive approaches to the bony structures force the surgeon to perform much more manipulation on the medullary tissues. In order to avoid this condition and to prevent medullary swellings, we prefer to perform a bilateral laminectomy, and only in very selected cases a laminotomy with laminoplasty (pediatric age). For those patients with rostral cervical tumors (C1) extended cranially up to the foramen magnum or with a clear bulbar involvement, together with a laminectomy, it is necessary to perform a small median suboccipital craniectomy/craniotomy to better dominate the apical pole of the tumor [2]. Nowadays, an intraoperative control might be performed with spinal neuronavigation or with ultrasounds. The advantages of the overlapping of the two technologies (MRI and ultrasonography) are evident also after the dural and arachnoid opening. CSF drainage is responsible for a reduced accuracy for "shift" phenomenon, and ultrasonography allows a real-time visualization and a correction of this aberration. At this point of the procedure, the use of operating microscope and neurophysiological monitoring is mandatory. The dural incision is performed with a scalpel along the midline, in craniocaudal direction, with particular care to not determine arachnoid opening or vascular damages.

25.8 Tumor Removal and Neurophysiological Monitoring

The majority of the intramedullary tumors have a dorsal effacement: a median posterior myelotomy or bulbotomy is then commonly performed. Even if the lateral medullary margin might appear as infiltrated by the tumor, a not centered myelotomy might lead to dorsal columns and vessels damages. Ultrasonography can identify medullary distortion and provide useful information on transversal and longitudinal axis and to identify the dentate ligament. The posterior median septum and the entry zones of the small dorsal nerve roots bilaterally are considered as a referral to perform a correct median incision. Myelotomy is centered on the most voluminous part of the tumor (bulky zone) and then extended to the entire length of the lesion. It is commonly performed with an arachnoid blade. Pial sutures are placed to realize a slight countertraction and to avoid any trauma on the nervous tissue. In case of an ependymoma, the presence of caudal or rostral cysts is a common finding, with a little prevalence of rostral pole cysts. It is necessary to cauterize the afferent vessels of the tumor, in order to mobilize and remove the tumor that is anchored by the same vessels to the surrounding parenchyma. For small tumors, once the correct plan of dissection has been identified, an "en bloc" removal might be performed, with an "outside-in" technique. In most cases, in particular for very large and infiltrating tumors, an intracapsular debulking performed with ultrasonic aspirator might be preferred, until the interface with the medullary tissue is identified ("inside-out" technique). The internal removal should be reduced to the minimum, in order to avoid a piecemeal resection due to a superficial fragmentation of the tumor and the loss of the cleavage plane.

Hemangioblastomas are commonly located on the medullary or bulbar dorsal or dorsolateral pial surface, and only occasionally require a myelotomy/bulbotomy. Their aspect is the one of well-encapsulated vascular masses with many superficial vessels feeding the tumor. An optimal resection is related to the control of the tumor vascularization. The cleavage plane is easily identified. The target for the removal of this kind of tumors is a gross total resection, aiming to preserve the draining veins. The ventral dissection is the most difficult and challenging step: the volume occupied by the tumor is the main obstacle to an optimal visualization of the medullary-tumor interface, and often the dissection is challenging despite the delicate pial countertraction [20, 21].

Nowadays the surgical resection of these tumors is more efficient thanks to the use of intraoperative neurophysiological monitoring, such as motor evoked potentials (MEP), somato-sensitive evoked potentials (SSEP), electromyography (EMG), and cranial nerves monitoring.

Since the performing of the myelotomy, SSEP are fundamental to identify the midline. The identification of the median raphe might be difficult in cases of anatomical alteration due to the presence of the tumor. Using the technique of the dorsal mapping, the physiological midline might be identified. The introduction of MEP, both muscular and epidural (D-wave), is considered as the gold standard for intramedullary tumors surgery. The fundamental role of the neuromonitoring is to interrupt the surgical dissection and avoid a neurological impairment. At the same time, it guarantees a safer and more radical resection. MEP modifications should invite the surgeon to interrupt the surgical manipulation, to irrigate the nervous tissue with tepid saline solution (that dilutes the extracellulary kalium and washes away metabolites and other irritating products), to apply papaverin and to create a moderate induced hypertension (papaverin and hypertension might prevent an ischemic damage). The cutoff for the D-wave reduction is 50%. The preservation of the D-wave above 50% has been evaluated as predictive for the long-term preservation of the voluntary control over the lower limbs. The loss of muscular MEP and the preservation of the height of the D-wave, a transient postoperative motor deficit. This condition has been described as "warning," a reversible phase in which the surgeon can modify the surgical strategy and manipulation before a permanent damage occurred. A difficult situation is observed when the referral value of MEPs is present and the D-wave is absent since the beginning. This occurs in about 30% of the patients and has been described as "D-wave desynchronization." Many authors have noticed the D-wave desynchronization to occur after radiation therapy intramedullary tumors associated to syringomyelia. Surgical radicality is influenced by many factors (histology, presence or absence of a cleavage plane, dimensions, anatomical localization), but the intraoperative modification of the potentials represents the main factor that might influence the surgeon to leave in place a small fragment of tumor [22, 23].

25.9 Discussion and Outcome

The first successful surgery for the resection of an intramedullary tumor was described by Elsberg and Beer in 1911 [20, 24]. After a century from that first surgical procedure, a lot of advancements in the pathology knowledge have been made: Guidetti and his co-workers, describing the long-term follow-up of a group of intramedullary gliomas treated between 1951 and 1978, analyzed the differences in terms of prognosis improvement related to the progression of the surgical techniques. The authors were able to identify an increase in gross total resection rate, a better functional outcome and recovery, and no intraoperative deaths only in the second part of their surgical experience, between 1967 and 1978, due to the technical advancements [20, 25].

The first papers describing intrinsic brainstem and CVJ tumors have been published in 1980, thanks to the contribution of some authors such as Epstein, McCleary, and Wisoff [26, 27]. They described the first results of their surgical experience in the treatment of this subgroup of patients and analyze their main characteristics. The analysis of the first two series, 35 brainstem gliomas and 20 CVJ intramedullary tumors, emerges that surgery was a sustainable and effective treatment option, and the worse results were mainly associated with aggressive forms of tumors. CVJ intramedullary tumors presented as a variegated oncological category, and the first examined series showed a characteristic melting pot of different pathologies with alternation of typically spinal histotypes and typical brainstem tumors. Tumors originating from the most cranial portion of the brainstem often show a higher histological malignity. On the other side, tumors of the caudal portion (bulb) are most similar to the low grade tumors (gliomas) typical of the spinal cord [27–30].

Patients with a clinical presentation represented by cervical pain and/or symptoms related to the impairment of the pyramidal tracts are probably more representative of a solid nucleus neoplasm in the cervical spinal cord, with a cystic component extended to the brainstem. This last kind of tumors have an aspect and a behavior similar to medullary astrocytomas, and are often associated to voluminous cystic components adherent to the cranial or caudal pole of the neoplasm [26, 28–34].

Even in the nomenclature we can appreciate this difference, distinguishing **cranio-spinal** and **spino-cranial** tumors. The first group is for tumors with a major extension in the cranial region; the second group has a major extension in the spinal compartment. Probably the portion of more representation of the tumor defines the region of origin of the neoplasm solid nucleus.

According to some authors, the spatial growth of these neoplasms follows a characteristic growth pattern defined as "stereotypical" and suggestive for an indolent behavior [35–37]. These neoplasms have the capability to grow in respect of the white matter fascicles pathways, so that, when the tumor grows in proximity of the pyramidal decussation or of the dorsal columns, the growth is interrupted by the pyramidal fascicles and by the medial lemniscus, grows in the dorsal direction an exophytical behavior in the cisterna magna or cranially in the IV ventricle.

The growth of these tumors often proceeds with a circumferential pattern around the pial structures and is led towards the interface with the white matter fascicles:

therefore it is rare to observe tumors extending beyond the pons-medulla oblongata junction [37, 38].

This restrictive growth pattern often delineates a good interface plan with the tumor, allowing an "easier" excision [39, 40]. The biological behavior of many "low-grade tumors" of the CVJ seems to mimic, as suggested by Daumas-Duport (in a particular topographic variant), the category called Neuroepithelial Dysembryoplastic Tumors [35, 41]. Neoplasms with a particularly favorable behavior are associated to a long history of preoperative symptoms and a favorable neurological outcome. In this subgroup of tumors, the tendency to develop a recurrence after a subtotal resection appears to be minimal.

A further typical feature of CVJ intramedullary tumors is the evidence that surgical treatment, often with gross total resection, is a feasible and effective treatment strategy. Surgery arrests the biological growth of most of those astrocytomas or low grade neoplasms, assuming an important therapeutic value [26].

For brainstem astrocytomas with growth above the medulla oblongata (pons and mesencephalon), the gross total resection is achieved in limited and occasional cases. Tumors with high grade of malignancy are associated with a different development: despite a gross total resection, the early recurrence, an infiltrating behavior towards the nervous structures, and the limited survival configure them as a subgroup with unfavorable prognosis, not similar to the majority of the tumors of the CVJ. The majority is represented by low grade gliomas and astrocytomas, despite the characteristics of those histotypes are well known, the literature does not express guidelines on the surgical timing and alternative treatment strategies. They are often scarcely responsive tumors to radiotherapic and chemotherapic treatments, so that surgical treatment with a maximally cytoreductive surgery remains the treatment of choice. The scarce response to adjuvant treatments has been attributed to a low proliferation index related to the poor malignancy of the most represented histotypes.

When the neurological deterioration related to the mass effect on the adjacent tissues becomes progressive and evident, it is common opinion that the surgical treatment is the only strategy to limit the damage or the complete loss of the neurological function. Surgical resection remains the best treatment option to obtain pathological tissue for a histological examination, to optimize a neurological recovery and to eradicate the tumor [20].

There are no codified guidelines on surgical indication, but only recommendations shared by the scientific community. For this specific tumoral subset (asymptomatic patients), the most approved indication is the radiological monitoring with systematic MRI scan controls (wait and see) [20]. Aghakhani, in a study on intramedullary ependymomas, compared the post-surgical results between a group of symptomatic patients and a group treated in absence of symptoms [20, 42]. The analysis of this series demonstrated that the surgical procedure was associated with a certain grade of neurological morbidity, without major differences in the two groups of patients (10% of postoperative neurological symptoms in both groups). Considering that the risk of neurological impairment [32, 42–51] related to the surgical procedure is not absent, the author underlines that for asymptomatic patients surgery is only a treatment option [20].

Patients with slow symptom onset before the diagnosis are often associated to a progressive neurological improvement and long-term survival. Weiner and co-workers reported a clinical course before the diagnosis of 24 weeks [35]. In patients with slow tumor growth and low grade tumors, even if the resection was subtotal, the clinical outcome was favorable [26]. On the other side, the neurological condition of fast growing neoplasm and acute onset symptoms, independently from the resection grade achieved, was not favorable. A symptom onset in the last 15 weeks was associated to a shorter progression free survival (PFS) at 5 years follow-up (Weiner describes a 46% PFS in patients with symptoms duration of less than 15 weeks, compared to the 72% more than 15 weeks). The second component able to conditionate the neurological status and the global survival is the tumor grade to the histopathological diagnosis [26]. The survival of patients treated for high grade gliomas was not superior to 6–9 months. On the other side, low grade tumors showed 5 years survival rate of 89% [35].

Very frequently, most of the studies demonstrate that preoperative neurological status is the most significative factor influencing the neurological and functional status of the patients in postoperative period [32, 35, 44, 49, 50, 52, 53]. Early surgical resection of intramedullary tumors is often recommended in order to maintain a good neurological condition and to avoid a severe deterioration. Malignant astrocytomas (WHO grade 3 and 4) are the only intramedullary tumors in which there is not a correlation between early surgery and neurological preservation or survival. In conclusion, the surgical resection has to be performed in all the patients with progressive neurological impairment because preoperative neurological status remains the most influencing predictive factor on the postoperative status [20]. The guide principle for the surgical resection of intramedullary tumors is traditionally based on the identification of an interface between tumor and adjacent parenchymal surface, defined as plane of dissection (POD). Benign tumors such as ependymomas and hemangioblastomas often show a clear plane of dissection and this facilitates the resection [54–56]. The presence of this plane has always encouraged the surgeons to perform a gross total resection [54, 55, 57]. The surgical treatment of malignant intramedullary neoplasms is still controversial [58, 59]. For infiltrating tumors such as astrocytomas, the absence of a plane of dissection has often led the surgeons to perform a subtotal resection or sometimes a simple biopsy in order to avoid aggressive manipulations that might cause neurological impairment [54, 60]. Garcés-Ambrossi and co-workers described the surgical experience of more than 100 patients; in the majority of cases they obtained a gross total resection but the good results were associated to the dimensions of the tumors and to the presence of a POD. The authors noticed that a clinical improvement during follow-up was associated to the presence of a POD in patients with an early postoperative improvement [40]. Gross total resection is often associated to a favorable outcome, mostly in low grade tumors such as ependymomas [61, 62] and hemangioblastomas [40, 63, 64]. The analysis of single and small case numbers suggest that a gross total resection is independent by the tumor dimensions; many authors, on the other hand, sustain that small tumors with a well-recognizable POD allow a gross total resection and an en bloc resection. The presence of a well-recognizable POD is one of the most important aspects for a safe and aggressive surgical resection. Many authors, as Schwartz and McCormick [65], emphasized this factor and suggested a more extended myelotomy to minimize the debulking maneuvers and an aggressive hemostasis to efficiently identify the different planes [40, 61, 66].

The vast majority of the literature on intramedullary tumors affirms that the presence or absence of a POD is histology related [52, 66–68], Garcés-Ambrossi affirms that there is a wide interindividual variability in the same histotype, and the presence of a POD is the element to be primarily considered to evaluate the entity of the resection. Any histotype might present a high variability if a POD is present or absent. The presence of a POD, independently from the grade of malignancy, is a positive prognostic factor to evaluate the biological behavior of the tumor and the recurrence rate [40].

In the study of Karikari, it is the histopathology that assumes a predictive value towards the presence of a POD and the resection grade [54]. Karikari obtained a gross total resection in 96.4% of cases, and in all cases a clear POD was identified. About 50% of patients with recurrence had not a clear POD. Similar results were obtained for hemangioblastomas and other tumors. None of the astrocytomas presented a clear POD, so that it did not report any gross total resection on this kind of tumor [54]. These data appear to be in contrast with what has been reported by Garcés-Ambrossi, that described gross total resection in 25%, 40%, and 44% of pilocytic astrocytomas, grade II, and malignant, respectively. This extreme diversity in the results in the different series makes it difficult to formulate recommendations for the management of intramedullary astrocytomas [40]. McGirt, for example, in his study, reported that gross total resection in intramedullary astrocytomas might not be associated to a statistically significant survival increase, and the surgical invasiveness is associated to a motor impairment [54, 58]. Unsatisfactory results in terms of short survival associated to astrocytomas surgery have been also described in Minehan's retrospective study, underlining the uncertainty for an optimal treatment [69]. Therefore, the surgical resection of astrocytomas without a clear POD should be influenced by factors such as the patient's will, the surgeon experience, and the intraoperative modifications of intraoperative motor and sensory evoked potentials. On the other hand, for benign tumors with intraoperative evidence of a POD, a gross total resection should be attempted due to the significant impact on the recurrence rate [54].

Another interesting aspect is the neurological status in the early and late follow-up. As reported by Garcés-Ambrossi, in one-third of the patients there is a neurological deterioration, and half of those have a consistent recovery during the following month. Most of the treated patients, therefore, presented an improvement of the preoperative neurological impairment, with a stable improvement maintained during follow-up [40].

An estimation of the postoperative neurological deterioration after intramedullary tumor resection is of about 20% in most of the series of the literature [52, 67, 70]. The only independent factors associated with an acute deterioration are the advanced age and an unfavorable MEP alteration during the surgical maneuvers [54, 71–73].

In the series of Garcés-Ambrossi, about a half of the patients with postoperative neurological deterioration returned to the preoperative neurological function in about 30 days from surgery [40].

Many authors describe a 60% improvement of the motor impairment 6 weeks after surgery [40, 64, 74].

Even if many authors affirm that the primary aim of intramedullary tumors surgery is to maintain the preoperative neurological status [44, 65, 75] and suggest to perform surgery before a neurological deterioration, other authors advocate that many patients might neurologically ameliorate and maintain this result event years after surgery [40, 44, 50, 52, 66, 76–79].

According to some authors, the strongest predictive factors that might influence the neurological outcome are the preoperative neurological status and the tumor histology, with a stability in maintaining the preoperative neurological status [54].

Authors such as Xu and co-workers describe a 77.6% rate of neurological improvement in the long-term follow-up [70]. Also in this point the results appear to be discordant with the results obtained by Karikari, that reported 20% of ependymomas had a neurological improvement, 69% maintained the same preoperative status, and 10.9% had a worsening. Even worse are the results obtained with astrocytomas: only 4.8% had a neurological improvement, 47.6 remained stable, 47% had a worsening.

In astrocytomas evaluation, the neurological impairment might be associated to a multifactorial aetiogenesis: sometimes as the result of a too aggressive surgery (early impairment in the postoperative period), but more often by the recurrence, responsible for a long-term neurological deterioration [54].

The anatomical location has been often associated to different neurological conditions during follow-up [50, 52, 54, 55]. Different conclusions might be analyzed about PFS, an aspect extremely variable and dependent by histology. Many studies analyze PFS with a recurrence rate between 34 and 54% [43, 66, 79], and according to some authors the association between adjuvant therapy and radiotherapy does not seem to be independently associated to survival [40, 80–82].

For the majority of the papers, histology is the most important predictive factor of PFS [66, 79]. The Garcés-Ambrossi study adds an interesting perspective. It affirms that the presence of a clear POD has a role in conditioning PFS with a value even higher than neoplasm histology, reporting an increasing PFS in each histotype. At 48 months the survival in ependymomas was 86% against 50% (absence of POD), at 48 months the survival of hemangioblastomas was 93% against 0% (absence of POD), at 24 months the survival of grade II astrocytomas was 100% against 43% (absence of POD); at 6 months the survival of a high grade astrocytoma was 50% against 25% (absence of plane) [40].

The association between PFS and gross total resection has been also described for hemangioblastomas and ependymomas, probably because the postoperative inflammation might eliminate and neutralize the microscopical residues [83, 84]. This same association is not so clear in the evaluation of astrocytomas [40, 43, 78, 85, 86].

25.10 Our Results/Institutional Findings

Our department describes its own surgical experience on intramedullary tumors of the CVJ through the results obtained in the resection of 28 neoplasms in the period between 1990 and 2016. All the patients had been treated with surgery, in the attempt of a gross total resection. Our series comprehended a 78.5% of low grade or benign tumors and a 21.5% of high grade tumors. The population included: 18% low grade astrocytomas, 14% hemangioblastomas, 11% low grade ependymomas, 36% cavernomas, 18% high grade astrocytomas, 3% high grade ependymomas.

This retrospective study analyzed all the intrinsic tumors involving the medulla oblongata (43%), the cervical spinal cord in its rostral portion (from C1 to C4 with involvement of the foramen magnum area, 25%), and cervicomedullary tumors (32%). Analyzing the growth pattern of the low grade tumors emerged a stereotypical pattern; also in our experience these tumors did not extend beyond the limit of the ponto-bulbar junction, and in 25% of the cases they extended cranially into the IV ventricle.

The duration onset of the symptoms was very long, with a mean value of 22, 8 weeks before the diagnosis. About 64% in the series showed a slowly progressive symptom onset, of more than 6 weeks. The long clinical history did not seem to be related (in a statistically significant manner) to a better long-term outcome. About 89% of the patients complained for sensitive or motor impairment and involvement of the pyramidal tracts, 43% had cranial nerves impairment (IX, X, XI, and XII cranial nerves), 11% had respiratory and cardiac disturbances, 21% pain, and 14% symptoms related to hydrocephalus.

All the patients who underwent surgery were symptomatic. In 61% of the patients, we performed a median suboccipital approach with the removal of C1 posterior arch (median tumors with main posterior development); in 35.5% of median suboccipital approaches, the extension to the IV ventricle imposed an adjunctive surgical route: transvermian in two cases and telovelar in four cases. In 18% of patients, a postero-lateral approach was performed (neoplasms with main anterior or anterolateral component) and with C1 posterior arch removal.

In 21% of patients, a posterior median cervical approach with laminectomy (83%) or laminotomy (17%) frequently associated with a small median suboccipital craniectomy to allow a better control of the foramen magnum area (intramedullary cervical tumors). Since the introduction of the neurophysiological examination, all patients underwent surgery with the possibility to control SSEP, MEP, EMG monitoring, and also cranial nerves.

In our series, a gross total resection was obtained in 54% of the patients, a subtotal resection (>90%) in 14%, and a partial resection (between 50 and 90%) in the remaining 32%. In 71% of our patients, a POD was clearly identified. The POD presence increased in a statistically significant manner ($P = 0.0004$) the possibility to perform a gross total resection, and this influenced a better neurological status during follow-up ($P < 0.0001$ al KPS, P 0.0004 MC). In our series, the presence of a POD was not statistically related to the histological subgroup. Gross total resection was influenced, in a statistically significant manner ($P < 0.0001$), by the histotype: in 100% of cavernomas and 75% of hemangioblastomas, a gross total resection was obtained; in 100% of high grade astrocytomas, a subtotal resection was achieved.

A high variability in maximal cytoreduction for all the low grade astrocytomas (low grade gliomas and ependymomas showed in 78% of the cases gross total resections or subtotal resections).

The gross total removal of the neoplasm seemed to be statistically significant on a better long-term outcome: 73% of the patients had a KPS > 70 (P 0.0012) or I grade MC (P 0.031) during late follow-up.

This result confirms that, in absence of intraoperative alterations in the neurophysiological monitoring, the target in tumor removal should be a total resection. In our experience, the gross total resection was not associated to a further neurological impairment.

The early neurological postoperative morbidity was 25%: 7% had a de novo cranial nerve impairment, 11% had a worsening in sensory and motor impairment, 7% had a de novo cardiac and respiratory impairment. The aforementioned morbidity was compatible with the procedure-related risk.

Despite the functional eloquence of this anatomical region, surgery allows an important stability of the preoperative symptoms.

During the 5.6 years follow-up (range 11 days–14 years), the neurological status was evaluated in a more accurate fashion, with an evaluation of the functional status with Karnofsky performance score (KPS) and McCormick grade (MC).

The preoperative evaluation, in 54% of the population, was KPS > 70, and 46% had a KPS ≤ 70 (32% MC grade I, 61% MC grade II, 7% MC grade III). At the end of follow-up, 79% of patients had a KPS > 70, while only 21% had a KPS ≤ 70 (75% MC grade I, 17% MC grade II, 8% MC grade III).

The late clinical worsening, defined as tardive morbidity, was evidenced in 21% of patients; in 84% of cases it was related to disease progression, with consequent neurological impairment in high grade gliomas. The overall survival rate was relevantly influenced by histology: low grade or benign tumors had 7 years overall survival and high grade gliomas showed 11.7 months survival.

The identification of a clear POD ($P < 0.0001$), the possibility of a gross total resection or a semi-total resection (P 0.0012), a preoperative functional status with a KPS > 70 or MC grade I (P 0.0012), the histological typization (hemangioblastomas, low grade gliomas, cavernomas), the use of intraoperative neuromonitoring and the advanced imaging (P 0.05), and the absence of tardive morbidity ($P < 0.0001$) were related to a statistically significant better tardive follow-up (KPS > 70 and MC grade I).

The possibility to maintain an optimal functional status during the follow-up was a prognostic positive factor on OS and PFS. About 94% of patients with tardive KPS > 70/MC grade I survived at the late follow-up and had a very low recurrence rate.

25.11 Conclusions

CVJ intramedullary tumors are rare neoplasms of the transition area between spinal cord and brainstem, for many years scarcely described in the literature.

The majority of these tumors are histologically benign, with a slow growth pattern, and a typical long-term onset of the symptoms before the diagnosis; they are considered suitable for a radical surgical resection. They have a stereotypical growth pattern, with the tendency to respect the white matter pathways. The goal of the surgical treatment is to reach, with the help of the neurophysiological monitoring, a maximal cytoreduction with a minimal postoperative risk of neurological damage.

This patient subgroup has many similarities with the pure intramedullary tumors. The total tumor resection is possible only with a clear POD between tumor and parenchyma, despite the functional eloquence of the anatomical area. In absence of a POD, it is recommended a submaximal resection in order to preserve the neurological function. These tumors show an indolent behavior, and are associated with a reduced rate of recurrence/regrowth, even if a gross total removal is not performed.

Obtaining a gross total resection is related to a better late functional outcome (evaluated with KPS and McCormick). Surgery is not free of risks. Those tumors are characterized by a good functional outcome, but not the high grade tumors, that are less represented and associated to an unfavorable biological and growth pattern.

The evaluation of late KPS and MC allowed to observe that the favorable outcome was often associated to: specific histological subgroups (hemangioblastomas, low grade gliomas/ependymomas and cavernomas), the presence of a POD, the achievement of a gross total or a subtotal resection, a good preoperative neurological condition, the use of intraoperative neuromonitoring and advanced imaging, the absence of late morbidity. An optimal functional outcome is a relevant element for an augmented overall survival and a good PFS (Fig. 25.1).

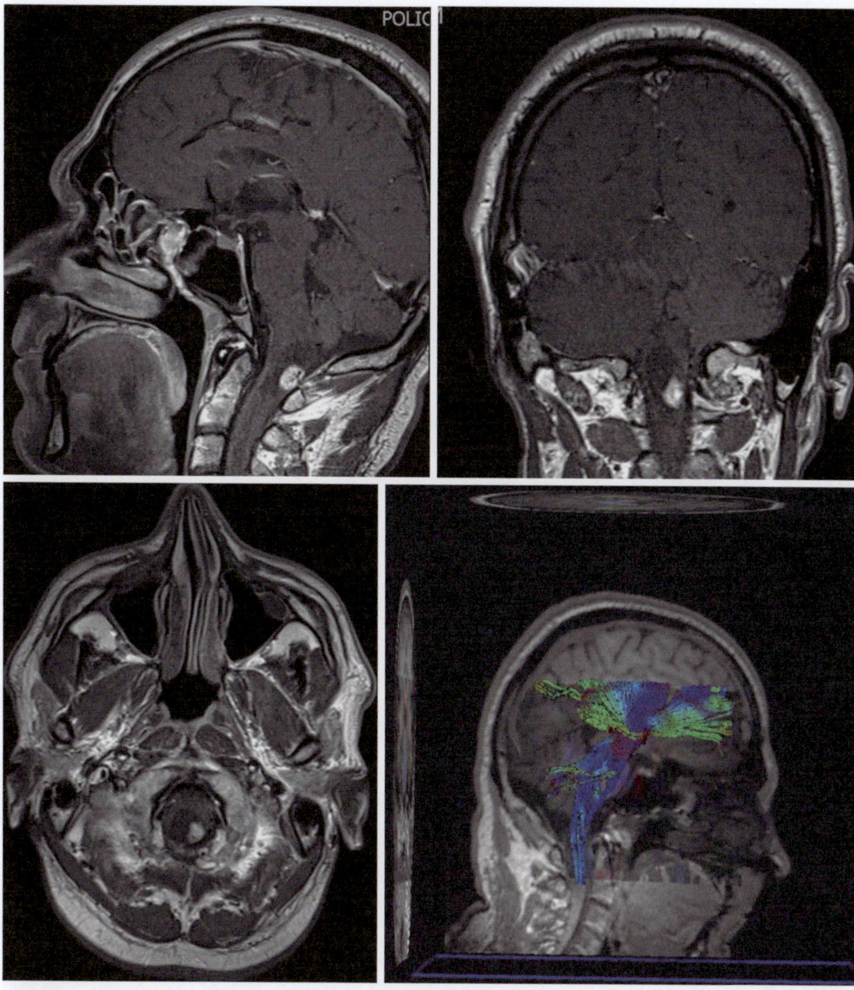

Fig. 25.1 (1) Sagittal scan, (2) coronal scan, and (3) axial scan of preoperative MRI: T1-weighted sequences with gadolinium that show a cervicomedullary pilocytic astrocytoma in a young man (34 years old). (4, 5) Sagittal scans (T2-weighted sequences) with fibers tracking reconstruction in preoperative MRI: cervicomedullary pilocytic astrocytoma (young man—34 years old) displacing anteriorly white matter. (6) Sagittal scan, (7) coronal scan, and (8) axial scan of postoperative MRI: T1-weighted sequences with gadolinium that show complete removal of a cervicomedullary pilocytic astrocytoma in a young man (34 years old). (9) Sagittal scan and (10) axial scan in T1-weighted sequences with gadolinium; (11) sagittal scan and (12) axial scan in T2-weighted sequences: preoperative MRI of medullary hemangioblastoma in adult woman (56 years old). (13) Sagittal scan and (14) axial scan in T2-weighted sequences; (15) sagittal scan and (16) axial scan in T1-weighted sequences with gadolinium: postoperative MRI that shows complete removal of a medullary hemangioblastoma in adult woman (56 years old)

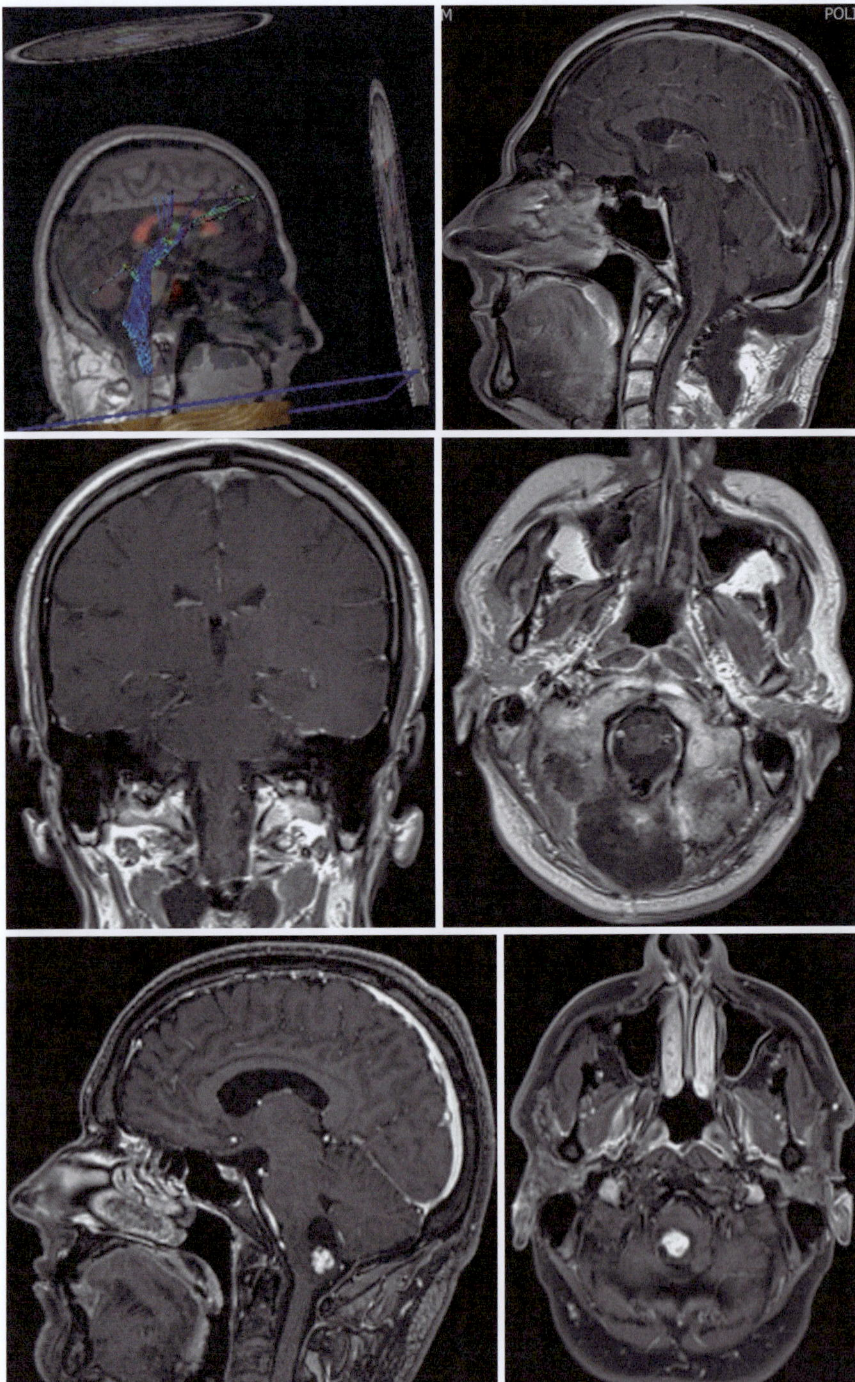

Fig. 25.1 (continued)

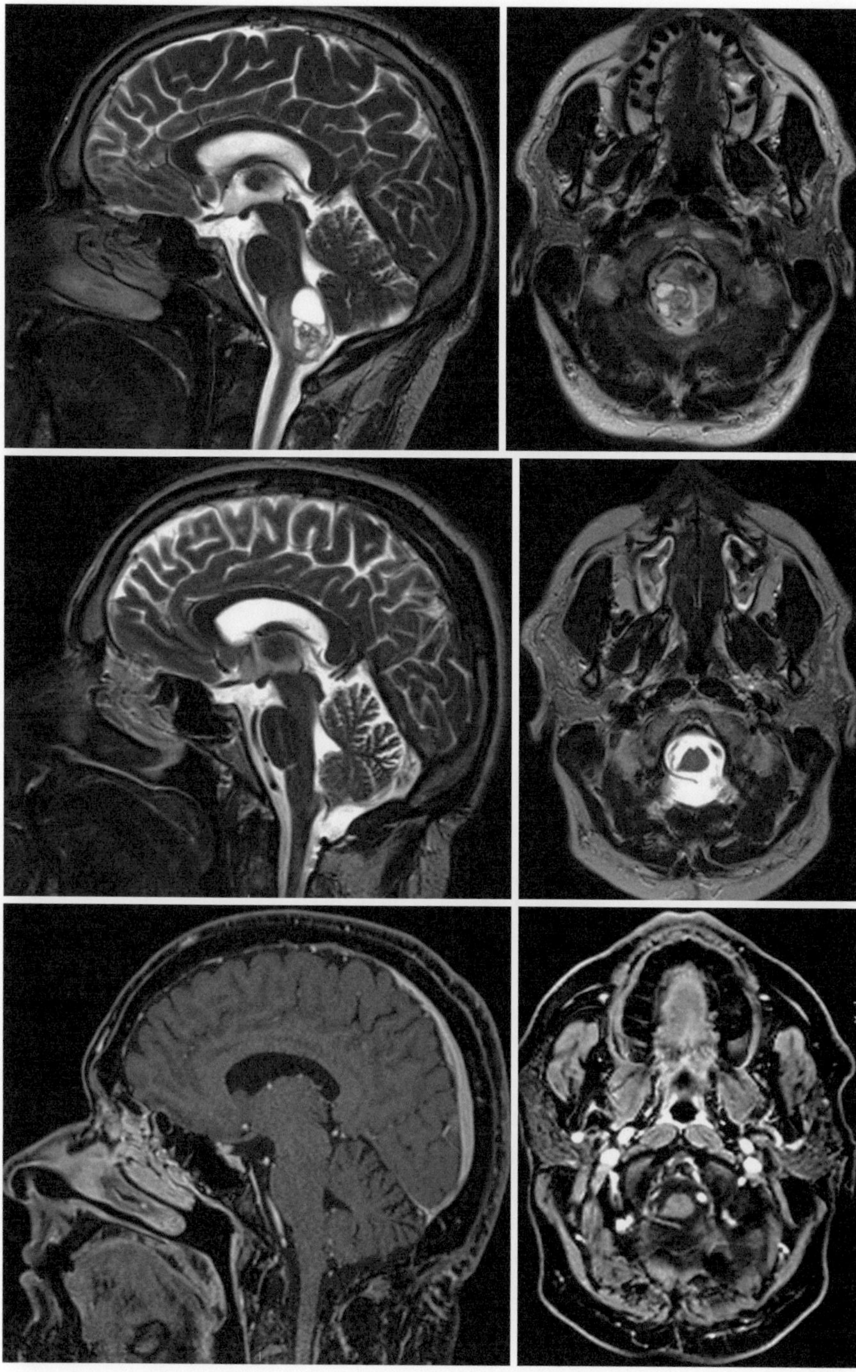

Fig. 25.1 (continued)

References

1. Nair AP, Mehrotra A, Das KK, Srivastava AK, Sahu RN, Kumar R. Clinico-radiological profile and nuances in the management of cervicomedullary junction intramedullary tumors. Asian J Neurosurg. 2014;9(1):21–8.
2. Samartzis D, Gillis CC, Shih P, O'Toole JE, Fessler RG. Intramedullary spinal cord tumors: part I-epidemiology, pathophysiology, and diagnosis. Global Spine J. 2015;5(5):425–35.
3. Krishnaney A, Modic MT. Chapter 18: Radiology of the spine. In: Winn HR, MD Copyright © 2011, 2004, 1996, 1990, 1982, 1973 by Saunders, an imprint of Elsevier Inc. Youmans neurological surgery. 6th ed. ISBN: 978-1-4160-5316-3.
4. Diagnostic imaging brain Anne G. Osborn text—Copyright Anne G. Osborn MD 2004 Composition by Amirsys Inc, Salt Lake City, Utah Printed by Friesens, Altona, Manitoba, Canada ISBN: 0-7216-2905-9.
5. Karam YR, Menezes AH, Traynelis VC. Posterolateral approaches to the craniovertebral junction. Neurosurgery. 2010;66(Suppl 3):A135–40.
6. Setzer M, Murtagh RD, Murtagh FR, Eleraky M, Jain S, Marquardt G, Seifert V, Vrionis FD. Diffusion tensor imaging tractography in patients with intramedullary tumors: comparison with intraoperative findings and value for prediction of tumor resectability. J Neurosurg Spine. 2010;13(3):371–80.
7. Landi A, Palmarini V, D'Elia A, Marotta N, Salvati M, Santoro A, Delfini R. Magnetic resonance diffusion tensor imaging and fiber-tracking diffusion tensor tractography in the management of spinal astrocytomas. World J Clin Cases. 2016;4(1):1–4.
8. Matsushima T, Inoue T, Inamura T, Natori Y, Ikezaki K, Fukui M. Transcerebellomedullary fissure approach with special reference to methods of dissecting the fissure. J Neurosurg. 2001;94(2):257–64.
9. Cohen AR, editor. Surgical disorders of the fourth ventricle. Cambridge: Blackwell Science; 1996. p. 147–60.
10. Kempe LG. Operative neurosurgery, vol. 2. New York: Springer; 1970. p. 1–13.
11. Kempe LG. Operative neurosurgery, vol. 2. New York: Springer; 1970. p. 14–33.
12. Sekhar LN. Midline and paramedian posterior fossa approaches to cerebellar and brainstem lesions. In: Sekhar LN, de Oliveira E, editors. Cranial microsurgery: approaches and techniques. New York: Thieme; 1999. p. 378–99.
13. Tanriover N, Ulm AJ, Rhoton AL Jr, Yasuda A. Comparison of the transvermian and telovelar approaches to the fourth ventricle. J Neurosurg. 2004;101(3):484–98.
14. Dandy WE. The brain. Practice of surgery. Hagerstown. In: Lewis D, editor. WF Prior; 1966. p. 452–8.
15. Kawashima M, Tanriover N, Rhoton AL Jr, Ulm AJ, Matsushima T. Comparison of the far lateral and extreme lateral variants of the atlanto-occipital transarticular approach to anterior extradural lesions of the craniovertebral junction. Neurosurgery. 2003;53(3):662–74; discussion 674–5.
16. Wen HT, Rhoton AL Jr, Katsuta T, de Oliveira E. Microsurgical anatomy of the transcondylar, supracondylar, and paracondylar extensions of the far-lateral approach. J Neurosurg. 1997;87:555–85.
17. Kyoshima K, Kobayashi S, Hirohiko GMO, Kuroyanagi T. A study of safe entry zones via the floor of the fourth ventricle for brain-stem lesions. J Neurosurg. 1993;78:987–93.
18. Cantore G, Missori P, Santoro A. Cavernous angiomas of the brain stem. Intra-axial anatomical pitfalls and surgical strategies. Surg Neurol. 1999;52(1):84–93; discussion 93–4.
19. Bricolo A, Turazzi S. Surgery for gliomas and other mass lesions of the brainstem. Adv Tech Stand Neurosurg. 1995;22:261–341.
20. Harrop JS, Ganju A, Groff M, Bilsky M. Primary intramedullary tumors of the spinal cord. Spine (Phila Pa 1976). 2009;34(22 Suppl):S69–77.
21. Samartzis D, Gillis CC, Shih P, O'Toole JE, Fessler RG. Intramedullary spinal cord tumors: part II—management options and outcomes. Global Spine J. 2016;6(2):176–85.
22. Sala F, Bricolo A, Faccioli F, Lanteri P, Gerosa M. Surgery for intramedullary spinal cord tumors: the role of intraoperative (neurophysiological) monitoring. Eur Spine J. 2007;16(Suppl 2):S130–9. Review.

23. Kothbauer KF. Intraoperative neurophysiologic monitoring for intramedullary spinal-cord tumor surgery. Neurophysiol Clin. 2007;37(6):407–14.
24. Elsberg CA, Beer E. The operability of intramedullary tumors of the spinal cord. A report of two operations with remarks upon the extrusion of intraspinal tumors. Am J Med Sci. 1911;142:636–47.
25. Guidetti B, Mercuri S, Vagnozzi R. Long-term results of the surgical treatment of 129 intramedullary spinal gliomas. J Neurosurg. 1981;54(3):323–30.
26. Epstein F, Wisoff J. Intra-axial tumors of the cervicomedullary junction. J Neurosurg. 1987;67(4):483–7.
27. Epstein F, McCleary EL. Intrinsic brain-stem tumors of childhood: surgical indications. J Neurosurg. 1986;64(1):11–5.
28. Epstein F, Epstein N. Intramedullary tumors of the spinal cord. In: American Association of Neurological Surgeons, editor. Pediatric neurosurgery. Surgery of the developing nervous system. New York: Grune & Stratton; 1982. p. 529–39.
29. Epstein F, Epstein N. Surgical management of extensive intramedullary spinal cord astrocytomas in children. In: American Society for Pediatric Neurosurgery, editor. Concepts in pediatric neurosurgery 2. Basel: Karger; 1982. p. 29–44.
30. Epstein F, Epstein N. Surgical management of holocord intramedullary spinal cord astrocytomas in children. Report of three cases. J Neurosurg. 1981;54(6):829–32.
31. Epstein F. Surgical treatment of extensive spinal cord astrocytomas of childhood. In: Raimondi AJ, editor. Concepts in pediatric neurosurgery 3. Basel: Karger; 1983. p. 157–69.
32. Epstein F, Epstein N. Surgical treatment of spinal cord astrocytomas of childhood. A series of 19 patients. J Neurosurg. 1982;57(5):685–9.
33. Epstein F, Wisoff J. Spinal cord astrocytomas of childhood: surgical considerations. In: Long DM, editor. Current therapy in neurological surgery, 1985-1986. Philadelphia: BC Decker; 1984. p. 159–61.
34. Raghavendra BN, Epstein F, McCleary L. Intramedullary spinal cord tumors in children: localization by intraoperative sonography. AJNR Am J Neuroradiol. 1984;5(4):395–7.
35. Weiner HL, Freed D, Woo HH, Rezai AR, Kim R, Epstein FJ. Intra-axial tumors of the cervicomedullary junction: surgical results and long-term outcome. Pediatr Neurosurg. 1997;27(1):12–8.
36. Abbott R, Ragheb J, Epstein FJ. Brainstem tumors: surgical indications. In: Cheek WR, Marlin AE, McLone DG, Reigel DH, Walker ML, editors. Pediatric neurosurgery: surgery of the developing nervous system. 3rd ed. Philadelphia: Saunders; 1994. p. 374–82.
37. Epstein FJ, Farmer JP. Brain-stem glioma growth patterns. J Neurosurg. 1993;78(3):408–12.
38. Squires LA, Constantini S, Miller DC, Epstein F. Diffuse infiltrating astrocytoma of the cervicomedullary region: clinicopathologic entity. Pediatr Neurosurg. 1997;27(3):153–9.
39. McAbee JH, Modica J, Thompson CJ, Broniscer A, Orr B, Choudhri AF, Boop FA, Klimo P Jr. Cervicomedullary tumors in children. J Neurosurg Pediatr. 2015;16(4):357–66.
40. Garcés-Ambrossi GL, McGirt MJ, Mehta VA, Sciubba DM, Witham TF, Bydon A, Wolinksy JP, Jallo GI, Gokaslan ZL. Factors associated with progression-free survival and long-term neurological outcome after resection of intramedullary spinal cord tumors: analysis of 101 consecutive cases. J Neurosurg Spine. 2009;11(5):591–9.
41. Daumas-Duport C. Patterns of tumor growth and problems associated with histological typing of low-grade gliomas. In: Apuzzo MLJ, editor. Benign cerebral glioma, vol. 1. Washington: American Association of Neurological Surgeons Publications; 1995. p. 125–47.
42. Aghakhani N, David P, Parker F, Lacroix C, Benoudiba F, Tadie M. Intramedullary spinal ependymomas: analysis of a consecutive series of 82 adult cases with particular attention to patients with no preoperative neurological deficit. Neurosurgery. 2008;62(6):1279–85; discussion 1285–6.
43. Cooper PR. Outcome after operative treatment of intramedullary spinal cord tumors in adults: intermediate and long-term results in 51 patients. Neurosurgery. 1989;25(6):855–9.
44. Epstein FJ, Farmer JP, Freed D. Adult intramedullary spinal cord ependymomas: the result of surgery in 38 patients. J Neurosurg. 1993;79(2):204–9.

45. Ferrante L, Mastronardi L, Celli P, Lunardi P, Acqui M, Fortuna A. Intramedullary spinal cord ependymomas—a study of 45 cases with long-term follow-up. Acta Neurochir (Wien). 1992;119(1–4):74–9.
46. Garcia DM. Primary spinal cord tumors treated with surgery and postoperative irradiation. Int J Radiat Oncol Biol Phys. 1985;11(11):1933–9.
47. Jallo GI, Danish S, Velasquez L, Epstein F. Intramedullary low-grade astrocytomas: long-term outcome following radical surgery. J Neurooncol. 2001;53(1):61–6.
48. Jallo GI, Freed D, Epstein F. Intramedullary spinal cord tumors in children. Childs Nerv Syst. 2003;19(9):641–9.
49. Samii M, Klekamp J. Surgical results of 100 intramedullary tumors in relation to accompanying syringomyelia. Neurosurgery. 1994;35(5):865–73; discussion 873.
50. Sandalcioglu IE, Gasser T, Asgari S, Lazorisak A, Engelhorn T, Egelhof T, Stolke D, Wiedemayer H. Functional outcome after surgical treatment of intramedullary spinal cord tumors: experience with 78 patients. Spinal Cord. 2005;43(1):34–41.
51. Shrivastava RK, Epstein FJ, Perin NI, Post KD, Jallo GI. Intramedullary spinal cord tumors in patients older than 50 years of age: management and outcome analysis. J Neurosurg Spine. 2005;2(3):249–55.
52. Cristante L, Herrmann HD. Surgical management of intramedullary spinal cord tumors: functional outcome and sources of morbidity. Neurosurgery. 1994;35(1):69–74; discussion 74–6.
53. Innocenzi G, Raco A, Cantore G, Raimondi AJ. Intramedullary astrocytomas and ependymomas in the pediatric age group: a retrospective study. Childs Nerv Syst. 1996;12(12):776–80.
54. Karikari IO, Nimjee SM, Hodges TR, Cutrell E, Hughes BD, Powers CJ, Mehta AI, Hardin C, Bagley CA, Isaacs RE, Haglund MM, Friedman AH. Impact of tumor histology on resectability and neurological outcome in primary intramedullary spinal cord tumors: a single-center experience with 102 patients. Neurosurgery. 2011;68(1):188–97; discussion 197.
55. Hoshimaru M, Koyama T, Hashimoto N, Kikuchi H. Results of microsurgical treatment for intramedullary spinal cord ependymomas: analysis of 36 cases. Neurosurgery. 1999;44(2):264–9.
56. Merchant TE, Kiehna EN, Thompson SJ, Heideman R, Sanford RA, Kun LE. Pediatric low-grade and ependymal spinal cord tumors. Pediatr Neurosurg. 2000;32(1):30–6.
57. Kochbati L, Nasr C, Frikha H, Gargouri W, Benna F, Besbes M, Daoud J, Bouaouina N, Ben Abdallah M, Maalej M. Primary intramedullary ependymomas: retrospective study of 16 cases. Cancer Radiother. 2003;7(1):17–21.
58. McGirt MJ, Goldstein IM, Chaichana KL, Tobias ME, Kothbauer KF, Jallo GI. Extent of surgical resection of malignant astrocytomas of the spinal cord: outcome analysis of 35 patients. Neurosurgery. 2008;63(1):55–60; discussion 60–1.
59. Kane PJ, el-Mahdy W, Singh A, Powell MP, Crockard HA. Spinal intradural tumors: part II–intramedullary. Br J Neurosurg. 1999;13(6):558–63.
60. Constantini S, Miller DC, Allen JC, Rorke LB, Freed D, Epstein FJ. Radical excision of intramedullary spinal cord tumors: surgical morbidity and longterm follow-up evaluation in 164 children and young adults. J Neurosurg. 2000;93(2 Suppl):183–93.
61. Hanbali F, Fourney DR, Marmor E, Suki D, Rhines LD, Weinberg JS, McCutcheon IE, Gokaslan AL, et al. Neurosurgery. 2002;51(5):1162–72; discussion 1172–4.
62. McCormick PC, Torres R, Post KD, Stein BM. Intramedullary ependymoma of the spinal cord. J Neurosurg. 1990;72(4):523–32.
63. Cristante L, Herrmann HD. Surgical management of intramedullary hemangioblastoma of the spinal cord. Acta Neurochir (Wien). 1999;141(4):333–9; discussion 339–40.
64. Lonser RR, Weil RJ, Wanebo JE, DeVroom HL, Oldfield EH. Surgical management of spinal cord hemangioblastomas in patients with von Hippel-Lindau disease. J Neurosurg. 2003;98(1):106–16.
65. Schwartz TH, McCormick PC. Intramedullary ependymomas: clinical presentation, surgical treatment strategies and prognosis. J Neurooncol. 2000;47(3):211–8.
66. Constantini S, Miller DC, Allen JC, Freed D, Ozek MM, Rorke LB, et al. Radical excision of intramedullary spinal cord tumors: surgical morbidity and long-term follow-up evaluation in 164 children and young adults. J Neurosurg. 2000;93:183–93.

67. Brotchi J, Dewitte O, Levivier M, Balériaux D, Vandesteene A, Raftopoulos C, Flament-Durand J, Noterman J. A survey of 65 tumors within the spinal cord: surgical results and the importance of preoperative magnetic resonance imaging. Neurosurgery. 1991;29(5):651–6; discussion 656–7.
68. Epstein FJ, Farmer JP, Freed D. Adult intramedullary astrocytomas of the spinal cord. J Neurosurg. 1992;77(3):355–9.
69. Minehan KJ, Brown PD, Scheithauer BW, Krauss WE, Wright MP. Prognosis and treatment of spinal cord astrocytoma. Int J Radiat Oncol Biol Phys. 2009;73(3):727–33.
70. Xu QW, Bao WM, Mao RL, Yang GY. Aggressive surgery for intramedullary tumor of cervical spinal cord. Surg Neurol. 1996;46(4):322–8.
71. Constantini S, Houten J, Miller DC, Freed D, Ozek MM, Rorke LB, Allen JC, Epstein FJ. Intramedullary spinal cord tumors in children under the age of 3 years. J Neurosurg. 1996;85(5):1036–43.
72. Kelleher MO, Tan G, Sarjeant R, Fehlings MG. Predictive value of intraoperative neurophysiological monitoring during cervical spine surgery: a prospective analysis of 1055 consecutive patients. J Neurosurg Spine. 2008;8(3):215–21.
73. Kothbauer K, Deletis V, Epstein FJ. Intraoperative spinal cord monitoring for intramedullary surgery: an essential adjunct. Pediatr Neurosurg. 1997;26(5):247–54.
74. Goh KY, Velasquez L, Epstein FJ. Pediatric intramedullary spinal cord tumors: is surgery alone enough? Pediatr Neurosurg. 1997;27(1):34–9.
75. Roonprapunt C, Houten JK. Spinal cord astrocytomas: presentation, management, and outcome. Neurosurg Clin N Am. 2006;17(1):29–36.
76. Chang UK, Choe WJ, Chung SK, Chung CK, Kim HJ. Surgical outcome and prognostic factors of spinal intramedullary ependymomas in adults. J Neurooncol. 2002;57(2):133–9.
77. Cooper PR, Epstein F. Radical resection of intramedullary spinal cord tumors in adults. Recent experience in 29 patients. J Neurosurg. 1985;63(4):492–9.
78. Innocenzi G, Salvati M, Cervoni L, Delfini R, Cantore G. Prognostic factors in intramedullary astrocytomas. Clin Neurol Neurosurg. 1997;99(1):1–5.
79. Raco A, Esposito V, Lenzi J, Piccirilli M, Delfini R, Cantore G. Long-term follow-up of intramedullary spinal cord tumors: a series of 202 cases. Neurosurgery. 2005;56(5):972–81.
80. Bouffet E, Pierre-Kahn A, Marchal JC, Jouvet A, Kalifa C, Choux M, Dhellemmes P, Guérin J, Tremoulet M, Mottolese C. Prognostic factors in pediatric spinal cord astrocytoma. Cancer. 1998;83(11):2391–9.
81. Eyre HJ, Crowley JJ, Townsend JJ, Eltringham JR, Morantz RA, Schulman SF, Quagliana JM, al-Sarraf M. A randomized trial of radiotherapy versus radiotherapy plus CCNU for incompletely resected low-grade gliomas: a Southwest Oncology Group study. J Neurosurg. 1993;78(6):909–14.
82. Fisher BJ, Bauman GS, Leighton CE, Liard A, Zomosa G, Menei P, et al. Low-grade gliomas in children: tumor volume response to radiation. Neurosurg Focus. 1998;4(4):E5.
83. Jarnagin WR, Zager JS, Klimstra D, Delman KA, Malhotra S, Ebright M, Little S, DeRubertis B, Stanziale SF, Hezel M, Federoff H, Fong Y. Neoadjuvant treatment of hepatic malignancy: an oncolytic herpes simplex virus expressing IL-12 effectively treats the parent tumor and protects against recurrence-after resection. Cancer Gene Ther. 2003;10(3):215–23.
84. Koebel CM, Vermi W, Swann JB, Zerafa N, Rodig SJ, Old LJ, Smyth MJ, Schreiber RD. Adaptive immunity maintains occult cancer in an equilibrium state. Nature. 2007;450(7171):903–7.
85. Minehan KJ, Shaw EG, Scheithauer BW, Davis DL, Onofrio BM. Spinal cord astrocytoma: pathological and treatment considerations. J Neurosurg. 1995;83(4):590–5.
86. Sandler HM, Papadopoulos SM, Thornton AF Jr, Ross DA. Spinal cord astrocytomas: results of therapy. Neurosurgery. 1992;30(4):490–3.

26 The Anterior (Endoscopic Endonasal) Approach and Outcomes for Foramen Magnum Tumors

Nathan T. Zwagerman, Juan C. Fernandez-Miranda, Eric W. Wang, Carl H. Snyderman, and Paul A. Gardner

26.1 Introduction

Disorders of the ventral cranio-vertebral junction are rare and, depending on the pathology, present because of neural element compression or pain. The classic description of foramen magnum syndrome involves weakness in one arm, followed by the ipsilateral leg, contralateral leg, and finally the contralateral upper extremity. More commonly, lesions in this area can present slowly with varying degrees of myelopathy, weakness, and cranial nerve deficit which are often indolent in nature leading to delayed diagnosis. Many of these patients present initially with posterior head and neck pain similarly to those classically associated with Chiari malformation. The treatment for diseases in this region depends largely on the pathology noted. Small, asymptomatic lesions found incidentally may be managed conservatively, whereas large symptomatic lesions require surgical intervention. Given the proximity to cranial nerves, vasculature, and the brain stem/cervical cord, traditional

N. T. Zwagerman
Department of Neurological Surgery, University of Pittsburgh School of Medicine, Pittsburgh, PA, USA
e-mail: nzwagerman@mcw.edu

J. C. Fernandez-Miranda · P. A. Gardner (✉)
Department of Neurological Surgery, University of Pittsburgh School of Medicine, Pittsburgh, PA, USA

UPMC Center for Cranial Base Surgery, Pittsburgh, PA, USA
e-mail: drjfm@stanford.edu; gardpa@upmc.edu

E. W. Wang · C. H. Snyderman
Department of Otolaryngology, University of Pittsburgh School of Medicine, Pittsburgh, PA, USA

UPMC Center for Cranial Base Surgery, Pittsburgh, PA, USA
e-mail: wangew@upmc.edu; snydermanch@upmc.edu

E. Tessitore et al. (eds.), *Surgery of the Cranio-Vertebral Junction*,
https://doi.org/10.1007/978-3-030-18700-2_26

approaches to this region inevitably require some degree of neurovascular manipulation. The operative approach must be catered to the specific goals of surgery and location of the pathology. Lesions located medial to the cranial nerves and above the nasopalatine line may be approached through the endoscopic endonasal route. In this chapter, we will present a case of a foramen magnum lesion, discuss the differential diagnosis, describe the surgical approach and present the current literature.

26.2 Case Illustration

A 51-year-old woman presents with significant neck pain as well as numbness in both of her arms for several months. The patient's symptoms have progressed so that she is having difficulty walking secondary to imbalance and gait instability. Imaging was performed and can be seen in Fig. 26.1. Her past medical history was unrevealing and she had not had prior surgery. Examination of the patient confirmed bilateral upper extremity weakness and dense myelopathy of the upper and lower limbs. She suffered from a wide-based gait with inability to walk heel to toe. She had bilateral Hoffman's sign as well as several beats of clonus. Her cranial nerve exam was intact. Formal speech evaluation was performed and no signs of dysphagia were noted. Given the progressive nature of the disease and imaging characteristics, she was diagnosed with a meningioma and surgical resection was recommended.

26.2.1 Differential Diagnosis

The differential diagnosis of extra-axial foramen magnum lesions can be broad but may be narrowed down based on the clinical history as well as the imaging

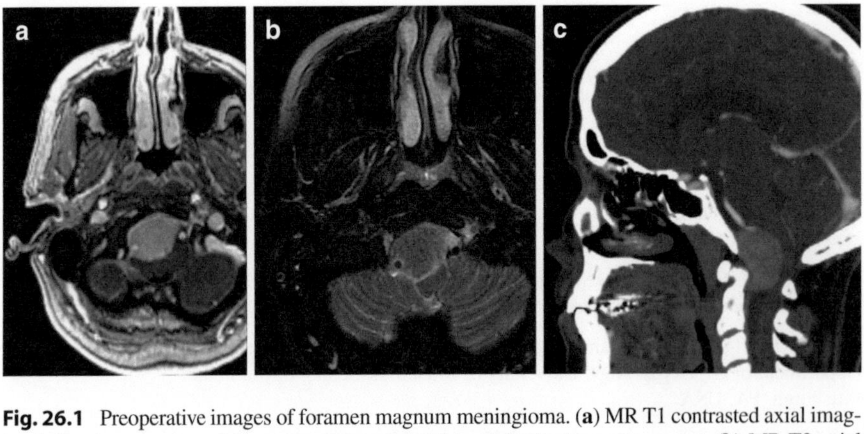

Fig. 26.1 Preoperative images of foramen magnum meningioma. (**a**) MR T1 contrasted axial imaging indicating severe medulla compression and right vertebral artery encasement. (**b**) MR T2 axial without contrast indicating signal change around the tumor and in the medulla. (**c**) CT with contrast, sagittal imaging indicating location at the foramen magnum and minimal bone involvement

Table 26.1 Differential diagnosis of extra-axial pathology at the foramen magnum

Neoplastic	Non-neoplastic
Meningioma	Odontoid pannus
Chordoma	Ectatic vertebral artery
Schwannoma	Aneurysm
Epidermoid tumor	Synovial cyst
Chondroma	
Chondrosarcoma	
Plasmacytoma	
Metastasis	

characteristics. The most common lesion at the cranio-vertebral junction is meningioma which is seen 78% of the time [1]. Other pathologies include chordoma (often involving or extending behind the dens), schwannoma, epidermoid, chondroma, chondrosarcoma, plasmacytoma, and metastasis. Non-neoplastic lesions must also be entertained which include ectasia/aneurysm of the vertebral artery, odontoid pannus in rheumatoid patients, or synovial cyst of the quadrate ligament (see Table 26.1).

Prior to treatment, it is important to refine the differential diagnosis as accurately as possible. When treating an odontoid pannus, there should not be a large dural defect, whereas the treatment for a meningioma requires a careful, multilayer, vascularized reconstruction to prevent postoperative complications. A chordoma would require a complete resection but leaving a small amount of residual tumor may be unavoidable. As a result, thorough review of the imaging characteristics of these lesions, which can be very specific, is critical for surgical planning.

26.2.2 Surgery

Surgical resection was recommended via the endoscopic endonasal approach (EEA). Care was taken during the preoperative planning to evaluate the location of the vertebral arteries as well as to identify the location of the cranial nerves. Pre-positioning somatosensory evoked potentials were performed to identify if any changes occurred during patient positioning. Image guidance was used to help facilitate intraoperative orientation and exposure planning. The patient was positioned in a neutral head position, with the vertex slightly pointed to the left and the head slightly turned to the right. Electromyography of bilateral cranial nerves IX–XII as well as bilateral auditory evoked potentials were monitored. The otolaryngology team performed the initial exposure and raised an extended nasoseptal flap (including the nasal floor mucosa). The maxillary crest/spine was reduced with a drill down to the level of the hard palate to gain more inferior access to the C1/C2 junction. The sphenoid sinus was opened and the septations removed. This allowed placement of the flap into the sphenoid until the end of the case. The nasopharyngeal mucosa, basopharyngeal fascia, and rectus capitis muscles were removed to expose the bottom of C1 and the base of the odontoid. This was carried out laterally to resect as much of the rectus capitis muscle as possible, limited by the parapharyngeal internal carotid arteries (ICAs). The landmarks for the parapharyngeal ICA, the Eustachian tubes, were preserved and mobilized laterally.

Bone removal was carried out by drilling the floor of the sphenoid sinus and then extending inferiorly. This extended laterally to the foramen lacerum and petroclival fissure bilaterally. The inferolateral exposure was extended to the proximal portion of the hypoglossal canals which were not opened. The clival bone was removed to expose the underlying dura. The inferior extent of exposure included drilling the superior half of the arch of C1 as well as the odontoid tip. Care was taken to preserve the body of the odontoid as well as the transverse ligament to preserve stability.

Once the dura was exposed, it was widely coagulated to devascularize the tumor. All visible dura was cauterized taking note to identify the interdural vertebral arteries to avoid incidental injury. The dura was then opened with a linear incision in the middle of the tumor. Microsurgical technique was used to debulk the lesion. At first the "two-suction" technique was employed; however, due to the fibrous nature of the lesion, an extended tip ultrasonic aspirator had to be used to accomplish any significant debulking. Once debulked, sharp dissection was used to remove the tumor from the bilateral vertebral arteries as well as the brain stem. The plane between the tumor and the brain stem was maintained by a layer of arachnoid. The nerves were preserved and small amounts of the tumor were left attached to the right vertebral artery for fear of injury. Once tumor resection was completed, the process of closing the defect began.

26.2.3 Closure

For closure of large clival defects, fascia lata is harvested from the ipsilateral leg which is prepped before draping. Superficial fat is also harvested from the leg to be used in the construct. An intradural collagen matrix is placed to serve as the first layer of closure. This was secured behind the dura with slits to allow for the exit of nerves and the dural entry of the vertebral arteries. Next, fascia lata is used to lay over the dural defect and is large enough to cover the defect, foramen lacerum, and is tucked behind the nasopharyngeal soft tissue to prevent cerebrospinal fluid leakage. A fat graft is used on top of this layer to provide for a buttress, fill in the space between ICAS, and provide a flat surface on which the nasoseptal flap will be laid. The nasoseptal flap covers the entire defect from the sphenoid sinus to the remaining arch of C1. Our current method is to suture the bottom edge of the fascia to the nasopharyngeal tissue to form a water tight closure. Nasal packing is left in place for 5–7 days to provide a buttress for wound healing. Often, nasal splints are used to prevent postoperative scarring. Lumbar drainage of cerebrospinal fluid is used for 72 h to prevent postoperative cerebral spinal fluid leaks. This is used for large anterior or posterior cranial defects and has been shown to reduce CSF leaks in a randomized controlled trial [2].

26.2.4 Postoperative Course

The patient did well and was extubated on postoperative day 1 with no new cranial nerve defects and only complaining of some postoperative headache. She was discharged from the intensive care unit on postoperative day 2 to a neurosurgical stepdown floor. Her lumbar drain was removed on postoperative day 4 and her nasal packing was removed on postoperative day 6. She was seen by physical therapy and cleared for discharge to home. She passed a bedside swallow evaluation without difficulty. She had full motor strength in her arms. She was discharged after her packing was removed. She suffered from no new cranial nerve defects. At her 6 month follow-up evaluation, her gait had improved and she stated her neck pain was gone. Her postoperative imaging revealed no obvious residual tumor (Fig. 26.2).

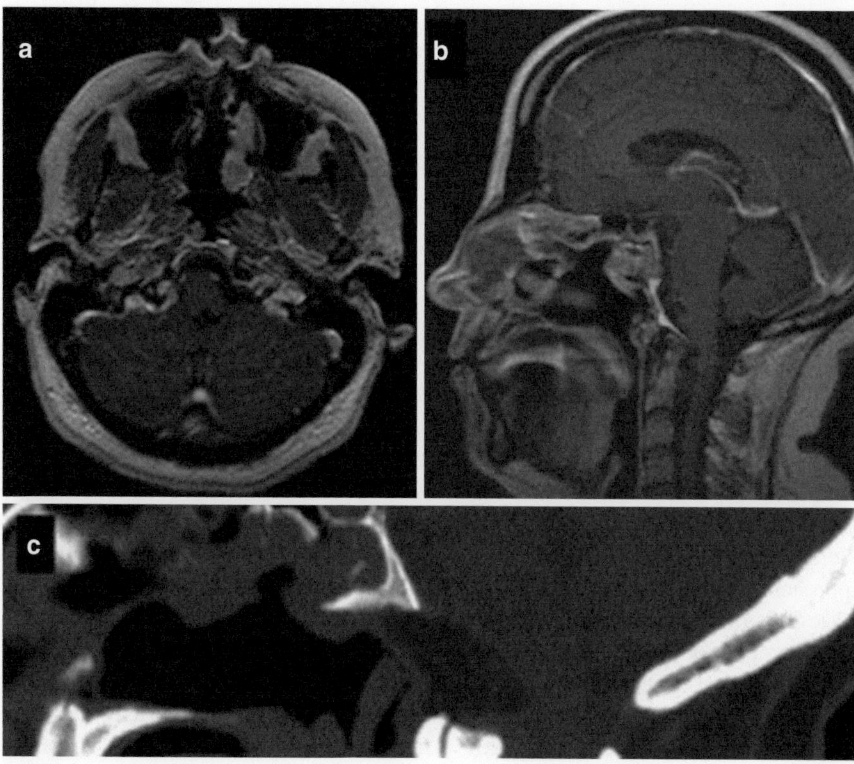

Fig. 26.2 Postoperative images of foramen magnum meningioma. (**a**) MR T1 contrasted axial imaging indicating complete resolution of brain stem compression and patent vertebral arteries. (**b**) MR T1 sagittal with contrast complete resection of the tumor and resolution of brain stem compression. (**c**) CT without contrast, axial imaging indicating fat graft in place and boney resection

26.3 Discussion

Traditional approaches to foramen magnum lesions initially included posterior midline approaches; however, these were associated with significant morbidity associated with retraction [1]. Later, posterolateral approaches were employed and provided a safe and effective route for anterior tumor resection; however, these approaches have limitations due to working between and around the lower cranial nerves and limited access to contralateral tumor expansion [3, 4]. The first anterior route was transoral; however, this approach was limited by cerebrospinal fluid leak with high rates of infection and spinal instability [5, 6]. Moreover, retraction of the soft palate has been known to cause velopharyngeal insufficiency in up to half of patients who undergo maneuvers such as splitting of the soft palate [7]. More recently, the anterior route to the foramen magnum through the endoscopic endonasal approach has been described by several authors [8–13]. In particular, this approach has been used with success in large series of 34 patients who underwent endoscopic endonasal odontoid resection [14]. This series indicates the safety and feasibility of regularly reaching the cranio-vertebral junction. The lower extent of approach is predicted by the nasopalatine line which has proven to be simple and practical for preoperative planning [15]. Lesions with expansion below this level should be approached using an alternative route. Several biomechanical studies indicated that with 50–75% occipital condyle resection, the occipital cervical joint becomes hypermobile [16, 17]. This corresponds to a retrospective review by Kooshkabadi who found that an inflexion point for cranio-vertebral instability occurs at 75% condyle resection [18]. Regardless, care must be taken to avoid destabilization of the cranio-vertebral junction. A recent report by Wang et al. performed an anatomical study on cadavers indicating only one fifth of the medial occipital condyle was needed to be drilled to provide access to the ventral foramen magnum [11].

Outcomes after the endoscopic endonasal approach to the cranio-vertebral junction and foramen magnum are limited to a few case series and reports. As mentioned, a series of 34 patients undergoing odontoidectomy avoided significant morbidity and velopalatal insufficiency [14]. A series of five patients who underwent EEA for foramen magnum tumors is being followed without cranio-vertebral insufficiency at an average 18 months of follow-up and demonstrates similar efficacy to the far lateral approach (in press, Operative Neurosurgery). No large series of the EEA for intradural lesions of the ventral foramen magnum currently exist, but several case reports including one by Wang, et al. indicate the safety and efficacy of the approach [11]. Given the novel development of this technique and the rarity of the lesions, it will take time to determine the limitations of this approach; however, the EEA does provide several added benefits including direct tumor access, minimal or no nerve manipulation, no brain stem/spinal cord retraction, and no velopalatal insufficiency compared with other approaches.

One of the major criticisms of this approach has the increased risk of CSF leak associated with other lesions (chordoma, olfactory groove meningioma) which has ranged as high as 30% [19, 20]. As a result, reconstruction is paramount for success when using the endoscopic endonasal approach. There have been many different closure techniques which include collagen grafts, fat grafts, and fascia lata, but the most important has been the use of the vascularized nasoseptal flap [21]. Our technique is to perform a multilayer closure with an in-lay collagen matrix, followed by an on-lay fascia lata graft. This is held in place by a fat graft which also helps to avoid pontine encephalocele formation [22] and fills in the space deep to the nasopharyngeal mucosa. This is covered by the nasoseptal flap. All patients with posterior fossa defects undergo postoperative lumbar drain placement based on a randomized controlled trial which found that the CSF leak rate drops from 32 to 9% with lumbar drainage [2].

26.4 Conclusion

The endoscopic endonasal approach for resection of foramen magnum lesions has significant promise as a direct approach to ventral lesions with no brain stem/spinal cord or cranial nerve manipulation. Several studies have indicated its feasibility and reports have indicated limited success. More studies are needed to document long-term tumor control rates and surgical morbidity.

References

1. Meyer FB, Ebersold MJ, Reese DF. Benign tumors of the foramen magnum. J Neurosurg. 1984;61(1):136–42.
2. Zwagerman NT, Wang EW, Shin SS, Chang YF, Fernandez-Miranda JC, Snyderman CH, Gardner PA. Does lumbar drainage reduce postoperative cerebrospinal fluid leak after endoscopic endonasal skull base surgery? A prospective, randomized controlled trial. J Neurosurg. 2018;1:1–7. [Epub ahead of print].
3. George B, Lot G. Anterolateral and posterolateral approaches to the foramen magnum: technical description and experience from 97 cases. Skull Base Surg. 1995;5(1):9–19.
4. Heros RC. Lateral suboccipital approach for vertebral and vertebrobasilar artery lesions. J Neurosurg. 1986;64(4):559–62.
5. Mummaneni PV, Haid RW. Transoral odontoidectomy. Neurosurgery. 2005;56(5):1045–50; discussion 1045–1050.
6. Crockard HA, Sen CN. The transoral approach for the management of intradural lesions at the craniovertebral junction: review of 7 cases. Neurosurgery. 1991;28(1):88–97; discussion 97–98.
7. Kingdom TT, Nockels RP, Kaplan MJ. Transoral-transpharyngeal approach to the craniovertebral junction. Otolaryngol Head Neck Surg. 1995;113(4):393–400.
8. Morera VA, Fernandez-Miranda JC, Prevedello DM, et al. "Far-medial" expanded endonasal approach to the inferior third of the clivus: the transcondylar and transjugular tubercle approaches. Neurosurgery. 2010;66(6 Suppl Operative):211–9; discussion 219–220.
9. Kassam AB, Gardner P, Snyderman C, Mintz A, Carrau R. Expanded endonasal approach: fully endoscopic, completely transnasal approach to the middle third of the clivus, petrous bone, middle cranial fossa, and infratemporal fossa. Neurosurg Focus. 2005;19(1):E6.
10. Frank G, Sciarretta V, Calbucci F, Farneti G, Mazzatenta D, Pasquini E. The endoscopic transnasal transsphenoidal approach for the treatment of cranial base chordomas and chondrosarcomas. Neurosurgery. 2006;59(1 Suppl 1):ONS50–7; discussion ONS50–57.

11. Wang W-H, Abhinav K, Wang E, Snyderman C, Gardner PA, Fernandez-Miranda JC. Endoscopic endonasal transclival transcondylar approach for foramen magnum meningiomas. Surgical anatomy and technical note. Oper Neurosurg. 2016;12(2):153–62.
12. Kassam A, Snyderman CH, Mintz A, Gardner P, Carrau RL. Expanded endonasal approach: the rostrocaudal axis. Part II. Posterior clinoids to the foramen magnum. Neurosurg Focus. 2005;19(1):E4.
13. Fernandez-Miranda JC, Morera VA, Snyderman CH, Gardner P. Endoscopic endonasal transclival approach to the jugular tubercle. Neurosurgery. 2012;71(1 Suppl Operative):146–58; discussion 158–159.
14. Zwagerman NT, Tormenti MJ, Tempel ZJ, et al. Endoscopic endonasal resection of the odontoid process: clinical outcomes in 34 adults. J Neurosurg. 2018;128(3):923–31.
15. de Almeida JR, Zanation AM, Snyderman CH, et al. Defining the nasopalatine line: the limit for endonasal surgery of the spine. Laryngoscope. 2009;119(2):239–44.
16. Little AS, Perez-Orribo L, Rodriguez-Martinez NG, et al. Biomechanical evaluation of the craniovertebral junction after inferior-third clivectomy and intradural exposure of the foramen magnum: implications for endoscopic endonasal approaches to the cranial base. J Neurosurg Spine. 2013;18(4):327–32.
17. Vishteh AG, Crawford NR, Melton MS, Spetzler RF, Sonntag VK, Dickman CA. Stability of the craniovertebral junction after unilateral occipital condyle resection: a biomechanical study. J Neurosurg. 1999;90(1 Suppl):91–8.
18. Kooshkabadi A, Choi PA, Koutourousiou M, et al. Atlanto-occipital instability following endoscopic endonasal approach for lower clival lesions: experience with 212 cases. Neurosurgery. 2015;77(6):888–97; discussion 897.
19. Koutourousiou M, Gardner PA, Tormenti MJ, et al. Endoscopic endonasal approach for resection of cranial base chordomas: outcomes and learning curve. Neurosurgery. 2012;71(3):614–25.
20. Koutourousiou M, Fernandez-Miranda JC, Wang EW, Snyderman CH, Gardner PA. Endoscopic endonasal surgery for olfactory groove meningiomas: outcomes and limitations in 50 patients. Neurosurg Focus. 2014;37(4):E8.
21. Hadad G, Bassagasteguy L, Carrau RL, et al. A novel reconstructive technique after endoscopic expanded endonasal approaches: vascular pedicle nasoseptal flap. Laryngoscope. 2006;116(10):1882–6.
22. Koutourousiou M, Filho FV, Costacou T, et al. Pontine encephalocele and abnormalities of the posterior fossa following transclival endoscopic endonasal surgery. J Neurosurg. 2014;121(2):359–66.

Foramen Magnum Tumours: Posterior Approaches and Outcome

27

Karl Schaller

Tumours at the foramen magnum are exceedingly rare. They are divided in *intradural tumours*, such as meningiomas, schwannomas, or neurofibromas, with foramen magnum meningiomas (FMMs) representing the majority among them. *Extradural tumours* include chordomas and chondrosarcomas, or metastases, with lower clival chordomas representing the most frequent entity of this group. Depending on size and extension a variety of surgical approaches to this region has been proposed, extending from endonasal endoscopic approaches to the anterior rim of the foramen magnum to far lateral trans-/paracondylar approaches with/without transient transposition of the vertebral artery (VA) to otherwise extended retrosigmoid approaches with additional opening of the foramen magnum—and to variations of the standard posterior midline approach [1–11].

FMMs originate from the dura of the foramen magnum proper, thereby accounting for less than 3% of intracranial meningiomas in large clinical series [12]. Epidemiologically they don't differ from meningiomas in other localizations, with a mean age of >50 years and a female predominance. They share with other intra- or extradural lesions of this particular region that they may reach a considerable size prior to diagnosis—despite their delicate localization close to critical neurovascular structures at the cranio-cervical junction. Most FMMs arise from the anterior or anterolateral aspect of the foramen magnum, that is anterior to the denticulate ligament. Likewise in FMMs and in other tumours, the relationship between the tumour and the V3 and V4 segments of the vertebral artery, with CN IX–XII, the posterior inferior cerebellar artery (PICA), and the brainstem are decisive for the surgical strategy. This anatomical complexity renders treatment of such tumours a challenge—despite all contemporary technology and techniques for diagnosis and for surgical treatment.

K. Schaller (✉)
Neurosurgical Unit, Geneva University Hospitals, Geneva, Switzerland
e-mail: karl.schaller@hcuge.ch

E. Tessitore et al. (eds.), *Surgery of the Cranio-Vertebral Junction*,
https://doi.org/10.1007/978-3-030-18700-2_27

27.1 Symptoms

Symptomatology includes spontaneous head and neck pain in the occipital and suboccipital region, and painful limitation of head movements in flexion, extension and on rotation [2, 5, 7, 9–11]. Subtle neurological deficits such as mild to moderate lower cranial nerve palsies may go unnoticed. For example, especially elderly patients may present with long-standing dysphagia, hoarseness, or with deviation of their tongue, problems which they may have attributed to more generalized aspects of ageing. Depending on the site of dural attachment, precise localization, and size, other symptoms include unilateral or bilateral long-tract signs such as spasticity and gait ataxia [2, 5, 7, 9–11].

27.2 Diagnosis

Adequate contemporary diagnostic workup includes not only thorough clinical examination and standard imaging, but video oesophago- and tracheoscopy and X-rays or MRI of the swallowing act as well. MR imaging of the whole neuraxis is recommended to exclude multiplicity of lesions. That is, elderly patients in particular who are presenting with uni- or bilateral long-tract signs may have suffered from previous stroke, or they may suffer from additional cervical spondylotic myelopathy (CSM), the latter of which has to be taken into account when it comes to positioning for surgery. MRI should include not only native and injected standard sequences, but MR venography in addition, because, especially in large FMMs, there may be involvement of the sigmoid sinus. A persisting occipital venous sinus should be ruled out as well, as this may represent a major source for surgical complications during the early phases of craniotomy and dural opening. High-resolution CT of the cranio-cervical junction is equally recommended: this helps to assess the degree of calcification of the FMMs and its potentially hyperostotic root, to understand the bony relationship with the occipital condyles and the transverse processes of C1, with the jugular tubercle, and to prepare for the case that instability may ensue due to (partial) drilling of the C0-C1 joints. Should involvement or encasement of the vertebral artery (typically segments C3 and C4) be suspected from the MRI, then performance of CT angiography is recommended. This may influence the surgical strategy, i.e. by preparation for vascular repair.

27.3 Classification

There are several classifications for FMMs (Lit) [3, 9, 13]. A more recent one was proposed by Bernard George's group from Paris, which is based on three main criteria: the compartment which contains the majority of the tumour mass, the site of dural insertion, and the degree of vertebral artery involvement. The tumours can be localized strictly intradurally (anterior, lateral, or posterior), combined intra-extradurally, or extradurally [3]. The latter two types are localized antero- or posterolaterally. An additional criterion concerns the relationship between the tumour and the VA: the FMMs may be localized above or below, or combined above and below with subsequent encasement of the VA.

27.4 Presurgical Considerations

In this author's view, it doesn't make sense to be apodictic about the approach to these lesions: posteriorly located FMMs are approached by a posterior midline approach anyway. When it comes to the surgical resection of antero- or posterolaterally located FMMs, different neurosurgical schools apply different rules. This includes patient installation in semi-sitting, or in supine, or in park-bench positions, and the practice of far lateral, or trans- and paracondylar approaches with varying degrees of drilling of the C0-C1 joints and the jugular tubercle [1, 2, 12, 14–17]. The vast majority of FMMs may be accessed by a posterior midline approach, however [12, 15, 18, 19].

27.5 Technique of Dorsal Midline or Paramedian Approach

The dorsal midline approach to FMMs is performed in the following steps:

1. Surgeon should assure herself/himself that adequate haemostatic material is available on the scrub nurse's table (i.e. Gelfoam™, Tachosil™, Surgiflo™, aneurysm clips in case of involvement of the VA).
2. In case of large FMMs and presence of additional CSM: Placement of monitoring tools and devices PRIOR to definitive patient positioning. This includes standard MEP and SEP monitoring to/from arms and legs (median nerve and tibial nerves, and corresponding specific muscles, respectively).
3. Prone position, the head in flexion (Concorde).
4. Linear incision, normally from inion to C3 (depending on extent of caudal tumour growth). Palpating the inion and the spinous processes of C2 and lower mxfhelps to draw an appropriate line on the skin.
5. Placement of one curved self-retaining retractors with the handle pointing cranially at the level of the posterior fossa, which follows the anatomical shape of the suboccipital region as to avoid interference with the surgeon's hands and hindering convenient access to the target region. A second self-retaining retractor may be used in reverse sense, its handle pointing caudally, depending on the necessity and extent of cervical exposition and possible need for resection of posterior arches C1 and C2. Resection of extradural tumours such as chordomas may end at this stage—with resection and drilling of affected bony structures around the FM.

6. Haemostasis, placement of cotton patties, and rinsing of the surgical field.
7. In a midline approach, and depending on the cranial extension of the tumour, it is advised to place two burr holes at the same horizontal level, on either side of the midline, and as far lateral as possible. Posterior fossa exposition is notoriously limited and easily misjudged in the beginning, and each millimetre of exposition counts. These twin burr holes are connected by a blunt dissector. Care must be taken not to run into a possible large venous lacuna or a persisting occipital venous sinus. In that case, drilling of the bone to complete the craniotomy may be safer than the blunt use of a craniotome for the connection of these two burr holes. Adequate haemostatic material and dural titanium clips should be ready to be used if deemed necessary.
8. The posterior atlanto-occipital membrane can be thickened and extremely cumbersome to be separated from the occipital bone.
9. Dural incision is performed in a way which leaves a 2–3 mm rim around the entrance zone of the vertebral artery, so as to have enough room for watertight dural closure at the end of the procedure and to minimize the risk for occurrence of a CSF fistula.
10. Upon dural opening, and in case of direct visibility of an aspect of the tumour it may be advisable to perform direct electrical stimulation of the exposed capsule in order to avoid to miss and to cut through a thinned and stretched CN.
11. If possible, the capsule of the tumour is followed toward its site of insertion. If being confronted with whitish fibres, which cannot be clearly attributed to CN or to denticulate ligament, then direct electrical stimulation is performed again. At the anterolateral insertion site, bipolar coagulation is performed for consequent devascularization of the tumour.
12. In most intradural tumours with no history of previous surgical or radiosurgical treatment, it is possible to find and to define an arachnoidal plane between their capsule and critical neurovascular structures such as CN or the brainstem. It is of utmost importance to guard this plane as it will help during tumour dissection from its surrounding structures. Large tumours may be debulked from internally first, thus facilitating manipulation of residual tumour and its capsule. The situation can be different and far more challenging in recurrent tumours where it might be advisable to leave a thin layer of tumour on CN or the brainstem rather than trying to peel it completely off and thereby causing structural damage and consecutive neurological worsening.
13. In most instances, the zone of dural attachment is resected in this late stage of the surgical procedure. If this concerns dura overlying the clivus, this does not require subsequent duroplasty. If the insertion site was more lateral or posterior, then bovine pericard can be used for duroplasty. It is advised to cover the dura with fibrinoid material at the end of the procedure (i.e. with Tachosil™).

27.6 Technique of Dorsal Paramedian Approach

Alternatively, and for a strictly lateralized approach, the skin incision should be placed on a line halfway between the posterior midline and the virtual projection of the lateral border of the patient's head ("mid of the mid"). Subcutaneous and transmuscular dissection will equally lead to the posterior fossa along its flattening aspect toward the foramen magnum, and laterally to the C0-C1 articulation and the basion.

27.7 Outcome

The posterior midline approach has been used for the treatment of FMMs since decades. This includes meningiomas of all sizes, calcified and non-calcified tumours, and antero-laterally and anteriorly localized FMMs. The rationale behind the use of (far) lateral approaches is the avoidance of traction-related neurological worsening, i.e. by placing retractors on the brainstem with direct impact on long white matter tracts and cranial nerve nuclei, or by transmitted traction on the cranial nerves themselves. Proponents of lateral approaches argue that there is better direct tumour exposition and local control of neurovascular structures around it by additional bone and C0/C1-joint drilling. This should then result in better clinical outcomes in large series of FMMs reported in the literature. In fact, this is not the case when different series from different neurosurgical centres are compared (with all the reservations with regard to such comparisons). The results which were obtained with the use of posterior approaches in respective clinical series of FMMs are as follows: permanent morbidities in the range of 5–10%, and mortality <5% [4, 9–11, 13, 15, 20–22]. This is not different from corresponding numbers for (far) lateral approaches with/without additional osteosynthesis of the cranio-cervical junction. In principle, these numbers show that surgery of tumours at the foramen magnum by experienced teams is entirely feasible. There seems to be an intrinsic rate of morbidity and mortality for the resection of these lesions, which is the same for both principally different types of approaches—dorsal vs. lateral. This is an argument in favour of the posterior approach, because it takes lesser time and resources—presumed that the results on long term are the same. Reported recurrence rates for either approach were similarly low, however [15, 20, 21, 23]. In addition, the application of simple posterior approaches without drilling of the C0/C1 joints does not require additional cranio-cervical osteosynthesis with all its inherent risks and complications (Figs. 27.1, 27.2, 27.3, 27.4, 27.5, 27.6, 27.7, and 27.8).

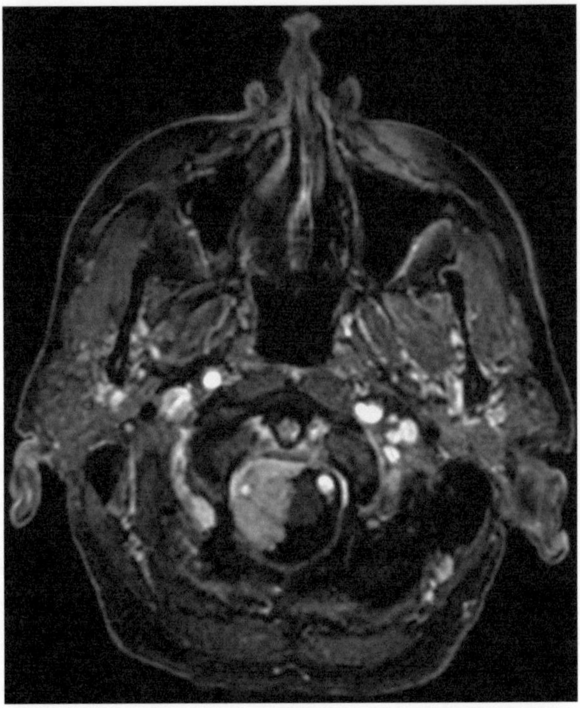

Fig. 27.1 Right-sided laterally localized FMM, with complete encasement of the (non-dominant) right vertebral artery in a 77-year-old female patient. This Gd-enhanced axial cut of a T1-weighted sequence allows to distinguish between the various involved neurovascular structures, the enhanced tumour, which takes approximatively up to 50% percent of the diameter at the level of the cranio-cervical junction. This tumour was approached via a standard midline incision, followed by a suboccipital craniotomy, resection of the posterior arch of C1, partial resection of the arch of C2—all more to the right side than to the left

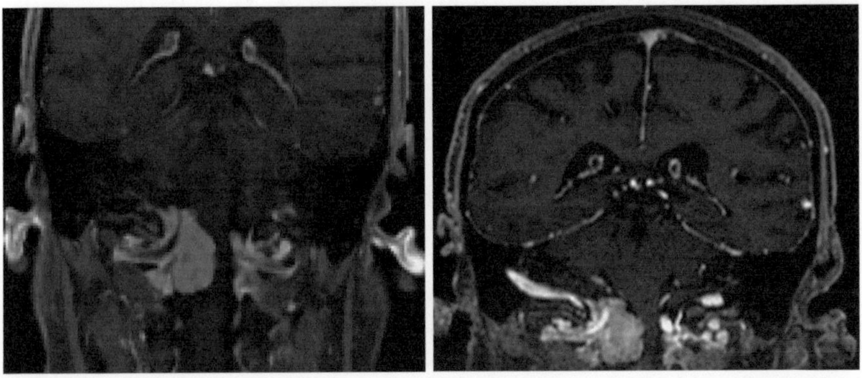

Fig. 27.2 Coronal view in same patient as in Fig. 27.1 of right-sided, laterally localized FMM, with complete encasement of the (non-dominant) right vertebral artery. T1-weighted Gd-enhanced imaging clearly shows the dural attachment and the venous sinuses. All this is relevant for planning of the surgical approach, and for preparation of material for vascular repair

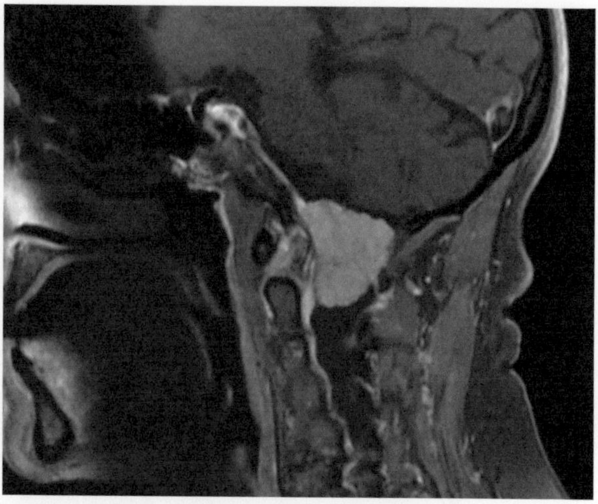

Fig. 27.3 Sagittal view in same patient as in Figs. 27.1 and 27.2 of right-sided, laterally localized FMM. This T1-weighted Gd-enhanced image is of particular value for assessment of the tumour size in the cranio-caudal direction and for presurgical planning, i.e. skin incision, resection of laminae C1 and C2, etc.

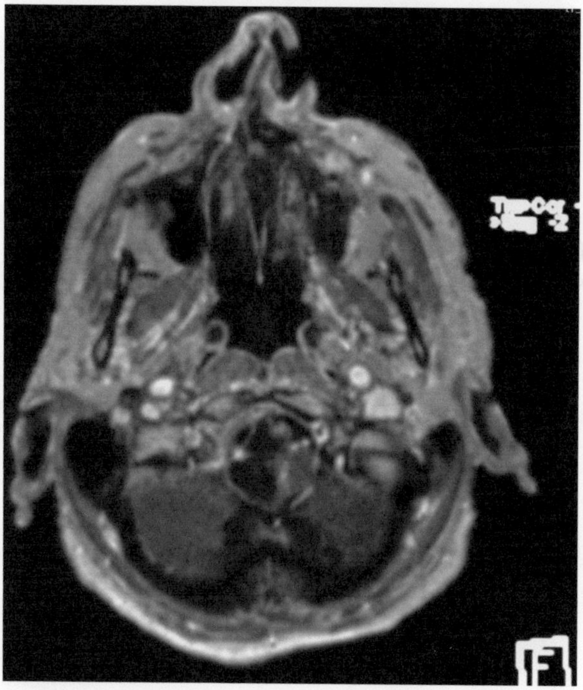

Fig. 27.4 Right-sided, anteriolaterally localized highly calcified meningioma in 67-year-old woman with known psychiatric disease and increasing walking difficulties. On this T1-weighted Gd-enhanced axial MR image, the tumours are mainly black. There is severe compression of the brainstem and partial encasement of the vertebral artery. The tumour was approached via a midline skin incision from the inion down to the spinous process of C2. Resection of the posterior arch of C1 and posterior enlargement of the foramen magnum by drilling the infero-posterior part of the occipital bones. This was followed by Y-shaped dural opening. Only subtotal removal was possible, because the tumour had to be drilled out partially, and a margin of security was left around the vertebral artery

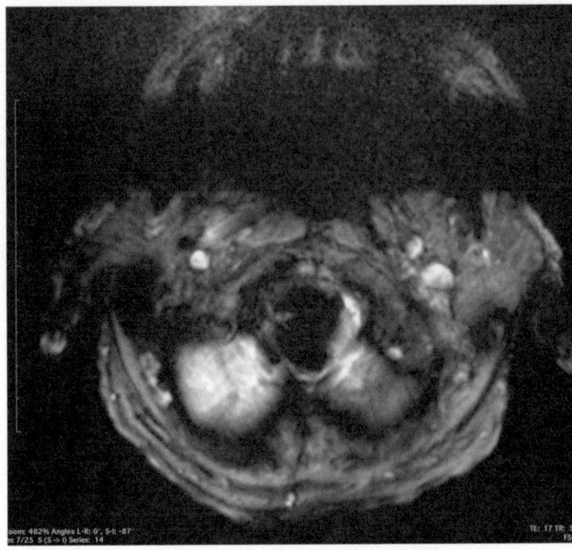

Fig. 27.5 Non-injected T2-weighted axial MR image of the same patient as in Fig. 27.4. The extent of the calcified process is better demarcated

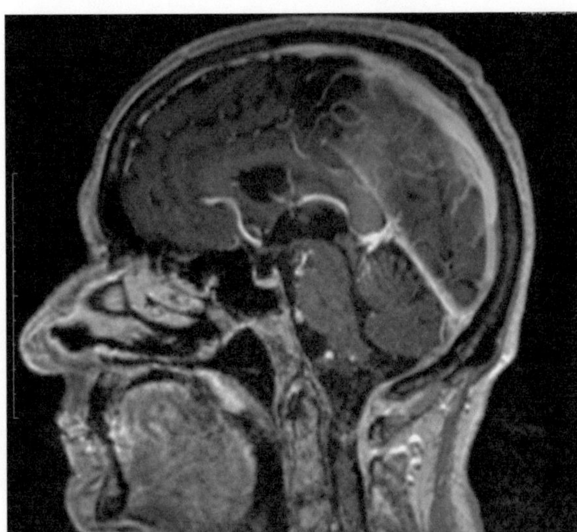

Fig. 27.6 Sagittal Gd-enhanced T1-weighted MR image of the same patient as in Fig. 27.4. The mass at the cranio-cervical junction can be seen as a mere "negative" defect of the medulla oblongata

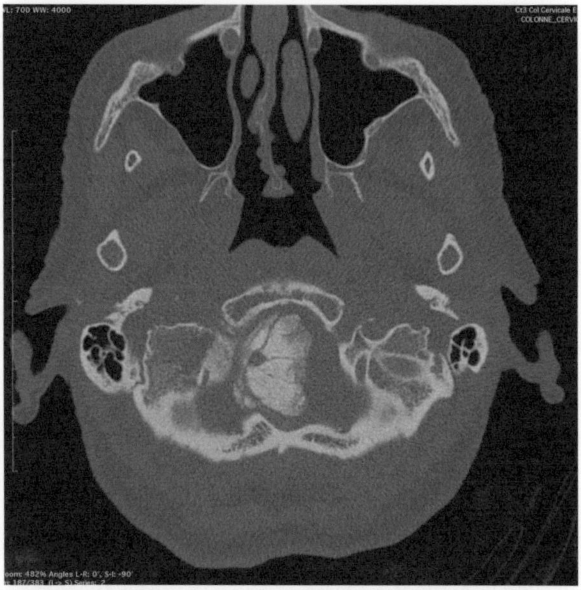

Fig. 27.7 Axial CT bone scan of the same patient as in Fig. 27.4. Extensive calcification can be seen obstructing the foramen magnum in a right-to-left direction

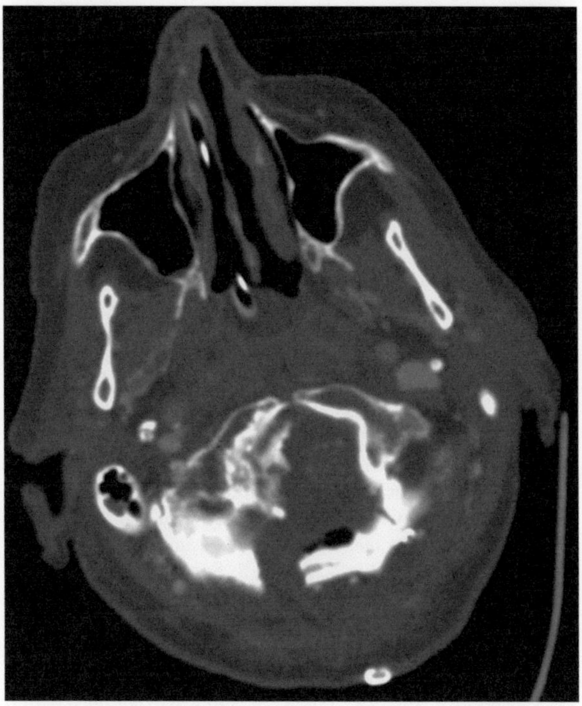

Fig. 27.8 Post-operative axial CT bone scan of the same patient as in Fig. 27.4. A hyperostotic shell is remaining along the dura and around the vertebral artery following subtotal removal of the calcified meningioma, which could be removed with extensive drilling only. Decompression of the brainstem has been achieved

References

1. Bruneau M, George B. Foramen magnum meningiomas: detailed surgical approaches and technical aspects at Lariboisière hospital and review of the literature. Neurosurg Rev. 2008;31:19–33.
2. Dobrowolski S, Ebner F, Lepski G, Tatagiba M. Foramen magnum meningioma: the midline suboccipital subtonsillar approach. Clin Neurol Neurosurg. 2016;145:28–34.
3. Bruneau M, George B. Classification system of foramen magnum meningiomas. J Craniovertebr Junction Spine. 2010;1(1):10–7.
4. Dahme R, Koussa S, Samaha E. C1 arch regeneration, tight cisterna magna, and cervical syringomyelia following foramen magnum surgery. Surg Neurol. 2009;72:83–6.
5. Meyer FB, Ebersold MJ, Reese D. Benign tumors of the foramen magnum. J Neurosurg. 1984;61:136–42.
6. Mostofi K. Foramen magnum meningioma: some anatomical and surgical remarks through five cases. Asian Spine J. 2015;9(1):54–8.
7. Pamir MN, Kilic T, Özduman K, Türe U. Experience of a single institution treating foramen magnum meningiomas. J Clin Neurosci. 2004;11(8):863–7.
8. Porras CL. Meningioma in the foramen magnum in a boy aged 8 years. J Neurosurg. 1963;20:167–8.
9. Roberti F, Sekhar L, Kalavakonda C, Wright DC. Posterior fossa meningiomas: surgical experience in 161 cases. Surg Neurol. 2001;56:8–21.
10. Talachi A, Biroli A, Soda C, Masotto B, Bricolo A. Surgical management of ventral and ventrolateral foramen magnum meningiomas: report on a 64-case series and review of the literature. Neurosurg Rev. 2012;35:359–68.
11. Wu Z, Hao S, Zhang J, Zhang L, Jia G, Tang J, Xiao X, Wang L, Wang Z. Foramen magnum meningiomas: experiences in 114 patients at a single institute over 15 years. Surg Neurol. 2009;72:376–82.
12. Della Puppa A, Rustemi O, Scienza R. The suboccipital midline approach to foramen magnum meningiomas. Acta Neurochir. 2015;157:869–73.
13. Li D, Wu Z, Ren C, Hao S-Y, Wang L, Xiao X-R, Tang J, Wang Y-G, Meng G-L, Zhang L-W, Zhang J-T. Foramen magnum meningiomas: surgical results and risks predicting poor outcomes based on a modified classification. J Neurosurg. 2016;13:1–16.
14. Bertalanffy H, Benes L, Becker R, Aboul-Enein H, Sure U. Surgery of intradural tumors at the foramen magnum level. Oper Tech Neurosurg. 2002;5(1):11–24.
15. Goel A, Desai K, Muzumdar D. Surgery on anterior foramen magnum meningiomas using a conventional posterior suboccipital approach: a report on an experience with 17 cases. Neurosurgery. 2001;49:102–7.
16. Moscovici S, Umansky F, Spektor S. "Lazy" far-lateral approach to the anterior foramen magnum and lower clivus. Neurosurg Focus. 2015;38(4):E14.
17. Samii M, Klekamp J, Gustavo C. Surgical results for meningiomas of the craniocervical junction. Neurosurgery. 1996;39(6):1086–95.
18. Kandenwein JA, Richter H-P, Antoniadis G. Foramen magnum meningiomas—experience with the posterior suboccipital approach. Br J Neurosurg. 2009;23(1):33–9.
19. Sohn S, Chung CK. Conventional posterior approach without far lateral approach for ventral foramen magnum meningiomas. J Korean Neurosurg Soc. 2013;54:373–8.
20. Bassiouni H, Ntoukas V, Asgari S, Sandalcioglu EI, Stolke D, Seifert V. Foramen magnum meningiomas: clinical outcome after microsurgical resection via a posterolateral retrocondylar approach. Neurosurgery. 2006;59:1177–87.
21. Samii M, Gerganov VM. Surgery of extra-axial tumors of the cerebral base. Neurosurgery. 2008;62(SHC Suppl 3):SHC1153–68.
22. Sanabria EA, Ehara K, Tamaki N. Surgical experience with skull base approaches for foramen magnum meningioma. Neurol Med Chir (Tokyo). 2002;42:472–80.
23. George B, Lot G, Boissonnet H. Meningioma of the foramen magnum: a series of 40 cases. Surg Neurol. 1997;47:371–9.

Surgery Involving the Vertebral Artery at the Cranio-vertebral Junction

28

Michael Bruneau and Bernard George

28.1 Introduction

The ability to surgically expose and control the vertebral artery (VA) in its third segment (V3) between C2 and the foramen magnum (FM), e.g., at the level of the cranio-vertebral junction (CVJ), is very useful as it permits to treat many problems; they include intrinsic occlusive VA diseases or extrinsic compression during particular movements of the head and neck, also named Bow Hunter's syndrome inducing vertebro-basilar ischemia, but also and mainly, many tumors that are also better treated using surgical approaches in which the VA exposure is part of the technique: FM, CVJ, and Jugular Foramen (JF) tumors [1–8].

All these pathologies need surgical approaches that include VA exposure but also specific techniques. In this chapter, the surgical exposure of the VA will be first described, and then the associated specific techniques necessary to treat all the previously mentioned pathologies will be reported.

For a better understanding, the reader is invited to previously read the chapter: Anatomy of the VA third segment.

M. Bruneau (✉)
Erasme Hospital, Department of Neurosurgery, Free University of Brussels, Brussels, Belgium
e-mail: mbruneau@ulb.ac.be

B. George
Lariboisiere Hospital Department of Neurosurgery, University Paris Descartes, Paris, France

E. Tessitore et al. (eds.), *Surgery of the Cranio-Vertebral Junction*,
https://doi.org/10.1007/978-3-030-18700-2_28

28.2 VA Exposure

The VA at the CVJ level can be exposed by two surgical approaches: the posterolateral and the anterolateral approach [2, 9]. After the initial description [10], they were published with some variations under different names, especially the far lateral and the extreme lateral [11–20].

28.2.1 Posterolateral Approach

The posterolateral approach (Fig. 28.1a) is a lateral extension of the standard midline posterior approach. The patient is most of the time placed in the prone position but some surgeons sometimes favor the lateral or the sitting position. The midline skin incision extends from the occipital protuberance down to the C4-C5 level and curves laterally along the superior occipital crest more or less toward the mastoid process following the size and shape of the neck. Some surgeons prefer a paramedian or an oblique straight or S shape incision. The advantage of the midline and superiorly curved skin incision is to start by a midline exposure which is familiar to everyone; then the muscles are detached from the superior occipital crest and are retracted inferiorly and laterally in one big layer with the skin. The occipital bone, the posterior arches of atlas (PAA), and the spinous process and laminae of C2 are subperiosteally exposed just like in the standard midline approach. The exposure of the PAA is then extended laterally starting by the inferior edge, next by the superior edge which in fact is the posterior limit of the VA groove. This groove extends from the transverse foramen (TF) to a step at the end of the groove where the height of

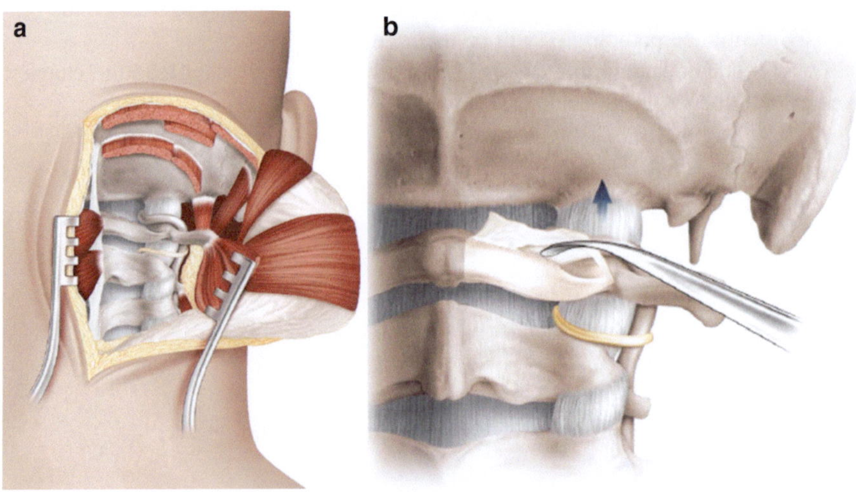

Fig. 28.1 The posterolateral approach. (**a**) Patient position, skin incision, and approach to the vertebral artery. (**b**) Subperiosteal dissection. (*From Pathology and Surgery around the Vertebral Artery. George B, Bruneau M, Spetzler RF (eds), Springer 2011*)

the PAA increases markedly (Fig. 28.1b). The subperiosteal exposure is a crucial point as it preserves the periosteal sheath surrounding the VA and its venous plexus. Therefore no troublesome bleeding is to be expected; however, some venous connections may exist between the VA venous plexus and the posterior condylar vein or the C1-C2 intervertebral plexus around the C2 nerve root. These connections can be easily coagulated and if necessary, the posterior condylar vein is controlled by Surgicel® and bone wax.

The posterolateral approach provides an easy and safe access and control to the VA segment above C1 from the transverse foramen to the FM dura. However, the vertical segment between the C2 and C1 TF is more difficult to reach in most cases. In fact, the posterolateral approach is essentially designed for the exposure of the VA horizontal segment above C1.

28.2.2 Anterolateral Approach

28.2.2.1 Exposure of the Two Vertical and Horizontal VA Segments

The anterolateral approach (Fig. 28.2a) at the CVJ level is basically similar to the one used lower in the neck to expose the VA in its V2 segment; it opens the field between the internal jugular vein (IJV) medially and the sterno-mastoid muscle (SM) laterally.

The patient is in the supine position with the head slightly extended, tilted down, and rotated toward the opposite side; in fact as C1 is rotating over C2 during head rotation the transverse process (TP) of atlas is projected anteriorly and the anterior arch is brought away.

The skin incision follows the medial edge of the SM in its superior part up to the tip of the mastoid process (MP), then curved along the superior occipital crest more or less toward the occipital protuberance following the size and shape of the neck. The posterior muscles are separated from the occipital bone and the MP including the tendon of the SM. They are then progressively retracted inferiorly and laterally. The IJV is next controlled in the inferior part of the field and progressively up to the skull base, moving up toward the MP and the digastric muscle. Between the IJV medially and the SM laterally, the depth of the field is filled by a fatty layer in which runs the accessory nerve (CN XI). This nerve should be identified and dissected free out of this fat layer that is then rolled around the nerve so as to retract the nerve inferiorly and medially. At this time of the approach, the field between the SM laterally, the IJV medially, and the digastric muscle superiorly is widely opened. About 15 mm below the tip of the MP, the tip of the TP of atlas can be palpated; it is connected with the occipital bone and C2 by several little muscles (levator scapulae, oblique and rectus muscles) which are now detached and retracted progressively giving view to the two VA segments: the vertical one between C2 and C1 and the horizontal segment in the groove of the PAA. This exposure must be achieved slowly so as to preserve the periosteal sheath of the VA and hence to avoid any troublesome bleeding. There is no landmark along the muscles resection except the anterior branch of the second cervical nerve root, which crosses the inferior part of the C1-C2 segment. In between the two VA segments and parallel to them is the PAA. As in the posterolateral approach, the PAA must be exposed subperiosteally, first on its posterior aspect then on its superior one, e.g., on the VA groove. The VA may be followed all along the VA groove until the step at the end of this groove is reached. From this point, the VA runs obliquely and superiorly toward the FM dura. There is often a muscular branch originating at the corner between the horizontal and oblique VA segments.

Again the main trick in this exposure is to work out of the periosteal sheath encircling the VA and the venous plexus.

28.2.2.2 Opening of the Transverse Foramen of Atlas and VA Transposition

Whenever the transverse foramen (TF) of atlas needs to be opened and furthermore when it is useful to transpose the VA out of this foramen, the preservation of the

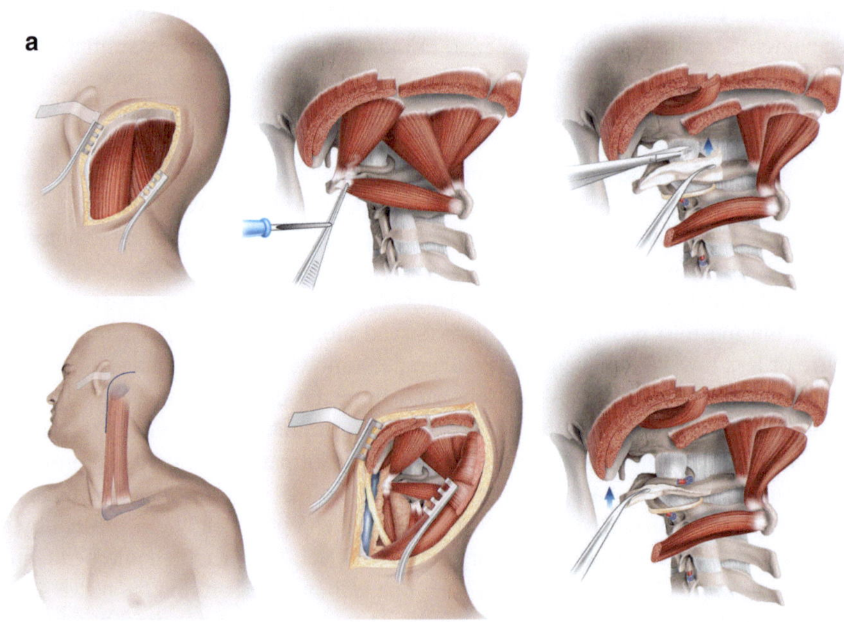

Fig. 28.2 (**a**) The anterolateral approach. A. Patient position and skin incision. B. Approach to the vertebral artery: superficial muscles exposure. C. Approach to the vertebral artery: deep muscles exposure. D. Section of the muscles inserting on the C1 transverse process. (**b**) Vertebral artery exposure and transposition. A. Subperiosteal dissection along the C1 posterior arch. B. Exposure of the VA V3 segment above C1. C. Subperiosteal dissection inside the C1 transverse foramen. D. Opening of the C1 transverse foramen by resection of the posterior branch of the C1 transverse process. E. Section of the ligament at the upper aspect of the vertebral artery, covering the occipital condyle. F. After unroofing of the vertebral artery at the level of the transverse foramen, the artery is transposed. (*From Pathology and Surgery around the Vertebral Artery. George B, Bruneau M, Spetzler RF (eds), Springer 2011*)

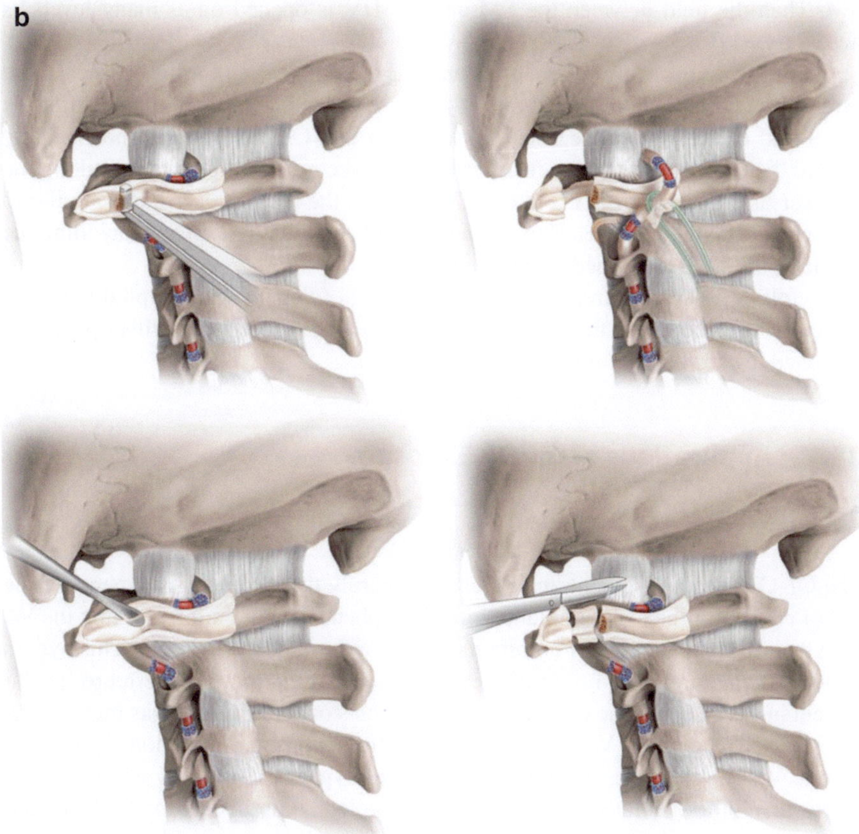

Fig. 28.2 (continued)

periosteal sheath is even more crucial (Fig. 28.2b). To achieve the opening of the C1 TF, the periosteum at the entrance and the exit of the TF must be elevated with a smooth spatula; then the heel of a Kerrison Rongeur is pushed in between the bone and the periosteum inside the TF to bite the bone covering the VA from both sides of the TF. To clear the field, the tip of the TP of atlas may be resected, as it is generally a huge piece of bone.

To transpose the VA out of the TF, the VA periosteal sheath must be split from the bone all around the VA inside the TF. Before pulling out the VA, the bone in the concavity of the loop formed by the two VA segments must be resected as much as possible. In fact, the VA may be torn during this maneuver if the tip of the PAA is not properly removed.

28.2.3 Extension Upstream and Downstream

The VA can be followed upstream as low in the neck as necessary using the anterolateral approach. For this, the skin incision is extended along the medial edge of the

SM. Then the field between the SM and the IJV is opened on as many levels as necessary.

The course of the VA between C2 and C3 is complex with a first corner at the level of the C2 TP and a second one at the base of the C2 vertebral body. After the lower end of the vertical segment between C1 and C2, the VA runs horizontally toward the C2 vertebral body and after the second corner vertically down along the transversary segment from C3 to C6. The work at the level of each TP is similar to the one done at the C1 level. The TP must be subperiosteally exposed including the inside of the TF if they need to be unroofed.

To follow the VA upstream on its V4 intradural segment, the occipital bone has to be opened; the upper the VA must be exposed, the more lateral this opening is extended toward the MP and the jugular tubercle.

28.3 Applications of the VA Exposure

28.3.1 VA Revascularization

The C1-C2 vertical segment and much more rarely the horizontal segment are the site of choice for the distal implantation of a saphenous vein graft bypassing the VA with the external, internal, or common carotid, or the subclavian artery. This bypass indication was pretty common 30 years ago to revascularize the vertebro-basilar system in case of multiple cervical vessels stenosis or occlusion. It was more rarely used to exclude cervical VA aneurysm and arterio-venous malformations by occluding the VA below the distal implantation of the bypass followed by embolization. However, all these indications have almost completely disappeared with the extensive development of endovascular techniques. It remains few indications in selected cases of tumor encasing a dominant VA when complete removal is contemplated and vessel preservation is not possible (Fig. 28.3). The VA must be completely exposed and controlled inside the periosteal sheath which hence needs to be opened. Obviously the venous plexus has to be controlled by bipolar coagulation. Most of the time the space between the C1 and C2 TF is quite sufficient to apply clips at both ends of this segment and to permit to suture the vein graft in between them. However if necessary the space may be enlarged by the opening of the C1 TF.

28.3.2 Extrinsic Compression of the VA; Bow Hunter Syndrome

This syndrome is rare but must be clearly identified since an appropriate and very efficient treatment can be proposed. It corresponds to an intermittent and severe compression of the VA in its V3 segment during a particular movement of the head and neck; this movement must always be the same and must induce a severe stenosis or an occlusion as demonstrated on any exam. Today angiography is no more necessary; Doppler ultrasound study and angio-CT are quite demonstrative and less invasive. The compression may be due to a bony or tendinous anomaly. Bony

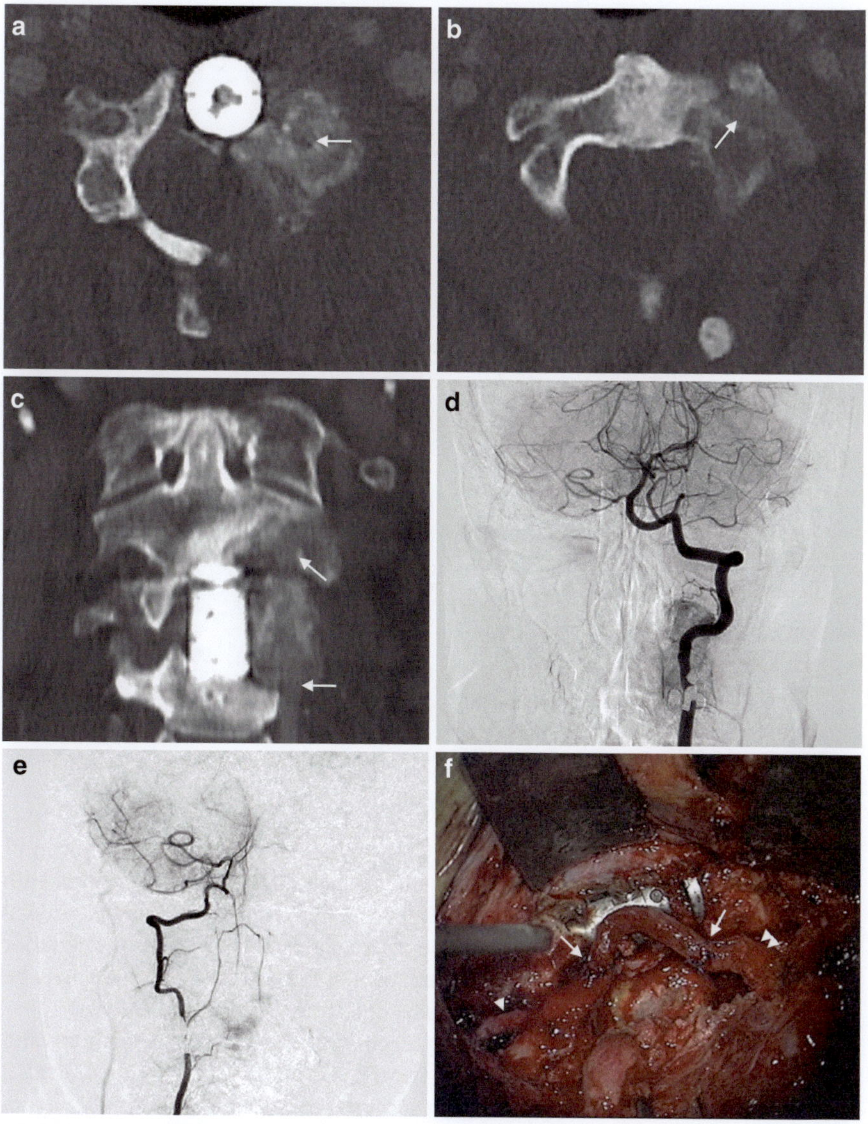

Fig. 28.3 Vertebral artery reconstruction by a C2-C4 bypass in a case of recurrent osteoblastoma. (**a**) This woman was already operated on twice in another institution with partial resection of the tumor and C2-C4 reconstruction with a distractible cage. The tumor remnant was growing. The tumor completely encases the left vertebral artery (arrow). (**b**) The tumor extends up to the base of C2 in close relation with the area where the vertebral artery performs an acute lateral bend (arrow). (**c**) Coronal view showing the relations between the tumor and the vertebral artery (arrows). (**d**, **e**) The left vertebral artery is clearly dominant and vascularizes the tumor. The left vertebral artery can not be sacrificed. (**f**) Intraoperative view after complete resection and reconstruction of the vertebral artery with a saphenous graft bypass. Proximal (arrowhead) and distal vertebral artery control (double arrowhead) were gained early in the procedure; temporary clips were placed at this level during the bypass. (**g–j**) Postoperative angio-CT controls confirming complete tumor resection and bypass patency (arrows). (*With permission of Erasme Hospital, ULB*)

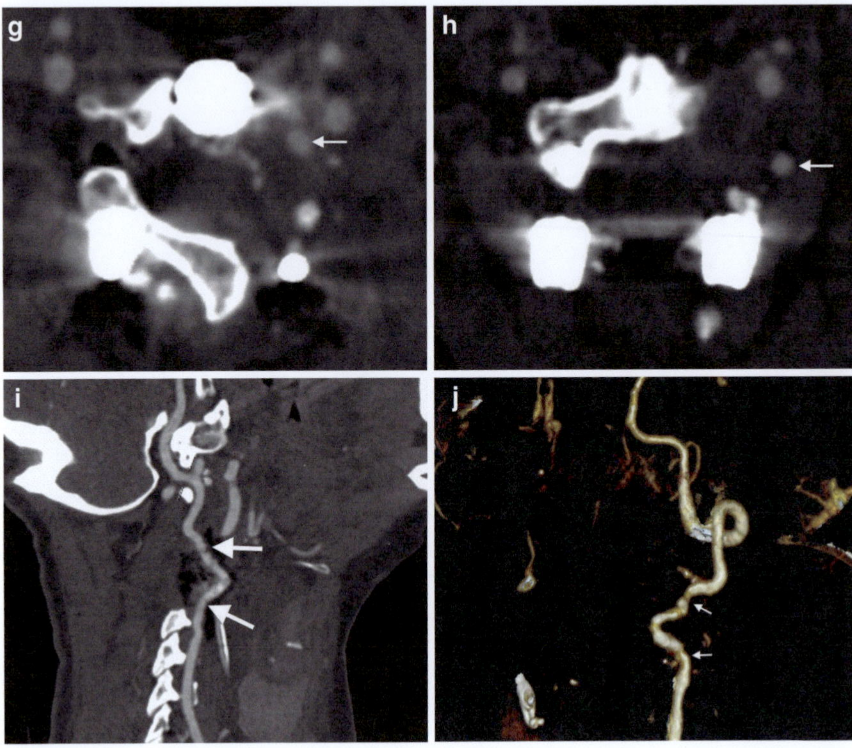

Fig. 28.3 (continued)

malformations are quite common at the CVJ including a supplementary piece of bone on the condyle or the lateral mass of atlas or a Klippel–Feil malformation with fusion between C1 and C2; it may be also tendon thickening either on the vertical (C1-C2) or the horizontal (above C1) segment. In our experience, the anterior branch of the C2 root crossing the anterior aspect of the VA C1-C2 segment may be part of the compression and had always to be cut.

The anterolateral approach is generally used with resection of the compressing element and very often the opening of the two TF (C1 and C2) and the cut of the C2 root. Some authors have also proposed to suppress the offending movement by an arthrodesis but this strategy can have a significant impact on head rotation and the quality of live [5, 7, 21].

28.3.3 FM Tumors

FM tumors and especially, by much the most frequent ones, meningiomas are best treated using the posterolateral approach. FM meningiomas are classified based on their compartment of development, their dural insertion, and their relation to the vertebral artery (Fig. 28.4). The bone opening is more or less extended following the

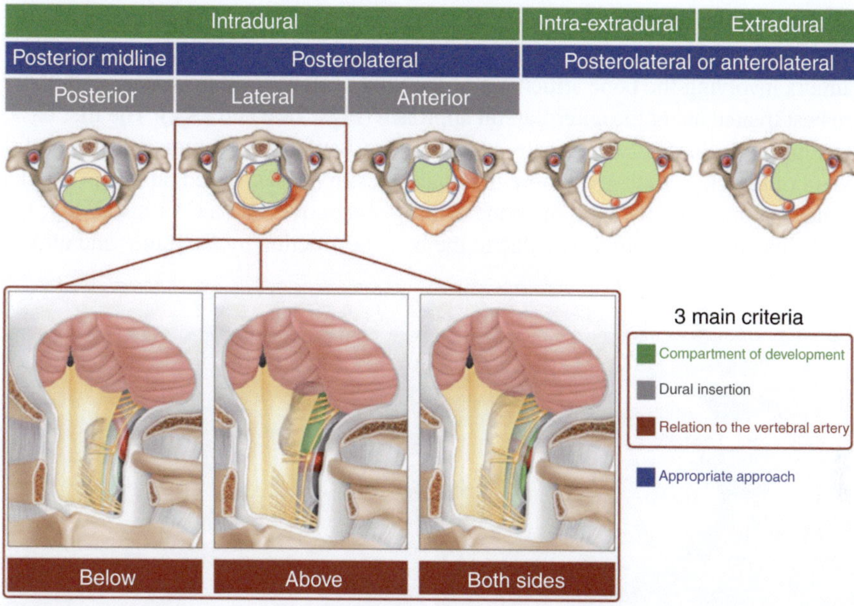

Fig. 28.4 Classification system of foramen magnum meningiomas. This classification system allows for determining preoperatively the adequate surgical strategy by determining the appropriate surgical approach and anticipating the modified position of vital neurovascular structures. FMMs are first classified by their compartment of development: purely intradural tumors, intra-extra-dural tumors, and purely extradural lesions. Intradural meningiomas are then subdivided according to their base of insertion and their relation with the VA, determining, respectively, the tumor position in the horizontal and vertical plane. According to their base of insertion, FMMs can be classified into anterior if its base of insertion is observed on both sides of the midline, lateral if it takes its origin between the midline and the dentate ligament, and posterior if found behind this ligament. According to their relation with the vertebral artery, FMMs are able to develop below, above, or on both sides of the VA. When located below the VA, the lower cranial nerves are always displaced cranially and posteriorly. If the meningioma grows above or on both sides of the VA, the position of the lower cranial nerves cannot be anticipated. (*From Pathology and Surgery around the Vertebral Artery. George B, Bruneau M, Spetzler RF (eds), Springer 2011*)

tumor location; anterior ones attached on both sides of the anterior midline need as lateral an extension as possible while lateral ones attached between the anterior midline and the denticulate ligament need a limited lateral opening. In fact with the posterolateral approach as described above (Sect. 28.2.1), it is never useful to drill far laterally either the occipital condyle or the lateral mass of atlas.

In case of involvement of the dura at the level of the VA penetration, it is safer to cut the dura at some distance around the VA so as to leave a cuff of dura because of the interconnection between the dura and the VA adventitia (see chapter anatomy).

The posterolateral approach is essentially designed for any intradural FM tumors (Fig. 28.5) but may be also applied on some extradural pathologies located inside the bone limits of the CVJ.

28.3.4 CVJ Tumors

Tumors involving the bone structures of the CVJ or developed in contact with them are best treated using the anterolateral approach (Figs. 28.6 and 28.7). The first basic principle is to perfectly delineate on the image workup the tumor and the useful extent of resection to drill no more than the necessary bone. Based on this principle, in the vast majority of cases, the bone drilling must not create a CVJ instability; the instability should essentially be due to the bone destruction by the tumor and almost

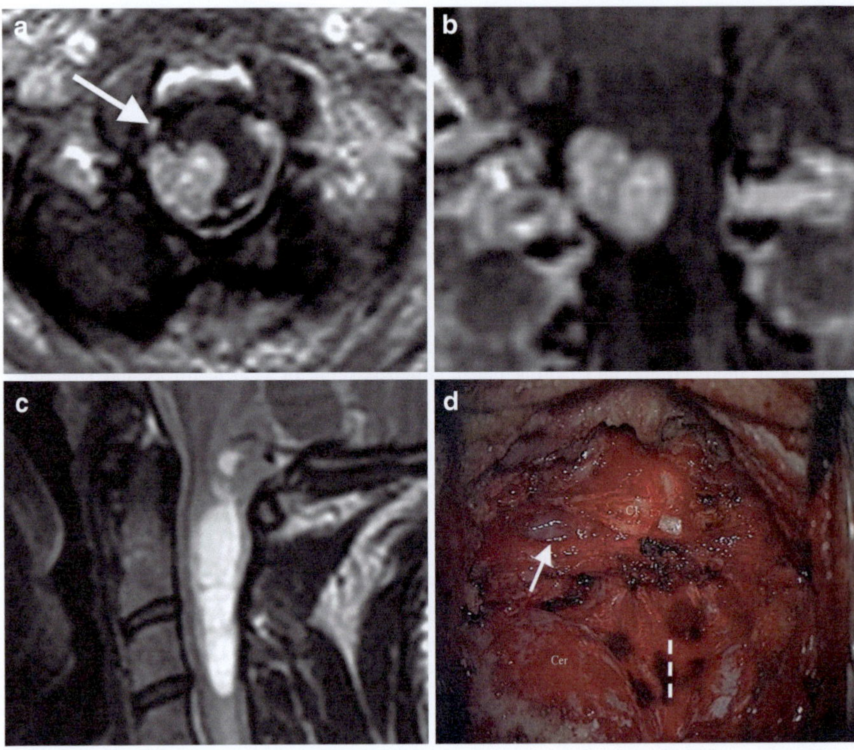

Fig. 28.5 Bulbomedullar hemangioblastoma. (**a**) The tumor is laterally located, close to the intradural segment (V4) of the vertebral artery. (**b**) Coronal view at the foramen magnum level. (**c**) The tumor is responsible for a syringomyelia. (**d**) View after the bilateral suboccipital craniotomy, more extended on the right side, exposing the cerebellar dura matter (Cer). The midline is showed with dotted line. The horizontal portion of the right vertebral artery V3 segment is visible above the C1 posterior arch (arrow). (**e**) Subperiosteal exposure of the horizontal portion of the vertebral artery V3 segment above the C1 posterior arch through a postero-lateral approach. (**f**) The control of the V3 segment allows to resect the C1 posterior arch laterally up to the C1 lateral wall and then to retract the dura matter more laterally. By doing this, the tumor can be exposed safely without any risk of tumor disruption to achieve a complete en-bloc resection and avoid profuse bleedings. The intradural segment of the vertebral artery (arrow) and the lower cranial nerves are controlled at the beginning of the procedure. (**g**) View at the completion of the complete resection. Neurological examination remained unchanged. (*With permission of Erasme Hospital, ULB*)

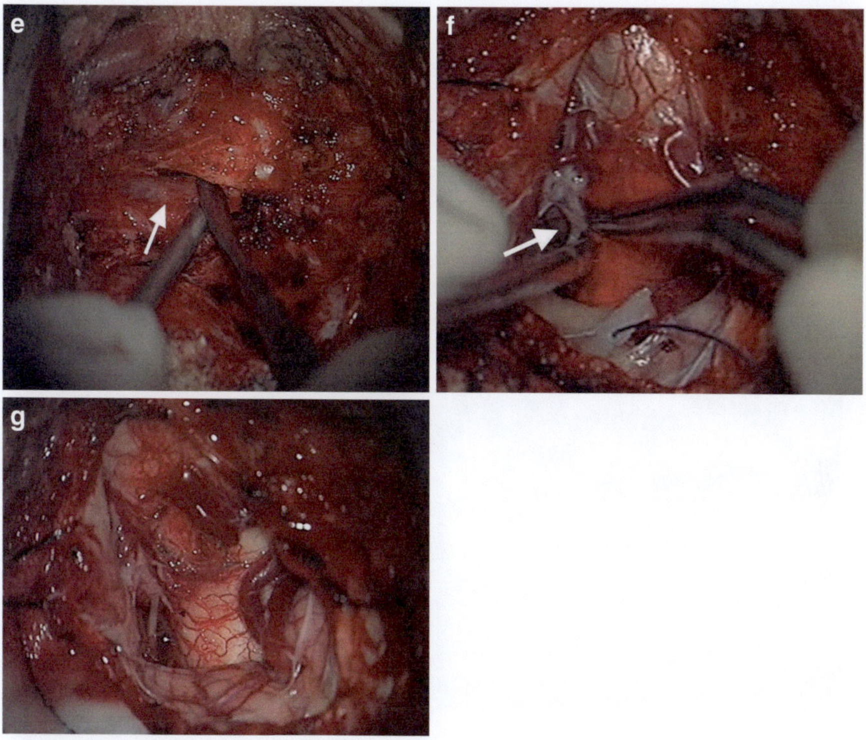

Fig. 28.5 (continued)

never to the surgical drilling. Following these points, an occipito-cervical fusion may have to be considered preoperatively and rarely postoperatively. In very particular cases, a bone graft, occasionally screwed, can be placed as a fixation.

The second basic principle is, before all, to control the VA on both sides of the tumor. Then if the VA is encased by the tumor, its size must be appreciated and a balloon occlusion test asked if a dominant VA has to be sacrificed or is at risk during the surgery.

28.3.5 JF Tumors

JF tumors include essentially paragangliomas (glomus tumors), neurinomas, and meningiomas [3, 22].

Especially for glomus tumors, the VA is one of the vasculo-nervous elements that need to be controlled in a first step before considering the tumor resection. Moreover, its control is necessary to gain a postero-inferior access to the JF without the need for any petrous bone drilling. This technique called the juxtacondylar approach is an extension of the anterolateral approach. The first step is the VA exposure, followed by the

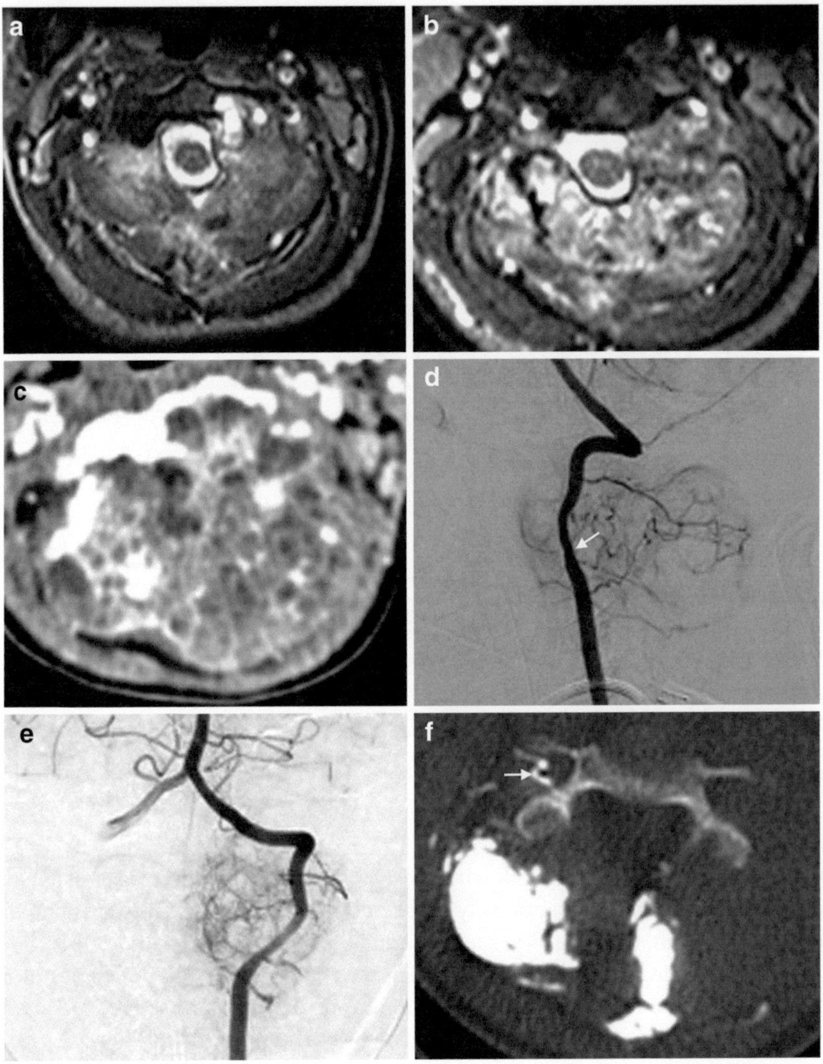

Fig. 28.6 Aneurysmal bone cyst quickly growing in a 6-year-old girl. (**a**, **b**) Preoperative MRI showing the tumor involving the posterior elements and the C2 vertebral body and C2-C3 intervertebral foramen on the left side. (**c**) Six weeks later, the tumor has grown significantly and compresses the spinal cord. Despite the compression, the neurological status remains normal. (**d**, **e**) The left vertebral artery vascularizes the tumor through several branches. The artery was compressed by the tumor (arrow). (**f**) The tumor was preoperatively embolized through direct transcutaneous punctures. The procedure was interrupted when observing some embolization material in the right vertebral artery (arrow). (**g**) The patient was operated on through a left lateral approach and then a posterior approach. The postoperative angio-CT shows the patent left vertebral artery (white arrow), the bone graft placed inside the C2 dens (black arrow), the bone graft between the C1 posterior arch and the C3 lamina on the right side (arrowhead). (**h**) After 6 months, the C2 bone graft was completely integrated (arrowheads). (**i**) View at the level of C2 showing the bone graft and reconstruction of the C2 lamina using bone chips. (**j**) Postoperative stabilization was achieved with C1 lateral mass screws and C3-C4 hooks due to the small size of the facets in this child. (**k**) MRI at 6 months confirms the complete resection. (*With permission of Erasme Hospital, ULB*)

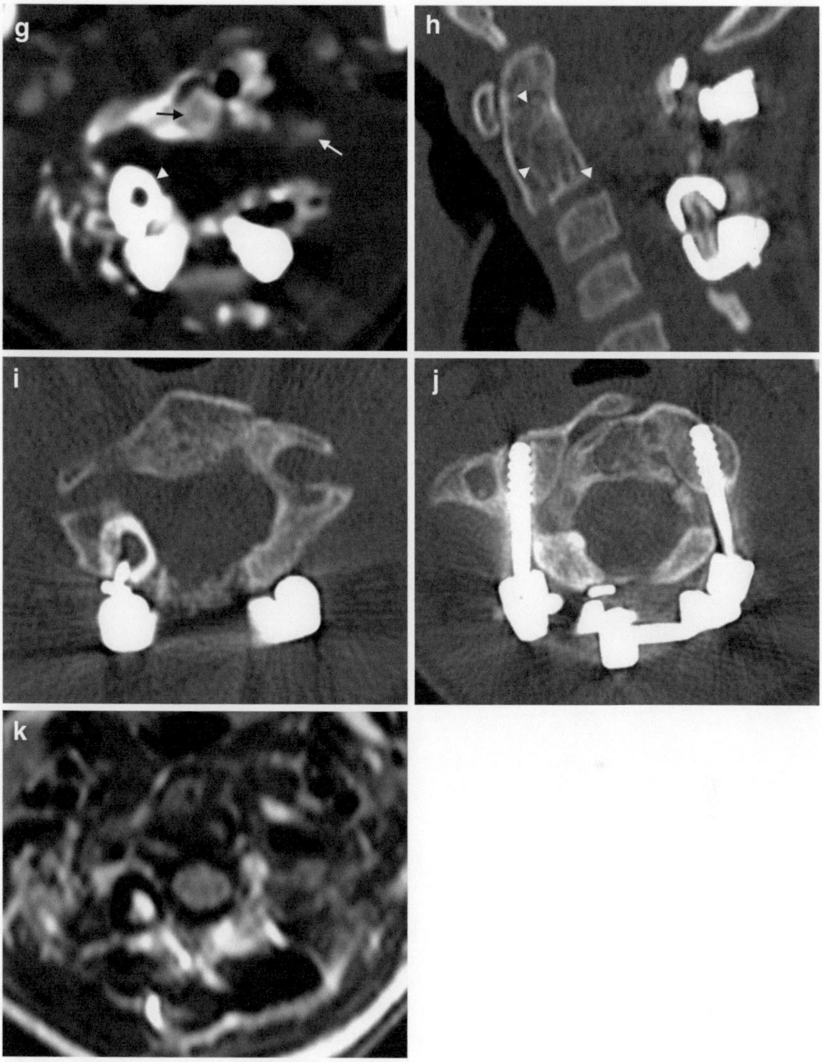

Fig. 28.6 (continued)

control of the vasculo-nervous cervical elements as needed: the internal and external carotid arteries; the IX, X, XI, and XII cranial nerves; and the sympathetic chain. Then a retrosigmoid opening is realized including a mastoidectomy exposing the last centimeters of the sigmoid sinus (SS). At this point it remain some bone covering the JF between the upper part of the IJV and the end of the SS. Unroofing the JF is rather easy in most cases since the JF is much enlarged by the tumor, the bone cover is thin, and the SS is generally occluded. Therefore this approach is quite sufficient for any tumor developed inside the bony limits of the JF. This is generally the case of neurinomas. Conversely in cases of tumors overtaking these bony limits and extending into the petrous bone, the bone drilling must follow these extensions but can be limited.

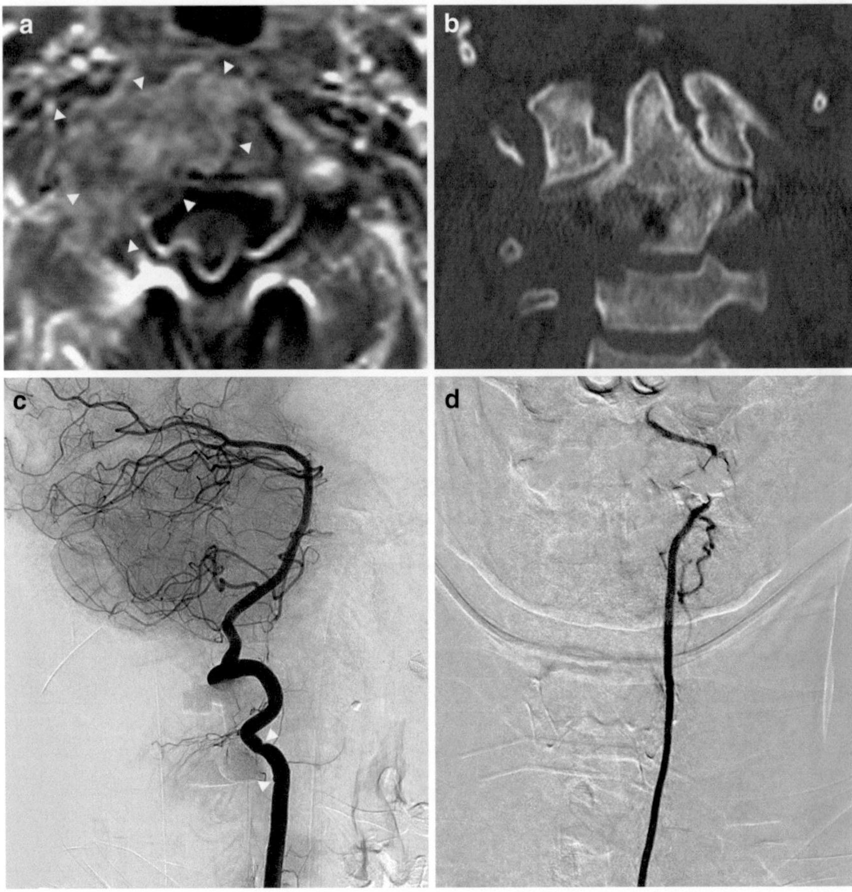

Fig. 28.7 The patient suffered from a right-sided C2 chordoma. The patient has already had a biopsy and a posterior fixation elsewhere. (**a**) The tumor (arrowheads) destructed the C2 vertebral body and the C2-C3 facet joint, and extended to the surrounding soft tissues, including the C2-C3 intervertebral foramen. (**b**) Coronal view showing also the extension to the uncus of C3. (**c**) The right vertebral artery was dominant. Note that the artery irregular to the compression by the tumor (arrowheads). (**d**) The contralateral vertebral artery was hypoplastic. (**e**) The tumor has been resected through a right-sided lateral approach. Note the exposure of the spinal accessory nerve (black arrow). The vertebral artery was first controlled at the level of the C1 transverse foramen (arrow) and then at the C3 level. (**f**) The vertebral artery is visible at the C2 level, showed by the forceps. (**g**) View after tumor resection extended up to normal bone. The vertebral artery is visible inside the periosteal sheath (arrow). (**h, i**) MRI confirmed the complete resection of the tumor and showed the right vertebral artery (arrow) after its dissection. (**j**) Bone stabilization was achieved using a distractible cage filling the bone defect and a 2-screw lateral plate. (*With permission of Erasme Hospital, ULB*)

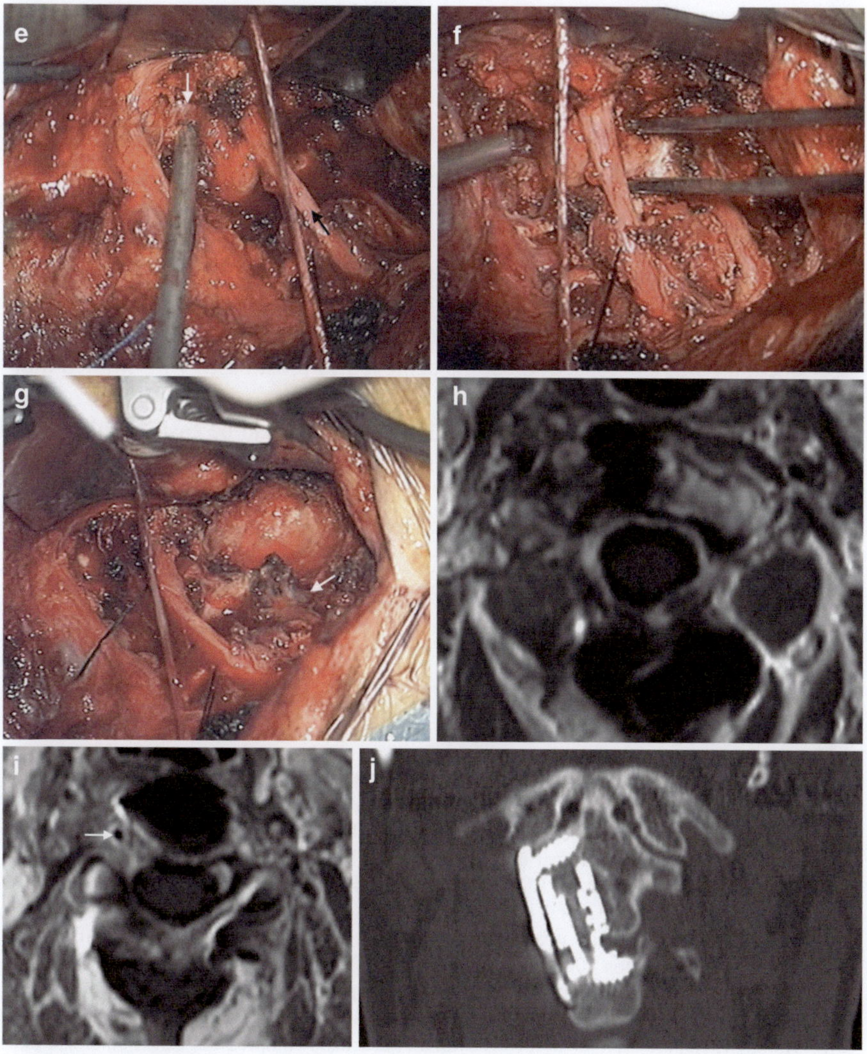

Fig. 28.7 (continued)

28.4 Risks and Hazards of the VA Exposure

The VA exposure in the neck from its origin to the FM dura penetration is a well-defined technique applied in our experience in more than 1700 cases including more than 400 at the CVJ (V3 level). Mortality and morbidity related to the VA exposure is very limited. There is no mortality, and morbidity is limited to some damages to the accessory nerve in three cases with painful stiffness of the SM resolving in 2 or 3 months. It can be explained by a too strong retraction of the SM. In our experience, no tear of the VA occurred.

28.5 Conclusions

The VA in its V3 segment at the CVJ level can be exposed and controlled using two well-defined techniques: the posterolateral approach essentially useful for intradural FM tumors and the anterolateral approach for VA revascularization, release of extrinsic intermittent compression, and resection of CVJ and JF tumors. In our experience, a complete resection can be achieved in most cases with limited morbidity and mortality.

The VA exposure is a well-defined technique, which can be easily applied after some training. The main trick is to preserve the periosteal sheath surrounding the VA and its venous plexus. Overall the VA control permits to extend the access around the CVJ without inducing in most cases a CVJ instability, avoiding unnecessary petrous bone drilling, and generally permitting a safe and radical tumoral resection. Moreover, the VA can be followed upstream in the lower neck and downstream inside the posterior fossa.

References

1. Bruneau M, George B. Foramen magnum meningiomas: detailed surgical approaches and technical aspects at Lariboisière hospital and review of the literature. Neurosurg Rev. 2008;31:19–32; discussion 32–3. https://doi.org/10.1007/s10143-007-0097-1.
2. Bruneau M, George B. Surgical approaches to the V3 segment of the vertebral artery. In: George B, Bruneau M, Spetzler RF, editors. Pathology and surgery around the vertebral artery. Paris: Springer; 2011. p. 329–60.
3. Bruneau M, George B. The juxtacondylar approach to the jugular foramen. Neurosurgery. 2008;62:75–8; discussion 80–1. https://doi.org/10.1227/01.neu.0000317375.38067.55.
4. Bruneau M, Cornelius JF, George B. Antero-lateral approach to the V3 segment of the vertebral artery. Neurosurgery. 2006;58:ONS29–35; discussion ONS29–35
5. Morimoto T, Nakase H, Sakaki T, Matsuyama T. Extrinsic compression Bow hunter's stroke. In: George B, Bruneau M, Spetzler RF, editors. Pathology and surgery around the vertebral artery. Paris: Springer; 2011. p. 473–87.
6. Bassiouni H, Ntoukas V, Asgari S, et al. Foramen magnum meningiomas: clinical outcome after microsurgical resection via a posterolateral suboccipital retrocondylar approach. Neurosurgery. 2006;59:1177–85; discussion 1185–7. https://doi.org/10.1227/01.NEU.0000245629.77968.37.
7. Matsuyama T, Morimoto T, Sakaki T. Comparison of C1-2 posterior fusion and decompression of the vertebral artery in the treatment of Bow hunter's stroke. J Neurosurg. 1997;86:619–23. https://doi.org/10.3171/jns.1997.86.4.0619.
8. Yang T, Tariq F, Duong HT, Sekhar LN. Bypass using V2-V3 segment of the vertebral artery as donor or recipient: technical nuances and results. World Neurosurg. 2014;82:1164–70. https://doi.org/10.1016/j.wneu.2014.02.034.

9. Bruneau M, George B. Chapter 26: Surgical technique for the resection of tumors in relation with the V3 and V4 segments of the vertebral artery. In: George B, Bruneau M, Spetzler RF, editors. Pathology and surgery around the vertebral artery. Paris: Springer; 2011. p. 362–405.
10. George B, Lot G. Anterolateral and posterolateral approaches to the foramen magnum: technical description and experience from 97 cases. Skull Base Surg. 1995;5:9–19.
11. Nanda A, Vincent DA, Vannemreddy PS, et al. Far-lateral approach to intradural lesions of the foramen magnum without resection of the occipital condyle. J Neurosurg. 2002;96:302–9. https://doi.org/10.3171/jns.2002.96.2.0302.
12. Lanzino G, Paolini S, Spetzler RF. Far-lateral approach to the craniocervical junction. Neurosurgery. 2005;57:367–71; discussion 367–71
13. Sharma BS, Gupta SK, Khosla VK, et al. Midline and far lateral approaches to foramen magnum lesions. Neurol India. 1999;47:268–71.
14. Spektor S, Anderson GJ, McMenomey SO, et al. Quantitative description of the far-lateral transcondylar transtubercular approach to the foramen magnum and clivus. J Neurosurg. 2000;92:824–31. https://doi.org/10.3171/jns.2000.92.5.0824.
15. Kratimenos GP, Crockard HA. The far lateral approach for ventrally placed foramen magnum and upper cervical spine tumours. Br J Neurosurg. 1993;7:129–40.
16. Rhoton AL. The far-lateral approach and its transcondylar, supracondylar, and paracondylar extensions. Neurosurgery. 2000;47:S195–209.
17. Babu RP, Sekhar LN, Wright DC. Extreme lateral transcondylar approach: technical improvements and lessons learned. J Neurosurg. 1994;81:49–59. https://doi.org/10.3171/jns.1994.81.1.0049.
18. Sen CN, Sekhar LN. An extreme lateral approach to intradural lesions of the cervical spine and foramen magnum. Neurosurgery. 1990;27:197–204.
19. Salas E, Sekhar LN, Ziyal IM, et al. Variations of the extreme-lateral craniocervical approach: anatomical study and clinical analysis of 69 patients. J Neurosurg. 1999;90:206–19.
20. Acikbas SC, Tuncer R, Demirez I, et al. The effect of condylectomy on extreme lateral transcondylar approach to the anterior foramen magnum. Acta Neurochir. 1997;139:546–50.
21. Morimoto T, Kaido T, Uchiyama Y, et al. Rotational obstruction of nondominant vertebral artery and ischemia. Case report. J Neurosurg. 1996;85:507–9. https://doi.org/10.3171/jns.1996.85.3.0507.
22. Bruneau M, Makiese O, Cornelius JF, et al. Chapter 44: The juxtacondylar approach to the jugular foramen. In: George B, Bruneau M, Spetzler RF, editors. Pathology and surgery around the vertebral artery. Paris: Springer; 2011. p. 641–68.

Management of Aneurysms and AVMs at the Cranio-vertebral Junction

29

Paolo Di Russo, Erez Nossek, and Amir R. Dehdashti

29.1 Aneurysms

Posterior circulation aneurysms account for 5–10% of all intracranial aneurysms, with the most common location at the basilar artery bifurcation (about 50% of cases), followed by vertebral artery–posterior inferior cerebellar artery (VA–PICA) aneurysms (about 10% of cases).

Intracranial aneurysms harboring in the posterior circulation have been considered difficult to manage, since first reports. They are usually deep located, close to the brainstem, and interposed between cranial nerves, always representing a surgical challenge for vascular neurosurgeons. Furthermore, the natural history of these aneurysms is also considered poorer, with higher risk of rupture when compared with other localizations in the anterior circulations.

Aneurysms at the cranial-vertebral junction are located in the lower third of posterior cranial fossa and they usually involve the vertebral artery and the PICA. Both saccular and dissecting aneurysms can occur at this level. They can be classified into two groups: vertebral artery–PICA aneurysms and distal PICA aneurysms.

In this context, VA–basilar artery aneurysms (or vertebrobasilar junction aneurysms) are located more cranially and farther from the CVJ.

P. Di Russo
Department of Neurosurgery, I.R.C.C.S Neuromed, Pozzilli, Italy

E. Nossek
Department of Neurosurgery, NYU School of Medicine, New York, NY, USA

A. R. Dehdashti (✉)
Department of Neurosurgery, North Shore University Hospital, Northwell Health, Manhasset, NY, USA

E. Tessitore et al. (eds.), *Surgery of the Cranio-Vertebral Junction*,
https://doi.org/10.1007/978-3-030-18700-2_29

29.1.1 Vertebral Artery–PICA Saccular Aneurysms

29.1.1.1 Introduction

The most common aneurysm arising at the CVJ is the VA–Posterior Inferior Cerebellar Artery (PICA) aneurysm, accounting for 0.5 to 3–4% of all intracranial aneurysms in different series. They can present both as saccular and fusiform/dissecting aneurysms.

Before the expansion of endovascular techniques, VA–PICA aneurysms were surgically approached and even considered relatively straightforward to access when addressed by expert neurosurgeon. The PICA lies into the cerebello-pontine angle cistern and the neurosurgeon confident with the neurovascular anatomy of the area can identify the VA–PICA convergence and gently dissect the neck and dome of the aneurysm for clipping.

In spite of this, the progressive development and refinement of endovascular treatment of intracranial aneurysms led the number of cases treated with surgical clipping to consequently decrease during years. Nevertheless, the common nature of small caliber of PICA, the small size of some PICA aneurysms, and also the broad neck of the aneurysm might favor a surgical clipping instead of endovascular treatment for some aneurysms. Furthermore, the lack of endovascular treatment in obtaining a high rate of complete occlusion of the aneurysms (reported rate of recanalization around 20–30%), as reported in several studies, emphasizes the matter that direct clipping is still an important option for treatment of these challenging lesions. Also complex cases, like large or giant aneurysms or the involvement of perforating vessel or important arterial branches, might sometimes be more suitable for surgical treatment.

29.1.1.2 Clinical Presentation

Patients with vertebral artery–PICA aneurysms usually present with subarachnoid hemorrhage (SAH), commonly with a high Fisher scoring, due to the presence of intraventricular hemorrhage (IVH), with real possibility of acute hydrocephalus. Otherwise, they also can be discovered occasionally as unruptured aneurysms or they can present with symptoms of cranial nerves or brainstem compression or ictus. VA–PICA aneurysm can also be incidentally diagnosed, in patients with multiple aneurysms, with a slight prevalence for the association with middle cerebral artery (MCA) aneurysms.

29.1.1.3 Neuroradiological Assessment

After computed tomography (CT) evidence of SAH, digital subtraction angiography (DSA) is still the gold standard method for diagnosing the presence of intracranial aneurysms. All the details of the aneurysm, like the shape, size, and location, can be observed with DSA. Nevertheless, also a less invasive exam like computed tomography angiography (CTA) identifies the presence of the aneurysm and furthermore allows to better relate the relationship of the aneurysm with important bony landmarks that can be used to plan the cranial or caudal extension of the craniotomy and dural opening. These structures are the edge of the foramen magnum, the occipital condyle, and the jugular tubercle. In fact, adjunctive bony work like partial drilling of the occipital condyle or the jugular tubercle could be necessary in some cases to enhance the surgical corridor.

29.1.1.4 Anatomy of VA–PICA Convergence and PICA

Posterior inferior cerebellar artery is the largest branch from the vertebral artery and presents the most variable and tortuous course of the cerebellar arteries. In about 90% of cases, PICA origins within 1 cm above the CVJ and 1 cm below the VA–basilar junction. Usually it has an intradural origin from the posterior or lateral aspect of the VA (V4 segment), anterior to the inferior olive and directed posteriorly and medially toward the cerebellomedullary fissure. Before reaching the fissure, along its course into the lateral part of the cisterna magna, the artery meets the lower cranial nerves. At this level, the artery first pass antero-lateral to medulla (*anterior medullary segment*) and in close relation with the rootles of hypoglossal nerve (XII c.n.). After, it curves at the level of the postero-lateral aspect of the medulla (*lateral medullary segment*) where it crosses glossopharyngeal (IX c.n.), vagus (X c.n.) and accessory (XI c.n.) nerves. Once passed lower cranial nerves, PICA enters the fissure and makes a caudal loop around the ipsilateral cerebellar tonsil (*tonsillomedullary segment*). Then, the artery takes an ascending course becoming very close to the roof of the fourth ventricle (*telovelotonsillary segment*) and looping again around the superior pole of the tonsil. Finally, the artery leaves the groove between the vermis and tonsil and bifurcates into two trunks giving off cortical branches (*cortical segment*), supplying vermis and cerebellar hemisphere on the suboccipital surface. Perforating vessels are important small arteries directed to the brainstem and they usually arise from the first three segments of the PICA.

The origin of the PICA could vary along the course of the VA, being next to the initial part of V4 (intradural segment of VA) or very close to vertebral-basilar junction, necessitating different surgical approaches when an aneurysm is sited. In a low number of cases, the origin of PICA is below the foramen magnum and even more rarely it comes off from the extradural VA. This anatomical variation can be preoperatively analyzed with DSA and CTA.

29.1.1.5 Aneurysm's Anatomical Features

The so-called PICA aneurysm is instead a truly VA aneurysm, with PICA usually originating from or close to the neck of the aneurysm. According to the origin of the neck, distally or cranially to the origin of the PICA on the VA, the aneurysms can be considered pre-PICA or post-PICA. Post-PICA have been reported as more common. Thus, in most cases, the neck of the aneurysm is wide and the origin of the PICA is included. The dome of the aneurysm can be directed cranially or caudally, and also medially toward the brainstem or laterally away from the brainstem. In most of cases, the dome has a cranial direction. Usually the medium size of VA–PICA aneurysms is 5–8 mm and giant aneurysms are seldom reported.

29.1.1.6 Preoperative Management

Depending on patient's level of consciousness, preoperative neurological examination is performed to rule out the presence of lower cranial nerve deficits or other symptoms. In the setting of subarachnoid hemorrhage and after CTA, most patients undergo an external ventricular drainage (EVD) placement. The patient is then transferred to neurosurgical intensive care unit (NICU) and a treatment between clipping and coiling is decided upon according to the angio-anatomy of the aneurysm and characteristics of a given patient. When surgical clipping is preferred, the timing of treatment depends on general clinical situation of the patient. Our policy is to perform surgery within 24 h of subarachnoid hemorrhage, to reduce the rate of early re-bleeding and poor outcome.

29.1.1.7 Surgical Approaches

The main goal of surgery for VA–PICA aneurysms follows the principles of aneurysm surgery. Obtaining an early proximal control, a direct view of the neck of the aneurysms and a comfortable surgical maneuverability for arachnoid dissection are all important key-points when dealing with these aneurysms. Different surgical approaches are suitable for this purpose. The choice of the approach depends on the origin of the PICA (and the aneurysm) along the VA and also on the surgeon preference.

Posterior-Lateral Approaches

The *far-lateral transcondylar approach* represents the work-horse for surgery around the CVJ and our preferred approach for PICA aneurysms. This approach allows an early identification of the extradural segment of the VA (V3) and a good exposure of the anterior-lateral aspect of the brainstem and upper cervical cord. Conventional far-lateral approach includes a lateral suboccipital craniotomy extended to the foramen magnum, C1 hemilaminectomy, and some drilling (10–30%) of the medial occipital condyle. Extension of the far-lateral approach has been proposed, according to the location of the lesions. Sometimes, the presence of a big tumor (e.g., foramen magnum meningioma) naturally increases the working space. Instead, in vascular cases, different amount of bony work could be helpful in order to obtain a better surgical maneuverability for aneurysm dissection and clipping or to gain space for temporary clipping if necessary or to manage cases with vascular anatomical variations. For instance, the posterior third of the occipital condyle can be drilled to a further extent (more than 30%) when a tortuous VA gives off a PICA closer to the midline. Moreover, the jugular tubercle can be drilled in cases of higher origin of the PICA closer to the vertebral-basilar junction (*trans-tubercular approach*). The entry point of VA into the dura of the CVJ is at the level of the occipital condyle, so the C1 hemilaminectomy increases the work space for safe identification and possible transposition of the VA if necessary. This is even more crucial when the origin of PICA is closer to the point where the VA pierces the dura. Usually it is not necessary to expose the transverse-sigmoid sinus junction, except for when the PICA has a much higher origin on the VA. These different scenarios can be preoperatively identified with CTA and DSA.

A three-quarter prone (park bench) position is used, with (1) the head inferiorly flexed, (2) rotated toward the floor (about 30–45°), (3) laterally tilted (about 20°), and (4) elevated above the heart level. Before the skin incision, neurophysiological monitoring of lower cranial nerves, somatosensory and motor evoked potentials are set up. A slightly curved skin incision is performed two finger breadth behind the base of the mastoid, using mastoid tip, C1 tubercle, and zygomatic arch as anatomical landmarks. The end of the incision curves toward the midline to identify the C2 spinous process during the dissection. C1 tubercle is a reliable landmark that can be palpated from outside and thus can be used for both planning of skin incision (which remains two finger breadth behind) and during the muscular dissection for identification of VA. The C2 spinous process helps in better identification of midline when the head is rotated in park bench position. Posterior-lateral muscles are dissected together with the bovie, leaving a small cuff just below the superior nuchal line, at the inferior nuchal line where superior oblique and rectus capitis posterior major (RCPMj) muscles attach. These two muscles together with inferior oblique muscle form the suboccipital triangle. In the depth of this triangle, the vertebral artery (V3 segment) can be identified. Superior oblique and RCPMj always need to be dissected bluntly with small periosteal elevators to allow performance of the craniotomy including opening of the foramen magnum. Detachment of the inferior oblique muscle exposes the underlying C1 lamina. After all muscles have been dissected in a subperiosteal fashion and the extradural vertebral artery is identified, a C1 hemilaminectomy followed by a low lateral suboccipital craniotomy (extended to the foramen magnum inferiorly and sigmoid sinus and jugular bulb laterally) is performed. At this point, the medial and posterior aspect of the occipital condyle is drilled to achieve a flat lateral surface of skull base. Usually 10–30% drilling is enough. Mobilization and transposition of the VA is not necessary unless a tumor anatomy dictates so or if the VA is used as a donor for a bypass graft.

The dura mater is opened in a linear fashion parallel to the skin incision from the upper extension of the craniotomy to the CVJ, as far caudal as bone removal (depending on C1 hemilaminectomy). The cut proceeds from above in a slight curvilinear shape, then becomes close to the later edge of the craniotomy (occipital condyle and jugular tubercle) and finally gently bends medially and down to the limit of bone removal beyond the foramen magnum and at the craniocervical junction. Particular attention must be made to not to injure the VA at the dura entry point, hence the importance of identification of VA before dural incision. Once the dura is opened, gentle arachnoid dissection together with egress of the cerebral-spinal fluid (CSF) allows to obtain a complete view of the lateral brainstem-upper medulla anatomy. Only the lateral edges of the dura need to be retracted with sutures. Lower cranial nerves, V4 and PICA lie in the lateral cerebellum-medullary cistern and the knowledge of neurovascular anatomy of this location easily allows the surgeon to identify the VA–PICA convergence. The dentate ligament can be cut at the level of the foramen magnum and C1, to reduce the tension on the brainstem if necessary. Its white tensioning fibrous structure distinguishes itself from the lower cranial nerves. The intradural segment of the VA is then identified and traced up to the PICA origin and the aneurysm is recognized. The whole approach is done in a retractorless fashion.

Retro-Sigmoid Approach

Different modifications of retro-sigmoid approach have been proposed and tailored according to specific neurovascular pathologies in the cerebellum-pontine angle. Surgical clipping of VA–PICA aneurysms through a retro-sigmoid craniotomy has also been described. Considering the already narrow corridor, this approach could further impact and reduce the space disposable to comfortably work in between cranial nerves. This will result in less surgical view and maneuverability, necessity of cerebellum retraction, and higher risk of cranial nerve injuries. In our opinion, retro-sigmoid approach should not be considered for these aneurysms.

Endoscopic Extended Endonasal Approach

During the past decade, the endoscopic endonasal skull base surgery has shown important improvements. Thus, expert skull base surgeons started to report clipping of posterior circulation aneurysms with pure extended endoscopic endonasal approaches (EEA). Few cases have been described, using a trans-clival route with only one successful attempt to clip a VA–PICA ruptured aneurysm. These small series underlined some limitations of the EEA in tackling such aneurysms. The higher risk of CSF leak, more restricted surgical maneuverability especially in the lateral direction, and suboptimal control for handling an intraoperative rupture are among serious limitations. For these reasons, despite the wide experience of the senior author (A.D.) in using EEA, we do not recommend an EEA for clipping of CVJ aneurysms or removal of AVMs.

29.1.1.8 Clipping Technique

Different clipping techniques have been described. The goal of surgery is to completely exclude the aneurysm from the circulation and to preserve blood flow inside the PICA. The patency of PICA could be compromised with improper visualization of distal PICA or the wrong choice of a clip type.

PICA is the most anterior structure in the surgical field and therefore the surgical depth is significant. Furthermore, the presence of numerous lower cranial nerve rootlets (IX, X, XI, XII c.n.) complicates the surgical maneuverability between them. The XII c.n. exits from the medulla at the anterior-lateral sulcus and passes over the PICA directed laterally toward the hypoglossal canal. Nevertheless, considering that the origin of the aneurysm is most of the times from the posterior or lateral aspect of the VA, the hypoglossal nerve can be located at the same level of the VA–PICA aneurysm in the surgical field. Therefore, sometimes XII c.n. is located laterally to the aneurysm and other times can even be located anterior and deeper in the surgical field hidden by the aneurysm. Instead, the accessory root of the XI c.n. runs with an inferior-superior direction and passes inside the foramen magnum to reach the IX, X, and XI c.n. rootlets before entering the jugular foramen. This nerve root can be adherent to the upper spinal cord and medulla or more lateral in the cistern obstructing the view of the neck. In these cases, it needs to be gently dissected medially or laterally to expose the aneurysm neck for clipping. In most cases, rootlets of IX, X, and XI CNs are cranial to the VA–PICA junction. Only in cases of higher PICA origin or large aneurysms, the superior aspect of the dome can be in relation with these nerves. Nevertheless, manipulation of lower cranial nerves should be as least as possible, to reduce the rate of postoperative related complication.

These anatomical details suggest that the best clipping technique should allow to clip aneurysm's neck, together with sparing cranial nerves rootlets and PICA origin. Considering this, the most common clipping technique is usually with the use of a fenestrated clip. First, a fenestrated clip encircling the PICA and/or lower cranial nerves (in most of cases spinal root of accessory nerve) is placed parallel to the VA axis (Illustrative Case 1). A second clip, usually straight, can be added over the first one completing the exclusion of the aneurysm. However, if the anatomy dictates, a straight or ballonet clip can be used instead of the first fenestrated clip. Also the direction of the dome of the aneurysms needs to be carefully evaluated preoperatively, because it can affect the surgical strategy. Most PICA aneurysms have a superior projection, along the axis of the VA. This feature highlights the importance of tandem clipping with fenestrated clip. When dealing with large aneurysm, usually the patient presents with symptoms due to compression medulla or lower cranial nerves. Consecutively, after clipping, incision and reduction of the aneurysm dome is an important step for decompression. During dissection and clipping of VA–PICA aneurysms, particular attention needs to be paid to avoid damage or occlusion of perforating arteries arising at the first three medullary segments of PICA. Particular assessment of the clips blade position must be done to not to injure the hypoglossal nerve rootles hidden behind the aneurysm dome.

29.1.1.9 Complications and Outcome

Despite the meticulous microsurgical technique and continuous intraoperative neurophysiological monitoring, complications leading to lower cranial nerves palsies (LCNP) are not uncommon. The onset of new LCNP after surgery is reported to be around 20–40%. LCNP are responsible for dysphagia and aspiration pneumonia. In the majority of cases, LCNP are partial and temporary, with complete recover after 3–9 months. The rate of permanent LCNP is about 10%. These patients present with persistent dysphagia, hoarseness, and need for prolonged tracheostomy.

The presence of a postoperative lateral medullary syndrome (Wallenberg syndrome) is usually related to the occlusion of perforating arteries during surgical manipulations or to the sacrifice of PICA proximal to the telovelotonsillary segment. This can result in permanent neurological deficits, e.g., mild or severe hemiparesis, ataxia, and swallowing difficulties.

The occurrence of hydrocephalus is more common in ruptured posterior circulation aneurysms, and even more for VA–PICA aneurysms, accounting for about 20–30% of cases. This is probably due to the proximity of the bleeding origin to the foramen of Luschka (mostly for aneurysms proximal on the VA) and consequently the presence of blood inside the fourth ventricle (about 80% of ruptured VA–PICA aneurysms). Many of these patients will require ventricular-peritoneal shunt placement.

Patients with poor grade SAH who survive are at a higher risk of worse and permanent LCNP (commonly present also before surgery), prolonged stay in the ICU, worse quality of life, and 1-year mortality rate of 20–30%.

29.1.2 Distal PICA Saccular Aneurysms

Distal PICA aneurysms are defined as aneurysms not involving the VA–PICA origin. They are less frequent than VA–PICA aneurysms (incidence is about 0.2–1.4%) and they can arise on each of five segments of PICA, showing prevalence for telovelotonsillary segment. Frequentely, hemodynamic stress factors contribute to the genesis of these aneurysms. Indeed, not rarely they are detected in presence of posterior fossa arteriovenous malformations (AVMs), as pre- or post-nidus aneurysms, or in case of absence of contralateral PICA. The anatomy of different segments of the PICA has already been discussed earlier.

Depending on the course and tortuosity of PICA and on the location of the aneurysm, all these aneurysms can be located and addressed with different surgical approaches toward the CVJ. Aneurysms arising in the first two segments of PICA are located in the cerebellum-medullary cistern and require a more lateral exposure (far lateral), as for VA–PICA aneurysms. Aneurysms on the last three segments of PICA lie in the paramedian area inside the Vallecula of Reil, which is a narrow space between the tonsils that interconnect the cisterna magna with the fourth ventricle and a midline suboccipital approach is favored. Considering their proximity to the cerebellar tonsils, they can also present with intracerebellar hematoma. More peripheral aneurysms instead lie on the cerebellar surface, and most of the times are far away from the CVJ.

As discussed for VA–PICA aneurysms, far-lateral approach is the best surgical option for aneurysms arising on the *anterior medullary* and *lateral medullary segment*. Most of the times, drilling of the occipital condyle is only very minimal because of the more medial location of these aneurysms. A temporary clip can be positioned on the proximal PICA before the aneurysmal segment. For aneurysms located on the *telovelotonsillar* or on *cortical segments*, a standard midline suboccipital craniotomy including the foramen magnum is suggested. After dissecting the cerebellomedullary and uvulo-tonsillar fissures, one or both tonsils can be displaced and retraced depending on the position of the aneurysm. Instead, for the *tonsillomedullary segment (and whenever an access to both proximal and detail PICA is needed)*, an approach combining a lateral and medial suboccipital craniotomy usually allows the surgeon to obtain enough space for proximal control and clipping. Also in these cases, according to the position and dimension of the aneurysms, tonsils can be retracted or in few cases partially resected if necessary to gain space for clipping. C1 laminectomy is not always necessary in this instance although we do prefer to do it for better maneuverability.

Distal PICA aneurysms are usually located more superficial than lower cranial nerves or relatively away from them. Thus, lower cranial nerve complications described for VA–PICA aneurysms are less frequent with more distal aneurysms.

29.1.3 Non-saccular VA and VA–PICA, Distal PICA Aneurysms

Dissecting and fusiform aneurysms are not infrequent at the VA–PICA junction or on distal PICA itself. The rate of these aneurysms at this level is higher when compared to other locations, accounting for about one-third of all VA–PICA and PICA aneurysms. They frequently involve a long tract of the VA across the CVJ, sometimes including the PICA origin. They usually present with ischemic symptoms (both dissecting and fusiform aneurysms) or SAH (dissecting aneurysms). Proximal VA dissecting aneurysms are routinely treated with endovascular occlusion leaving the PICA origin intact if possible. Revascularization options should be considered if PICA origin is planned to be sacrificed. For fusiform PICA aneurysms, due to non-clippability and the importance of preserving PICA, especially in the first three segments, a bypass strategy is favored. Bypass options are described in another chapter.

29.2 Arteriovenous Malformations

Brain arteriovenous malformations (AVMs) present an estimated prevalence close to 10/1,00,000 in general population. They are complex vascular lesions to manage and surgery plays a primary role in treatment.

Deep brainstem AVMs are rare (2–3% of all AVMs) and considered more challenging to treat. Spetzler–Martin grading is not helpful in this particular location and these AVMs are seldom addressed for surgery due to high rate of complications deriving from brainstem potential injury. In this area, also radiosurgery (RS) and embolization are not free of morbidity. For this reasons, in the past, observation with radiological follow-up has been advocated for this AVMs. Nevertheless, they are more aggressive when compared with supratentorial ones, with annual hemorrhages rate of 15–20%. Thus, even if affected by high complication rate, a tentative to cure these AVMs should be suggested, considering both single and multimodality treatment strategies.

In this context, AVMs fed by vertebral artery and posterior inferior cerebellar artery, with nidus located on the anterior or lateral aspect of the *medulla oblongata*, are considered to be related to the Craniovertebral Junction. During discussion, we refer also to AVMs located at the cervical-medullary junction, considering the same vascular anatomy (feeding arteries and draining veins) and surgical approaches required.

29.2.1 Anterior and Lateral Medullary and Cervical-Medullary Junction AVMs

29.2.1.1 Introduction

According to the location of the nidus, brainstem arteriovenous malformations have been recently classified into six different types: anterior and posterior midbrain, anterior and lateral pons, anterior and lateral medulla. AVMs located around the CVJ are those with nidus sitting on anterior medulla, lateral medulla, and cervico-medullary junction. They account for 4–30% of brainstem AVMs in different series. Lateral medullary AVMs are more common ones.

29.2.1.2 Clinical Presentation and Neuroradiological Assessment

AVMs located at the cranial-vertebral junction usually present with subarachnoid hemorrhage (SAH) with or without intraparenchymal hemorrhage (IPH), detected on computed tomography (CT) scan. After acute onset with headache, nausea, and vomiting, patients usually show up with severe life-threatening symptoms, like decreased consciousness and cranial nerve deficits. About 80% of patients present with SAH. Others with cervical-medullary AVMs present with venous drainage into spinal veins, and potentially progressive cervical myelopathy.

CTA (CT Angiography) and diagnostic angiogram are both necessary for decision-making regarding treatment of such AVMs.

During pre-treatment planning, magnetic resonance imaging (MRI) is always performed, as it shows the exact anatomical location of the nidus on the surface of the medulla and defines the extension at the cervico-medullary junction. MRI is also fundamental in distinguishing a pial from a parenchymal AVM. Pial AVM is a signal-void lesion both in T_1 and T_2, with exophytic growth in the anterior or lateral medullary cistern. Parenchymal AVM presents the same magnetic signal but is surrounded by brainstem tissue.

29.2.1.3 Regional Vascular Anatomy

Vertebral artery (VA) pierces the dura mater less than 1 cm below the CVJ, after running inside a groove over C1 lamina (sulcus arteriosus) in lateral to medial and caudal to cranial direction. VA gives off several intradural branches in the region of the foramen magnum: PICA (already described in this chapter), posterior and anterior spinal arteries. Extradural branches (meningeal arteries) will be discussed later in this chapter.

Posterior spinal arteries can arise both intra- or extradurally from the VA and they are usually embedded into the same dural ring of the VA (at V3–V4 junction). They present an ascending and descending branch, taking blood supply to dorsal structures of medulla and spinal cord.

Anterior ventral spinal arteries are the last (most cranial) branches of VA, with an intradural origin close to VA–basilar junction. They join together into the anterior spinal artery that descends through the foramen magnum along CVJ, supplying ventral-lateral aspect of the medulla and spinal cord.

Venous drainage in the region of the foramen magnum is guaranteed by several intradural veins connected with dural sinuses by bridging veins. Veins of the medulla and upper cervical spinal cord anastomose at the CVJ into longitudinal plexiform channels. These veins run into longitudinal sulci of the medulla and upper spinal cord, taking the name from them: median anterior and posterior spinal and median anterior and posterior medullary veins, lateral anterior and posterior spinal and lateral anterior and posterior medullary veins. Transverse venous channels interconnect longitudinal vessels (transverse medullary and transverse spinal veins). Vein of the cerebellum-medullary fissure also participates in draining this region.

29.2.1.4 AVM's Anatomical Features

Anterior medullary AVM is located below the ponto-medullary sulcus, between the anterior-lateral sulcus and hypoglossal nerve rootles. It is usually supplied by radiculomedullary branches of VA (often bilaterally) and anterior spinal artery. Median anterior medullary vein drains these AVMs. Lateral medullary AVM is always located below the ponto-medullary sulcus, lateral to the anterior-lateral sulcus and between rootles of LCNs (IX, X, XI, and XII CNs). Arterial feeders comes from the branches of VA unilaterally (lateral spinal artery and radiculomedullary branches) and from the ipsilateral PICA. Venous drainage is taken by lateral medullary vein, median anterior medullary vein, and transverse pontine vein. AVMs with extension below the cervico-medullary junction drained also through the anterior spinal vein.

Brainstem AVMs can present with two different types of nidus. *Pial AVMs* present with exophytic nidus, growing from pial surface of the brainstem toward the facing cistern. *Parenchymal AVMs* are instead embedded inside the brainstem presenting pial involvement. Pial nidus is more frequent for lateral medullary AVMs, presenting with growth into the cerebellum-medullary cistern.

29.2.1.5 Preoperative Management

Generally patients with ruptured medullary or cervico-medullary AVMs present a lower level of consciousness and orotracheal intubation is useful in order to control and stabilize blood pressure and other vital parameters. When it is possible, pre-intubation neurological examination is performed to depict potential lower cranial nerve deficits or other symptoms. When intraventricular blood or hydrocephalus is shown in the CT scan, external ventricular drainage (EVD) is placed in the frontal horn of lateral ventricle.

Considering their complexity, multidisciplinary team evaluation is always required. Indeed, morphology and location and most importantly the mode of presentation (ruptured vs. unruptured) of the AVM strongly influence treatment decision. Surgery, radiosurgery, and endovascular treatment might all have a significant role, alone or in combination for treatment of these lesions.

When surgery is indicated and considered for the specific case, we will delay the surgery by 10–14 days after hemorrhage to carefully evaluate and perform all preoperative necessary tests if possible. Only when the brainstem is compressed by intraparenchymal hematoma, the surgery is performed emergently.

29.2.1.6 Surgical Approach

Far-lateral approach is our preferred approach for these specific AVMs, mostly for lateral medullary brainstem locations. Anterior medullary brainstem AVMs are rare lesions and can still be approached through the same route. Surgical procedures are performed in the same way as previously described in this chapter. Transcondylar approach and eventually combined with trans-tubercular addition are often necessary in order to increase the working space and the line of sight over the anterior midline, and to control feeders coming off anteriorly. The use of intraoperative ICG (indocyanine green) angiography is helpful in better defining the AVM characteristics.

29.2.1.7 Exclusion Techniques

In contrast to AVMs located elsewhere in the brain (supratentorial or cerebellar AVMs), surgical experience for brainstem AVMs has been limited. As mentioned before, surgery presents a high rate of up-front complications due to brainstem manipulation and direct surgical insult. Thus, less invasive treatment strategies are often preferred. Among them, radiosurgery presents a relatively appealing option with an occlusion rate of about 40–60% in different series. Nevertheless, in the absence of other less invasive treatment options, microsurgical resection of the AVM could be suggested, for more superficial lesions, with reasonable outcome especially in the context of a ruptured AVM.

After opening the dura, ICG angiography is performed to better understand the anatomy of the AVM. Extensive arachnoid dissection inside the cerebellum-medullary cistern allows to easily identify feeding arteries between lower cranial nerves. Thus, feeders are disconnected or clipped, while preserving en-passage arteries and venous channels. Red draining vein clearly changes color to dark blue and ICG-VA is used to confirm change in blood flow. During dissection, LCNs manipulation should be as minimal as possible as already described to reduce postoperative palsies. After that, the nidus is explored and observed to distinguish between parenchymal and pial AVMs.

When the nidus shows an exophytic growth inside the lateral medullary cistern (*pial AVMs*), extensive coagulation and circumferential dissection of the nidus can be performed without entering the brainstem. Then the nidus is resected and removed as for supratentorial or cerebellar AVMs. Instead, when the nidus is highly embedded into the brainstem (*parenchymal AVMs*), the surgery is much more challenging. If the surgical decision is made based on the ruptured status and angioarchitecture of the AVM, the AVM will be resected through the closest pial surface with the same technique. However, if there is a gradual change in neuromonitoring, minimal or partial removal of the nidus is preferred to limit postoperative deficit. In these cases, the so-called "occlusion in situ" technique is used. Circumferential pial dissection is performed without or with minimal resection of the nidus, in order to not violate the brainstem. When a brainstem hemorrhage is present, it makes the road to the nidus and further resection potentially less risky. Residual nidus left in the brainstem is then selected for observation or further additional treatments (RS or embolization). We do not have personal experience with this last scenario. Benefits and complications of multimodalities treatments or observation need to be carefully evaluated.

29.2.1.8 Complications and Outcome

Complication rate is relatively high for surgery of brainstem AVMs (around 25% in different series) with a high mortality rate (around 5–6%). Usually, serious preoperative symptoms after acute onset strongly affect patient quality of life.

Moreover, postoperative hemiparesis, hemorrhage, and cranial nerve palsies further worsen patient's course and quality of life. Lateral medullary (together with lateral pontine) AVMs present the best outcomes, probably for the relatively easier surgical access.

AVM obliteration rate reaches 60–80% in different reports and depends on the possibility to excise the AVM or to completely close all arterial feeders. Multimodality treatment (endovascular + surgery treatment followed by radiosurgery if residual nidus is identified) is sometimes proposed to increase the probability of AVM's occlusion. The potential cumulative risks of multiple treatments should be considered before suggesting a more complex treatment plan.

29.3 Dural Arteriovenous Fistulas

Dural arteriovenous fistulas (DAVFs) can involve both brain and spine. They are pathological vascular connections between an extradural artery and an intradural vein inside the dura mater, without a nidus between artery and vein. They can be related (*sinusal DAVF, Borden type I and II*) or not (*extra-sinusal, Borden type III*) with venous sinuses.

DAVFs showing a retrograde venous drainage (RVD) into cortical veins necessitate treatment in most cases. Nowadays, endovascular treatment (trans-arterial or trans-venous embolization) and if not possible surgery share the primary role in DAVFs management, with different rates of occlusion and complications for the two procedures reported in different series coming from neurosurgical or interventional radiology groups.

29.3.1 Dural Arteriovenous Fistulas at the Craniovertebral Junction

29.3.1.1 Introduction

Dural AV fistulas at the CVJ are rare lesions, and they account for 2% of all DAVFs.

Confounding nomenclature has been used in literature for CVJ dural AV fistulas. They have been classified both into cranial and spinal dural AV fistulas. According to the site of connection inside the dura between the artery and vein, they can be sub-divided in: DAVFs of the foramen magnum, hypoglossal canal fistulas, jugular foramen fistulas, and marginal sinus fistulas. These sub-types present some common features and some differences in management strategies.

29.3.1.2 Clinical Presentation and Neuroradiological Assessment

DAVFs at the CVJ can equally present with acute or chronic myelopathy, or with SAH. Rarely they present with brainstem edema and related dysfunction. It is not the site of AV connections, but the direction of the retrograde venous drainage (RVD) which causes different clinical presentations. DAVFs with an ascending RVD into an intracranial vein are usually associated with venous varices and present with SAH. Instead, a descending RVD results in spinal venous hypertension and spinal cord dysfunction with myelopathy. Orbital symptoms (chemosis and diplopia) are common presentations of hypoglossal canal DAVFs, due to the connections with cavernous sinus and orbital veins. Also continuous tinnitus is common in those cases with progressive onset.

CT scan is first performed in those cases presenting with acute onset, to diagnose SAH. The absence of aneurysm on CT angiogram suspects the presence of a vascular malformation. CTA and MRI are helpful in localizing the exact location of the DAVF connection if visualized. In those patients presenting with sudden progressive neurological symptoms (like cervical myelopathy), the evidence of cervical spinal venous engorgement or spinal cord hyperintensity on MRI suggest the presence of DAVF and prompting further investigation. In both cases, DSA is mandatory to confirm the suspicion of a DAVF.

29.3.1.3 Regional Vascular Anatomy

Before piercing the dura mater, VA–V3 segment gives off anterior and posterior meningeal branches taking blood supply to the dura of the clivus and foramen magnum region and also to the dura covering the posterior fossa and to the tentorium. Also meningeal arteries coming from external carotid artery circulation (ascending pharyngeal artery and occipital artery) participate in vascularizing this area, often with anastomosis between them and VA meningeal branches. One of two branches of the ascending pharyngeal artery passes through the hypoglossal canal (HC), and the other one penetrates the jugular foramen (JF). Meningeal branches coming from occipital artery are inconstant.

Internal jugular vein (IJV) and its tributaries form an important drainage system of the brain at the CVJ. IJV originates at the jugular foramen and descends caudally into posterior-lateral cervical region. Vertebral artery venous plexus surrounds the VA and communicates through the posterior condylar emissary vein (PCV) with the sigmoid sinus (SS). The venous plexus of the hypoglossal canal (HC) connects with the marginal sinus, which encircles the foramen magnum. Venous plexus of the HC has other important communications through the anterior condylar vein (ACV) with: IJV, PCV, internal carotid artery venous plexus, marginal sinus, inferior petrosal sinus, and cavernous sinus. Moreover, marginal sinus (MS) presents several connections with other important venous structures of the skull base like basilar sinus (anteriorly), occipital sinus (posteriorly), vertebral artery venous plexus and deep cervical veins (inferiorly).

29.3.1.4 DAVF's Anatomical Features

Three major components of DAVFs are: dural artery, fistulous point inside dura mater, and vein of drainage.

In most cases, meningeal branches coming from vertebral artery, ascending pharyngeal artery or occipital artery participate in DAVFs at the CVJ.

The point of fistula can be located on the posterior or lateral (or anterolateral) aspect of the dura mater covering the cervical-medullary junction, at the level of the foramen magnum (involving or not the marginal sinus), or lower closer to C1 vertebra or at the level of specific anatomic structures like hypoglossal canal or jugular foramen.

DAVFs with *ascending venous drainage* usually use longitudinal venous channels of the medulla oblongata ending into a major dural sinus like marginal sinus, superior and inferior petrous sinus, cavernous sinus, or transverse-sigmoid sinus. In most cases, a venous varix is present along the course of the draining vein. The combination of DAVF and pill AVF of the CV junction should be considered among possible angiographic configurations (Illustrative Case 2).

Instead, longitudinal venous channels of the cervical spine are involved in DAVFs with *descending venous drainage*, causing venous hypertension into the spinal cord.

HC–DAVFs are usually fed by neuro-meningeal division of the ascending pharyngeal artery or trans-mastoid branches of occipital artery. The fistulous point is located at the level of ACV. Considering the wide venous connections in this area, RVD can show different patterns toward cavernous sinus and orbital veins or toward the IJV.

JF–DAVFs present an arterial supply by the other division of the ascending pharyngeal artery, a fistulous point inside the dura close to the JF, and a venous drainage through lateral medullary vein both ascending (toward inferior petrous sinus and cavernous sinus) or descending (toward deep cervical veins) (Illustrative Case 3).

29.3.1.5 Preoperative Management

Patients presenting with SAH receive the same preoperative investigations already described for ruptured VA–PICA aneurysms and CVJ AVMs.

Depending on the rupture status or presence or absence of myelopathy, a treatment between endovascular occlusion and surgical obliteration of fistula is decided.

Our preferred approach is an endovascular obliteration of the fistula through trans-arterial embolization, and rarely transvenous (the latter has not been our group experience).

However, often the access to the fistula is difficult or embolization cannot achieve complete obliteration of the fistula, with remaining flow through the RVD, and therefore a surgical disconnection of the fistula is indicated.

29.3.1.6 Surgical Approach

Dural AV fistulas at the CVJ are usually approached through a posterolateral or far-lateral approach as they are located at the lateral or posterolateral edge of the dura. Details of the procedure have already been described in this chapter. For foramen magnum DAVFs, C1 hemilaminectomy is always necessary to expose a wide area of the dura covering the cervical-medullary junction. Hypoglossal canal dura AV fistulas always require a transcondylar approach. If more than one-third of occipital condyle needs to be drilled to expose the fistulous point, occipital-cervical fusion might become necessary to avoid future cranial-cervical instability. A supracondylar approach through the jugular tubercle is necessary for dural AV fistulas located close to the jugular foramen.

29.3.1.7 Exclusion Techniques

The main advantage of microsurgical treatment for DAVFs at the CVJ is the high obliteration rate. The reported obliteration rate with surgery is about 98% versus about 60% with embolization alone. Furthermore, the presence of multiple arterial feeders coming from VA, occipital artery, and ascending pharyngeal artery makes endovascular treatment more challenging and less effective. Even with a good initial embolization, there is a high chance for new feeders recruitment at follow-up. For single channel AV fistulas fed by ascending pharyngeal artery, there is a high risk of lower cranial nerves (LCNs) palsy with trans-arterial embolization, due to vasa vasorum involvement. Conversely, DAVFs involving the marginal sinus are well suitable for trans-venous embolization, presenting various routes for access due to wide venous connections of the MS. HC–DAVFs, usually approached with surgery, have been recently treated also with trans-venous embolization with similar results in terms of obliteration of the fistulous channel. Transient or permanent hypoglossal nerve palsy due to compression of the nerve inside its canal is one of the possible complications after trans-venous embolization.

As for other location of DAVFs, microsurgical obliteration of the fistula at the CVJ is based on the ligation or coagulation of the draining vein at the fistulous point. The disconnection between the artery and the vein at the fistulous point represents the most efficient way to treat the dural AV fistulas.

A hypertrophic meningeal artery coming from VA or occipital artery is usually visible over the dura mater. Branches coming from ascending pharyngeal artery are seldom visible because of their deeper origin hidden by bony structures. After opening the dura and wide arachnoid dissection, one or more large tortuous veins come into view, in strict relation with the VA dural entry point (foramen magnum DAVFs) or more lateral (HC or JF dural AV fistulas). Color of the vein is usually turned to red. Then, ICG-VA is performed showing an arterial flow pattern inside the vein and confirming the exact position of the dural fistulous point. Now, the draining vein is coagulated or clipped at its point of origin from the dura and transected. Red vein rapidly changes color into blue. At the end, we use again the ICG-VA to make sure of complete exclusion of the anomalous shunt. ICG-VA during temporary clipping of the feeding artery or of the draining vein could also be helpful before definitive coagulation of the point of fistula, in those cases presenting with complex vascular shunts (with multiple arterial feeders or draining veins).

29.3.1.8 Complications and Outcome

As previously described, surgery around this region could be affected by different complications, e.g., LCNs palsies, CVJ instability, motor/sensory deficits, and hydrocephalus. With regard to DAVFs treatment, the outcome is usually better than for ruptured aneurysms and AVMs in this location. In fact, in a symptomatic or ruptured situation, both preoperative condition of the patient and postoperative complications are generally less severe. Good recovery is achieved in more than 75% of patients presenting with SAH or intraparenchymal hematoma (it is typically mild in DAVFs of CVJ). Interestingly, patients presenting with advanced progressive myelopathy present poorer outcome after treatment, with a moderate disability in more than 50%. Indeed, long-term venous hypertension could result in permanent damage to the spinal cord. For HC–DAVFs, cranial-cervical instability could be a concerning issue if more than one-third of the occipital condyle is resected to unhidden the fistulous point. This will require subsequent occipital-cervical fusion.

29.4 Case Illustrations

Case 1: Ruptured PICA Aneurysm

Fifty-five-year-old female presenting with a ruptured large (1.1 cm) right PICA aneurysm underwent initial balloon assisted coiling of the aneurysm due to incorporation of the PICA at the base of the aneurysm (Fig. 29.1a, b). The procedure was aborted after subtotal coiling of the aneurysm (Fig. 29.1c) and emboli in the PICA

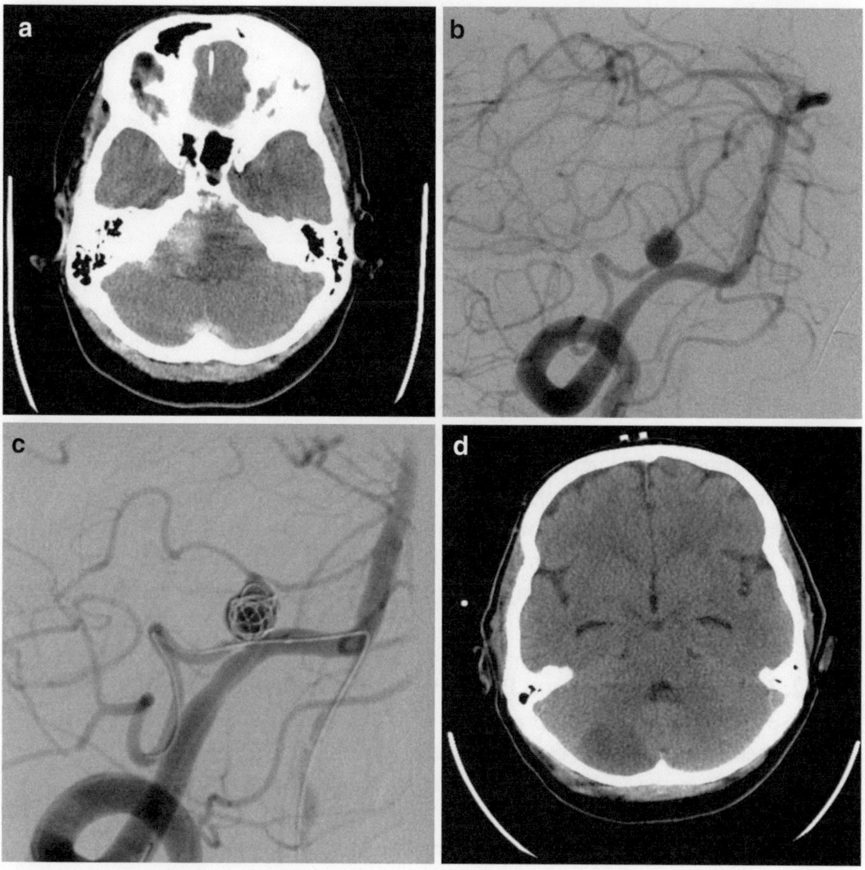

Fig. 29.1 (**a**) Computed tomography (CT) scan showing subarachnoid hemorrhage (SAH) with a clot in the right cerebellopontine angle (CPA). (**b**) Digital subtracted angiogram (DSA) showing a large (1.1 cm) right VA-PICA aneurysm. (**c**) DSA demonstrating an incomplete obliteration of the dome of the aneurysm after initial balloon coiling. (**d**) Post-procedure CT revealing a moderate PICA territory stroke scan due to emboli during the endovascular procedure. (**e**, **f**) Intraoperative pictures showing the exposure of the aneurysm through a far-lateral craniotomy. (**g**) Clipping of the aneurysm with a fenestrated clip incorporating the PICA inside the fenestration. (**h**) Postoperative DSA confirming complete exclusion of the aneurysm and patency of PICA

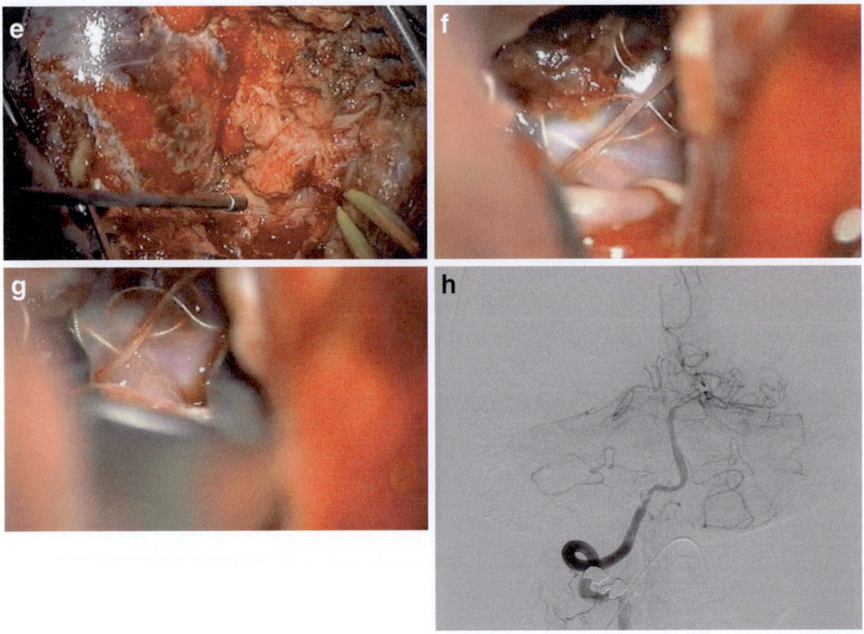

Fig. 29.1 (continued)

during the procedure. Patient recovered from the initial treatment despite a moderate PICA territory stroke (Fig. 29.1d) and underwent surgical clipping of the aneurysm after the vasospasm period. Intraoperative picture shows the exposure of the aneurysm through a far-lateral craniotomy (Fig. 29.1e, f). Clipping of the aneurysm with a fenestrated clip incorporating the PICA inside the fenestration (Fig. 29.1g), and postoperative angiogram confirming complete exclusion of the aneurysm and patency of the PICA (although diminished in caliber) (Fig. 29.1h). The patient needed a temporary tracheostomy but recovered to mRS score of 1 at 3 months follow-up.

Case 2: Concurrent DAVF and Pial Arteriovenous Fistula of the CV Junction
Thirty-seven-year-old female presented with sudden onset headache and the CT shows a hemorrhage inside the fourth ventricle (Fig. 29.2a). CTA and angiogram reveal a DAVF at the CV junction fed by meningeal branches of vertebral artery draining into a perimedullary arterialized vein (Fig. 29.2b). There was also the association with a pial arteriovenous fistula harboring an aneurysm at the fistulous point (Fig. 29.2c). Due to patient young age and lack of adequate endovascular access to the fistulous point, a left far lateral transcondylar trans-tubercular approach was selected, aneurysm and fistula exposed (Fig. 29.2d, e), and the aneurysm was resected which led to interruption of the pial arteriovenous fistula (Fig. 29.2f) and the DAVF (identified with ICG, Fig. 29.2g) clipped (Fig. 29.2h). Intraoperative angiogram confirms complete obliteration of the fistula (Fig. 29.2i).

Case 3: Ruptured Jugular Foramen DAVF

Seventy-two-year-old male presented with right medullary hemorrhage (Fig. 29.3a). A DAVF of the right jugular foramen was identified. The fistula was fed by branches of external carotid artery (right occipital, ascending pharyngeal, and middle meningeal) (Fig. 29.3b) and meningeal branches of the vertebral artery (C1 and C3 odontoid arch) (Fig. 29.3c). Two sessions of embolization was performed through different afferent feeders but there was a remaining faint shunt which recruited new feeders including contralateral falx cerebelli (Fig. 29.3d, e) at 9 months follow-up. Patient

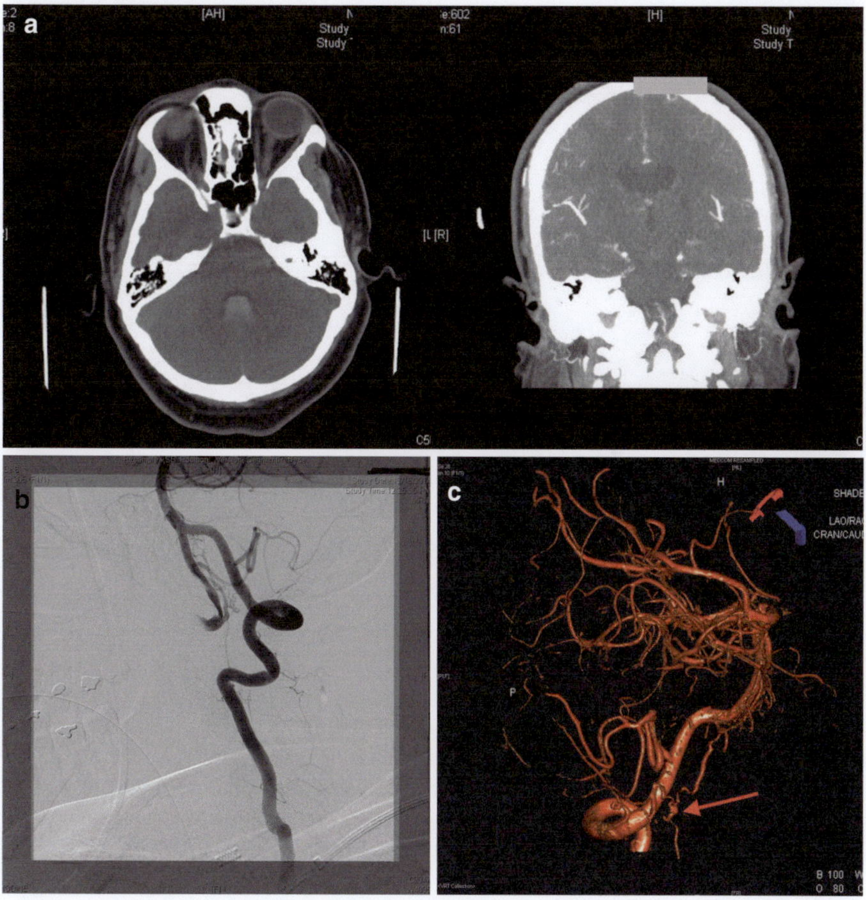

Fig. 29.2 (**a**) CT scan and CT angio showing intraventricular hemorrhage in the fourth ventricle. (**b**) DSA revealed a DAVF at the CVJ fed by meningeal branch of VA and draining into a perimedullary arterialized vein. (**c**) *Red arrow* indicates the concomitant presence of a pial AV fistula harboring an aneurysm at the fistulous point. (**d**, **e**) Intraoperative pictures of left far lateral transcondylar trans-tubercular approach. (**f**) Exposure and resection of the aneurysm with interruption of the pial AV fistula. (**g**) Intraoperative indocyanine green (ICG) video fluoroangiography helped to identify the DAVF. (**h**) Clipping of the fistulous point of the DAVF at the CVJ. (**i**) Intraoperative DSA confirms complete obliteration of the fistula

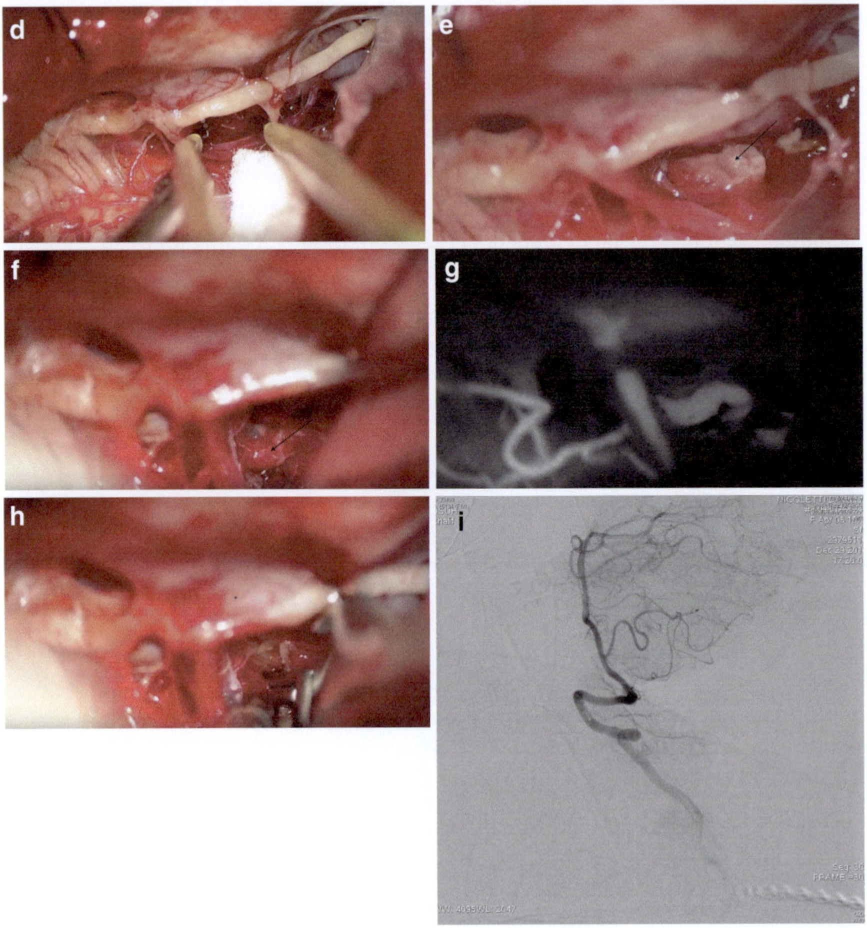

Fig. 29.2 (continued)

was operated through a far-lateral transcondylar approach (Fig. 29.3f, g) and the fistula was identified below the jugular foramen, confirmed by ICG videoangiography and disconnected (Fig. 29.3h, i). Postoperative angiogram confirmed absence of any remaining shunt or abnormal pial cortical venous drainage (Fig. 29.3j).

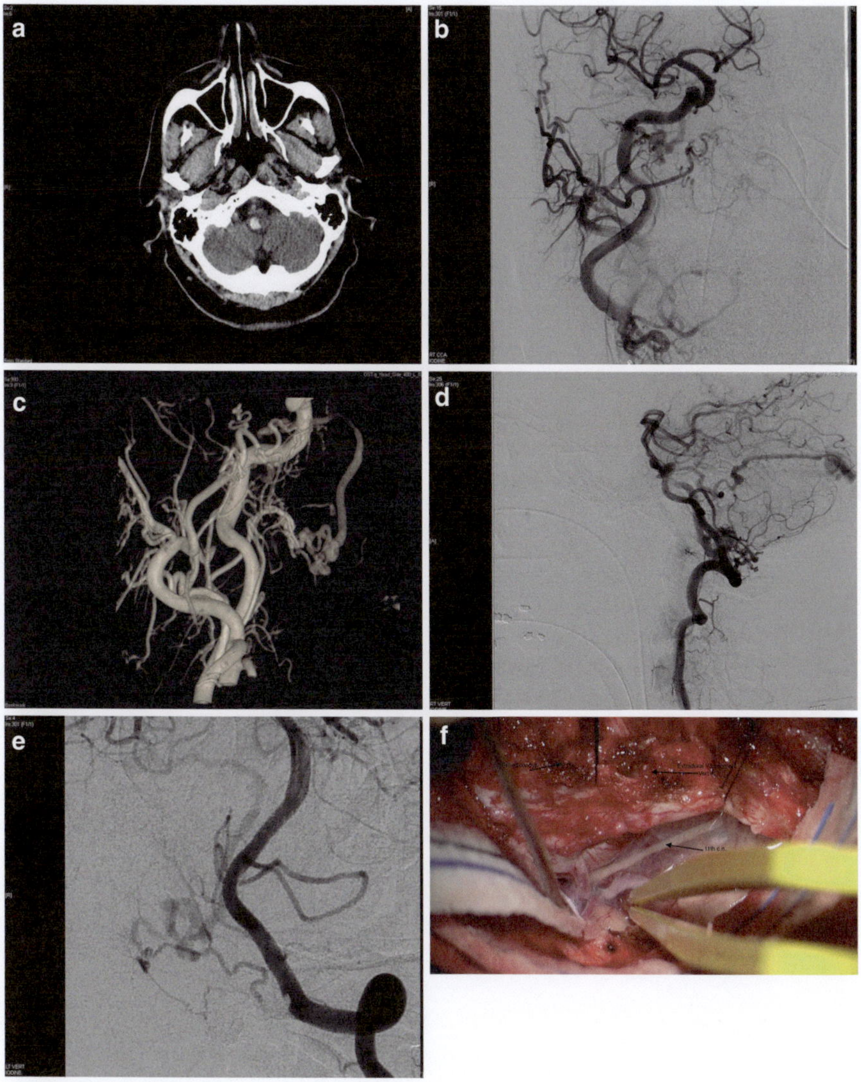

Fig. 29.3 (**a**) CT scan showing a right medullary hemorrhage. (**b**, **c**) DSA identified a DAVF of the right jugular foramen, fed by branches of external carotid artery (right occipital, ascending pharyngeal, and middle meningeal) and meningeal branches of the vertebral artery (C1 and C3 odontoid arch). (**d**, **e**) CT scan at 9 months follow-up after endovascular procedure, demonstrating persistent fistula which recruited new feeders. (**f**, **g**) Intraoperative captures of the fistula, exposed below the level of the jugular foramen through a far-lateral transcondylar approach. (**h**, **i**) Intraoperative view and ICG videoangiography confirmation after disconnection of the fistula. (**j**) Postoperative DSA confirmed absence of further shunts or abnormal pial venous drainage

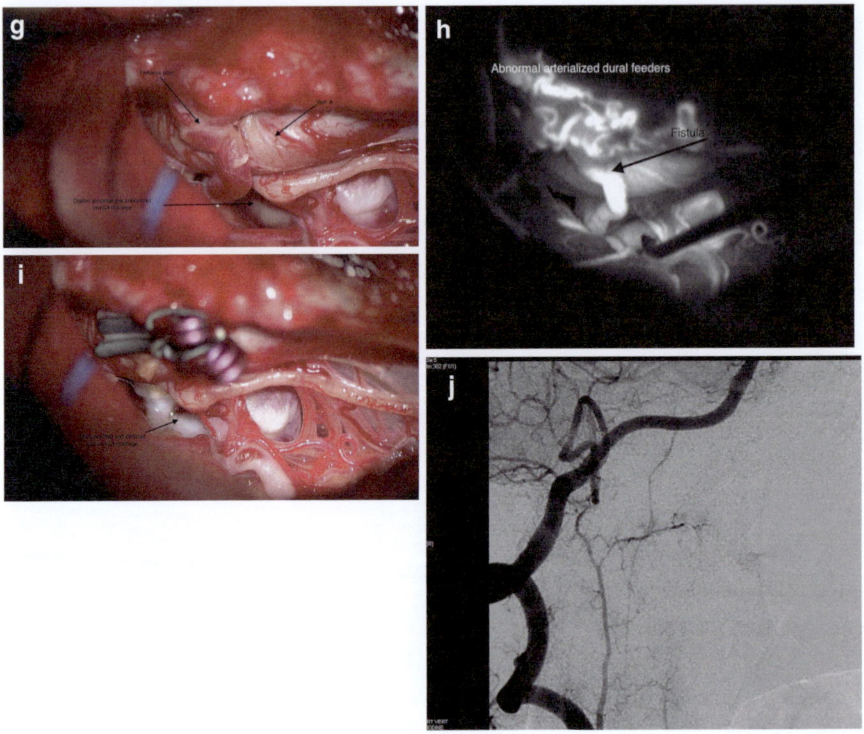

Fig. 29.3 (continued)

Posterior Fossa Revascularization Options at the Cranio-vertebral Junction

30

Erez Nossek and Amir R. Dehdashti

30.1 Bypass Techniques

PICA-PICA Bypass (Side to side, end to end, re-implantation).

30.1.1 Background

Whenever a PICA sacrifice is considered especially in the first three segments (antero-medullary, latero-medullary, and tonsillomedullary), the revascularization of PICA is recommended. Although there are alternatives for PICA-PICA end to end or side to side bypass, e.g., occipital artery-PICA bypass or radial artery jump graft from vertebral artery to PICA, the end to end or side to side PICA-PICA bypass are the most elegant and rational alternatives, as long as there is enough redundancy for an end to end bypass, or in case of a side to side bypass, if the donor PICA has sufficient size and the distance between the two PICA caudal loops after release of all arachnoid adhesions is not more than 5–6 mm.

30.1.2 Posterior Inferior Cerebellar Artery in Situ Bypass Options

The PICA is divided into five segments: (1) the anterior medullary segment, which extends posteriorly from the origin of the PICA at the vertebral artery to the inferior olivary prominence and passes near the hypoglossal nerve, (2) the lateral medullary segment, from the inferior olive to the origins of lower cranial nerves, (3) the

E. Nossek
Department of Neurosurgery, NYU School of Medicine, New York, NY, USA

A. R. Dehdashti (✉)
Department of Neurosurgery, North Shore University Hospital, Northwell Health, Manhasset, NY, USA

E. Tessitore et al. (eds.), *Surgery of the Cranio-Vertebral Junction*, https://doi.org/10.1007/978-3-030-18700-2_30

tonsillomedullary segments, from the lower cranial nerves to the caudal loop, (4) the telovelotonsillar segment, from the caudal loop to the cranial loop, and (5) the cortical segment which extends to the cerebellar vermis and hemisphere. Because the first three segments, and occasionally the proximal part of the fourth segments, might have critical perforators to the brainstem, their sacrifice might cause debilitating stroke, and therefore, a strategy for revascularization should be considered if lesions to be treated are proximal to the telovelotonsillar segment and that the treatment involves sacrifice of the segment, e.g., in dissecting vertebral artery-PICA aneurysms. Although other alternatives including occipital artery to PICA bypass and vertebral artery to PICA bypass using radial artery graft exist, the side to side PICA-PICA is more attractive due to a lower risk of bypass occlusion and the avoidance of tedious harvesting of the occipital artery or other type of graft.

There might be tiny brainstem perforators at the junction of the tonsillomedullary and telovelotonsillary segments of PICAs on the side wall of the arteriotomy. Those perforators should be separately clipped and preserved before arteriotomy and their sacrifice should be avoided. Attention to details including the type of temporary clip used, the exact location of the arteriotomy on the vessel, the type of suture and needle used, and the length of the suture is crucial to perform.

If the donor PICA size is less than 1 mm, or the distance between the two caudal loops of PICAs is more than 5 mm after liberation of arachnoid adhesions, then the PICA-PICA side to side bypass might not be an appropriate option. If the flow measured by the flow probe is significantly lower in the donor PICA, another revascularization alternative should be considered, and, therefore, the option of OA-PICA bypass should always exist as the plan B during the procedure and the patency and anatomy of the occipital artery should be thoroughly evaluated.

30.1.3 Description of the Technique

Patients are put on aspirin 325 mg the night before the procedure. Under general anesthesia, the patient is monitored for motor, sensory, and brainstem evoked potentials and positioned in a prone concord (or alternatively, a park-bench position which favors a far lateral approach if needed). The trajectory of the occipital artery on the side of affected PICA is identified with a handheld Doppler and marked on the skin in case an OA-PICA bypass is decided upon. A midline incision, caudal to the nuchal line down to C2 spinous process, is performed. Suboccipital bone and C1 lamina are exposed in a subperiosteal fashion. An oval suboccipital craniotomy (4 × 3 cm, exposing the foramen magnum) and a C1 laminectomy are performed. Dura is opened in a Y-shaped fashion and the cerebellomedullary fissure is exposed.

Under microscopic vision, the arachnoid of the tonsillomedullary fissure is incised, cerebellar tonsils are gently retracted, and the two PICAs are separated from their adhesions just below the obex. The two tonsillomedullary and telovelotonsillar segments of the PICA are freed from arachnoid adhesions and mobilized and approximated for side to side bypass. The caudal loop which is the transition between the tonsillomedullary segment and the telovelotonsillar segment is the only suitable location for this particular bypass. The baseline PICA flow can be measured with a flow probe. Two 5 mm mini clips are used for proximal clipping of both PICAs and two 3 mm straight or slightly curved clips are used for distal vessels. Approximately 1 cm of both vessels at the caudal loop of both PICAs ideally with the least amount of perforators should be available between the clips. The part of the caudal loop which is easier to mobilize is selected. The patient receives 3000 iu of heparin at this time. It is crucial that the arteriotomy be placed at 10 and 2 o'clock on each vessel, respectively, and be exactly the same length of approximately 4–6 mm (at least double the diameter of the larger PICA). Methylene blue is used to mark the arteriotomy line. Arteriotomy is performed using a back-cutting micro knife (APEX Inc.) or a 27 gauge needle and extending with microscissors. The choice of suture and needle is fundamental. A 10-0 Ethilon nylon monofilament V75-3 needle has the appropriate size and needle curvature for performance of this bypass. It has to be cut to 5 cm for each wall of the arteriotomy. The first knot is very important. The apices (distal end) of both arteriotomies are approximated with the first stitch going outside-inside of one apex and coming out inside-outside of the other apex. After making the knot on the backside of the arteriotomy, the needle has to be passed underneath the knot to keep it outside the lumen and a running closure of the inferior wall is performed with the first passage being outside-inside and then inside-outside of the other side, and so on. Once the inferior wall is sewed all the way to the proximal ends, the suture is tightened after the last pass of the suture from inside to outside, to keep the knot outside the arteriotomy lumen. Then the front wall is closed in a running fashion. Suture loops are tightened with the aid of a microhook and the last suture is tied on its own just before the initial knot. The lumen is irrigated with heparinized saline and a final interrupted suture is added to close the opening between the superior (or front) wall closure and the very first knot.

Preparing for revascularization, a tiny piece of gelfoam is positioned in the back wall of the arteriotomy to protect against any potential ooze in an area which is difficult to visualize. Temporary occlusion time is about 45 min. The distal clips first, and the proximal clips on PICA next, are removed to allow recirculation. With the running suture technique, the leakage should be minimal. The author uses a flow probe Doppler to measure the flow in the PICAs before and after anastomosis. If there is a dramatic drop in the flow of either PICA, or obvious occlusion of the bypass, the anastomosis is reopened for inspection. An ICG videoangiography is performed to confirm patency of the bypass while leaving a clip on the proximal segment of the recipient PICA. Attention is paid to retrograde flow into the recipient PICA proximally.

The closure is performed similar to a standard closure of a midline suboccipital craniotomy. A postoperative good quality CTA or angiogram is performed to confirm patency of the bypass. Patients will receive aspirin 325 mg once daily after surgery for at least 1 year.

Alternative to PICA-PICA side to side bypass is an end to end bypass. Interestingly, this would be the most favorable bypass option if there is enough PICA redundancy to exclude the diseases segment and to reconstruct the PICA with end to end anastomoses. The limitations for this bypass are: (1) absence of PICA redundancy, (2) presence of critical brainstem perforators at the level of the aneurysmal segment precluding the option of complete aneurysm segment sacrifice, (3) significant length of the diseased segment not allowing approximation of the two PICA ends, and (4) first segment PICA aneurysms.

The technical details are those of an end to end bypass. We usually start at the lower wall, approximating the two ends together and then the exact opposite at 180° is approximated with an interrupted suture. Then, each remaining side is closed with interrupted or running fashion. 10-0 or 9-0 BV100-3 sutures are suitable for this type of bypass.

One other option is to re-implant the proximal part of the distal PICA on the vertebral artery, if there is enough redundancy. In our practice, this has not been a common scenario but the surgeon should consider this alternative for some very redundant PICA where direct re-implantation on vertebral artery seems reasonable. Furthermore, using a jump graft (radial artery, occipital artery, etc.) to be used as interposition and connect the proximal and distal PICA together (in a nonredundant PICA, where the disease segment can be resected without sacrifice of the perforators) could be considered as another rare but potential alternative for PICA revascularization (Fig. 30.1).

30.2 Occipital Artery to PICA

30.2.1 Background

In cases where sacrifice of the proximal three segments of the PICA is deemed necessary, we plan a bypass procedure. Our first choice in these cases is the in situ option of a PICA-PICA bypass due to its high patency rate and the avoidance of the necessity of an extracranial donor vessel. Whenever the PICA-PICA end to end is not feasible, or the contralateral donor PICA is unavailable (i.e., when the distance between the two PICAs is above 5 mm or there is presence of a hypoplastic or absent contralateral PICA), we perform an OA-PICA bypass. We always prep the radial artery as a backup plan for the third option (VA-PICA bypass), only if the OA-PICA plan fails or if it is not feasible due to poor quality or size of the donor.

A complete cerebral angiogram is performed prior to the bypass procedure. The caliber of the OA should be at least 0.8 mm and the PICA should be a similar caliber. Preoperative angiographic assessment includes assessment of the specific course of the OA in order to accomplish successful harvesting of the donor artery. Aspirin (325 mg) is administered the night before the procedure or even 3–5 days prior to surgery, once daily.

The OA has a high (13%) rate of spasm and occlusion, thus a backup plan must be in place, consisting of either a PICA-PICA bypass or a vertebral-PICA jump graft, using the radial artery or a saphenous vein. Dissection of the OA may be challenging, especially in its transitional segment. We favor the use of the surgical microscope and repetitive microdoppler evaluations in order to avoid damage to the vessel. Attempts should be made to handle the vessel adventitia rather than the vessel wall itself, as this will decrease the risk of spasm and intra-luminal thrombosis.

With regard to the PICA itself, ideally, a perforator-free segment in the tonsillomedullary segment should be selected for anastomosis. If there are small microperforating arteries from the backside of the PICA's arteriotomy site, they must be temporarily clipped and completely preserved.

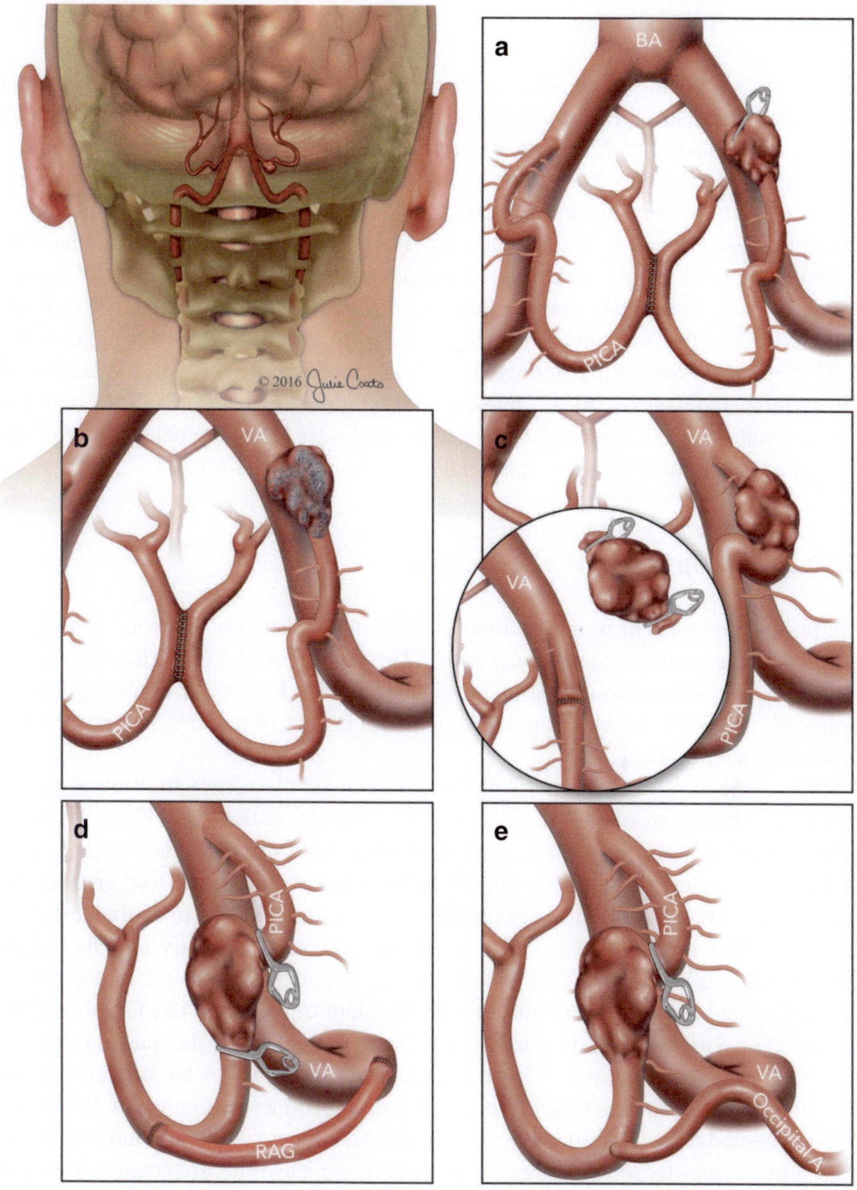

Fig. 30.1 Artist rendering of different PICA revascularization scenarios and options. (**a**) Side to side bypass and proximal trapping of a dysplastic PICA aneurysm. (**b**) Side to side bypass and proximal coiling of a dysplastic PICA aneurysm. (**c**) End to end anastomoses and resection of the aneurysmal segment considering that no critical perforator is involved in the aneurysm segment. (**d**) VA-PICA bypass using a jump radial artery graft and trapping of the aneurysm considering there is no perforator involved in the aneurysmal segment. (**e**) OA-PICA bypass and proximal clipping of the aneurysm due to perforators involved directly in the aneurysm segment

30.2.2 Occipital Artery

The OA originates from the posterior aspect of the external carotid artery. It travels along the medial surface of the digastric muscle. Under the mastoid groove, the OA turns posteromedially. Near the external occipital protuberance, the OA turns upwards and terminates in one or two main terminal trunks. The OA, distal to the posterior belly of the digastric muscle, may be divided into three segments: intramuscular, transitional, and subcutaneous. The intramuscular segment of the OA, from the digastric groove to the superior edge of splenius capitis muscle (SPC), runs in a single fatty connective tissue layer between the SPC and the semispinalis capitis muscle (SSC). The transitional segment of the OA, from the superior edge of the SPC to the superior nuchal line (SNL), travels superficially through the tendon of the sternocleidomastoid (SCM) muscle and the galea aponeurotica. This segment crosses multiple vertically superimposed tissue layers. The subcutaneous segment is located above the SNL and superficial to the galea aponeurotica.

30.2.3 Description of the Technique

We place the patient in prone position in a Sugita head frame. Flexion of the head without airway compromise is mandatory. The pinning of the calvarium should be carefully assessed to allow creation of the hockey stick incision without any limitations. We use the handheld Doppler to mark the course of the OA. A hockey stick incision is then utilized.

We use the microscope to perform the donor vessel dissection after initial superficial incision is performed. The subcutaneous segment of the OA is dissected from an epigaleal layer, the transitional segment is dissected from multiple muscle layers, and the intramuscular segment is further harvested down to the mastoid groove. We leave a peri-adventitial cuff along the OA in order to avoid spasm of the vessel. A large muscular branch of the OA is often encountered proximally and should be coagulated and sectioned. This vessel can be anticipated from the preoperative angiogram and must not be confused with the main trunk itself. The OA should be dissected proximally until its entrance into the muscular bed at the mastoid groove. Although Atez et al. found a 58 mm mean length of OA to be suitable for an OA-PICA bypass on a cadaveric study; we recommend a total length of 10–12 cm to be dissected to reach to the site of anastomosis so as to avoid any tension in the region of the anastomotic sutures. At this point, we leave the dissected OA in situ and perform the craniotomy and preparation of the recipient artery.

An oval suboccipital craniotomy (4 × 3 cm, with exposure of the foramen magnum) or a far lateral approach that includes drilling of 20% of the medial occipital condyle (in cases where control over the proximal PICA or over the vertebral artery is deemed necessary) is performed, proceeded by a C1 laminectomy. Under microscopic vision, the dura is then opened over the foramen magnum in a linear fashion and subsequently this opening is curved laterally and superiorly towards the cerebellar hemisphere. The PICA's caudal loop and its more proximal segments (anterior and lateral medullary segment) are then exposed (Fig. 30.2). The arachnoid of

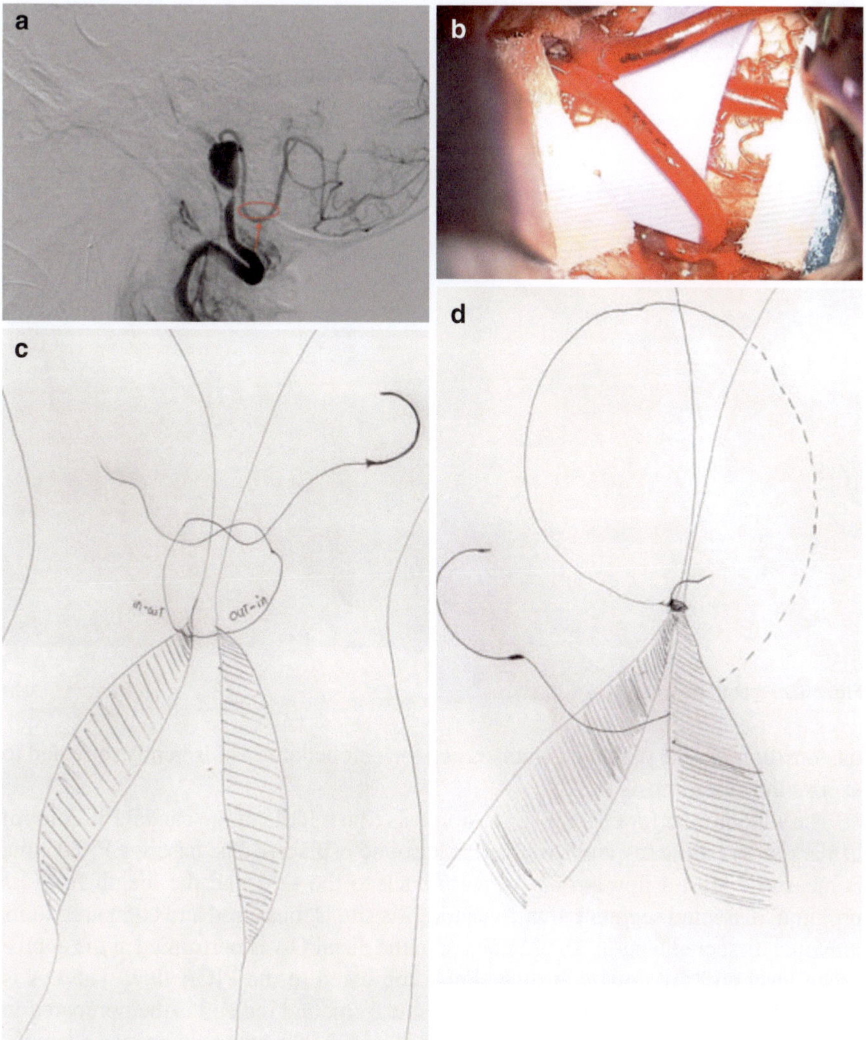

Fig. 30.2 PICA side to side bypass: (**a**) A ruptured dissecting first segment PICA aneurysm not amenable to a direct constructive treatment approach. (**b**) Exposure of bilateral PICA through a midline suboccipital craniotomy. Notice the location and similar size and extension of the arteriotomy lines. (**c**–**e**) Drawings showing the key portion of the side to side bypass. The first knot bringing the two distal ends together. The suture is passed behind the vessel to keep the knot outside the lumen, and then running sutures on the deep anastomoses layer are performed (out-in, in-out as it is shown). At the proximal end of the deep layer bypass, the suture configuration should be "in-out" and a knot is made outside the lumen. Then, the superficial layer of the bypass is done in a running fashion as described in the technique. (**f**) Completion of the PICA-PICA side to side bypass. (**g**) Postoperative angiogram confirming patency of the bypass (arrow)

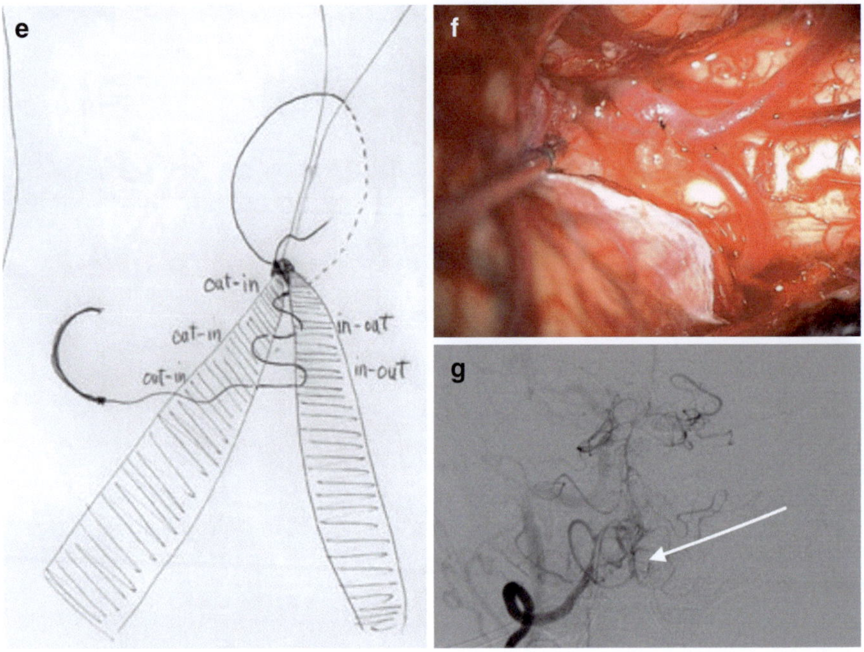

Fig. 30.2 (continued)

the tonsillomedullary fissure is incised and the cerebellar tonsil is gently retracted to expose the anastomosis site.

The suitable site for OA-PICA anastomosis (the middle of the caudal PICA loop) is marked with blue ink and a rubber background is placed. The baseline PICA flow is measured with a flow probe. We turn back to the OA, and the length from its proximal dissected segment to the anastomosis site is measured and compared to its maximal dissected length. An oblique cut in the distal OA is performed at the appropriate level and the flow is evaluated and compared to the PICA flow. The OA is prepared and cleaned of adventitia for the last 2 cm, and the end is then prepared in a "fish mouth" fashion. The vessel is flushed with heparinized saline and a temporary clip is applied to its proximal segment. One 5 mm mini-clip is used for proximal clipping of the PICA and one 3 mm straight or slightly curved clip is used for distal PICA. 3000 iu of heparin is then administered to the patient. We use the back-cutting knife (Apex Inc.) for the arteriotomy. The vessel is then irrigated with heparinized saline. The size of the arteriotomy is about 2.5–3 times the diameter of larger vessel (donor or recipient).

A 9-0 Ethilon nylon monofilament needle (V75-3) is suitable for the performance of this anastomosis. We first perform the two knots at the two lateral apices of the anastomosis in an outside-inside, inside-outside fashion. We then proceed to the placement of interrupted stitches at 12 and 6 o'clock. Then, the front side anastomosis, which is technically less challenging, is completed with interrupted sutures (generally two interrupted stitches between previously placed knots, starting with the periapical stitch on each side). Once the front wall is sewn, then the back wall is closed in the same interrupted fashion on either sides of the 12 o'clock stitch. Doing the easier front side first makes the more difficult backside suturing easier to perform. The lumen is irrigated with heparinized saline before the final stitch is tied. We first remove the temporary clip from the distal PICA, followed by the release of the temporary clip from the proximal PICA. The temporary clip is then removed from the OA. If any bleeding at the anastomotic site occurs, it will generally stop with the application of warm saline irrigation and gelfoam. In cases of a high flow opening in the anastomosis, an additional suture is added. In order to evaluate the patency and flow through the bypass, we utilize the microdoppler, the flow probe, and ICG videoangiography (Figs. 30.3, 30.4, and 30.5).

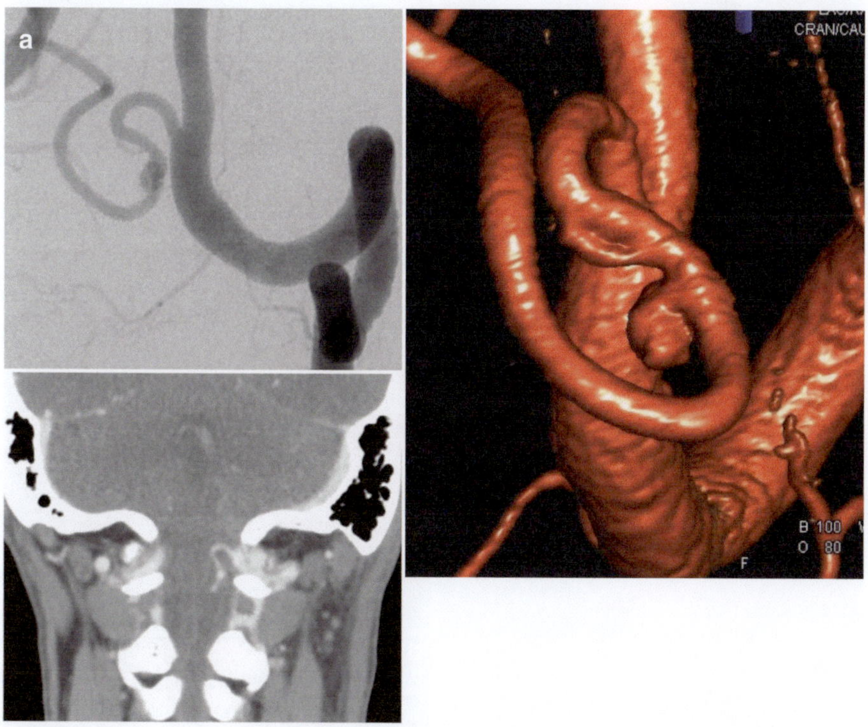

Fig. 30.3 PICA end to end bypass: (**a**) Dysplastic fusiform second segment ruptured PICA aneurysm initially treated by endovascular coiling. (**b–d**) The aneurysm regrew/recurred with rebleed after coiling. Surgical exposure at the foramen magnum showing the resection of the aneurysmal segment (note the extracranial origin of PICA, and absence of perforators involved in the aneurysm segment). The aneurysm segment resected and end to end bypass performed. (**e**) Patency confirmed with intraoperative ICG videoangiography

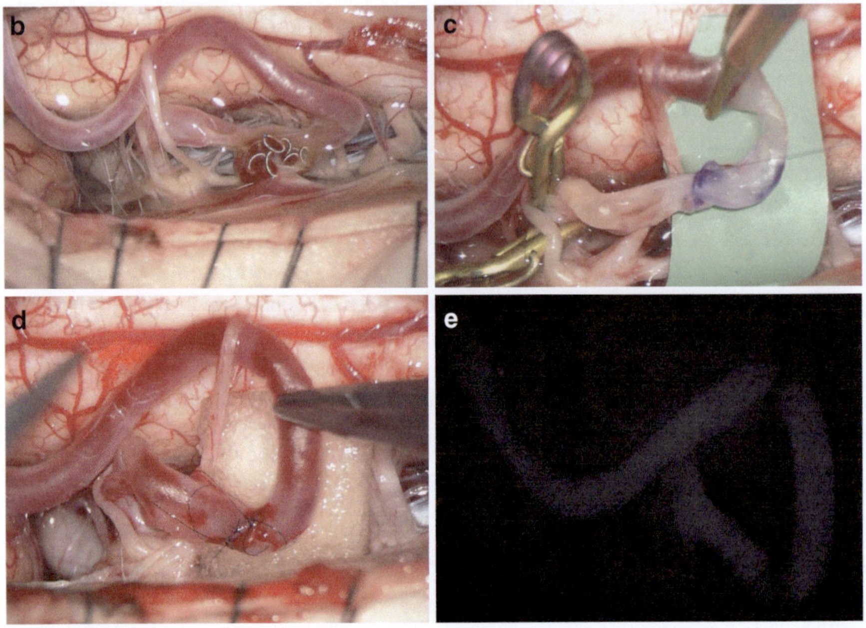

Fig. 30.3 (continued)

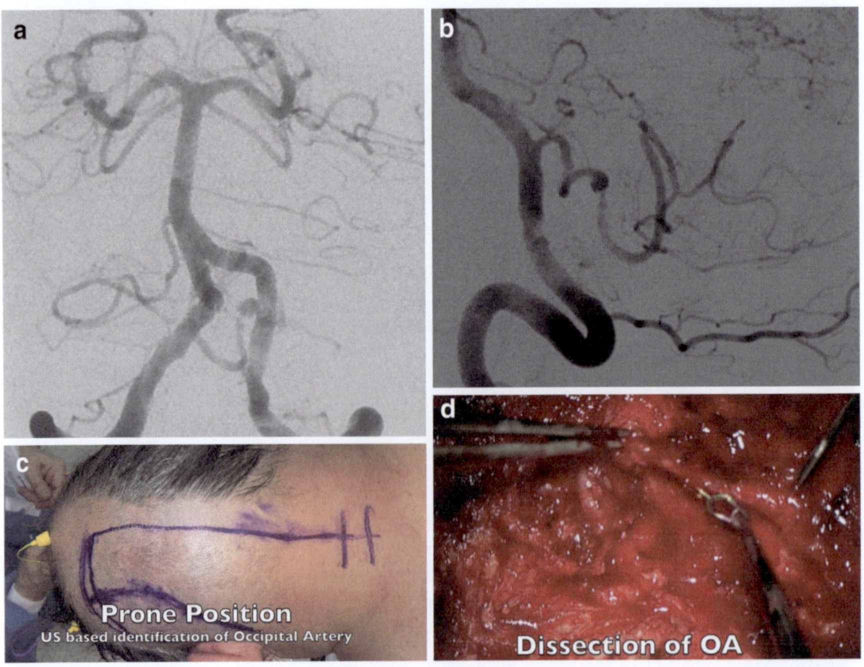

Fig. 30.4 OA-PICA bypass: (**a**, **b**) a ruptured fusiform third segment PICA aneurysm identified on cerebral angiogram. (**c**) Surface identification of occipital artery. (**d**–**h**) Dissection of occipital artery, exposure of the caudal loop (tonsillomedullary segment of the PICA), arteriotomy, and end to side bypass from OA to PICA. Finally trapping and resection of the dissecting aneurysm (arrow) as there is no involved critical brainstem perforators in the aneurysmal segment

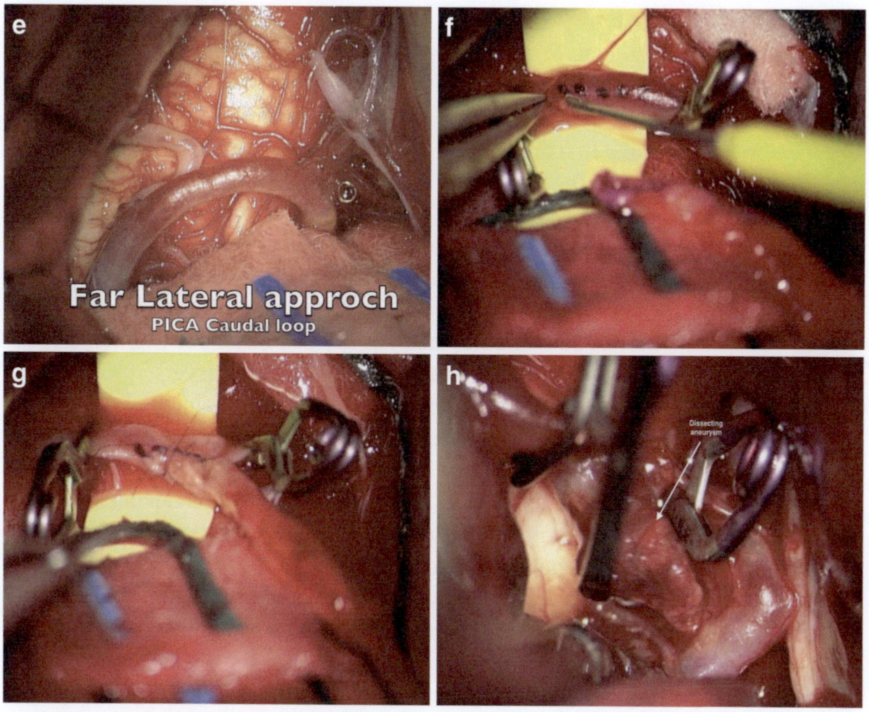

Fig. 30.4 (continued)

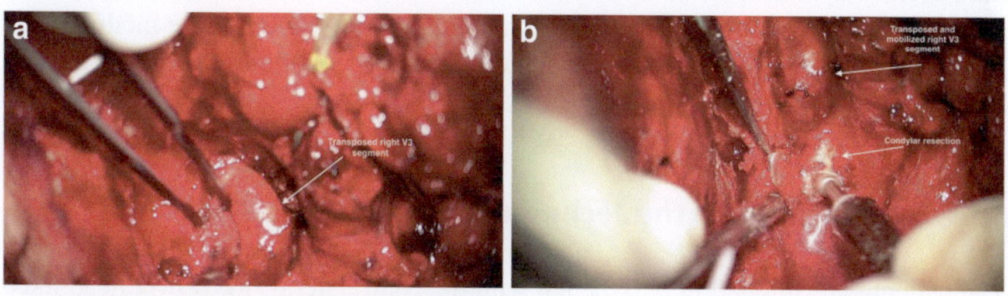

Fig. 30.5 (**a**) Exposure of extracranial V3 segment of the vertebral artery for VA-PICA bypass (arrow). (**b**) Transcondylar approach by drilling about 20% of the medial condyle and transposition of the vertebral artery

The closure is performed similar to a standard closure of a suboccipital craniotomy and great attention is directed at the OA at its entrance into the dura. Because of the inherent non-watertight dural closure that is necessary to keep the bypass under zero tension, the muscle and subcutaneous closure should be performed very cautiously to decrease the risk of postoperative CSF leak.

A postoperative CTA or angiogram is performed to confirm patency of the bypass. Patients receive aspirin 325 mg once daily after surgery for at least 1 year.

30.3 Vertebral Artery-PICA

30.3.1 Vertebral Artery Anatomy

The vertebral artery is the first and largest artery off the subclavian artery. The artery usually transverse through the transverse processes of the upper six cervical vertebrae, then it passes posterior and around the lateral mass of the occipital condyle and penetrates the dura at the level of the foramen magnum lateral and anterior to the medulla. The vertebral artery then joins the contralateral vertebral artery to form the basilar artery.

The extracranial part of the vertebral artery is divided into three segments. V1 is the first segment from the subclavian up to the level of C6 transverse process. The takeoff of the artery is usually from the cranial and posterior segment of the subclavian artery. This segment is situated posterior to the jugular vein and just anterior to the transverse process of the C7 vertebra. The second (V2) segment ascends through the transverse foramina of the upper six vertebrae. This segments deviates laterally at the level of C2 to reach a more lateral location of the C1 transverse foramina.

The third (V3) segment extends from the transverse foramen of C1 up to where it passes through the dura matter at the level of the foramen magnum. This segment is divided into three portions: vertical portion through the foramina of C1, horizontal segment course in the groove of the superior portion of the posterior arch of C1, and an oblique portion that transverse through the dura. This last segment passes medially and behind the lateral mass of the C1 and the atlanto-occipital joint.

The intradural segment (V4) begins at the lateral dual foramina, and this thick dura creates a funnel of dural sleeve where the artery crosses intradurally. The artery then ascends from lower lateral to upper anterior surface of the medulla, and it then crosses the pyramids to join the contralateral vertebral artery to form the basilar artery.

30.3.2 Description of the Technique

The patient is positioned in park bench with the contralateral side down, head fixed in the Sugita holder, 40° towards the floor in slight flexion. The right arm was prepped for the harvest of a brachiocephalic vein or radial artery. A retromastoid incision is performed two fingerbreadths behind the mastoid process and extended medially towards the midline. We usually perform a C1 laminectomy all the way to the lateral mass of C1. We identify the vertebral artery and its venous plexus which was microsurgically dissected, packed, and separated. The V3 segment is isolated for a length of about 2–3 cm and taken out from the C1 groove to have a comfortable position for trapping. A retrosigmoid craniotomy is performed inclusive of opening of the foramen magnum with identification of the sigmoid sinus and its connection to the jugular bulb laterally. We drilled at the level of the condyle, and then bring the microscope in, and further drilled the condyle (about 10–20%) to have a full far lateral approach. Mastoid cells are identified and sealed with bone wax at this point.

The dura is opened in a linear fashion from the cisterna magna. Microsurgical tack-up sutures are added in the periphery of the dura, and microsurgical dissection under high magnification was performed to identify the vertebral artery intracranially, origin of PICA, and the distal PICA. Identification of small perforators incorporated feeding the posterior part of the spinal cord is crucial.

We identify the distal PICA the area for appropriate anastomosis, which is then microsurgically separated, and prepared. We then return to the V3 segment of the vertebral artery extracranially, which was microsurgically transposed and dissected away to be ready for trapping and bypass.

We choose approximately a 5 cm length of graft vessel (radial artery or brachiocephalic vein) with the correct orientation, and we perform initially the distal anastomosis by temporarily trapping the distal PICA. An arteriotomy is performed with a back-cutting knife under high magnification, and the bypass is performed with interrupted sutures, starting the toe and the heel of the anastomosis and then periapical sutures and other sutures are added as needed. Alternative to periapical sutures would be do the 12 and 6 o'clock sutures after the first two anchoring stitches, and leave the periapical and paramedian knots for last.

We then performed a back flow to the graft which shows good flow, and a clip is positioned just above the distal anastomosis. When good flow to the PICA with no oozing from the bypass is demonstrated, we proceed with a proximal anastomosis by performing a trapping of the vertebral artery, and an arteriotomy of appropriate size. We perform a suture to the vertebral artery with an 8.0 monofilament at the toe and the heel of the anastomosis and then continue with either a running suture (preferable due to larger vessel size) or interrupted sutures on either side to finalize the bypass on this artery.

Then, we release the clips over the vertebral artery, first distally and then proximally and then removed the clip from the bypass. Verification of flow is performed with microdoppler, video ICG, or intraoperative cerebral angiogram.

30.3.3 Vertebral Artery Sacrifice and Jump Graft

There are rare situations where the vertebral artery is involved by a tumor and the resection of the tumor involves sacrifice or embolization of the vertebral artery. If the vertebral artery is dominant, or there is evidence based on a test occlusion or quantitative flow studies (e.g., NOVA MRA) that sacrifice as such will incur disturbed flow to the posterior circulation, a jump graft replacement of vertebral artery is performed. We have performed this procedure in a chordoma patient in whom a saphenous vain graft was used to reconstruct a new vertebral artery from C5 (V2 segment) to V3 segment, before a second stage removal of the tumor and resection of the involved vertebral artery.

30.4 Summary

PICA revascularization remains an important option in the armamentarium of cerebrovascular surgeons. The versatility of this vessel and the variety of bypass options in this limited region of the foramen magnum make the indications, choice of bypass options, rescue strategies, and technical details crucial to achieve a good surgical result and clinical outcome.

Management of Cavernous Malformation of the Cervicomedullary Junction

31

M. Neil Woodall and Peter Nakaji

Abbreviations

CSF	Cerebrospinal fluid
DVA	Developmental venous anomaly
EEG	Electroencephalography
MRI	Magnetic resonance imaging
PICA	Posterior inferior cerebellar artery
SSEP	Somatosensory evoked potential

31.1 Introduction

Cavernous malformations located at the cervicomedullary junction represent a challenging surgical problem. A cavernous malformation can be conceptualized as a benign vascular "tumor" made up of thinly veiled endothelial channels. Repetitive microhemorrhages may lead to growth of the cavernous malformation and a slowly worsening mass effect. Larger hemorrhages may also occur, leading to rapid expansion of the lesion and sudden neurological decline. The symptom complex caused by a particular cavernous malformation is dictated primarily by its location within the nervous system. Lesions involving the cervicomedullary junction have a tendency to cause dysfunction of the lower cranial nerve nuclei or long tracts traversing this region.

M. N. Woodall
Department of Neurosurgery, Barrow Neurological Institute, St. Joseph's Hospital and Medical Center, Phoenix, AZ, USA

P. Nakaji (✉)
Department of Neurosurgery, University of Arizona College of Medicine Phoenix, Phoenix, AZ, USA
e-mail: Neuropub@barrowneuro.org; nakaji@email.arizona.edu

E. Tessitore et al. (eds.), *Surgery of the Cranio-Vertebral Junction*,
https://doi.org/10.1007/978-3-030-18700-2_31

Counseling and treating patients with cavernous malformations of the cervicomedullary junction requires the surgeon to understand numerous factors. These include (1) the natural history of cavernous malformations and risks of treatments; (2) indications for treatment; (3) local neurovascular anatomy, including safe entry points to the brainstem; (4) bony anatomy and skull base approaches to the cranio-vertebral junction; and (5) microsurgical techniques unique to the resection of cavernous malformations.

A dense bundle of long tracts and nuclei is contained within the medulla and upper cervical spinal cord, complicating surgical excision of lesions in this location. This region is a transitional zone between the brainstem and spinal cord, and it therefore requires a combination of principles and approaches used for both cranial and spinal pathologies. A thorough understanding of regional bone, vascular, and neural anatomy is mandatory for the microsurgical treatment of any lesion involving the cervicomedullary junction. To make an adequate assessment of the risks and benefits of treatment versus conservative management and to counsel the patient, the neurosurgeon must review and weigh the natural history of cavernous malformations in the location particular to each case.

31.2 Natural History and Indications

In familial studies, rupture rates of cavernous malformations have been estimated at 0.6–2% per lesion per year (including asymptomatic hemorrhage). In sporadic cases, rupture rates have been estimated to be 0.7–3.1% per year, with re-hemorrhage rates as high as 22.9%. Brainstem cavernous malformations may have a re-hemorrhage rate as high as 35% per year (4.6% per patient-year preoperatively), but this number may be biased by referral center populations that are more likely to see progressive lesions with repetitive hemorrhages [1].

The surgical treatment of cavernous malformations of the brainstem and upper cervical spinal cord is typically reserved to patients who are symptomatic, who have a history of hemorrhage, or who have a lesion that presents to an ependymal surface. Asymptomatic lesions and lesions that would require navigation through significant neural tissue for resection of the lesion are typically recommended for conservative management. Clinical or radiographic evidence of prior hemorrhage is considered an indication for treatment if the lesion is thought to be surgically accessible. Some neurosurgeons argue that a history of recurrent hemorrhage should be required before offering surgical resection of brainstem cavernous malformations. Repetitive hemorrhage of brainstem cavernous malformations tends to produce a pattern of step-wise neurological decline. In our experience, patients with good functional status and minimal deficits tend to tolerate surgical resection better than those with more severe deficits. Therefore, we tend to recommend intervention at the first symptomatic hemorrhage rather than waiting for a second neurological decline [2, 3]. Certainly, any decision to offer treatment must consider individual patient factors that might increase the risk of surgical intervention and factors such as age and medical comorbidities. Current medical evidence indicates that microsurgical resection is the preferred treatment for cavernous malformations because stereotactic radiosurgery does not appear to be effective [4, 5].

31.3 Anatomy

The cranio-vertebral junction presents a conceptual challenge because treatment of this region requires an analysis of both cranial and spinal anatomy at their transition point. The bony confines of the cranio-vertebral junction are created by the clivus, anterior C1 arch, and odontoid process anteriorly. Posterolaterally, the occipital condyles, occipital bone, and cervical lamina guard the posterior fossa and spinal canal (Fig. 31.1). The paired vertebral arteries course through the C1 vertebral foramen and turn posteromedially in the sulcus arteriosus before piercing the dura (Fig. 31.2). Intracranially, the vertebral arteries give rise to the posterior inferior cerebellar arteries (PICA) and give rise to the anterior spinal artery just proximal to the vertebrobasilar junction. The anterior spinal artery runs in the midline of the ventral spinal cord. The paired posterior spinal arteries run along the dorsal aspect of the cervical cord and receive blood supply primarily from radicular branches arising from the vertebral arteries (Figs. 31.3 and 31.4) [6].

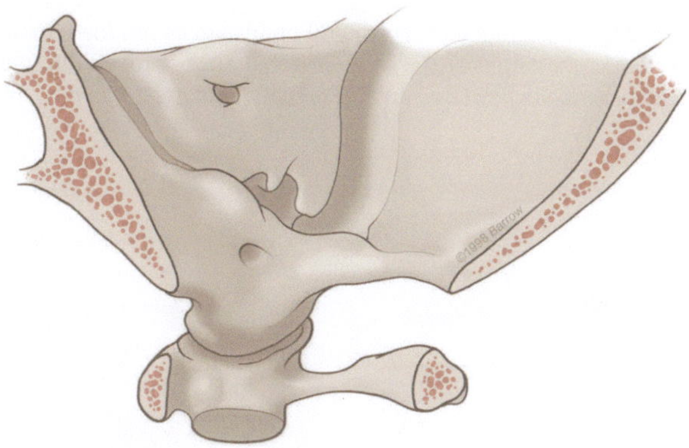

Fig. 31.1 Illustration demonstrates the bony anatomy of the cranio-vertebral junction. (*Used with permission from Barrow Neurological Institute, Phoenix, Arizona*)

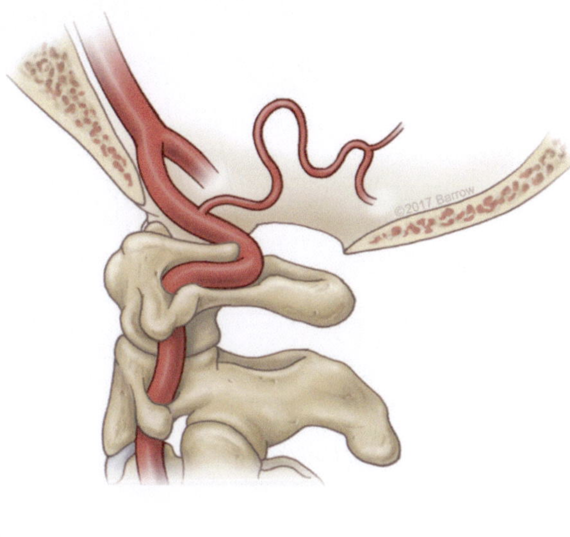

Fig. 31.2 The vertebral artery courses through the vertebral foramina of C1 and C2, the sulcus arteriosus, and finally pierces the dura to run intracranially. (*Used with permission from Barrow Neurological Institute, Phoenix, Arizona*)

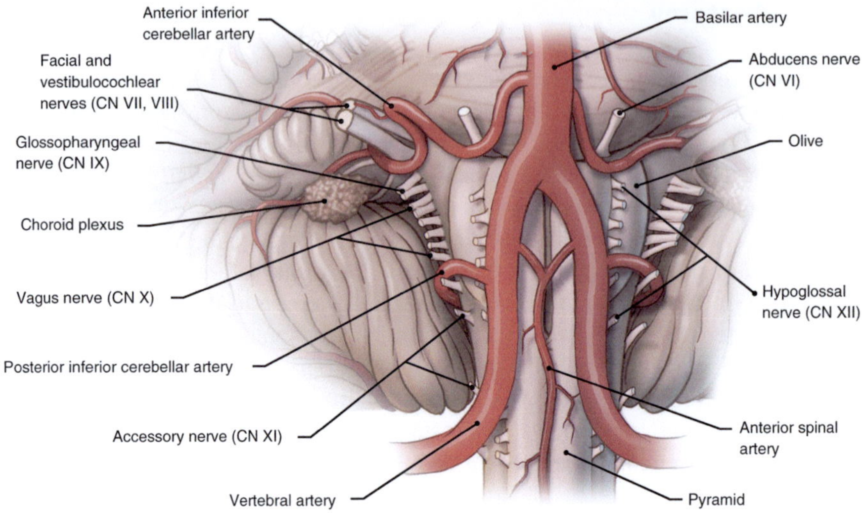

Fig. 31.3 Illustration of the ventral brainstem shows the relevant vascular and neural structures, including the origin of the anterior spinal artery proximal to the vertebrobasilar junction. (*Used with permission from Barrow Neurological Institute, Phoenix, Arizona*)

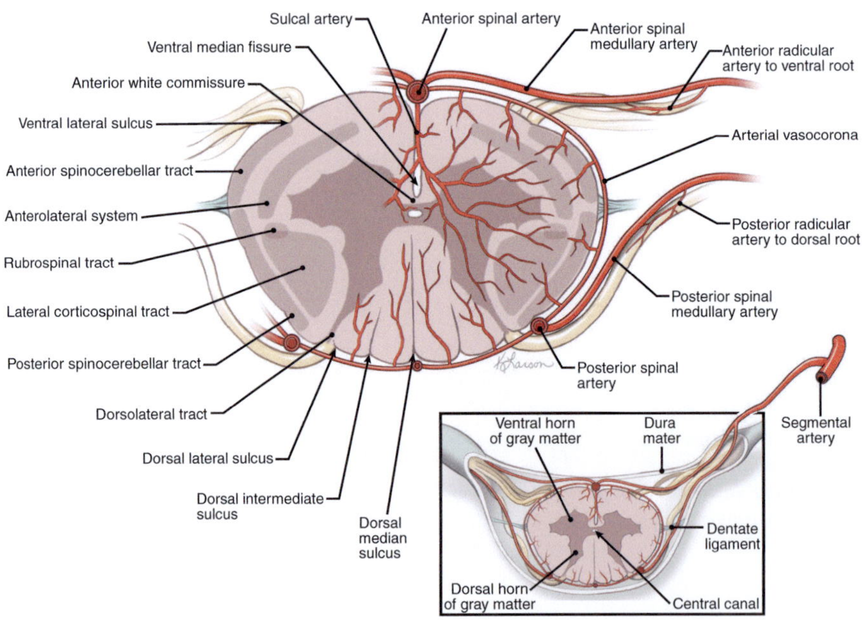

Fig. 31.4 Illustration depicts an axial section through the upper cervical spinal cord, showing the vascular arcades originating from the anterior and posterior spinal arteries. (*Used with permission from Barrow Neurological Institute, Phoenix, Arizona*)

Ideally, the lesion will present to an ependymal surface, which can serve as the entry point to the brainstem or spinal cord. If neural tissue must be traversed, safe entry zones to the brainstem should be used (Fig. 31.5). Those relevant to the craniovertebral junction include the peritrigeminal and lateral pontine safe entry zones, the anterolateral and posterior median medullary sulci, the olivary safe entry zone, and the lateral medullary safe entry zone. The peritrigeminal safe entry zone in the anterolateral pons, just anterior to the trigeminal nerve root safe entry zone (lateral to the corticospinal tract and anterior to trigeminal nerve nuclei), is an option for anterolaterally situated pontine lesions. The lateral pontine safe entry zone, which is located at the junction of the pons and middle cerebellar peduncle between cranial nerve V (trigeminal nerve) and the cranial nerve VII–VIII (facial and vestibulocochlear nerves) complex entry/exit zones, is the primary safe entry point for lesions of the pons and middle cerebellar peduncle. The anterolateral medullary sulcus lies lateral to the pyramid between the hypoglossal and C1 rootlets and can be used as an entry point for lesions in the ventral caudal medulla. The posterior median sulcus can be used below the obex to approach dorsal midline lesions in a fashion similar to the midline myelotomy approach used for spinal lesions. The olivary safe entry zone can be used for lesions in the anterolateral medulla up to an estimated depth of approximately 5 mm. The lateral medullary safe entry zone can be used to access the dorsolateral medulla. An incision is made in the inferior cerebellar peduncle via the foramen of Luschka just posterior to the origins of cranial nerves IX and X (spinal accessory and vagus nerves) [7].

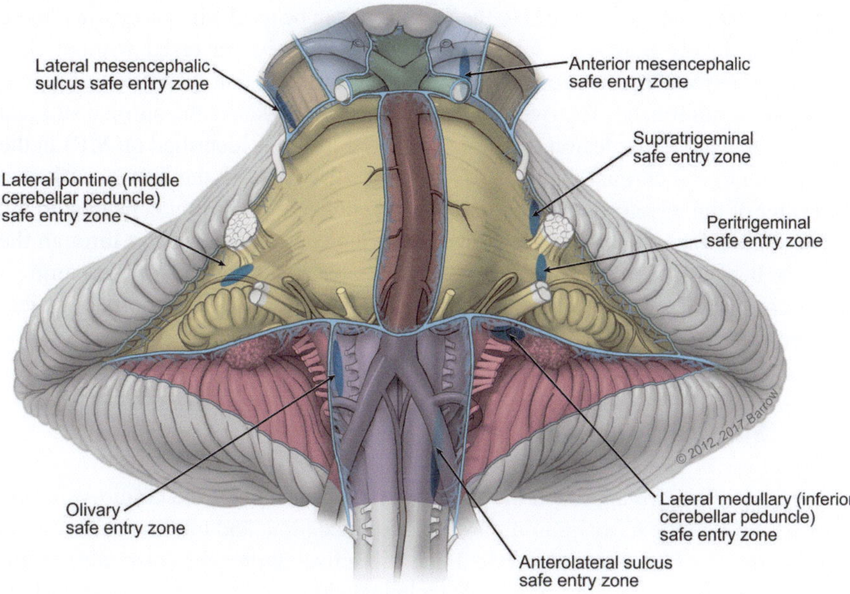

Fig. 31.5 Safe entry zones to the brainstem. (*Used with permission from Barrow Neurological Institute, Phoenix, Arizona*)

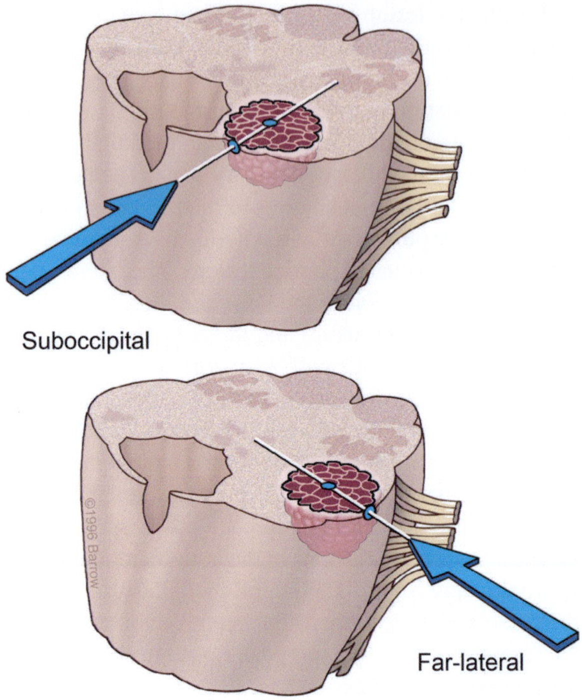

Fig. 31.6 The two-point method drives the choice of surgical approach between the suboccipital approach and the far-lateral approach in this example. (*Used with permission from Barrow Neurological Institute, Phoenix, Arizona*)

Although the safe entry zones to the brainstem can be used when necessary, there is no place in the brainstem where neural tissue can be traversed without risk. Ideally, lesions will present to an ependymal surface such that disruption of neural tissue can be minimized. The two-point method is used to select the optimal surgical approach to a particular lesion (Fig. 31.6) [8]. The lesion is identified on MRI in the axial, sagittal, and coronal planes. Two points are then placed: the first is marked at the center of the lesion, and the second is marked where the lesion is nearest to the ependymal surface. A line is then drawn from the center of the lesion through the point at the surface of the lesion, which dictates the direction of the surgical approach. A skull base approach is then selected that allows for the approach trajectory prescribed by the two-point method [8].

31.4 Surgical Approaches

At our institution, we approach the vast majority of lesions of the cranio-vertebral junction through the retrosigmoid, far-lateral suboccipital, and midline suboccipital approaches. The high anterior cervical and transclival approaches also are reasonable options to access this region. A technical description of each approach is beyond the scope of this chapter. Instead, we will discuss the view afforded by each approach and suitable approaches for each lesion location.

With the retrosigmoid approach, a craniotomy in the region of the transverse-sigmoid junction gives wide access to the cerebellopontine angle cistern, views of cranial nerves V–XI (trigeminal, abducens, facial, vestibulocochlear, glossopharyngeal, vagus, and spinal accessory nerves), and access to the root entry/exit zones of cranial nerves V and VII (trigeminal and facial nerves). The choroid plexus and flocculus of the cerebellum mark the location of the foramen of Luschka, which can also be accessed via the retrosigmoid approach (Fig. 31.7). We routinely skeletonize the sigmoid sinus so that the sinus can be retracted laterally to facilitate maximal exposure. Skeletonizing the sigmoid sinus maximizes a flat approach along the petrous bone and minimizes brain retraction, which allows the neurosurgeon an enhanced lateral view of the brainstem. The use of fixed retractors is rarely necessary for visualization; instead, dynamic retraction using the suction cannula and bipolar forceps is almost always sufficient. The retrosigmoid approach is suitable for lesions in the lateral or anterior pons and for lesions presenting to the lateral surface of the middle cerebellar peduncle. Lesions occurring at the pontomedullary junction are also often treated via a retrosigmoid approach. Ventral pontomedullary lesions that are centered in the pons are accessed through a retrosigmoid approach,

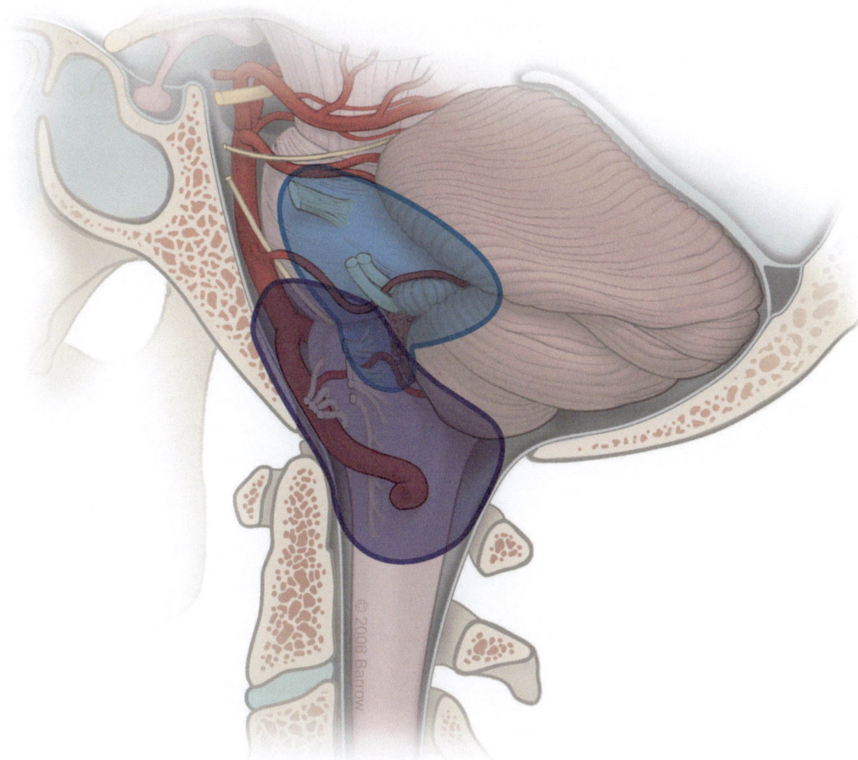

Fig. 31.7 Different exposures are afforded by the retrosigmoid approach (*blue*) and the far-lateral (*purple*) approach. (*Used with permission from Barrow Neurological Institute, Phoenix, Arizona*)

whereas pontomedullary lesions that occur mostly in the medulla are approached via a far-lateral craniotomy. Lesions with significant extension into the midbrain are not suitable for the retrosigmoid approach [9].

The far-lateral approach is performed via a lateral suboccipital craniotomy down to the level of the foramen magnum. The posterior portion of the occipital condyle is drilled to flatten the approach and to maximize lateral retraction of the dura. A C1 hemilaminectomy is usually performed to widen the opening of the dura and improve the surgical view. Several variations of the far-lateral approach have been described, including the transcondylar, supracondylar, and paracondylar extensions, which highlight the versatility of this approach for both intra- and extra-axial lesions occurring at the level of the foramen magnum. The far-lateral craniotomy provides access to the ipsilateral vertebral artery, PICA origin, jugular foramen, cranial nerves IX–XII (glossopharyngeal, vagus, spinal accessory, and hypoglossal nerves), and the lateral medulla (Fig. 31.7) [6]. The far-lateral approach is useful for ventral lesions situated at the pontomedullary junction that are centered in the medulla, whereas a retrosigmoid approach is more suitable for those centered in the pons. A far-lateral approach is useful for lesions located in the medulla or at the cervicomedullary junction that present to the ventral or lateral ependymal surface [2, 7].

The midline suboccipital approach, which is used for lesions presenting to the dorsolateral or dorsal surface of the brainstem, consists of a midline suboccipital craniotomy, including the foramen magnum, and a C1 laminectomy (Fig. 31.8). The cerebellar tonsils, the distal PICA, and the dorsal cervical cord can be visualized after the dura has been opened. The cerebellar tonsil can be gently elevated to expose the dorsolateral medulla. The arachnoid membrane between the vermis and

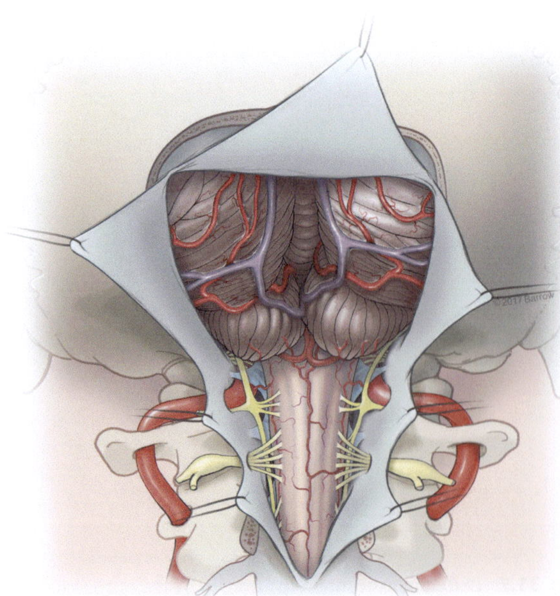

Fig. 31.8 Illustration demonstrates the exposure afforded by the midline suboccipital approach. (*Used with permission from Barrow Neurological Institute, Phoenix, Arizona*)

cerebellar hemisphere can be split to gain access to the fourth ventricle. This opening can be carried rostrally through the thin veil of the arachnoid membrane connecting the flocculus to the uvula (the telovelar approach) (Figs. 31.6, 31.9, and 31.10). This corridor provides access to the foramen of Luschka and lateral recess of the fourth ventricle, and it is useful for cavernous malformations presenting to the medial surface of the middle cerebellar peduncle. Lesions presenting to the floor of the fourth ventricle can be approached through the midline suboccipital approach (Fig. 31.11) [10].

The high anterior cervical approach exploits the retropharyngeal space to access the C1-3 region for decompression of the ventral spinal canal or access to intradural pathology at these levels. This approach is associated with significant dysphagia and often requires prolonged postoperative intubation, and it is therefore not favored in our practice [11]. An endoscopic transclival approach provides a direct route to

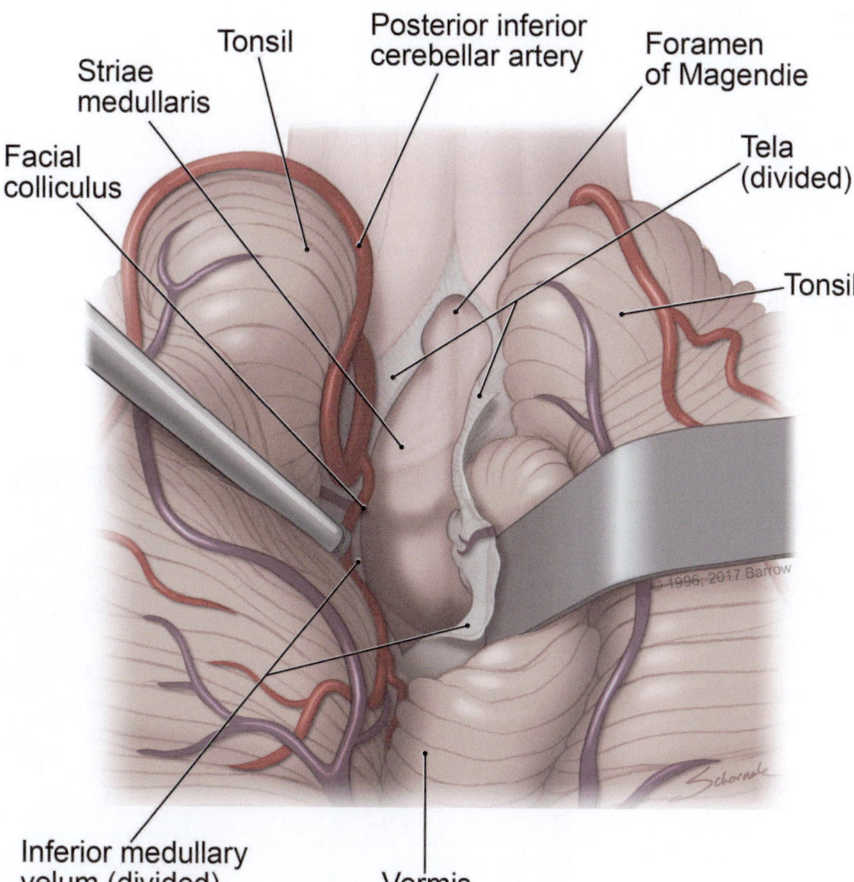

Fig. 31.9 In the telovelar approach, the tela and inferior medullary velum are divided. (*Used with permission from Barrow Neurological Institute, Phoenix, Arizona*)

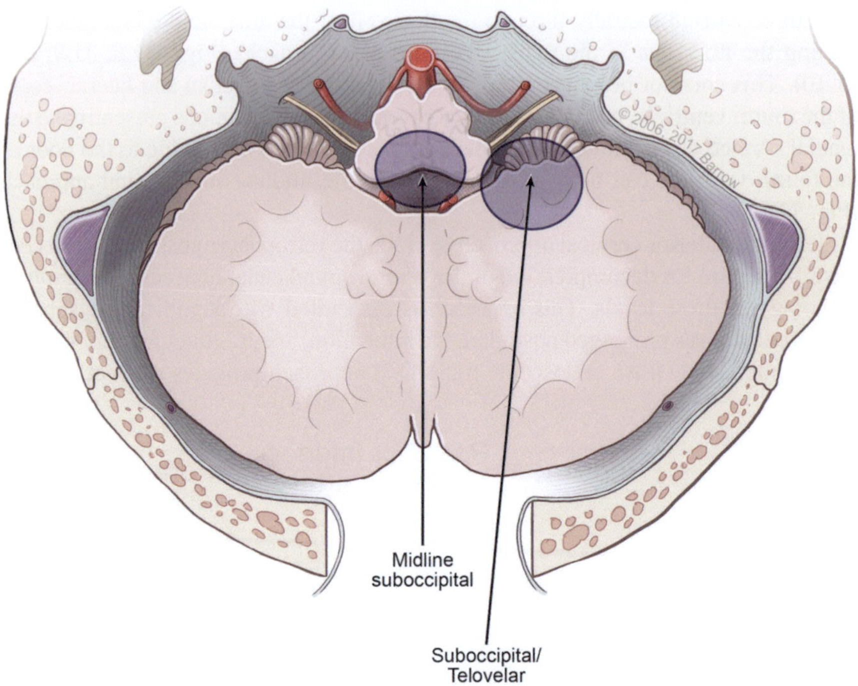

Fig. 31.10 Lesion location has an impact on the choice between a midline suboccipital approach and a telovelar approach. (*Used with permission from Barrow Neurological Institute, Phoenix, Arizona*)

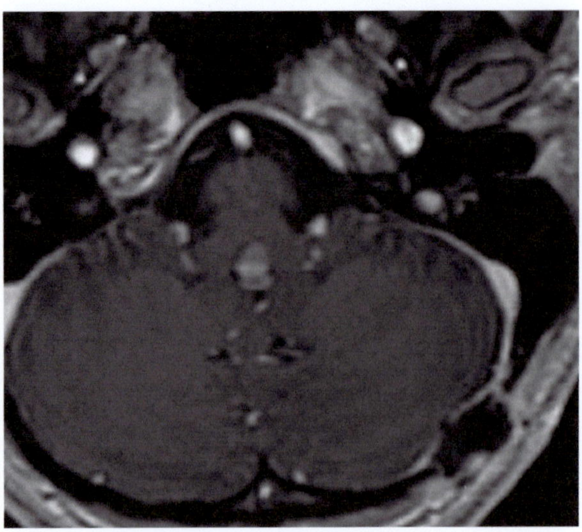

Fig. 31.11 Axial T1-weighted post-contrast magnetic resonance image shows a cavernous malformation situated in the midline of the fourth ventricle. (*Used with permission from Barrow Neurological Institute, Phoenix, Arizona*)

ventral pathology with excellent visualization. The midline transclival approach obviates the need to cross cranial nerves to access ventrally situated lesions [12]. Cerebrospinal fluid (CSF) leakage can be a troublesome complication of the transclival approach, but the rates of CSF leakage have improved for expanded endoscopic skull base approaches with the advent and widespread use of vascularized flaps [13]. Although the techniques employed using the endoscope are fundamentally microsurgical techniques, we believe that superior surgical fidelity can be achieved using the binocular vision of the operating microscope. Therefore, we favor a far-lateral suboccipital craniotomy for ventrally situated lesions at the cranio-vertebral junction.

31.5 Technique

The resection of cavernous malformations of the brainstem and spinal cord is technically similar to the resection of cavernous malformations located in non-eloquent sites in the brain, but it can be complicated by a sometimes deep and narrow exposure. Advances in microsurgical instrumentation, navigation, and our understanding of cavernous malformations have contributed to safer microsurgery for these lesions. Some of the considerations for the resection of cavernous malformations are outlined in the following sections.

31.5.1 Developmental Venous Anomaly

Cavernous malformations are often associated with a developmental venous anomaly (DVA). The DVA represents a confluence of veins that can have a candelabra or "caput medusae" appearance on angiography. The DVA provides venous drainage to healthy tissue and is therefore important to recognize and preserve. Inadvertent ligation of the DVA during resection of a cavernous malformation can potentially lead to venous infarction of the tissue drained by the DVA. The consistent relationship between cavernous malformations and DVAs has led some authors to postulate that these lesions represent entities along a disease spectrum rather than separate distinct processes. A DVA in the absence of an associated cavernous malformation does not pose a risk of spontaneous intracerebral hemorrhage [14].

31.5.2 Navigation

The use of frameless stereotactic navigation has become our standard practice in the treatment of brainstem cavernous malformations. Navigation allows for increased accuracy in planning the craniotomy and minimizing the skin incision length and the size of the bony opening. More importantly, the use of navigation that is co-registered with the operating microscope allows the surgeon to enter the parenchyma precisely where the lesion comes closest to the ependymal surface and to approach the lesion along an ideal trajectory. An entry point to the lesion can be preselected on the workstation using the preoperative imaging feature of the microscope. This feature allows the microscope to move into position automatically, aligning the surgeon's line of site along the desired trajectory that was planned preoperatively (Stealth Medtronic Sofamor Danek, Zeiss Pentero). The ideal entry point can typically be confirmed visually by yellow hemosiderin staining on the brainstem surface. Information provided by the image guidance system is complementary to the surgeon's firm understanding of regional 3-dimensional anatomy, for which there is no substitute.

31.5.3 Neurophysiological Monitoring

Intraoperative neurophysiological monitoring is another tool that can potentially increase the safety of surgery. The modalities used for a particular patient are largely dictated by the location of the lesion and patient-specific concerns regarding possible at-risk structures. Somatosensory evoked potentials (SSEPs) and electroencephalography (EEG) are monitored in every patient, regardless of lesion location. Changes in SSEPs can alert the operating room staff to peripheral nerve compression related to positioning (e.g., ulnar nerve compression and brachial plexus stretch) and may detect spinal cord compression related to manipulation of the neck during positioning. Early detection of SSEP changes allows for re-positioning of the patient and theoretical avoidance of a positioning-related neurological deficit. Changes in SSEP amplitude may also alert the surgeon to dorsal column dysfunction related to manipulation of the long tracts. The role of EEG is primarily to estimate the depth of anesthesia in these patients. It is our practice to induce EEG burst suppression to promote brain relaxation.

31.5.4 Microsurgical Instruments

The efficiency and safety of microsurgical resection of cavernous malformations have been enhanced through the development of specialized microsurgical instruments. Specialized micro bayonet forceps with teeth are invaluable during cavernous malformation resection (Figs. 31.12 and 31.13). These specialized forceps can be used to grasp the lesion and apply traction while gentle countertraction is applied to the adjacent tissue using the suction cannula in a sweeping motion. Spreading and dissecting with the bipolar forceps or micro bayonet forceps can further develop the dissection plane.

The deep and sometimes narrow exposure necessary to approach brainstem lesions can sometimes limit the illumination afforded by the operating microscope. Lighted instruments have been developed to eliminate these situations. Lighted suction cannulas and bipolar forceps are available that deliver light to the surgical bed, enhancing visualization in the deep aspect of the exposure (Figs. 31.14 and 31.15). The lighted suction cannula is used routinely because it tends to stay in the surgical

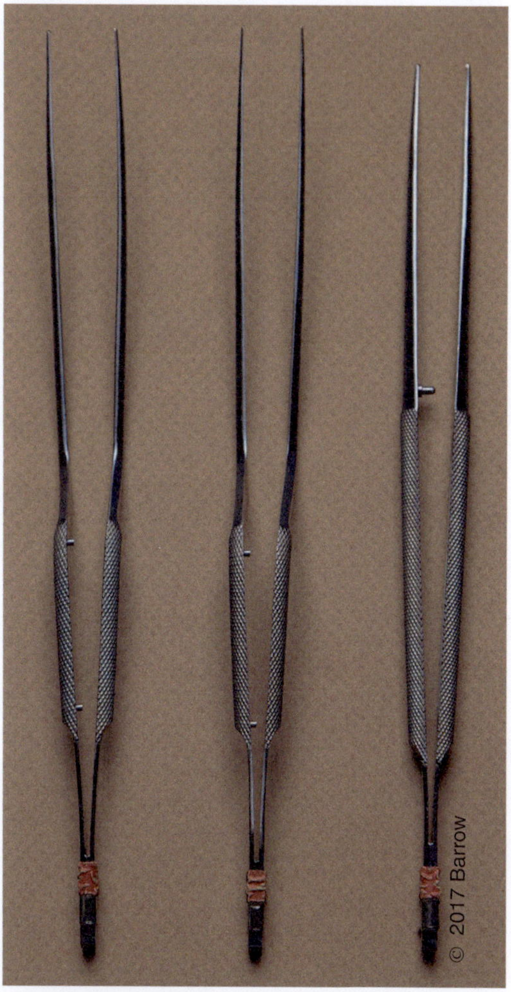

Fig. 31.12 Micro bayonet forceps with teeth facilitate resection of cavernous malformations. (*Used with permission from Barrow Neurological Institute, Phoenix, Arizona*)

field in the neurosurgeon's non-dominant hand throughout the resection while the bipolar forceps tend to be interchanged with other microsurgical instruments (dissectors, scissors, or bayonet forceps) in the dominant hand.

31.6 Conclusions

Treatment of cavernous malformations of the cranio-vertebral junction represents an exciting surgical challenge. Implementation of skull base techniques, microsurgery, navigation, neuromonitoring, and specialized microsurgical instruments have made microsurgical resection of these lesions safer now than in the past. Microsurgical resection remains the mainstay of therapy for symptomatic

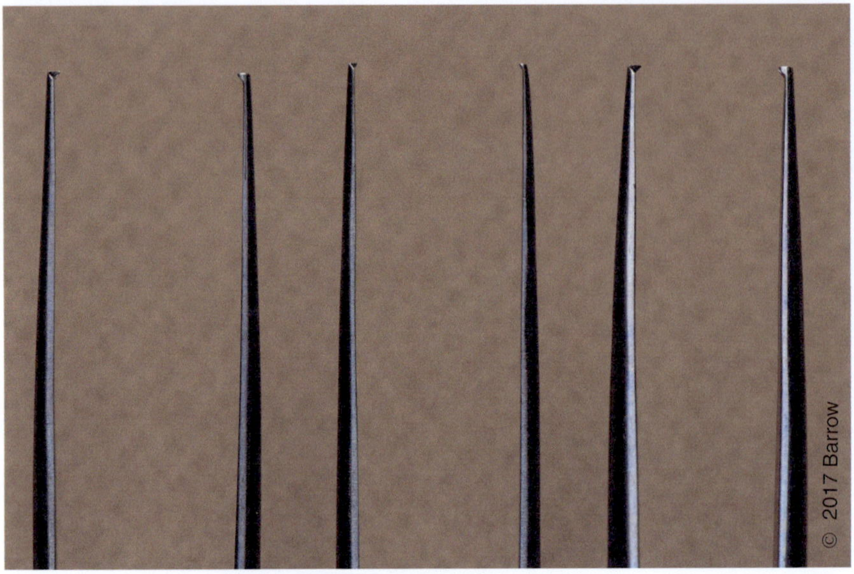

Fig. 31.13 Close-up photograph shows the teeth on the specialized micro bayonet forceps used for resection of cavernous malformations. (*Used with permission from Barrow Neurological Institute, Phoenix, Arizona*)

Fig. 31.14 A lighted suction cannula aids the resection of cavernous malformations. (*Used with permission from Barrow Neurological Institute, Phoenix, Arizona*)

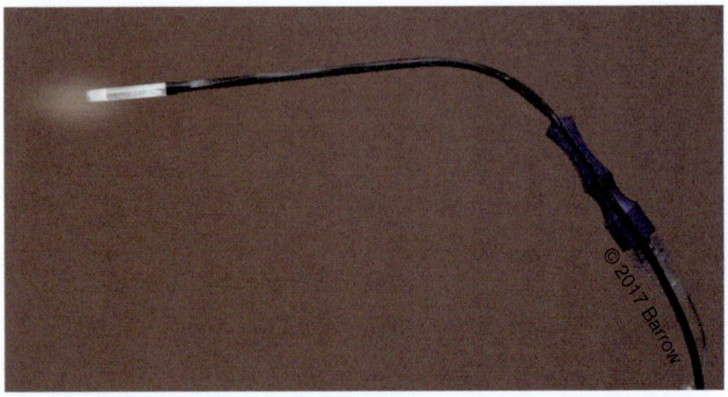

Fig. 31.15 Lighted bipolar forceps are typically used in resecting cavernous malformations. (*Used with permission from Barrow Neurological Institute, Phoenix, Arizona*)

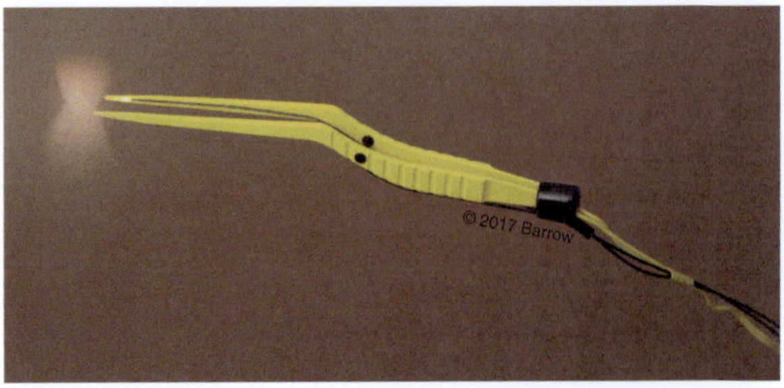

cavernous malformations. Despite technological advances, the surgeon's knowledge of local 3-dimensional anatomy remains the most valuable tool in the surgical armamentarium.

Acknowledgments The authors thank the Neuroscience Publications staff at Barrow Neurological Institute for assistance with the preparation of the manuscript and illustrations.

Disclosures: None.

Financial Support: None.

References

1. Abla AA, Spetzler RF. Cavernous malformations of the thalamus: a relatively rare but controversial entity. World Neurosurg. 2013;79:641–4.
2. Abla AA, Lekovic GP, Turner JD, De Oliveira JG, Porter R, Spetzler RF. Advances in the treatment and outcome of brainstem cavernous malformation surgery: a single-center case series of 300 surgically treated patients. Neurosurgery. 2011;68:403–14; discussion 414–5.
3. Abla AA, Spetzler RF. Brainstem cavernoma surgery: the state of the art. World Neurosurg. 2013;80:44–6.
4. Almefty KK, Spetzler RF. Management of brainstem cavernous malformations. World Neurosurg. 2015;83:317–9.
5. Davies JM, Kim H, Lawton MT. Surgical treatment of cerebral cavernous malformations. J Neurosurg Sci. 2015;59:255–70.
6. Rhoton AL Jr. The far-lateral approach and its transcondylar, supracondylar, and paracondylar extensions. Neurosurgery. 2000;47:S195–209.
7. Cavalcanti DD, Preul MC, Kalani MY, Spetzler RF. Microsurgical anatomy of safe entry zones to the brainstem. J Neurosurg. 2016;124:1359–76.
8. Brown AP, Thompson BG, Spetzler RF. The two-point method: evaluating brain stem lesions. BNI Quarterly. 1996;12:20–4.
9. Rhoton AL Jr. The cerebellopontine angle and posterior fossa cranial nerves by the retrosigmoid approach. Neurosurgery. 2000;47:S93–129.
10. Mussi AC, Rhoton AL Jr. Telovelar approach to the fourth ventricle: microsurgical anatomy. J Neurosurg. 2000;92:812–23.
11. Vender JR, Harrison SJ, McDonnell DE. Fusion and instrumentation at C1-3 via the high anterior cervical approach. J Neurosurg. 2000;92:24–9.
12. Gomez-Amador JL, Ortega-Porcayo LA, Palacios-Ortiz IJ, Perdomo-Pantoja A, Nares-Lopez FE, Vega-Alarcon A. Endoscopic endonasal transclival resection of a ventral pontine cavernous malformation: technical case report. J Neurosurg. 2017;127:553–8.
13. Kamat A, Lee JY, Goldstein GH, Newman JG, Storm PB, Palmer JN, Adappa ND. Reconstructive challenges in the extended endoscopic transclival approach. J Laryngol Otol. 2015;129:468–72.
14. Kalani MY, Zabramski JM, Martirosyan NL, Spetzler RF. Developmental venous anomaly, capillary telangiectasia, cavernous malformation, and arteriovenous malformation: spectrum of a common pathological entity? Acta Neurochir. 2016;158:547–50.

Management of Chiari Malformation

32

Giannantonio Spena and Marco Maria Fontanella

Abbreviations

BI	Basilar invagination
CMI	Chiari malformation type I
CSF	Cerebro-spinal fluid
GH	Growth hormone
IH	Intracranial hypotension
IIH	Idiopathic intracranial hypertension
MRI	Magnetic resonance imaging
Sym	Syringomyelia

32.1 Introduction

For CMI is commonly intended the type I of a class of four different malformative diseases which involve the rhombencephalon. The type I, II, and III present different degrees of the cerebellum, tonsils, and brainstem downward dislocation as well as other intracranial and spinal anomalies (hydrocephalus, corpus callosum agenesis, myelomeningocele). Type IV consists in severe agenesis of the cerebellum [1]. Further description of these entities is beyond the scope of this chapter. We will focus on CM type I, the most frequent type which is estimated to affect approximately 1 out of 1500 patients.

G. Spena
Unit of Neurosurgery, Department of Neurosciences, A. Manzoni Hospital, Lecco, Italy

M. M. Fontanella (✉)
Unit of Neurosurgery, Spedali Civili of Brescia, University of Brescia, Brescia, Italy
e-mail: marco.fontanella@unibs.it

E. Tessitore et al. (eds.), *Surgery of the Cranio-Vertebral Junction*,
https://doi.org/10.1007/978-3-030-18700-2_32

32.2 Pathophysiology

The most used definition for CMI is a descent of the cerebellar tonsils into the cervical canal due to a volumetric disproportion between the posterior fossa and cerebellar volumes. This definition takes into account just one mechanism of cerebellar tonsils descent, that of an embryological defect. In clinical routine, CMI is used as a synonym of cerebellar tonsils dislocation. However, mechanisms creating a sagging of the tonsils through the foramen magnum are varied and different, which are both congenital and acquired. Hence, the first concept to keep in mind is that cerebellar tonsils downward displacement is very often a radiological finding which does not define a pathophysiologic mechanism. All the efforts must be done to comprehend pathophysiology, since this is the basilar condition to give a patient the best chance to manage his or her pathology. Besides, when Hans Chiari first observed the protrusion of tonsils in cadaveric specimens, he understood that in one case tonsils were pushed out of the skull following an increase of intracranial pressure due to hydrocephalus; the other specimen presented instead an anomaly of the development of the posterior skull which reduced the volume of the posterior fossa forcing the tonsils beyond the foramen magnum [2].

Grossly, we can recognize some basilar mechanisms underlying the tonsils protrusion. In some cases, there is a state of increasing intracranial pressure which pushes posterior fossa content to slide through the foramen magnum; in other patients, a mismatch between content and container can be recognized, forcing the tonsils out of the cranium; in other words, a block at the level of the foramen magnum impedes the normal CSF flow from cranium to the spinal arachnoid space; also, rarely can a tethered cord pull the rhombencephalon from below; still, if a pressure gradient between the intracranial and spinal compartment takes place, tonsils can migrate because of a lack of sustainability from below. In this light, the modern conception of CMI comprehends several different mechanisms correlated to the tonsillar descent [3]. To complicate the matter, in some cases these mechanisms can gather, which makes diagnosis and treatment particularly intricate.

In more than one-third of cases, CMI is associated with syringomyelia (Sym), a cystic dilation of the spinal cord which can lead to debilitating myelopathy. It has been demonstrated that the obstruction of the cerebrospinal fluid flow at the level of the foramen magnum caused by the low-lying tonsils generates a pulsatile wave onto the spinal cord which favors the penetration of CSF from the subarachnoid space into the cord through the perivascular spaces of Virchow [4–6]. The understanding of the relationship between CMI and Sym has deeply changed the treatment's paradigms since the surgical resolution of CMI can very often cure Sym too (Fig. 32.1).

32.2.1 Intracranial Hypertension

All the conditions creating an increase in intracranial pressure can provoke tonsillar descent. Due to the shape of the posterior fossa which resembles that of a funnel, a constant pressure from above pushes the lower part of the rhombencephalon to slide

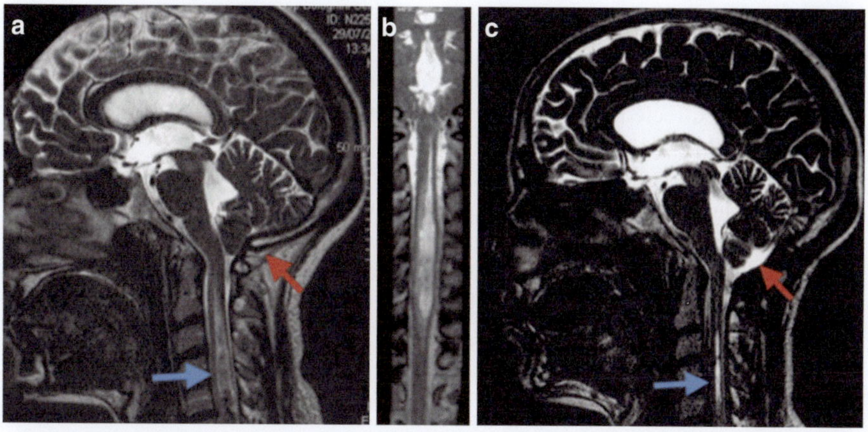

Fig. 32.1 (**a**) Preoperative MRI of a young lady with typical CMI associated with Sym. Note the presence of ventricular dilation. The patient did not complaint any symptoms related to intracranial hypertension but rather a left sided sensory syndrome and severe imbalance. (**b**) Coronal cut MRI demonstrating the left sided large Sym. (**c**) Osteo-dural decompression of the posterior fossa permitted to create a new cisternal magna and reduce the Sym volume. The patient returned to a fully active life in about 4 months. After 7 years, she still complaints dysesthesia at the left limbs

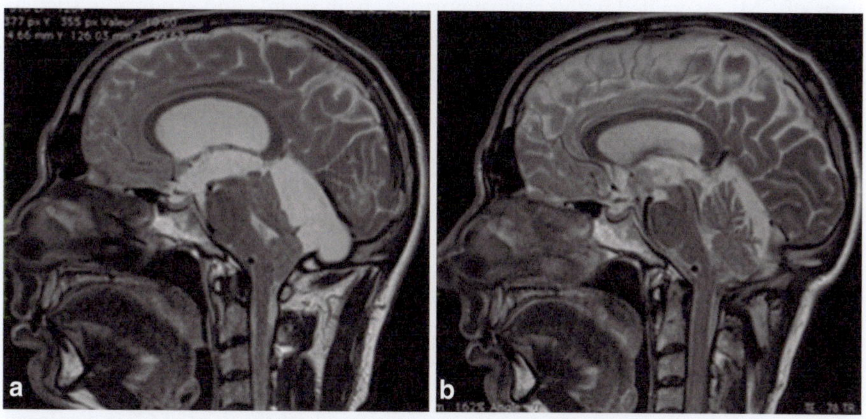

Fig. 32.2 (**a**) Preoperative MRI showing voluminous arachnoidal cyst of the posterior fossa provoking compression of the cerebellum and brainstem with subsequent tonsillar ectopia. Note the supratentorial hydrocephalus. Patients underwent posterior fossa decompression with cyst's fenestration and endoscopic third ventriculostomy. (**b**) 8 months later MRI demonstrated the disappearance of the cyst with re-expansion of the structures of the posterior fossa and resolution of the hydrocephalus

through the foramen magnum. This is typically found in the case of hydrocephalus or following the presence of tumor masses in both supra- and infratentorial spaces (Fig. 32.2) [7, 8]. Diagnostic and therapeutic implications are very relevant, particularly for hydrocephalus. It must be kept in mind that CMI is frequently associated with CSF circulation disturbances and in approximately 10% of patients, a clear hydrocephalus is also diagnosed. It is hence basilar to ascertain the causative role of CMI in generating hydrocephalus or, conversely, in being an effect of hydrocephalus. This distinction strongly influences surgical treatment which, in the latter case, should first be directed at correcting hydrocephalus through ventriculoperitoneal shunt or an endoscopic third ventriculostomy.

A CSF circulation impairment can be also found in the case of idiopathic intracranial hypertension (IIH) where ventricles are not dilated and tonsils can be sometimes low-lying. If IIH is suspected, it is mandatory to rule it out by excluding the presence of typical MRI (perioptic membranes dilation, empty sella, Meckel's cave enlargement) and ophthalmologic findings [9, 10]. The underestimation of CSF circulation problems can complicate the surgical outcome because of higher risk of CSF fistulas and pseudomeningocele.

32.2.2 Skull Deformities

Many abnormalities of the skull's development which can be associated with CMI have been described. All these diseases are explained by the mismatch between container and content. In other words, the cranial volume is reduced with subsequently reduced room for encephalon. The early closure of cranial sutures is at the basis of CMI associated with craniosynostosis, both simple and syndromic such as Crouzon, Apert, and Pfeiffer syndromes. Still, congenital deficiency in growth hormone (GH) can manifest with an underdevelopment of the posterior fossa volume and subsequent tonsillar descent [11].

With the same mechanism but acquired are those skull deformities related to thickening of the bone as it is found in Paget disease, rickets, osteopetrosis, erythroid hyperplasia, and acromegaly.

32.2.3 Cranio-cervical Junction Deformities

In this class falls a large group of congenital and acquired anomalies which can create a reduction of CSF spaces at the level of the foramen magnum region. The typical example is the basilar invagination (BI), a condition where the dens of C2 is displaced into the cranial space above the foramen magnum (trespassing the basion-opisthion line, the McRae's line). BI can be found in patients with congenital (osteogenesis imperfecta, achondroplasia) or acquired pathologies (rheumatoid arthritis, Paget's disease). A more frequent finding in pediatric patients is an odontoid retroflexion without BI, which implies a brainstem compression and reduction of CSF spaces. However, odontoid retroflexion can occasionally be detected in CMI diagnosis without any causative role. Achondroplasia, the most common cause of short-limbs dwarfism, is usually associated with stenosis of the foramen magnum with obliteration of cerebrospinal fluid spaces and the consequent block of the CSF circulation. Other cranio-cervical anomalies associated with CMI are platybasia and atlas assimilation.

The detection of these alterations in the context of a CMI is of uppermost importance as it can deeply modify the surgical strategy. It is mandatory to rule out a

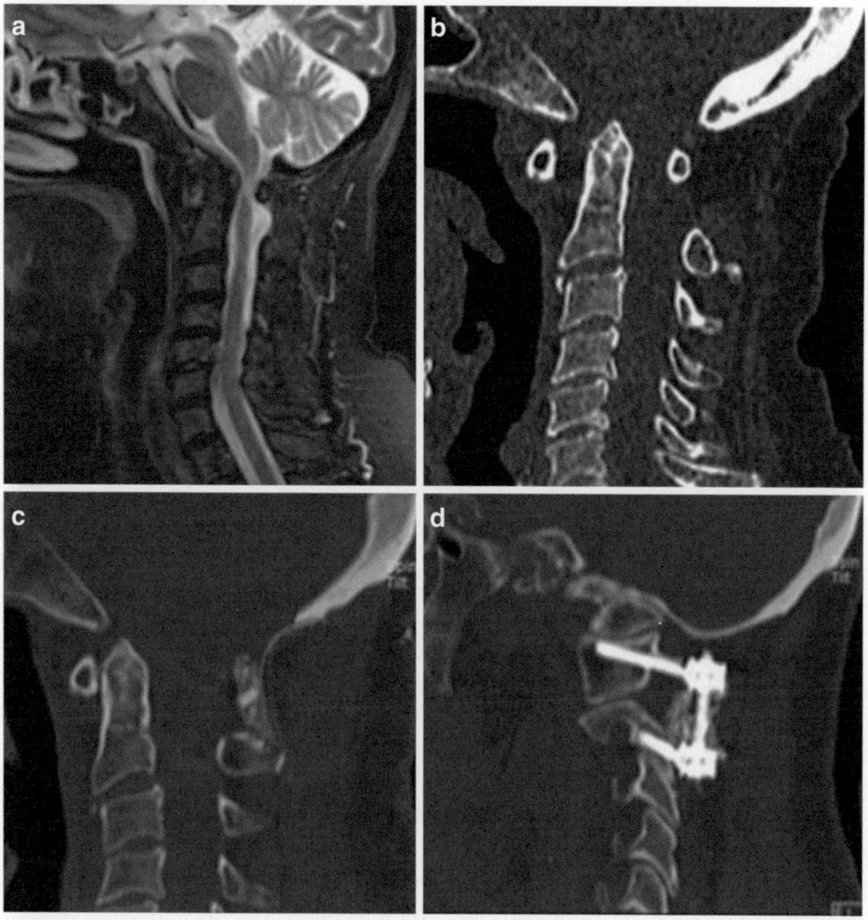

Fig. 32.3 This 64 years old female presented with intense occipital pain and severe myelopathy (paraparesis, swallowing, and phonetic difficulties). The preoperative MRI (**a** and **b**) showed a malformation of the posterior fossa with totally occluded cisterna magna associated with C1 subluxation and upper dislocation of the axis. (**c** and **d**) Surgery was addressed to intraoperative reduction of the luxation, stabilization with C1-C2 screw fixation, and C1 laminectomy. After 1 year, the patient is able to drive

cranio-cervical instability as well in order to decide for an cranio-cervical fusion surgery as an adjunct to posterior fossa decompression, or to consider a transoral or transnasal odontoid process resection [12–21] (Fig. 32.3).

32.2.4 "Typical" CMI

The classical conception of CMI is that of a congenital volumetric mismatch between a small posterior fossa and the neural content. At the basis of this alteration should be a defect into the embryology of the paraxial mesoderm generating the occipital somites with subsequent underdevelopment of occipital bone [1]. This pathophysiologic mechanism has been strongly supported following the seminal experiments by Marin-Padilla et al. [22] who described a small posterior fossa in rodents undergoing a teratogenic regimen of vitamin A in which a tonsillar descent was observed [1]. In that light, CMI is frequently classified as part of the spectrum of cranio-cervical junction abnormalities (see above). There have been described numerous morphological alterations associated with CMI, even though they are not always present and none is pathognomonic. The most frequent are short clivus and supraocciput; large foramen magnum (although many patients show a narrow foramen magnum); shallow posterior fossa; lower torcular Herophili with vertical straight sinus; thickened occiput occluding the cisternal magna space; occipital condyles deformities; and reduced volume of the posterior fossa [23–30].

32.2.5 Spinal Cord Tethering

Tethered cord is typically found in the type II CM, as part of a more complex syndrome associated with myelomeningocele or another form of spinal dysraphisms. However, rarely CMI can be associated with occult tethered cord and it is hypothesized that the traction from below could explain the low position of tonsils. If this is the case, the surgical strategy should be first addressed to freeing the filum terminale. This hypothesis justifies the completion of neuroimaging with brain and spine MRI not only to rule out syringomyelia but also cord tethering [31–33].

32.2.6 Intracranial Hypotension (IH)

Typical cranial MRI signs of IH are cerebellar tonsils ptosis, slit ventricle, downward displacement of the brainstem, and bright meningeal contrast medium uptake. IH can be secondary (following spinal surgery or lumbar punctures) or primary when an evident cause is not detected. Sometimes during spinal surgery, a dural tearing can happen with subsequent chronic CSF to leak. In those patients harboring a spino-peritoneal, over-drainage can sometimes manifest as sagging tonsils.

When CM is associated with some of the MRI signs mentioned above and the patient complaint of an orthostatic headache, it is mandatory to hypothesize IH and search for the eventual cause and address the treatment to first solve the hypotension [34].

32.3 Clinical Diagnosis

Before being an anatomical and radiological issue, CMI is peculiarly a clinical diagnosis. It is hard to recognize a paradigmatic CMI patient as symptoms can greatly vary and be complicated by the coexistence of other associated pathology (syringomyelia and all the above-mentioned diseases) as well as by the overlapping or mistaking of other not related pathologies. Hence it is first fundamental to ascertain that complaints concern to CMI.

Careful and detailed record of patient's history is of uppermost importance; symptoms can be grouped in those presenting very frequently and other more rarely or exceedingly rarely.

The most important complaint from almost all the CMI patients is a headache. This is sited in the occipito-nuchal region and is usually triggered by a cough, straining, running, and prolonged or extreme neck flexion. It can frequently irradiate to shoulders and dorsum. If the headache is the only symptom, it is mandatory to put into differential diagnosis also the cough headache. This latter tends to be the sole symptom referred and it lasts no longer than few seconds [35]. CMI occipital headache is more often long-lasting (from minutes to entire days) and is very frequently associated with other neurological symptoms (see below). The physiopathology of CMI headache is not completely understood. The most accredited theory calls the CSF block at the level of the foramen magnum which impedes the normal flow toward the spinal space during efforts creating a sudden increase of intracranial pressure [36].

On a regular basis, CMI patients complain of visual (diplopia, scotomas, retroocular pain, photophobia, visual filed alterations) and otoneurological symptoms (vertigo, tinnitus, sensation of pressure into the ears, hearing dysfunction). These disturbances are most probably due to the deformation and stretching of both cranial nerves and cerebellar peduncles/brainstem. Similarly, numbness or tingling in hands or arms can be frequently referred. Even though a clear pathophysiologic mechanism has not yet been described, patients often refer fatigue, concentration, and sleeping problems.

In more severe forms of brainstem compression, patients can show swallowing difficulties, short breath, nystagmus, the absence of gag reflex, facial hypoesthesia, and hemiatrophy of the tongue.

When associated with syringomyelia, clinical findings are mainly related to spinal cord damage and depend upon the extension and position of the Sym. The most typical complaint is dysesthesic pain to limbs or trunk; in more severe form, upper extremity weakness and atrophy and long-tract signs can be found.

32.4 Indications for Surgery

As stated, CMI patients represent a multifaceted universe of history, symptoms, and signs. More, it is worth noting that psychological aspects should be considered in the capacity to accept and bear the symptoms (especially pain) is different in every person. If it is quite straightforward to indicate surgery in a subject with cranial nerves impairment and 9 mm tonsils' descent on MRI, problems may arise with patients having an only headache, other subtle or vague disturbances, and tonsils few millimeters beyond the foramen magnum. Quite, unfortunately, the degree of tonsils' descent is not a sufficient criterion to indicate surgery. It has been acquired that there is no direct correlation between the degree of tonsils' descent and severity of

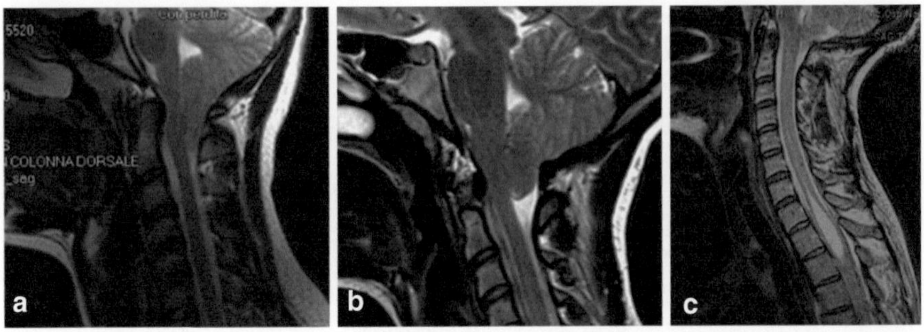

Fig. 32.4 These three examples demonstrate the lack of correlation with the severity of tonsils' descent and clinical presentation. The patients in A and B had evident tonsils ptosis (until C2). These patients were asymptomatic; in C, tonsils were just few millimeter beyond the foramen magnum and the patient complaint important neurological disturbances associated with cervico-thoracic Sym

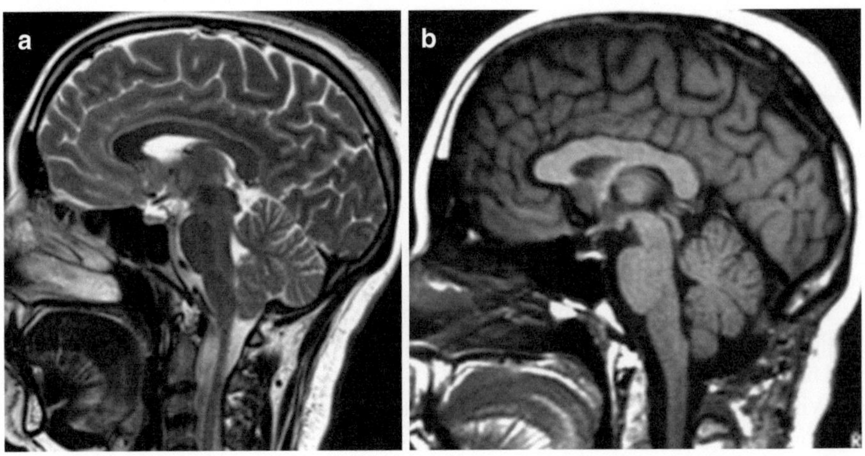

Fig. 32.5 (**a**) Preoperative MRI of a young female with intense occipital headache, hemifacial hypoesthesia, severe dizziness, and swallowing difficulties. Pay attention to the tonsils which slightly protrude through the foramen magnum. Note also how the occipital bone is thick with complete disappearance of the cisterna magna. (**b**) Postoperative MRI showing a satisfying posterior fossa decompression with duroplastic. Patient returned to work after 2 months

symptoms/signs nor to the risk of developing syringomyelia [37–39] (Figs. 32.4 and 32.5). Hence the classical 5 mm rule can lead to under- or overtreatment and physician's judgement based on physical examination and patient's history is the key for correct decision-making [3, 40]. Similarly, the widespread of MRI availability has risen the number of accidentally diagnosed tonsillar ectopia [41–44]. At present, there is a lack of evidence that any neuroradiological or neurophysiological exams can be conclusive in indicating surgery for patients with mild or suspect symptoms.

In the end, we can recognize some fundamental steps in the decision-making: (1) making correct correlation between imaging and clinical history/symptoms/signs;

(2) recognizing the overlapping diseases (i.e., migraine or cough headache, Meniere syndrome, cervical spondylosis, degenerative neurological diseases, etc.); (3) understanding the pathophysiology of the cerebellar descent and the role of other associated or causative conditions (see above); (4) comprehension of patient's expectations and conception of his/her CMI.

The association of CMI and Sym triggers in the most part of neurosurgeon the attitude for early intervention as the appearance of disturbance related to spinal cord injury should be irreversible. It is not clear if asymptomatic patients with CMI and Sym should be only followed up until an enlargement of Sym is detected or even subtle symptoms appear [45]. Actually, studies about the evolution in such patients are lacking [46].

32.5 Surgical Technique

The last two decades have seen a vivid discussion among neurosurgeons on some surgical nuances. It is nowadays assumed that the posterior fossa decompression with the aim of restoring a cisternal magna and CSF flow through the foramen magnum is the goal of surgery for both CMI and CMI plus syringomyelia [38]. Similarly, many other techniques such as arachnoid dissection, tonsils' coagulation, and plugging of the obex are now much less used. This has been a natural consequence of the better understanding of pathophysiology and the necessity to strongly reduce any kind of complication [47, 48]. One of the main surgical issues is the necessity to create a duroplasty as further enlargement of the space for the cisternal magna. The literature is rich of works dealing with this matter; the most recent meta-analyses and reviews give the indication that clinical results between duroplasty or craniotomy alone are not statistically different. However, on the long run, patients without duroplasty can show higher rates of redo surgery because of the formation of compressive scars. On the other hand, patients undergoing duroplasty show higher rates of perioperative CSF leaks and pseudomeningocele [49–52]. In our center, we indicate duroplasty in all the patients especially young adults. In rarest cases of elderly patients, we prefer not to open the dura in trying to eliminate any possible risk of surgery. Similarly, in pediatric patients where the peculiar CSF circulation dynamics make the risk of leakage very high, we prefer to use the craniectomy with only outer dura layer dissection [53, 54].

32.5.1 Minimally Invasive Technique and Rationale

We routinely adopt the same strategy for both CMI and CMI plus Sym, that is an occipital craniectomy, C1 laminectomy, and duroplasty. It is our aim to perform the most minimally invasive approach possible in order to decrease complications, reducing the damage to nuchal muscles and enhancing the cosmetic results. Specifically, rectus capitis posterior major muscle, which connects the inferior nuchal line to the arch of C2, has been shown to have a role in the proprioceptive system and in controlling the balance of the atlanto-axial and occipito-axial articulations [55–57]. Respecting these muscles may help patients in recovering faster especially those with preoperative dizziness and imbalance (Fig. 32.6).

After the administration of intravenous antibiotics prophylaxis and positioning of pneumatic stockings, the patient is placed in prone position with the head fixed in the three-pin clamp and flexed until the vertex point the floor. The correct flexion of the head allows to widen the angle between occiput and cervical spine reducing the necessity of large skin incision (Fig. 32.7). Nuchal muscles dissection is started on

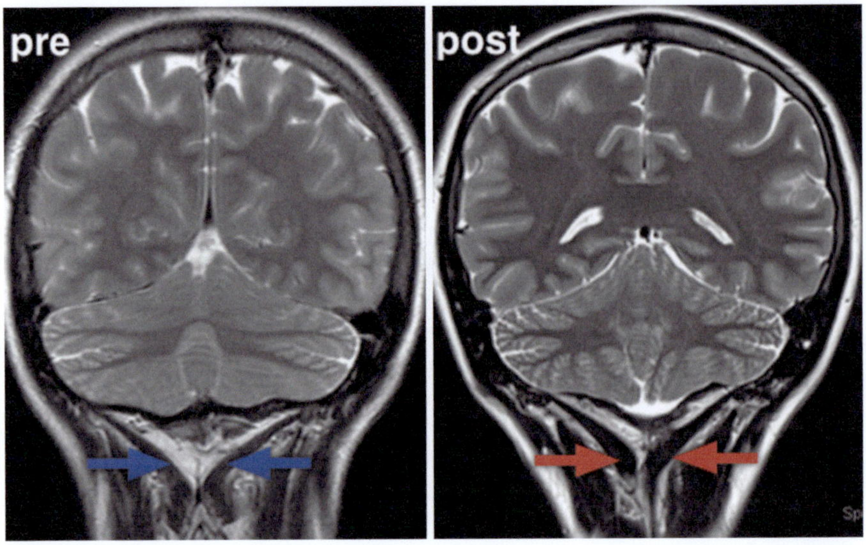

Fig. 32.6 This coronal MRI show the status of the rectus capitis posterior major before and after surgery. Note that postoperatively the muscle is in the same position as before. The cisternal magna is now visible

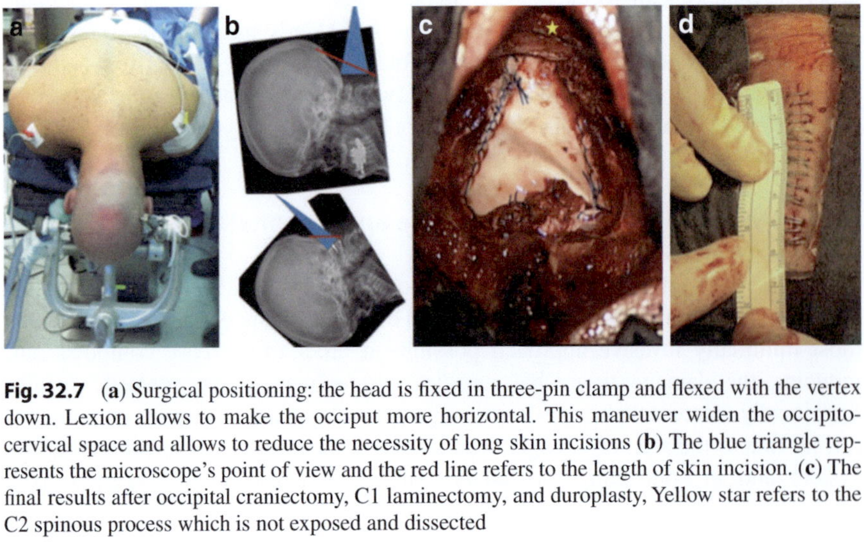

Fig. 32.7 (**a**) Surgical positioning: the head is fixed in three-pin clamp and flexed with the vertex down. Lexion allows to make the occiput more horizontal. This maneuver widen the occipito-cervical space and allows to reduce the necessity of long skin incisions (**b**) The blue triangle represents the microscope's point of view and the red line refers to the length of skin incision. (**c**) The final results after occipital craniectomy, C1 laminectomy, and duroplasty, Yellow star refers to the C2 spinous process which is not exposed and dissected

the midline in the avascular connective tissue until the posterior edge of the foramen magnum is under control as well as the posterior arch of C1 and the occipital plate onto the superior nuchal line and inion. C2 spinous process is left untouched along with muscles and ligaments. The resection of occiput is done by means of perforators or high-speed drills; the size of craniectomy should reach superiorly the inferior nuchal line and extend laterally for no more than 2.5 cm. An exceedingly large craniectomy can put the patient at risk of cerebellar sagging, a very rare surgical complication [58, 59]. The posterior arch of C1 is removed for a lateral extension of no more than 1.5 cm. The typical occipito-cervical band (which is frequently thick and adherent) should be removed completely. Under operating microscope vision, the dura is opened in a Y shape, trying not to violate the arachnoid. A correct dura opening should expose the tonsils, the cisterna magna, and the cervical spinal cord. We prefer to resect the dura flap in order to avoid any future scarring due to its strong osteogenic capacity. No attempt to dissect arachnoid, coagulate tonsils, and explore the obex is performed. Finally, a dural substitute is sutured with running stitches. It is mandatory not to cut the dura substitute too small in order to avoid excessive traction which could lacerate during head movement or coughing. We conclude the closure with collagen sponge and fibrin glue to cover the whole dural surface. Specific attention must be given to the muscles and subcutaneous closure with at least four different layers (deep muscles, superficial muscles, fascia, subcutaneous layers). Skin is closed with monofilament 3-0 running suture. The dressing should be compressive. The patient spends the night in the semi-intensive care room with the bed at 40° elevation of the thorax. Pain medications are arranged based on the need of the patient. After 48 h the patient can leave the bed and start walking with the help of the physical therapist. Once the skin is perfectly closed, we use to transfer the patient to our rehabilitation clinic to favor physical recovery, no matter the severity of preoperative neurological impairment. This period helps the patients to come back home with the best performance possible.

32.6 Surgical Complications

The described technique is related to the extremely low rate of complication. We have so far reported no cases of surgical site hematoma, cerebellar infarction, or neurological deterioration [39].

The only issue in the perioperative period is the CSF leak. Apart the good selection of patients (excluding CSF circulation anomalies on both MRI and patient examination), it is mandatory to dedicate time to dural closure by verifying intraoperatively the perfect water tightness of the suture (ask the anesthesiologist to perform repeated Valsalva maneuvers). In the postoperative period, the patient must avoid excessive mobilization and efforts (alvus must be free). If CSF leak should happen, we first try with adding sutures to the skin; if not sufficient, a lumbar drain is inserted for 4–5 days. It is extremely rare to take the patient to the operating room to restoring the dural patch. Another issue is the late pseudomeningocele which present weeks or months after surgery and can be silent in the majority of patients. If it represents only an MRI finding, there is no need for correction. However, when

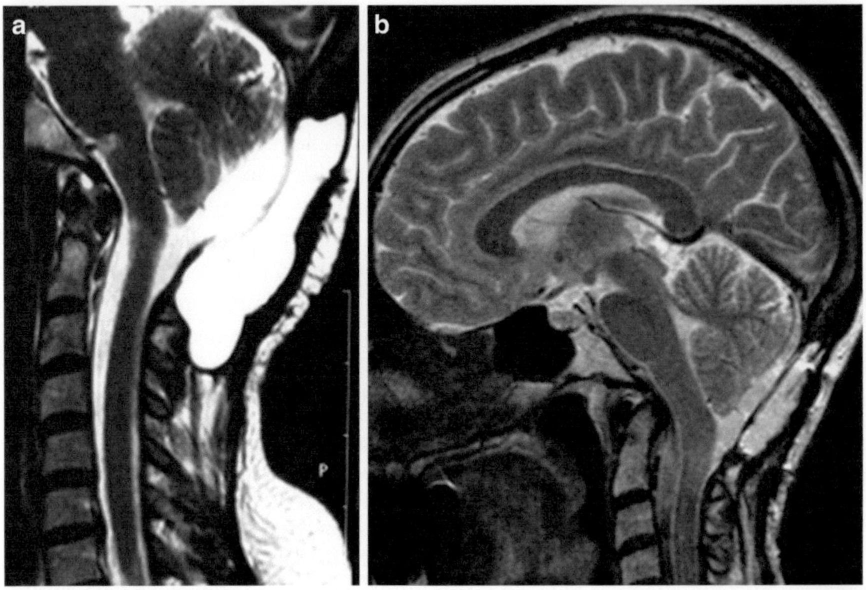

Fig. 32.8 (**a**) Postoperative MR showing a large and compressing pseudomeningocele. In this case, it was necessary a "redo" surgery and reconstructing dural patch with resolution of compressive effect (**b**)

it is compressive, painful and provokes the same disturbance as before surgical decompression, a new dural patch should be created. In those cases where pseudomeningocele do not heal with redo surgery on posterior fossa, it is advisable to consider ventriculoperitoneal shunting as most probably a CSF circulation alteration has been underestimated (Fig. 32.8).

Sometimes patients can have fever and headache after 2–3 days from surgery. Fever is typically not elevated (no more than 38 °C/100.4 °F). If no other cause of fever is found (urosepsis, for example), the most probable cause is aseptic meningitis which can be cured with steroids and analgesics. Of course, if fever is higher and accompanied by neurological deterioration, bacterial meningitis should be suspected and a spinal tap with cells count and culture is then performed.

32.6.1 What to Expect from Surgery and How to Manage Failures

The most important factors to consider in previewing the effect of surgery are: (1) correct diagnosis with imaging to clinical correlation; (2) severity of preoperative clinical state; (3) coexistence of associated pathologies. A CMI patient presenting with typical occipital headache and other minor symptoms has more than 85% of possibility to completely cure his/her problem. In general, headache is the symptom that resolves first and more than others. Other forms of a headache could coexist and hence persist after surgery. On the other hand, CMI plus Sym patients with long-lasting signs and symptoms of myelopathy have the lowest rate of resolution. Specifically, sensory loss, pain, and dysesthesia are symptoms which typically resolve less [60]. Disturbances related to myelopathy can persist even in the case of excellent Sym shrink on MRI. In fact, there is no correlation between postoperative Sym volume and the evolution of symptoms [39, 60]. Sometimes, a good clinical outcome can be coupled to a totally stable Sym on MRI, and vice versa.

The goal of surgery is to create a new cisternal magna, hence follow-up MRI should show the reappearance of CSF space around the tonsils and brainstem rather than the ascent of the tonsils [37].

In CMI, the persistence of preoperative symptoms especially neck pain or an occipital headache should first suggest the execution of MRI in order to ascertain the quality of decompression. If this is optimal, consider the possibility of other cause of a headache. Otherwise, it should also be taken into consideration the coexistence of CSF circulation alteration and a spinal tap with infusion and subtraction tests proposed. In the case where MRI show an incomplete decompression, redo surgery is the first procedure to adopt.

Concerning Sym, the clinical postoperative evolution can be detached from the MRI evolution. However, in the case of clinical worsening and large or evolving Sym with satisfying posterior fossa decompression, a direct surgery on Sym should be considered. In this rare instance, we prefer to perform syringo-subarachnoid shunt through laminotomy, myelotomy (in the thinnest part of the spinal cord corresponding to the larger section of the Sym), and insertion of a catheter into the cyst. Once again, this surgery can lead to the collapse of the Sym but this does not guarantee the resolution of disturbances.

32.7 Conclusions and Future Perspectives

The management of CMI and Sym has evolved through these last decades thanks to the better understanding of pathophysiology, the growing interest of researchers, and publication of numerous surgical series. Surgery can help a large part of patients if a scrupulous selection is made. More, a multidisciplinary team is needed to take care of the patient in the immediate postoperative period to enhance the recovery. However, there are still many patients which do not obtain the expected relief from surgery. Many surgical nuances are still under debate but it seems that the real problem resides in the understanding of subtle differences among patients. Actually, many issues are still obscure. Why patients with similar tonsils' position on MRI present completely different complaints (or none at all)? Why some patient obtains complete relief from surgery, whereas others take only partial advantage? Which patient is more prone to develop Sym and why?

A response to all these uncertainties will likely come from a more global approach to CMI patient not looking only to the base of the skull and posterior fossa. It is acquired that CMI concerns intracranial compliance, the ability of the body to manage a volume increase in the intrathecal CNS space without causing a pressure increase [61]. As mentioned, the different causes of obstruction to CSF flow at the foramen magnum are based on reduced compliance. Actually, evidence of obstruction may be present without an obvious [62] tonsils' descent as described in cases of so-called Chiari 0 or in those patients with typical CMI symptoms but with only mild cerebellar dislocation. MRI (both anatomical and phase-contrast) are usually performed with the patient in a state of relaxation. It should be considered the execution of MRI during Valsalva maneuvers in order to better understand the fate of the tonsils during intracranial pressure increase. Moreover, the absence of an association between the degree of hindbrain herniation and the spinal injury in syringomyelia [40] and between the posterior fossa size and the degree of cerebellar herniation in CMI [28] indicates that factors other than posterior fossa hypoplasia are influencing the degree of neural injury. Much less attention has been paid to the venous blood volume, for example, which could play a role in creating or at least facilitating the disequilibrium between intracranial and intraspinal pressures; in other words, a reduced compliance of the intracranial compartment related to a given alteration of CSF circulation at the level the posterior fossa cannot be balanced by an adequate venous volume outflow. Probably, a thorough functional exploration of the extracranial venous drainage system could add more hints in understanding the dark side of this complex and intriguing disease.

References

1. Bejjani GK. Definition of the adult Chiari malformation: a brief historical overview. Neurosurg Focus. 2001;11(1):E1.
2. Siasios J, Kapsalaki EZ, Fountas KN. Surgical management of patients with Chiari I malformation. Int J Pediatr. 2012;2012:640127.
3. Milhorat TH, Chou MW, Trinidad EM, et al. Chiari I malformation redefined: clinical and radiographic findings for 364 symptomatic patients. Neurosurgery. 1999;44:1005–17.
4. Bunck AC, Kroeger JR, Juettner A, et al. Magnetic resonance 4D flow analysis of cerebrospinal fluid dynamics in Chiari I malformation with and without syringomyelia. Eur Radiol. 2012;22(9):1860–70.
5. Heiss JD, Patronas N, DeVroom HL, Shawker T, Ennis R, Kammerer W, Eidsath A, Talbot T, Morris J, Eskioglu E, Oldfield EH. Elucidating the pathophysiology of syringomyelia. J Neurosurg. 1999 Oct;91(4):553–62.
6. Oldfield EH. Syringomyelia. J Neurosurg. 2001;95(Suppl 1):153–5.
7. Morioka T, Shono T, Nishio S, et al. Acquired Chiari I malformation and syringomyelia associated with bilateral chronic subdural hematoma. Case report. J Neurosurg. 1995;83(3):556–8.
8. Tachibana S, Harada K, Abe T, et al. Syringomyelia secondary to tonsillar herniation caused by posterior fossa tumors. Surg Neurol. 1995;43(5):470–5.
9. Fagan LH, Ferguson S, Yassari R, et al. The Chiari pseudotumor cerebri syndrome: symptom recurrence after decompressive surgery for Chiari malformation type I. Pediatr Neurosurg. 2006;42(1):14–9.
10. Istek S. Chiari type 1 malformation in a pseudotumour cerebri patient: is it an acquired or congenital Chiari malformation? BMJ Case Rep. 2014;2014. pii: bcr2013201845.
11. Tubbs RS, Beckman J, Naftel RP, et al. Institutional experience with 500 cases of surgically treated pediatric Chiari malformation type I. Clinical article. J Neurosurg Pediatr. 2011;7:248–56.
12. Aronson DD, Kahn RH, Canady A, et al. Instability of the cervical spine after decompression in patients who have Arnold–Chiari malformation. J Bone Jt Surg. 1991;73:898–906.

13. Behari S, Kalra SK, Kiran Kumar MV, et al. Chiari I malformation associated with atlanto-axial dislocation: focussing on the anterior cervico-medullary compression. Acta Neurochir. 2007;149(1):41–50.
14. Bollo RJ, Riva-Cambrin J, Brockmeyer MM, et al. Complex Chiari malformations in children: an analysis of preoperative risk factors for occipitocervical fusion. J Neurosurg Pediatr. 2012;10(2):134–41.
15. Fenoy AJ, Menezes AH, Fenoy KA. Craniocervical junction fusions in patients with hindbrain herniation and syringohydromyelia. J Neurosurg Spine. 2008;9(1):1–9.
16. Hankinson TC, Grunstein E, Gardner P, et al. Transnasal odontoid resection followed by posterior decompression and occipitocervical fusion in children with Chiari malformation type I and ventral brainstem compression. J Neurosurg Pediatr. 2010;5(6):549–53.
17. Ladner TR, Dewan MC, Day MA, et al. Evaluating the relationship of the pB-C2 line to clinical outcomes in a 15-year single-center cohort of pediatric Chiari I malformation. J Neurosurg Pediatr. 2015;15(2):178–88.
18. Martin MD, Bruner HJ, Maiman D. Anatomic and biomechanical considerations of the craniovertebral junction. Neurosurgery. 2010;66(suppl_3):A2–6.
19. Menezes AH. Craniovertebral junction abnormalities with hindbrain herniation and syringomyelia: regression of syringomyelia after removal of ventral craniovertebral junction compression. J Neurosurg. 2012;116(2):301–9.
20. Nishikawa M, Ohata K, Baba M, et al. Chiari I malformation associated with ventral compression and instability: one-stage posterior decompression and fusion with a new instrumentation technique. Neurosurgery. 2004;54(6):1430–4.
21. Salunke P, Sura S, Futane S, et al. Ventral compression in adult patients with Chiari 1 malformation sans basilar invagination: cause and management. Acta Neurochir. 2012;154(1):147–52.
22. Marin-Padilla M, Marin-Padilla TM. Morphogenesis of experimentally induced Arnold–Chiari malformation. J Neurol Sci. 1981;50(1):29–55.
23. Alperin N, Loftus JR, Oliu CJ, et al. Magnetic resonance imaging measures of posterior cranial fossa morphology and cerebrospinal fluid physiology in Chiari malformation type I. Neurosurgery. 2014;75(5):515–22.
24. Dagtekin A, Avci E, Kara E, et al. Posterior cranial fossa morphometry in symptomatic adult Chiari I malformation patients: comparative clinical and anatomical study. Clin Neurol Neurosurg. 2011;113(5):399–403.
25. Hwang HS, Moon JG, Kim CH, et al. The comparative morphometric study of the posterior cranial fossa: what is effective approaches to the treatment of Chiari malformation type 1? J Korean Neurosurg Soc. 2013;54:405–10.
26. Nishikawa M, Sakamoto H, Hakuba A, et al. Pathogenesis of Chiari malformation: a morphometric study of the posterior cranial fossa. J Neurosurg. 1997;86(1):40–7.
27. Noudel R, Jovenin N, Eap C, et al. Incidence of basioccipital hypoplasia in Chiari malformation type I: comparative morphometric study of the posterior cranial fossa. Clinical article. J Neurosurg. 2009;111(5):1046–52.
28. Tubbs RS, Elton S, Grabb P, et al. Analysis of the posterior fossa in children with the Chiari 0 malformation. Neurosurgery. 2001;48:1050–5.
29. Urbizu A, Poca MA, Vidal X, et al. MRI-based morphometric analysis of posterior cranial fossa in the diagnosis of chiari malformation type I. J Neuroimaging. 2014;24(3):250–6.
30. Yasuhara T, Miyoshi Y, Date I. Chiari malformation with thick occipital bone. Acta Med Okayama. 2011;65(1):59–61.
31. Chumas PD, Armstrong DC, Drake JM, et al. Tonsillar herniation: the rule rather than the exception after lumboperitoneal shunting in the pediatric population. J Neurosurg. 1993;78(4):568–73.
32. Glenn C, Cheema AA, Safavi-Abbasi S, et al. Spinal cord detethering in children with tethered cord syndrome and Chiari type 1 malformations. J Clin Neurosci. 2015;22(11):1749–52.
33. Milhorat TH, Bolognese PA, Nishikawa M, et al. Association of Chiari malformation type I and tethered cord syndrome: preliminary results of sectioning filum terminale. Surg Neurol. 2009;72(1):20–35.

34. Mea E, Chiapparini L, Leone M, et al. Chronic daily headache in the adults: differential diagnosis between symptomatic Chiari I malformation and spontaneous intracranial hypotension. Neurol Sci. 2011;32(Suppl 3):291–4.
35. Alperin N, Loftus JR, Oliu CJ, et al. Imaging-based features of headaches in Chiari malformation type I. Neurosurgery. 2015;77(1):96–103.
36. Stovner LJ. Headache associated with the Chiari type I malformation. Headache. 1993;33(4):175–81.
37. Heiss JD, Suffredini G, Bakhtian KD, et al. Normalization of hindbrain morphology after decompression of Chiari malformation type I. J Neurosurg. 2012;117(5):942–6.
38. Munshi I, Frim D, Stine-Reyes R. Effects of posterior fossa decompression with and without duraplasty on Chiari malformation-associated hydromyelia. Neurosurgery. 2000;46:1384–90.
39. Spena G, Bernucci C, Garbossa D, et al. Clinical and radiological outcome of craniocervical osteo-dural decompression for Chiari I-associated syringomyelia. Neurosurg Rev. 2010;33(3):297–303.
40. Elster AD, Chen MY. Chiari I malformations: clinical and radiologic reappraisal. Radiology. 1992;183:347–53.
41. Hofkes SK, Iskandar BJ, Turski PA, et al. Differentiation between symptomatic Chiari I malformation and asymptomatic Tonsilar Ectopia by using cerebrospinal fluid flow imaging: initial estimate of imaging accuracy. Radiology. 2007;245(2):532–40.
42. Killeen A, Roguski M, Chavez A, et al. Non-operative outcomes in Chiari I malformation patients. J Clin Neurosci. 2015;22(1):133–8.
43. Meadows J, Kraut M, Guarieri M, et al. Asymptomatic Chiari type I malformations identified on magnetic resonance imaging. J Neurosurg. 2000;92:920–6.
44. Morris Z, Whiteley WN, Longstreth WT Jr, et al. Incidental findings on brain magnetic resonance imaging: systematic review and meta-analysis. BMJ. 2009;339:b3016.
45. Rocque BG, George TM, Kestle J, et al. Treatment practices for Chiari malformation type I with syringomyelia: results of a survey of the American Society of Pediatric Neurosurgeons. J Neurosurg Pediatr. 2011;8(5):430–7.
46. Singhal A, Bowen-Roberts T, Steinbok P, et al. Natural history of untreated syringomyelia in pediatric patients. Neurosurg Focus. 2011;31(6):E13.
47. Blagodatsky MD, Larionov SN, Alexandrov YA, et al. Surgical treatment of Chiari I malformation with or without syringomyelia. Acta Neurochir. 1999;141:963–8.
48. Sakamoto H, Nishikawa M, Hakuba A, et al. Expansive suboccipital cranioplasty for the treatment of syringomyelia associated with Chiari malformation. Acta Neurochir. 1999;141:949–61.
49. Yilmaz A, Kanat A, Muscleman AM, et al. When is duraplasty required in the surgical treatment of Chiari malformation type I based on tonsillar descending grading scale? World Neurosurg. 2011;75:307–13.
50. Förander P, Sjåvik K, Solheim O, et al. The case for duraplasty in adults undergoing posterior fossa decompression for Chiari I malformation: a systematic review and meta-analysis of observational studies. Clin Neurol Neurosurg. 2014;125:58–64.
51. Krishna V, McLawhorn M, Kosnik-Infinger L, et al. High long-term symptomatic recurrence rates after Chiari-1 decompression without dural opening: a single center experience. Clin Neurol Neurosurg. 2014;118:53–8.
52. Xu H, Chu L, He R, et al. Posterior fossa decompression with and without duraplasty for the treatment of Chiari malformation type I-a systematic review and meta-analysis. Neurosurg Rev. 2017;40(2):213–21.
53. Durham SR, Fjeld-Olenec K. Comparison of posterior fossa decompression with and without duraplasty for the surgical treatment of Chiari malformation type I in pediatric patients: a meta-analysis. J Neurosurg Pediatr. 2008;2:42–9.
54. Genitori L, Peretta P, Nurisso C, et al. Chiari type I anomalies in children and adolescents: minimally invasive management in a series of 53 cases. Childs Nerv Syst. 2000;16(10–11):707–18.
55. Kato M, Nakamura H, Konishi S. Effect of preserving paraspinal muscles on postoperative axial pain in the selective cervical aminoplasty. Spine. 2008;33(14):E455–9.

56. Scali F, Pontell M, Enix D, et al. Histological analysis of the rectus wapitis posterior major's myodural bridge. Spine J. 2013;13:558–63.
57. Zhang J, Tsuzuki N, Hirabayashi S, et al. Surgical anatomy of the nerves and muscles in the posterior cervical spine. A guide for avoiding inadvertent nerve injuries during the posterior approach. Spine. 2003;13:1379–84.
58. Di X, Luciano MG, Benzel EC. Acute respiratory arrest following partial suboccipital cranioplasty for cerebellar ptosis from Chiari malformation decompression. Neurosurg Focus. 2008;25(6):E12.
59. Holly LT, Batzdorf U. Management of cerebellar ptosis following craniovertebral decompression for Chiari I malformation. J Neurosurg. 2001;94(1):21–6.
60. Wetjen NM, Heiss JD, Oldfield EH. Time course of syringomyelia resolution following decompression of Chiari malformation type I. J Neurosurg Pediatr. 2008;1(2):118–23.
61. Czosnyka M, Pickard JD. Monitoring and interpretation of intracranial pressure. J Neurol Neurosurg Psychiatry. 2004;75:813–21.
62. Sekula R, Jannetta PJ, Casey KF, et al. Dimensions of the posterior fossa in patients symptomatic for Chiari I malformation but without cerebellar tonsillar descent. Cerebrospinal Fluid Res. 2005;2:11.

Congenital Anomalies of Cranio-vertebral Junction

33

Jayesh C. Sardhara, Chaitanya Godbole, Pavaman Sindgikar, and Sanjay Behari

33.1 Introduction

The natural architectural axiom regards flexibility and stability as mutually exclusive events. The flexibility of the cranio-vertebral junction (CVJ) and the stability of rest of the spine are no exception to this axiom. While the complementing facetal surfaces of vertebrae provide stability to the spine with limited flexibility, the first (C1) and second cervical (C2) vertebral facet joints provide flexibility at the cost of stability. Congenital atlanto-axial dislocation (CAAD) is the natural corollary of this phenomenon. Before the tenth week of intrauterine life, genetic or developmental intrauterine insults may be responsible for one or all of the osseous and neural anomalies like congenital atlanto-axial dislocation, platybasia, occipitalized atlas, Klippel–Feil anomaly, basilar invagination (BI), Arnold Chiari malformation (ACM), and associated torticollis as well as various vascular anomalies. This chapter is an attempt to understand the genesis and management of CAAD with the overall focus being on its embryological basis, anatomy, clinical features, and nuances of surgical management. This complicated cause of high cervical myelopathy has the potential to cause severe myelopathy, respiratory difficulty, and even mortality.

J. C. Sardhara · C. Godbole · P. Sindgikar · S. Behari (✉)
Department of Neurosurgery, Sanjay Gandhi Postgraduate Institute of Medical Sciences, Lucknow, India

E. Tessitore et al. (eds.), *Surgery of the Cranio-Vertebral Junction*,
https://doi.org/10.1007/978-3-030-18700-2_33

33.2 Pathogenesis of AAD, BI, and Coexisting Congenital CVJ Anomalies: Embryological, Anatomical, and Biomechanical Considerations

The cranio-vertebral complex comprises two sets of joints, the occipito-atlantal and atlanto-axial joints. While the occipito-atlantal joints are very stable, the atlanto-axial joints are the most mobile of all the joints of the spine. Thus, the atlanto-axial joint is most susceptible to instability especially when there is a failure of the supporting ligaments (Fig. 33.1).

Congenital AAD very frequently coexists with assimilation of the atlas, basilar invagination, anomalous C2/C3 fusion, and platybasia, along with clival segmentation anomalies. Assimilation of the atlas may be unilateral, bilateral, focal, or segmental. Various etiologies have been speculated in literature for the genesis of CVJ anomalies including mechanical factors, embryological or genetic abnormalities, and viral infections [1–3]. One of the schools of thought suggested that bony instability at the CV junction occurs as a pure "mechanical" failure occurring by the slippage of C2 facets over C1 facets due to their congenital obliquity [4]. Others have proposed that it is a pure congenital or embryological phenomenon due to suboccipital dysplasia [3, 4]. Congenital occipital dysplasia results in coexistence of congenital AAD, BI, platybasia, ACM type 1, and rotational deformity due to the combined effects of deformed growth of the occipital primordium (causing basiocciput dysgenesis and manifesting as assimilated atlas and platybasia) and

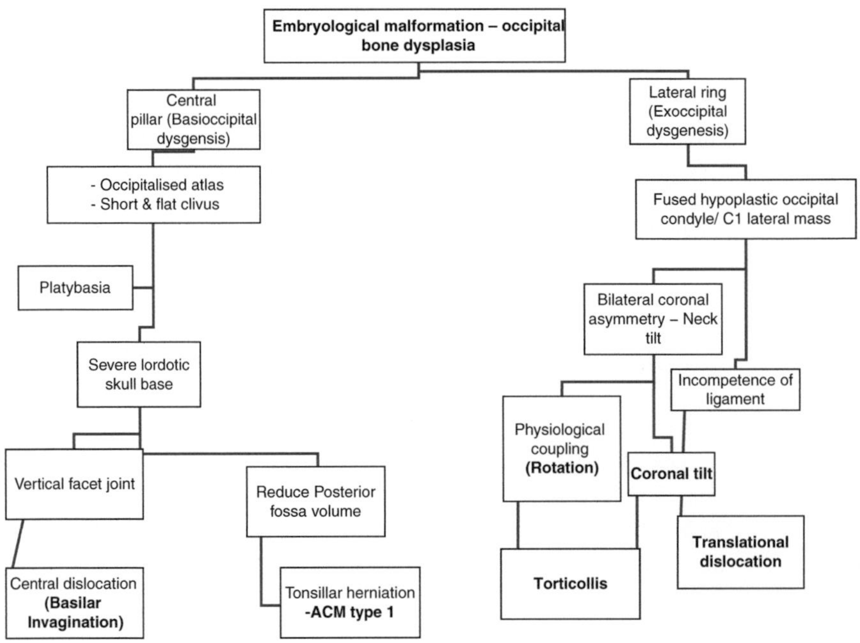

Fig. 33.1 Embryological considerations of CVJ anomalies. (original picture)

exoccipital dysgenesis (resulting in laterally assimilated atlas and condylar asymmetry) [2, 3]. The summated effect of a congenitally short and flat clivus (causing platybasia and assimilated atlas) is that later on, the basion is gradually raised above it and moves cranially. This forces the plane of the foramen magnum to tilt upwards at a lordotic angle taking with it the planes of the occipital condyle and C0-C articulation [3]. The fusion and chondrification of the basioccipital and exoccipital sclerotome also occurs slightly earlier than the C1-C2 re-segmentation [2, 3]. A severely lordotic skull-base angle consequently forces the emerging upper cervical sclerotomal column to bend upwards and backwards. This could probably be responsible for the vertical and asymmetrical facet joints between the assimilated atlas and C2 vertebra. In patients with central dislocation (BI), there is an upward dislocation of the axis due to the presence of nearly vertical C1-2 facet joint surfaces as compared to the relatively normal horizontal C1-2 facet joint alignment [5]. Thus, BI represents the vertical type of AAD. Congenital AAD in the presence of platybasia and occipitalized atlas have been often associated with rotational deformity and coronal tilt due to the presence of C0-C1 lateral mass asymmetry.

In the presence of exoccipital dysgenesis, where assimilated atlas with fused hypoplastic occipital condyle and C1 lateral mass coexist, the transverse and alar ligaments may become weaker on one or both the sides. The anomalous vertically oriented and often asymmetrical C1-2 facet joints may further facilitate both vertical and translational displacements. The physiological coupling movements may also cause rotational as well as lateral displacements of the C1-2 joints [1, 6]. Initially, the atlanto-axial instability will be reducible and because of the vertical joints, there is gradual upward dislocation of the axis, resulting in "reducible" BI in the pediatric population. According to Menezes, as the child grows, grooving occurs behind the occipital condyle, and later on, by the age of 14 to 16 years, the BI becomes irreducible [6]. Under these circumstances, the clivus tends to become horizontal and this also adds to the occurrence of complete irreducibility. The summated effects of the cranio-cervical kyphosis and raised clival angle lead to reduction in the posterior fossa volume (that is reduced from the normal by an average of 13.4 mL^3), further promoting tonsillar herniation (Arnold Chiari malformation) [7]. Thus, atlanto-axial instability is the prime mechanical basis for the occurrence of all types of BI but it occurs due to an anomalous bony development.

33.3 Various Classifications for CVJ Anomalies

CVJ anomalies are a combination of congenital, developmental, or acquired abnormalities. Menezes classified the congenital anomalies of CVJ into different malformations of occiput, atlas, and axis (Table 33.1) [1]. Atlanto-axial instability can be classified into the reducible (in the flexed position of the neck) and the irreducible varieties (in the extended position of the neck) [8]. Goel classified AAD into three types according to the direction of C1-2 facet joint dislocation as type 1 (anterior AAD), type 2 (posterior AAD), and type 3 (central dislocation without any atlanto-axial instability) [9]. Atlanto-axial dislocation [AAD] is traditionally defined as an

Table 33.1 Classification of congenital anomalies of CVJ [1]

A	Occipital bone anomalies 1. Manifestations of the occipital vertebra (a) Clivus segmentations (b) Remnants around the foramen magnum (c) Atlas variants (d) Dens segmentation anomalies 2. Basilar invagination 3. Condylar hypoplasia 4. Assimilation of the atlas
B	Atlas anomalies 1. Assimilation of the atlas 2. Atlanto-axial fusion 3. Aplasia of the atlas arches
C	Axis anomalies 1. Irregular atlanto-axial segmentation 2. Dens dysplasias (a) Ossiculum terminale persistens (b) Os odontoideum (c) Hypoplasia/aplasia 3. Segmentation failure of C2-C3

Based on: Menezes A, Ahmed R, Dlouhy B. Developmental anomalies of the craniovertebral junction and surgical management. In: Winn HR. Youman's neurological surgery. Philadelphia: Editora Saunders; 2003; p. 1856–70 [1]

abnormal increase in the atlanto-dental interval [ADI] of more than 3 mm in adults and more than 4.5 mm in the pediatric age group [10]. The ADI measures the displacement of the atlas relative to the axis in only a single two-dimensional plane, but as coupled movements of the occipital and cervical C1 and C2 complex occur in a three-dimensional plane based on the standard Cartesian coordinate system, dislocations in this region also usually occur in 3 different planes and are often seen in combinations. This also includes rotational dislocation and coronal tilt of the C1 and C2 vertebrae in different planes. We defined congenital AAD based on their three-dimensional dislocation in terms of the planes defined by the three Cartesian coordinates (Table 33.2), identified the different multiplanar C1-2 displacements occurring due to facet joint dislocations in all dimensions (based on the three-dimensional computed tomographic [3D CT] evaluation) and classified the AAD based on its various combinations (Table 33.3) (Fig. 33.2) [11]. Goel proposed a classification of basilar invagination based on the presence (Group A) or absence (Group B) of clinical and radiological instability [12]. Group B is usually associated with ACM type 1 (Fig. 33.3).

33.3.1 Vertebral Artery Anomalies

Variability in dimensions and course of the vertebral artery (VA) makes it highly vulnerable to injury during surgery for congenital AAD. An evaluation of 104 patients (65 with AAD; 39 controls) with a three-dimensional multiplanar

Table 33.2 Definition of congenital atlanto-axial dislocation based on the Cartesian coordinates

1. **Along Z coordinate: Translational dislocation [anteroposterior displacement occurring in XZ plane]** Atlanto-dental dislocation >3 mm in adult or >4.5 mm in pediatric population less than 9 years of age
2. **Along Y coordinate: Central dislocation [vertical displacement occurring in YZ plane]** Presence of basilar invagination based upon McCrae' line [the height of tip of the odontoid intersecting the line joining the basion (anterior margin of foramen magnum) to basion (posterior margin of foramen magnum)]
3. **Along X coordinate: rotational atlanto-axial dislocation and coronal tilt causing cervical torticollis [occurring in coronal XY plane]** (a) Presence of rotation of axis in relation to atlas (>5°) (b) Coronal tilt: Difference of atlanto-axial facet joint angle >10° bilaterally in coronal plane
4. **Combination of above (1, 2, 3)**

(The head is assumed to be in anatomical position with patient standing and the face facing anteriorly) [11]

Sardhara J, Behari S, Sindgikar P, Srivastava A, Jaiswal A, Sahu R, et al. Evaluating atlanto-axial dislocation based on Cartesian coordinates: Proposing a new definition and its impact on assessment of congenital torticollis. Neurosurgery. 2018;82(4):525–40. https://doi.org/10.1093/neuros/nyx196 [11]

Table 33.3 Types of congenital atlanto-axial dislocation based on the Cartesian coordinates found in our series [11]

No.	Type of AAD [According to *X*, *Y*, and *Z* Cartesian's axes]
Type I	Translational dislocation **(Along Z coordinate [anteroposterior dislocation occurring in XZ plane])**
Type II	Central dislocation [Basilar invagination] (**Along Y coordinate [vertical displacement occurring in YZ plane]**
Type III	Translational dislocation + central dislocation **[along Z + Y coordinates occurring in XZ and YZ planes]**
Type IV	Translational dislocation + rotational dislocation + coronal tilt **[along Z + X coordinates occurring in XZ and XY planes]**
Type V	Central dislocation (BI) + rotational dislocation + coronal tilt **[along Y + X coordinates occurring in ZY and XY planes]**
Type VI	Combined type of dislocation [Translation + central dislocation + rotation + coronal tilt] **[occurring along all three axes and in all three planes]**

Sardhara J, Behari S, Sidgikar P, Srivastava A, Jaiswal A, Sahu R, et al. Evaluating atlanto-axial dislocation based on Cartesian coordinates: Proposing a new definition and its impact on assessment of congenital torticollis. Neurosurgery. 2018;82(4):525–40. https://doi.org/10.1093/neuros/nyx196 [11]

computed tomographic (CT) angiography was performed to assess the anatomical variations in the VA size, course, and anomalous medial deviation as well as in the type of axial isthmus and rotational deformity/tilt at the CVJ [13]. Based on the dimensions and course of VA, anomalous variations of the VA were classified into 5 types (Table 33.4). A risk stratification score that measured the vulnerability of VA to injury was developed. The total score ranged from 5 to 9. If the overall score of the VA variation was 5 or less, it was labeled as a "low risk" situation, and if the

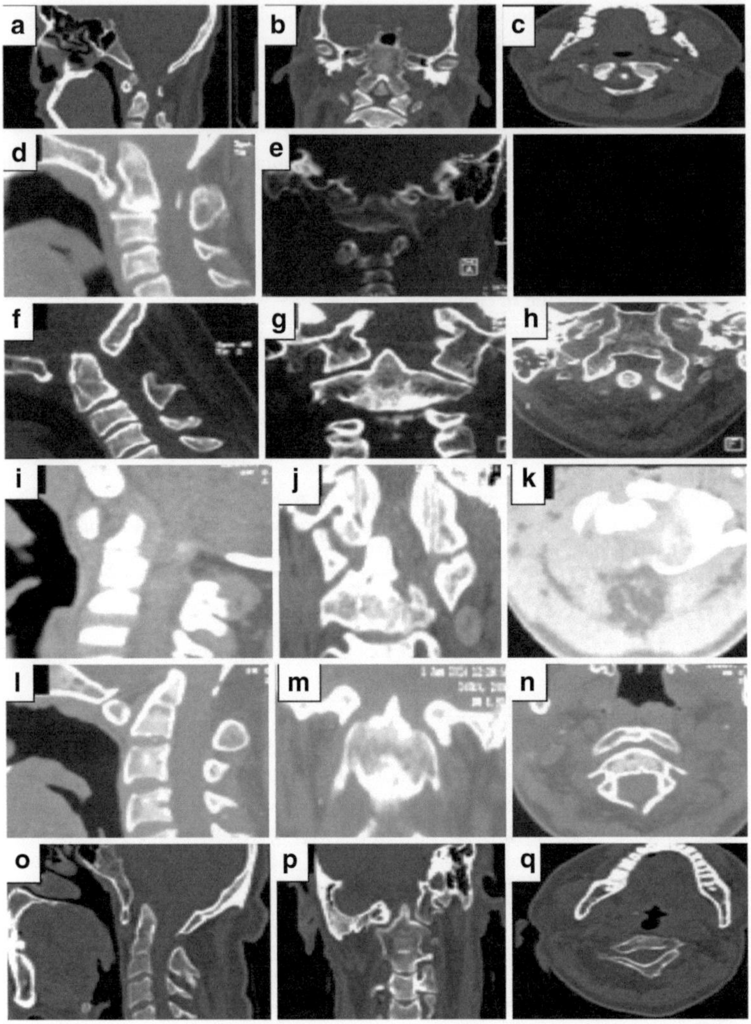

Fig. 33.2 CT CVJ with Type I AAD: (**a**) Sagittal reconstructed; (**b**) coronal; and (**c**) axial image showing an anteroposterior translational dislocation (with an os odontoideum and bifid C1 posterior arch) without basilar invagination, rotational deformity, or coronal tilt. Type 2 AAD: (**d**) Sagittal reconstructed CT image; and (**e**) coronal image showing a Type II C1-2 dislocation that consisted of pure vertical dislocation (BI) with a normal atlanto-dental interval, and without rotatory dislocation or a coronal tilt. Type 3 AAD: (**f**) Sagittal reconstructed CT image; (**g**) coronal image; and (**h**) axial image showing a translational anteroposterior with central (BI) dislocation but without rotatory dislocation/coronal tilt. Type 4 AAD: (**i**) Sagittal reconstructed CT image; (**j**) coronal image; and (**k**) axial image showing anteroposterior C1-2 dislocation with rotatory dislocation and coronal tilt but without vertical (BI) dislocation. Type 5 AAD: (**l**) Sagittal reconstructed CT image; (**m**) coronal image; and (**n**) axial image showing a central (BI) and rotational dislocation with coronal tilt but without anteroposterior dislocation. Type 6 AAD: (**o**) Sagittal reconstructed CT image; (**p**) coronal image; and (**q**) axial image showing a Type VI combined C1-2 dislocation, that is, translational anteroposterior, central (BI) and rotational dislocation with coronal tilt. (original picture)

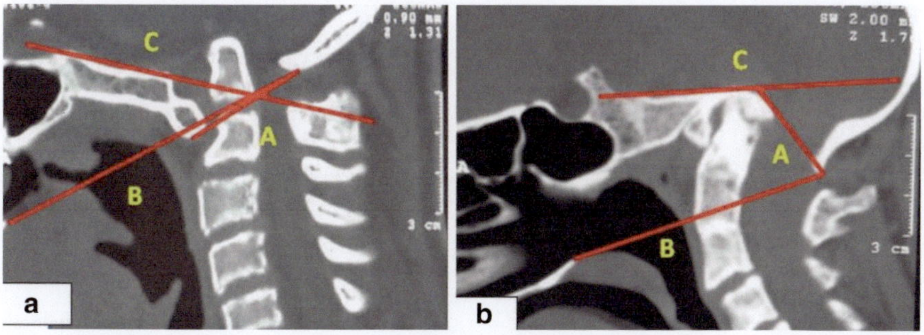

Fig. 33.3 Figure showing a patient with two types of basilar invagination. Group A (**a**): (1) Atlanto-dental interval (>3 mm), (2) tip of the odontoid process showing invagination into the foramen magnum and above the Chamberlain line (**b**), McRae line (**a**), and Wackenheim clival line (**c**); Group B (**b**): (1) Atlanto-dental interval is normal; (2) tip of the odontoid process is above the Chamberlain's line (**b**) (>5 mm); (3) tip of the odontoid is below the Wackenheim clival line (**c**) and the McRae's line (**a**). (original picture)

Table 33.4 Classification of vertebral artery anomalous variations at CVJ and scoring system for risk stratification of vertebral artery injury during surgery at CVJ [13]

Type	VA anomaly	Score[a]	Surgical implication
Type-1	Anomaly related to size		
1a	Bilateral equal in size	1	
1b	Bilateral asymmetry with unilateral dominance without hypoplasia/aplasia	1	
1c	Bilateral asymmetry with unilateral hypoplasia	1	Risk of vertebrobasilar insufficiency if injury occurs to dominant VA in 1c and 1d
1d	Bilateral asymmetry with unilateral aplasia	1	
Type-2	Anomalies associated with course of VA		
2a	Normal course	1	
2b	Cranial entry site from a congenital foramen in the occipitalized atlas and the occipital bone (representing C1 foramen transversarium)	1	Course of VA is often variable making it vulnerable to injury (if situated in an unanticipated position) Surgical dissection on the posterior arch of atlas is safe up to 2.5 cm laterally on either side
2c	Persistent first intersegmental artery	2	VA located posterior to C1-2 facet joint
2d	Fenestrated VA	2	
2e	Low-lying PICA	2	
Type-3	Anomalous medial deviation of V3 segment of VA		
3a	Absent	1	

(continued)

Table 33.4 (continued)

3b	Present	2	Lateral dissection and bony decompression of the occipital bone and occipitalized atlas at the foramen magnum or at the posterior arch of C1; or, odontoid and C2 body drilling during transoral decompression may render VA vulnerable to injury
Type-4	Anomaly related to VA groove at C2 vertebra		
4a	Wide and low	1	Transarticular, transpedicular, and translaminar screw placement is safe in 4a Transarticular or transpedicular screw placement is risky as the screws need to be placed through narrow isthmus (<4.5 mm) in 4b, 4c, and 4d
4b	Narrow and high (high riding VA)	2	Trans-pedicular or pars screw is risky in the presence of high riding VA
4c	Narrow and low	2	
4d	Wide and high	2	
Type-5	Anomalies related to rotational deformity or tilt at the occipito-C1-C2 region		
5a	Absent	1	
5b	Present	2	Medially deviated VA loop makes it more prone to injury during transoral odontoidectomy and lateral mass/pedicle screw fixation

Sardhara J, Behari S, Mohan BM, Jaiswal AK, Sahu RN, Srivastava A, et al. Risk stratification of vertebral artery vulnerability during surgery for congenital atlanto-axial dislocation with or without an occipitalized atlas. Neurol India. 2015;63:382–91 [13]

[a]A score of 2 was given when the risk of VA injury was anticipated due its anomalous course. All the other anatomical variations that did not pose an increased risk to the VA received a score of 1. The minimum score achieved was 5 and represented less vulnerability of the vertebral artery to injury during anterior or posterior access to the CVJ; a score of 6–9 represented an increased risk of VA injury during surgery. The risk of VA injury proportionately increased according to the score achieved. *C1* atlas; *C2* axis; *V3* third segment of vertebral artery; *VA* vertebral artery; *PICA* posterior inferior cerebellar artery; *CVJ* cranio-vertebral junction

score was between 6 and 9, it considered as a "high risk" situation with increased vulnerability of the VA to injury during either the transoral surgery or posterior distraction/stabilization procedures. Interestingly, in our cohort, 68% of the patients had a high risk of injury. Of them, 81% had an assimilated atlas.

33.3.1.1 Clinical Presentation

The clinical features of patients with congenital CVJ anomalies are highly variable and range from an asymptomatic presentation, to a slowly progressive spastic quadriparesis, or even a rapid neurological progression followed by sudden death.

The most common symptom of CVJ abnormalities is mild neck pain originating in the suboccipital region with radiation to the cranial vertex, that occurs in 85% of the patients. The most common neurological deficit in children with congenital CVJ anomalies is myelopathy. Klippel–Feil syndrome may manifest as a classic triad of abnormally low posterior hairline, limitation of neck motion, and short neck, often associated with facial asymmetry, neck webbing, and scoliosis [5]. It is not uncommon to see children with a small dysmorphic stature [5]. Sensory abnormalities usually manifest as neurological deficits related to posterior column dysfunction. The most common cranial nerve dysfunction is hearing loss, occurring in 25% of the cases, that is commonly found in patients with Klippel–Feil syndrome [1]. Vascular symptoms such as intermittent attacks of altered consciousness, transient loss of visual fields, confusion, and vertigo appear in 15% to 25% of patients with abnormalities of the CVJ. The phenomenon of basilar migraine, which affects about 25% of children with basilar invagination and medullary compression, usually involves compression of the vertebra-basilar arterial system. The other characteristic stigmata of CVJ anomalies include a short neck with a reduced neck-body ratio, a webbed neck, a high arched palate, atrophy of small muscles of the hand, and mirror movements.

33.3.1.2 Radiological Diagnosis

Patients presenting with upper cervical myelopathy or radiculopathy should be evaluated with an initial magnetic resonance imaging (MRI) of the cervical spine, to assess for both bony and soft tissue anomalies, and with dynamic cervical trans-table lateral radiographs to assess for C1/C2 instability. An increased atlanto-dental interval (ADI) > 3 mm in adult and ≥ 4.5 mm in pediatric patients (<9 years of age) demands conduction of a dynamic computed tomographic (CT) scan of the cranio-vertebral junction (CVJ) with sagittal and coronal reconstruction for a thorough evaluation of the bony anatomy. Patients with complex congenital CVJ anomaly have AAD coexisting with occipitalized atlas, basilar invagination (BI), rotational dislocation, and coronal tilt in the majority of cases [14–17]. Thus, it is imperative to assess for the three-dimensional dislocation of facet joints for planning for optimal surgical treatment [11, 18]. The simultaneous evaluation of ADI, severity of BI, torticollis, bilateral atlanto-axial joint angle and extent of their vertical positions relative to each other, the degree of rotational dislocation as well as coronal tilt provide complete information for the preoperative planning and combined correction of all the coexisting facet joint displacements, for correction of torticollis, and for surgical fusion in physiological bony alignment [11]. A CT angiography for vertebral artery evaluation at the CVJ to assess its course and also to determine the existence of one of its anomalous variations is also recommended [13]. A classification and scoring system for VA in relation to C1/C2 helps in risk stratification and prevention of vascular injury during instrumentation [13]. MRI is also useful to assess for the neuraxial anomalies like associated tonsillar herniation and syringomyelia.

For the purpose of understanding the basic concepts of the types of BI, its severity and its management, assessment of the following craniometric parameters are essential (Fig. 33.4).

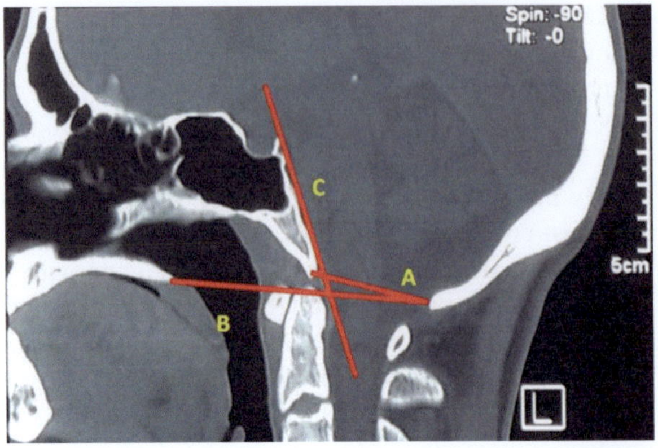

Fig. 33.4 Diagram depicting McRae's line (**a**), Chamberlain's line (**b**), and Wackenheim clival line (**c**) in normal patients. (original picture)

McRae line: It extends from the basion (anterior margin of foramen magnum) to opisthion (posterior margin of the foramen magnum). The tip of the odontoid should be below this line. BI is considered as present if the tip of the odontoid extends above the line. Narrowing of the foramen magnum in the sagittal plane to less than 19 mm is associated with the development of neurological deficits [19].

Chamberlain's line: It extends from the posterior most point of hard palate to the opisthion. In normal subjects, the odontoid process should be located below this line. BI is considered if the tip of the odontoid is extending >5 mm above this line [14, 20].

Wackenheim clivus baseline: This line passes tangential to the clivus extending to the upper cervical spinal canal. It should lie tangential to the posterior aspect of the tip of odontoid process [21]. If the tip of the odontoid crosses this line, it is indicative of BI.

33.3.2 Methods of Measurement of Severity of BI

Coronal inclination: BI is a progressive disease often related to the age of the patient. Measuring progressive changes in the joint indices, therefore, help in evaluating the severity of BI (Fig. 33.5). In coronal CT images, the angle between the intersection of the lines drawn along the edge of foramen magnum and C1 inferior surface measures the C1 coronal angle (Fig. 33.5a). It objectively measures the obliquity of the C1/C2 joint or coronal inclination [22]. Chandra et al. also analyzed and compared the coronal inclination between normal subjects with patients having BI and AAD. In their study, the normal value of coronal inclination was 110.3 ± 4.23°, and in patients with BI it was 121.15 ± 14.6°[22].

Cranio-cervical tilt: This angle is measured between the long axis of the odontoid process and the clivus. A line is drawn first along the anterior border of the odontoid process and extended upward. Next, a line is drawn along the anterior border of the clivus. The angle subtended between these two lines is called the cranio-cervical tilt (Fig. 33.5b). The value in normal subjects is 60.2 ± 9.2° and in patients with basilar invagination (BI) and atlanto-axial dislocation (AAD), it is

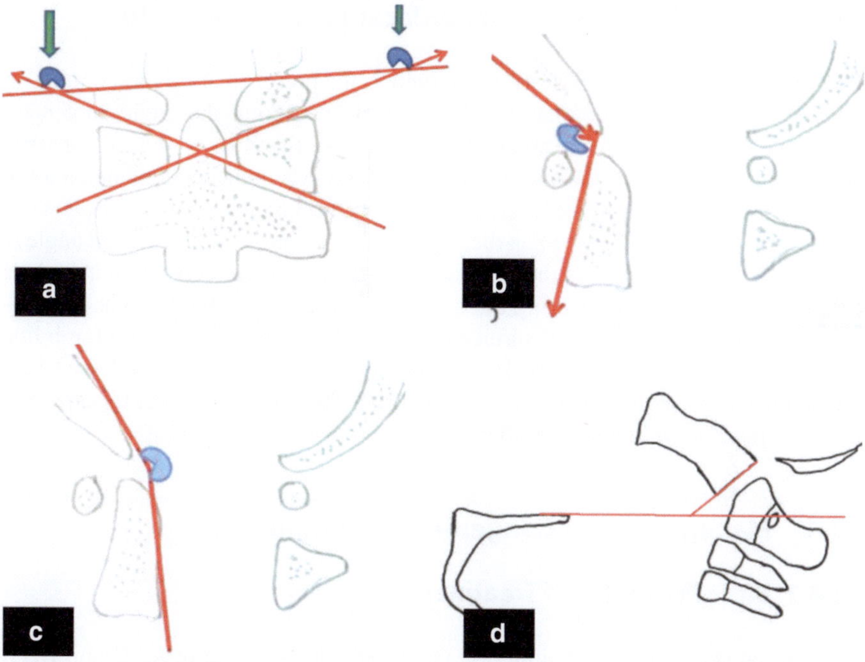

Fig. 33.5 Measurement of severity of BI: (1) Coronal inclination: In coronal CT image, the angle between the intersection of the line drawn along the lower margin of the foramen magnum and the inferior surface of the C1 facet joint measures the C1 coronal angle (**a**). It objectively measured the obliquity of the C1/C2 joint or coronal inclination. (2) Cranio-cervical tilt: This angle is subtended between the long axis of the odontoid process and the clivus. A line is first drawn along the anterior border of the odontoid process and extended upward. Next, a line is drawn along the anterior border of the clivus. The angle subtended between these two lines is called the cranio-cervical tilt (**b**). (3) Clivus-canal angle: The angle formed by the intersection of the line constructed along the posterior surface of the axis body and the Wackenheim clivus baseline is called the clivus-canal angle (**c**). (4) Inferior sagittal C1 facet angle: This is defined as the angle between the line joining the anterosuperior and posterior points of the hard palate and the line joining the anteroinferior and posteroinferior points of the C-1 facet in that sagittal section (**d**) (original picture)

84.0 ± 15.1° [22]. It provides information regarding the severity of upward and posterior invagination of the dens.

Clivus-canal angle: The angle formed by the intersection of the line constructed along the posterior surface of the axis body and the Wackenheim clivus baseline is called as clivus-canal angle (Fig. 33.5c). It normally ranges from 150 to 180°, changing about 30° in flexion and extension positions of the neck [14, 23] Cranio-cervical kyphosis is seen when the clivus-canal angle is less than 150°.

Inferior sagittal C1 facet angle: This is defined as the angle between the line joining the anterosuperior and posterior points of the hard palate and the line joining the anteroinferior and posteroinferior points of the C-1 facet in that sagittal section (Fig. 33.5d) [18]. In the normal population, these two lines remain almost parallel with an angle of nearly 180°. An inferior sagittal C-1 facet angle of more than 150° in the sagittal plane predicts reducibility of the C1-2 joints.

33.3.3 Evaluation of Rotational Dislocation and Coronal Tilt

Rotatory dislocation is considered when there is the presence of rotation of atlas in relation to axis of greater than 5° (assessed by measuring the angle subtended between a line drawn from the anterior to the posterior tubercles on the arch of atlas, and the line tangential to the anterior surface of the axis in the axial plane on a CT scan performed at the level of C1-2 level) [11] (Fig. 33.6).

Coronal tilt is considered when the difference of atlanto-axial facet joint angle is greater than 10° bilaterally in the coronal plane (the atlanto-axial facet joint angle is assessed bilaterally by measuring the angle of intersection of the line passing tangential to the superior articular surface of the C2 facet, and the vertical plumb line passing through the midpoint of inferior border of body of C2 and C3 vertebrae [along the y axis] in the midline) [11] (Fig. 33.7). The normal value of this angle in a control population according to our previous study is $117^0 \pm 6$ [13].

33.4 Management of Congenital CVJ Anomalies

33.4.1 Basic Principles of Treatment

The normal shape of the CV junction is "funnel" shaped, but in AAD and BI, it becomes "hourglass" shaped. The principle is either correction of the dislocation by cranio-cervical realignment or by removal of bone for generous three-dimensional decompression, i.e., anterior-posterior (z axis), transverse (x axis), and vertical (y axis), to make the CV junction funnel shaped and provide an optimal space for the cervicomedullary structures. The following steps are required:

1. Reduction of all types of dislocation focusing on the facet joints of C1/C2 vertebrae by the closed method (preoperative traction) or the open method (distraction between C1/C2 vertebrae or the occipitalized C1/C2 vertebrae by the anterior or posterior approach) can usually correct the associated AAD and/or BI.
2. An internal arthrodesis between C1 and C2 to make the correction permanent.
3. If optimal decompression is not feasible from a posterior approach, a ventral (transoral) decompression is required to decompress the neuraxis.
4. An associated ACM may also warrant a posterior fossa decompression by foramen magnum ± C1 posterior arch excision. If it is associated with AAD, then an additional posterior C1-2 stabilization is mandatory.

33.4.2 Preoperative Traction (Closed Reduction)

Traction provides some degree of alignment and stability for the spine during the shifting, intubation, and positioning of the patient and also helps in distraction of the C1-2 vertebrae (bringing the axis inferiorly in the case of BI, and

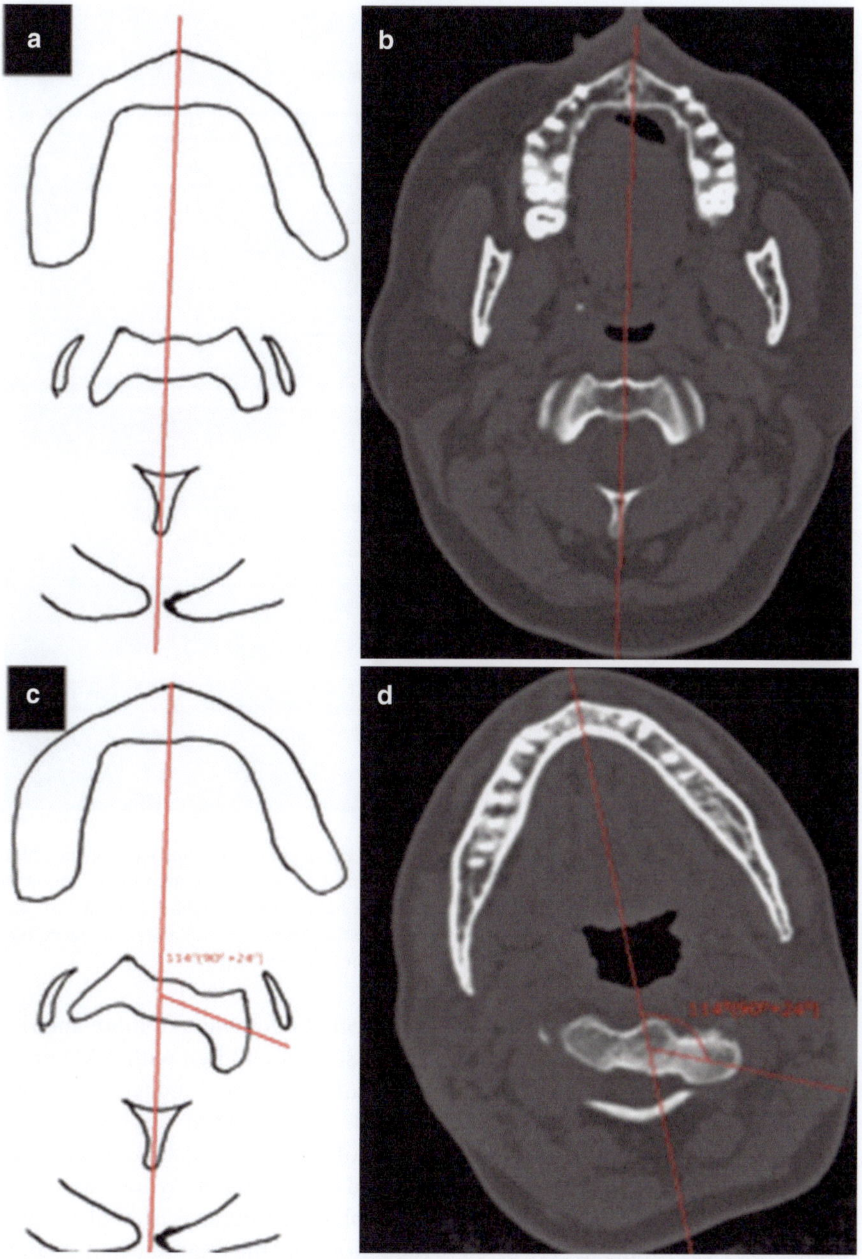

Fig. 33.6 A to D: Rotatory dislocation is considered when there is presence of rotation of atlas in relation to axis of greater than 5° (assessed by measuring the angle subtended between a line drawn from the anterior to the posterior tubercles on the arch of atlas, and the line tangential to the anterior surface of the axis in the axial plane on CT scan performed at the level of cervical 1–2 level). (original picture)

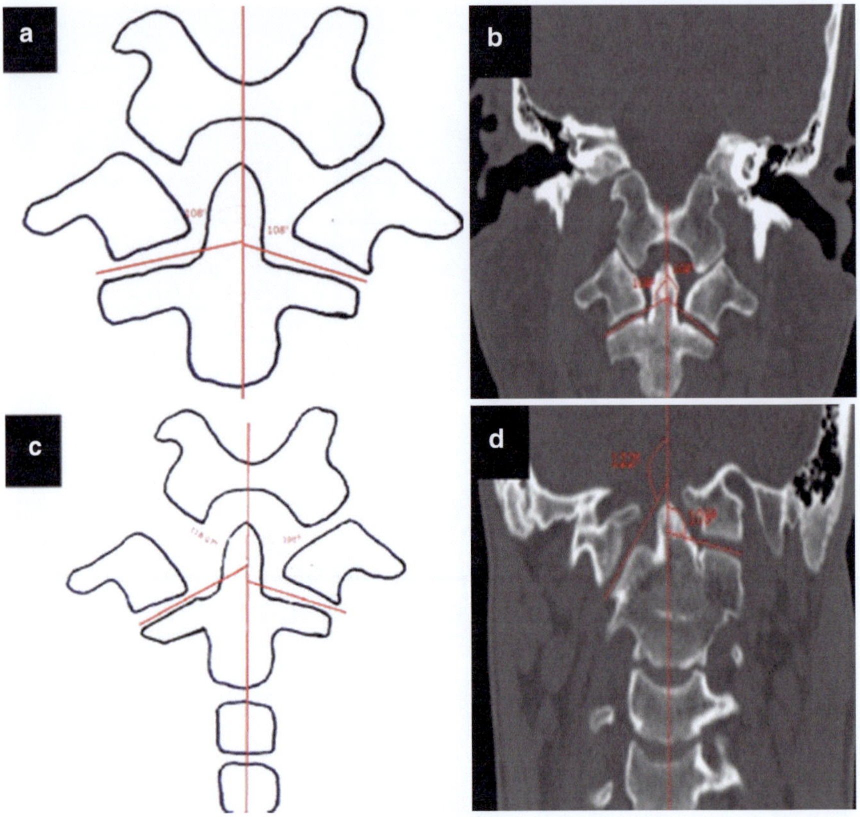

Fig. 33.7 (**a–d**) Atlanto-axial facet joint angle is formed by meeting of the line passing tangential to the superior surface of the C2 facet and vertical plumb line passing through the midpoint of inferior border of body of C2 vertebra and C3 vertebra (*y* axis) in the midline. In each case, the larger angle is considered. Coronal tilt is considered when the difference of atlanto-axial facet joint angle is greater than 10° bilaterally in the coronal plane. (original picture)

realigning the curvature of the posteriorly directed odontoid to a more anterior one to relieve the thecal compression). Up to 80% of children with AAD or BI below the age of 14 can have a significant realignment and reduction of their dislocation by a preoperative traction [12, 24]. The weight of cervical traction applied is dependent upon the age and weight of the patient. It should generally be initiated with 7–8% of the body weight and can be gradually increased to a maximum of 7 kg. Interval lateral cervical plain radiographs should be performed to assess for the degree of C1-2 reduction, and the requirement for additional weight supplementation until an optimal reduction is obtained (or until the subaxial distraction precludes the addition of further weights). Goel et al. have reported that out of 82 patients of BI without associated ACM, 82% patients improved instantaneously after application of the traction in comparison to only 1 patient (out of 20) of BI with ACM [12, 24].

33.4.3 Factor Influencing the Reducibility of Irreducible Atlanto-axial Dislocation with or Without Basilar Invagination

Clinical studies have demonstrated that the contraction of anterior muscles, ligaments, and capsules of the atlanto-axial joint, especially the osteophytes and scar tissue inside the atlanto-dens interspace prevent the complete reduction in IAAD and BI [25, 26]. Some of the factors which prevent the complete reduction and optimal decompression at the level of the C1-2 vertebrae are a high coronal inclination, a highly retroverted odontoid (severe cranio-cervical kyphosis) as well as, rotation and tilt of the axis in relation to atlas due to congenitally anomalous and asymmetrical facet joint orientation. An inferior sagittal C1 facet angle of more than 150° in the sagittal plane also predicted reducibility [18]. A preoperative assessment of the aforementioned radiological factors definitely helps in optimizing the surgical approach and in planning for management of BI.

33.4.4 Types of Approaches

1. **Combined approach**

   Since the last three decades, treatment of choice for irreducible AAD with or without BI was considered as transoral decompression followed by a posterior cervical C1/C2 or occipito-C2 fixation [25–33] (Fig. 33.8). In the recent era, although anterior approach for ventral decompression is rarely used for the routine irreducible AAD, it is still being used in the cases of a very high BI, or in the cases of irreducible AAD with BI with ventral compression associated with severe cranio-cervical kyphosis. In these cases, often the posterior-only distraction procedures are unable to achieve a significant reduction of the AAD and BI. Recently endoscopic transnasal, transoral, and even transcervical approaches have also been performed, followed by a posterior fusion in some centers [34–36]. The endoscopic transnasal odontoidectomy is a feasible approach for anterior decompression of the odontoid at the cervicomedullary junction, especially in selected cases presenting with some anomalous anatomical conditions related to the oral cavity like micrognathia, macroglossia as well as in the presence of a high retroverted position of the odontoid that is in a very high position in the case of BI [35, 36]. The advantages of the endoscopic approaches over the standard transoral odontoidectomy include elimination of the risk of tongue swelling and damage to the teeth due to the application of an oral traction, improvement of visualization of the posterior pharyngeal wall, alleviation of the need for a prolonged intubation, reduction of the need for enteral tube feeding, and less risk of compromised phonation [34, 36]. The minimally invasive access and faster recovery associated with this technique makes it a valid alternative to routinely practiced conventional transoral decompression of the odontoid.
2. **Posterior approach:** The spectrum of techniques described in literature for posterior cervical fixation range from utilization of a silk wire (1910) to C1-C2 translaminar screw methods described by Wright in 2004 [4]. The others are

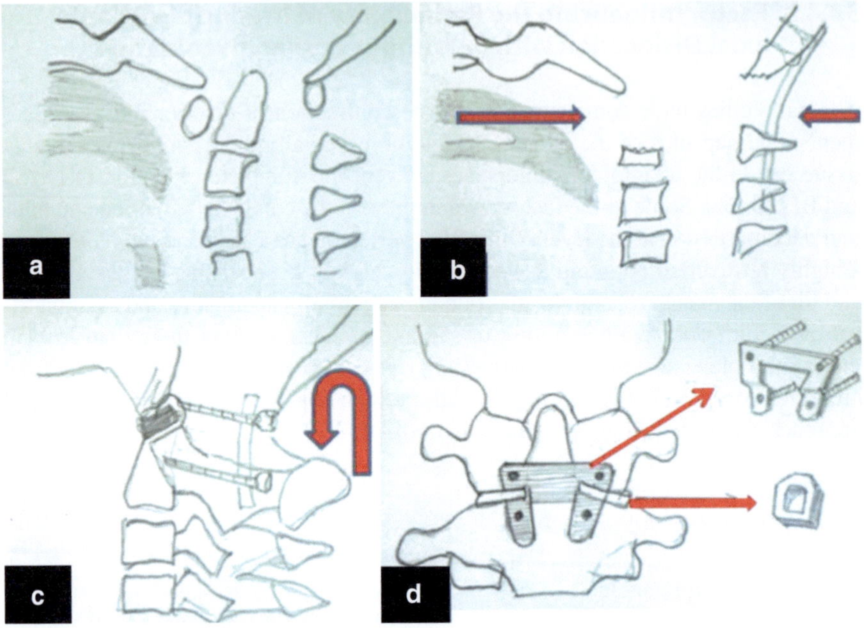

Fig. 33.8 Diagram showing the surgical approaches for CVJ anomalies: (1) Combined approach, that is, transoral decompression followed by posterior fusion by occipito-C2/C3 or C1/C2 lateral mass screw and rod (**a** and **b**). (2) Posterior approach: C1/C2 distraction followed by C1/2 fusion by screw and rod (**c**). (3) Anterior approach: C1/C2 distraction and fusion by transoral atlanto-axial reduction plate (TARP) and cage with C1/C2 lateral mass screw fixation (**d**). (original picture)

Gallie's posterior arch-C2 spinous wiring, Brook's C1-2 sublaminar wiring, Sonntag's wiring, and Magerl's C1/2 transarticular screw technique. A novel technique described by Goel as well as Harms in 2004 is the one most accepted and is now being considered as the standard treatment of choice for posterior fusion [24, 37]. This involves a C1 lateral mass with C2 pars interarticularis or pedicle screw fixation with rod (or plate) and screw technique. Recently, to alleviate the need for a two-stage transoral decompression and posterior fusion for irreducible AAD and/or basilar invagination, a single stage C1-2 facet distraction C1-2 facet joints is in vogue. It helps to reduce the irreducible AAD as well as basilar invagination by decreasing the degree of odontoid migration and re-establishes the cranio-cervical alignment with only the posterior approach [38–40]. A study shows an adequate cranio-cervical realignment and reversal of longstanding musculoskeletal changes like short neck, torticollis, cervical spondylotic myelopathy, and compressive myelopathy with the utilization of this technique [41]. Jian et al., in 2010, published a series of 27 patients successfully treated with direct intraoperative posterior occipito-C2 reduction using distraction over the occipito-C2 rods after occipital and C2 pedicle screw fixation in patients with BI [42]. Although this technique is equally effective in achieving a

CVJ realignment, its disadvantage is that it can lead to cranio-cervical fixation in flexion; the additional incorporation of the occipital bone in the fusion process in patients without atlantal assimilation leads to further loss of movements at the CVJ. Facet joint drilling to make it bilateral symmetrical for the purpose of reduction or manual distraction, compression, and reduction of facet joints has also shown good correction in literature [42–45]. Among the various techniques mentioned above, C1-2 transarticular screws, combined with a Sonntag type interlaminar wiring construct, have been shown to be superior to all other constructs in achieving a rigid fixation of the axis to atlas, based upon the biomechanical studies [46–48].

3. **Anterior only approach (anterior distraction techniques for BI)**

   The transoral atlanto-axial reduction plate (TARP) fixation has been introduced recently to achieve reduction, decompression, fixation, and fusion of C1–C2 through an anterior-only approach [49–51]. The approach could also be carried out using the retropharyngeal approach which has the advantage of bypassing the potentially infected oral cavity [52]. This device may increase stability and fusion rates, maintain or improve atlanto-axial fusion angle, as well as prevent bone graft collapse, excursion, re-sorption, and micro-motion. It not only provides stabilization and fusion, but also restores C1-C2 fusion angle. However, it may also be associated with potential disadvantages, including dysphagia and load shielding (disuse osteoporosis effect on the underlying bone graft as a result of the rigidity of the reconstruction plate) of the bone graft. To prevent the potential disadvantages related to TARP fixation, another novel transoral atlanto-axial fusion cage with integrated plate (cage and plate) device for stabilization of the C1-C2 segment has been designed. In one biomechanical study by Zhang et al. [53], the authors compare the biomechanical differences between cage and plate device and cage and TARP device for the treatment of BI with IRAAD. The results indicated that the novel cage and plate device may provide a lower biomechanical stability than the cage and TARP device in flexion, extension, and axial rotation; however, it may reduce stress shielding of the bone graft for successful fusion and also minimize the risk of postoperative dysphagia.

33.5 Surgical Management of BI with ACM and Syrinx Without AAD

It is an indisputable fact that in patients with Chiari malformation with AAD with or without basilar invagination, the anterior dislocation should be addressed first [54]. This could be in the form of posterior reduction with distraction of the AAD/BI or a direct transoral approach followed by a posterior fusion. However, the treatment for BI with Chiari malformation without atlanto-axial dislocation is still being debated. Some authors advocate posterior fossa decompression only [55–59]. Decompression procedures vary from subpial resection of tonsils, adhesinolysis, or only dural opening. Several studies have reported patients of BI operated

Table 33.5 Summary of major studies using combined approach (transoral decompression + posterior fusion by C1/C2 screw and rods) for treatment of CVJ anomalies

Studies	No. of patients (total no = 751)	Follow-up (months)	Postoperative neurological outcome
1. Goel et al. (1998) [24]	102	6–120 months	102 (100%) improved
2. Jain et al. (1999) [17]	74	47 (3–24 months)	Improved 26 (55%); same: 14(29.8%); deteriorated: 7(14.9%); deaths: 6 (poor respiratory reserve)
3. Behari et al. (2007) [16]	39 AAD, 19 BI with ACM (TOD + PF)	39 (3–85 months)	27 (70%) improved, 1 died (poor respiratory drive), 11—same
4. Menezes et al. (2008) [29]	220	6–96 months	220—improved; 5—velopalatine incompetence; 1—retropharyngeal infection
5. Perrini et al. (2009) [32]	34	28 (0.5–84 months)	Improved: 86%; same: 14%; deaths: 6%; morbidity 18%
6. Mouchaty et al. (2009) [31]	52 (BI-32) (TOD +PF)	33 (4–96 months)	Improved—46 (81%); 19.2% same or deterioration; morbidity—2 patients
7. Yerramneni (2011) [7]	100 (BI-87) TOD (n = 59), OCF (n = 69), C(1)-C(2) fusion (n = 22), occiput-C(2) wiring (n = 5), and FMD (n = 5)	138 (1–84 months)	Improved: 86%; same: 10%; deteriorated: 4% deaths: 5
8. Klekamp et al. (2015) [27]	46 (A: 31 with ventral compression (TOD + PF) and B:15 without ventral compression (only FMD))	46 (1–120 months)	A: 42 improved; 4 same B: 25% deteriorated in long-term follow-up

AAD atlanto-axial dislocation; *PF* posterior fusion; *BI* basilar invagination; *ACM* Arnold Chiari malformation; *TOD* transoral decompression; *FMD* foramen magnum decompression; *C(1)-C(2)* cervical; *OCF* occipito-cervical fusion

utilizing posterior fossa decompression with a good outcome. Goel et al. have, however, recommended only posterior atlanto-axial fixation and fusion without bony decompression for group patients with BI associated with ACM after a study of 65 patients in which 57 patients clinically improved significantly [60]. Worsening of the cranio-cervical kyphosis can exacerbate cervicomedullary compression over the odontoid.

In patients with a kyphotic clivus-canal angle (less than 130^0), the brainstem can suffer severe deformative stress, resulting in clinical deterioration. These patients may have clinical benefit with a cranio-cervical fusion in mild extension, improving clivus-canal angle up to 30^0 to decrease the brainstem deformity and stress [61].

Table 33.6 Summary of major studies used only posterior approach [(A) C1/C2 distraction followed by fusion and (B) Foramen magnum decompression only] for treatment of CVJ anomalies in literature

Method of posterior fusion	Studies	No. of patients (total = 782)	Follow-up (months)	Postoperative neurological outcome
(A) C1/C2 distraction followed by fusion	1. Goel et al. (2004) [38]	22 (PF with spacer and C1/C2 screw and rod)	28 months	Improved—22 (100%)
	2. Kim et al. (2004) [43]	11 BI and ACM (C1-2 plate and screw distraction and FMD)	11 (3–92 months)	Improved—9 (81%), 1 same, 1 worse
	3. Goel et al. (2009) [41]	170	5–60 months	Improved—170 (100%); in 85% patients torticollis and neck alignment improved
	4. Jian et al. (2010) [42]	28 (direct posterior reduction and distraction without spacer)	6–50 months	26 (92.9%) improved, 2 (7.1%) stable >50% reduction in 27/28 patients (96.4%)
	5. Yin et al. (2014) [40]	146	143 (6–48 months)	Improved—135/143 (94%)
	6. Salunke et al. (2015) [44]	19 (C1-2 facet drilling and distraction)	19	19(100%) improvement and 89% reduction (except in 2 patients with vertical joint and anomalous vertebral artery)
	7. Chandra et al. (2013) [39]	79 (C1-2 distraction, compression, extension, reduction)	69 (12–39 months)	100% improvement and 100% reduction
(B) Foramen magnum decompression only, without fusion	1. Goel et al. (1998) [24]	112 (with ACM) (PF in 28 patients)	6–120 months	Improved—112 (100%)
	2. Andrie et al. (2004) [53]	26 (PF in 10 patients)	26 (1–25 months)	Improved—22 (84%); Same— 4(15%); poor grade—1
	3. Goncalves da Silva et al. (2011) [57]	104 (51 with ACM)	104	Improved 10 (13%); 42 (100%)—rhinolalia; 14 (26%) paresthesia

AAD atlanto-axial dislocation; *PF* posterior fusion: *BI* basilar invagination; *ACM* Arnold Chiari malformation; *TOD* transoral decompression; *FMD* foramen magnum decompression

33.5.1 Debate: Anterior Vs. Posterior Approach

Unfortunately, the current literature is lacking in defining definitive criteria which would help to indicate the need for a pure anterior, a pure posterior, or a combined approach. Considering the studies that favored an anterior decompression prior to a posterior stabilization, as a general rule, AAD and BI that do not seem reducible have been treated with ventral decompression followed by posterior cervical stabilization. Menezes reported a series of 72 patients of BI operated by anterior decompression which included 15 patients of BI with associated ACM who were previously treated by only posterior decompression, and deteriorated in the postoperative period. Postoperative MRI was suggestive of an increase in the cranio-cervical kyphosis and ventral compression which required further anterior decompression and posterior fusion [30]. This was further substantiated in 2008 in 733 patients who underwent a transoral decompression. In a study of 100 cases of ACM, it was found that BI was an associated feature in 92% of cases, and 34% also had atlanto-axial instability which required an atlanto-axial fusion along with posterior fossa decompression as described by Menezes [62]. A study of 170 patients surgically treated with only posterior approach have also shown optimal results [41]. We have attempted to describe the outcome of different approaches and methods used in Tables 33.5 and 33.6. In the case of bony anomalies of the CVJ, it is essential to focus on the instability of facet joints, which are the prime factors responsible for the dislocation, for achieving an optimal outcome [63].

33.6 Conclusions

A detailed evaluation of the facet joint anatomy is essential to understand the etiology responsible for the irreducibility of AAD and BI with other bony and soft tissue coexisting anomalies. The algorithm for CVJ anomalies management must be individualized and should be based on the facet joint anatomy, presence or absence of instability, surgeon's personal experience and choice.

References

1. Menezes A, Ahmed R, Dlouhy B. Developmental anomalies of the cranio-vertebral junction and surgical management. In: Winn HR, editor. Youman's neurological surgery. Philadelphia: Editora Saunders; 2003. p. 1856–70.
2. Müller F, O'Rahilly R. Segmentation in staged human embryos: the occipitocervical region revisited. J Anat. 2003;203:297–315.
3. Pang D, Thompson DN. Embryology and bony malformations of the cranio-vertebral junction. Childs Nerv Syst. 2014;27:523–64.
4. Wright NM. Posterior C2 fixation using bilateral, crossing C2 laminar screws: case series and technical note. J Spinal Disord Tech. 2004;17:158–62.
5. Sardhara J, Behari S, Jaiswal AK, Srivastava A, Sahu RN, Mehrotra A, et al. Syndromic versus nonsyndromic atlantoaxial dislocation: do clinico-radiological differences have a bearing on management? Acta Neurochir. 2013;155:1157–67.

6. Menezes AH. Developmental and acquired abnormalities of the cranio-vertebral junction. In: VanGilder JC, Menezes AH, Dolan KD, editors. The cranio-vertebral junction and its abnormalities. New York: Futura; 1987. p. 109–58.
7. Yerramneni VK, Chandra PS, Kale SS, Lythalling RK, Mahapatra AK. A 6-year experience of 100 cases of pediatric bony cranio-vertebral junction abnormalities: treatment and outcomes. Pediatr Neurosurg. 2011;47:45–50.
8. Behari S, Bhargava V, Nayak S, et al. Congenital reducible atlantoaxial dislocation: classification and surgical considerations. Acta Neurochir. 2002;144:1165–77.
9. Goel A. Goel's classification of atlantoaxial "facetal" dislocation. J Craniovertebr Junct Spine. 2014;5:3–8.
10. Fielding JW, Cochran GV, Lawsing JF III, Hohl M. Tears of the transverse ligament of the atlas. A clinical and biomechanical study. J Bone Joint Surg Am. 1974;56:1683–91.
11. Sardhara J, Behari S, Sindgikar P, Srivastava A, Jaiswal A, Sahu R, et al. Evaluating atlanto-axial dislocation based on cartesian coordinates: proposing a new definition and its impact on assessment of congenital torticollis. Neurosurgery. 2018;82(4):525–40. https://doi.org/10.1093/neuros/nyx196.
12. Goel A. Basilar invagination, chiari malformation, syringomyelia: a review. Neurol India. 2009;57:235–46.
13. Sardhara J, Behari S, Mohan BM, Jaiswal AK, Sahu RN, Srivastava A, et al. Risk stratification of vertebral artery vulnerability during surgery for congenital atlanto-axial dislocation with or without an occipitalized atlas. Neurol India. 2015;63:382–91.
14. Smoker WR. Cranio-vertebral junction: Normal anatomy, craniometry, and congenital anomalies. Radiographics. 1994;14:255–77.
15. VanGilder JC, Menezes MI, Dolan KD. The cranio-vertebral junction and its abnormalities. New York: Futura; 1987.
16. Behari S, Kalra SK, Kiran Kumar MV, Salunke P, Jaiswal AK, Jain VK. Chiari I malformation associated with atlanto-axial dislocation: focussing on the anterior cervico-medullary compression. Acta Neurochir. 2007;149:41–50.
17. Jain VK, Behari S, Banerji D, Bhargava V, Chhabra DK. Transoral decompression for cranio-vertebral osseous anomalies: Perioperative management dilemmas. Neurol India. 1999;47:188–95.
18. Salunke P, Sharma M, Sodhi HB, Mukherjee KK, Khandelwal NK. Congenital atlanto-axial dislocation: a dynamic process and role of facets in irreducibility. J Neurosurg Spine. 2011;15:678–85.
19. McRae DL, Barnum AS. Occipitalization of the atlas. Am J Roentgenol Radium Ther Nucl Med. 1953;70:23–46.
20. Chamberlain WE. Basilar impression (platybasia). Yale J Biol Med. 1939;11:487–96.
21. Wackenheim A. Roentgen diagnosis of the cranio-vertebral region. New York: Springer; 1974.
22. Chandra PS, Goyal N, Chauhan A, Ansari A, Sharma BS, Garg A. The severity of basilar invagination and atlantoaxial dislocation correlates with sagittal joint inclination, coronal joint inclination, and cranio-cervical tilt: a description of new indices for the cranio-vertebral junction. Neurosurgery. 2014;10:ONS621–30.
23. Smoker WR, Khanna G. Imaging the cranio-cervical junction. Childs Nerv Syst. 2008;24:1123–45.
24. Goel A, Bhatjiwale M, Desai K. Basilar invagination: a study based on 190 surgically treated patients. J Neurosurg. 1998;88:962–8.
25. Wang C, Yan M, Zhou HT, Wang SL, Dang GT. Open reduction of irreducible atlantoaxial dislocation by transoral anterior atlantoaxial release and posterior internal fixation. Spine. 2006;31:E306–13.
26. Yang J, Ma X, Xia H, Wu Z, Ai F, Yin Q. Transoral anterior revision surgeries for basilar invagination with irreducible atlantoaxial dislocation after posterior decompression: a retrospective study of 30 cases. Eur Spine J. 2014;23:1099–108.
27. Klekamp J. Chiari I malformation with and without basilar invagination: a comparative study. Neurosurg Focus. 2015;38:E12.

28. Menezes AH. Surgical approaches: postoperative care and complications "transoral- transpalatopharyngeal approach to the cranio-cervical junction". Childs Nerv Syst. 2008;24:1187–93.
29. Menezes AH. Complications of surgery at the cranio-vertebral junction: avoidance and management. Pediatr Neurosurg. 1991;17:254–66.
30. Menezes AH, VanGilder JC. Transoral-transpharyngeal approach to the anterior craniocervical junction: ten-year experience with 72 patients. J Neurosurg. 1988;69:895–903.
31. Mouchaty H, Perrini P, Conti R, Di Lorenzo N. Cranio-vertebral junction lesions: our experience with the transoral surgical approach. Eur Spine J. 2009;18:13–9.
32. Perrini P, Benedetto N, Guidi E, Di Lorenzo N. Transoral approach and its superior extensions to the cranio-vertebral junction malformations: surgical strategies and results. Neurosurgery. 2009;64:331–42.
33. Zileli M, Cagli S. Combined anterior and posterior approach for managing basilar invagination associated with type I Chiari malformation. J Spinal Disord Tech. 2002;15:284–9.
34. Baird CJ, Conway JE, Sciubba DM, Prevedello DM, Quiñones- Hinojosa A, Kassam AB. Radiographic and anatomic basis of endoscopic anterior cranio-cervical decompression: a comparison of endonasal, transoral, and transcervical approaches. Neurosurgery. 2009;65:158–63.
35. Dasenbrock HH, Clarke MJ, Bydon A, Sciubba DM, Witham TF, Gokaslan ZL, et al. Endoscopic image-guided transcervical odontoidectomy: outcomes of 15 patients with basilar invagination. Neurosurgery. 2012;70:351–9.
36. Mazzatenta D, Zoli M, Mascari C, Pasquini E, Frank G. Endoscopic endonasal odontoidectomy: clinical series. Spine. 1976;39:846–53.
37. Harms J, Melcher RP. Posterior C1-C2 fusion with polyaxial screw and rod fixation. Spine. 2001;26:2467–71.
38. Goel A. Treatment of basilar invagination by atlantoaxial joint distraction and direct lateral mass fixation. J Neurosurg Spine. 2004;1:281–6.
39. Chandra PS, Kumar A, Chauhan A, Ansari A, Mishra NK, Sharma BS. Distraction, compression, and extension reduction of basilar invagination and atlantoaxial dislocation: a novel pilot technique. Neurosurgery. 2013;72:1040–53.
40. Yin YH, Yu XG, Qiao GY, Guo SL, Zhang JN. C1 lateral mass screw placement in occipitalization with atlantoaxial dislocation and basilar invagination: a report of 146 cases. Spine. 2014;39:2013–8.
41. Goel A, Shah A. Reversal of longstanding musculoskeletal changes in basilar invagination after surgical decompression and stabilization. J Neurosurg Spine. 2009;10:220–7.
42. Jian FZ, Chen Z, Wrede KH, Samii M, Ling F. Direct posterior reduction and fixation for the treatment of basilar invagination with atlantoaxial dislocation. Neurosurgery. 2010;66:678–87.
43. Kim LJ, Rekate HL, Klopfenstein JD, Sonntag VK. Treatment of basilar invagination associated with Chiari I malformations in the pediatric population: cervical reduction and posterior occipitocervical fusion. J Neurosurg. 2004;101:189–95.
44. Salunke P, Sahoo SK, Deepak AN, Ghuman MS, Khandelwal NK. Comprehensive drilling of the C1-2 facets to achieve direct posterior reduction in irreducible atlantoaxial dislocation. J Neurosurg Spine. 2015;23:294–302.
45. Salunke P. Artificial atlanto-axial joints. On the "move". Neurol India. 2016;64:275–8.
46. Menezes AH, Traynelis VC. Anatomy and biomechanics of normal cranio-vertebral junction (a) and biomechanics of stabilization (b). Childs Nerv Syst. 2008;24:1091–100.
47. Mummaneni PV, Haid RW. Atlantoaxial fixation: overview of all techniques. Neurol India. 2005;53:408–15.
48. Sindgikar P, Das KK, Sardhara J, Bhaisora KS, Srivastava AK, Mehrotra A, Jaiswal AK, Sahu RN, Behari S. Cranio-vertebral junction anomalies: when is resurgery required? Neurol India. 2016;64:1220–32.
49. Ai FZ, Yin QS, Xu DC, Xia H, Wu ZH, Mai XH. Transoral atlantoaxial reduction plate internal fixation with transoral transpedicular or articular mass screw of C2 for the treatment of irreducible atlantoaxial dislocation: two case reports. Spine. 2011;36:E556–62.

50. Jiang YW, Xia H, Wang ZY, Wu ZH, Ma XY, Wei GJ, et al. Variation of cranio-cervical junction volume as an effective parameter for basilar invagination treatment. Eur Rev Med Pharmacol Sci. 2015;19:1754–60.
51. Li X, Ai F, Xia H, Wu Z, Ma X, Yin Q. Radiographic and clinical assessment on the accuracy and complications of C1 anterior lateral mass and C2 anterior pedicle screw placement in the TARP-III procedure: study of 106 patients. Eur Spine J. 2014;23:1712–9.
52. Yadav YR, Ratre S, Parhihar V, Dubey A, Dubey NM. Endoscopic technique for single-stage anterior decompression and anterior fusion by transcervical approach in atlantoaxial dislocation. Neurol India. 2017;65:341–7.
53. Zhang BC, Liu HB, Cai XH, Wang ZH, Xu F, Kang H, et al. Biomechanical comparison of a novel transoral atlantoaxial anchored cage with established fixation technique-a finite element analysis. BMC Musculoskelet Disord. 2015;16:261.
54. Behari S, Kalra SK, Kiran Kumar MV, Salunke P, Jaiswal AK, Jain VK. Chiari I malformation associated with atlanto-axial dislocation: focusing on the anterior cervico-medullary compression. Acta Neurochir. 2007;149:41–50.
55. Di Lorenzo N, Fortuna A, Guidetti B. Cranio-vertebral junction malformations: clinicoradiological findings, long-term results, and surgical indications in 63 cases. J Neurosurg. 1982;56:603–8.
56. Fischer EG. Posterior fossa decompression for Chiari 1 deformity, including resection of the cerebellar tonsils. Childs Nerv Syst. 1995;11:625–9.
57. Alberto da Silva J, dos Santos AA Jr, Melo LR, de Araújo AF, Regueira GP. Posterior fossa decompression with tonsillectomy in 104 cases of basilar impression, Chiari malformation and/or syringomyelia. Arq Neuropsiquiatr. 2011;69:817–23.
58. Levy WJ, Mason L, Hahn JF. Chiari malformation presenting in adults: a surgical experience in 127 cases. Neurosurgery. 1983;12:377–90.
59. Logue V, Edwards MR. Syringomyelia and its surgical treatment: an analysis of 75 patients. J Neurol Neurosurg Psychiatry. 1981;44:273–84.
60. Goel A. Is atlantoaxial instability the cause of Chiari malformation? Outcome analysis of 65 patients treated by atlantoaxial fixation. J Neurosurg Spine. 2015;22:116–27.
61. Menezes AH. Primary cranio-vertebral anomalies and the hindbrain herniation syndrome (Chiari I): data base analysis. Pediatr Neurosurg. 1995;23:260–9.
62. Menezes AH, Fenoy KA. Remnants of occipital vertebrae: proatlas segmentation abnormalities. Neurosurgery. 2009;64:945–54.
63. Joaquim AF, Ghizoni E, Giacomini LA, Tedeschi H, Patel AA. Basilar invagination: surgical results. J Craniovertebr Junct Spine. 2014;5:78–84.

Infections at the Cranio-vertebral Junction

34

Andrea Barbanera, Vincenzo Grasso, Andrea Cattalani, and Matteo Vitali

34.1 Introduction

Spine infections, despite improvement of prognosis in recent years due to amelioration of antibiotic therapy, new diagnostic tools [Computed Tomography scan (CT scan), Magnetic Resonance Imaging (MRI)] and progress in surgical techniques, are life-threatening diseases with still high morbidity and mortality rates.

Early evidence of vertebral osteomyelitis was found in Egyptian mummies. While Hippocrates of Cos in his book (On Articulations) described spinal deformities similar to those of Pott's disease [1], Galen was the first physician who described the relationship between spinal deformity and infectious process [2].

Before the era of antibiotics, little knowledge was added to the Hippocratic/Galen school until 1779, when sir Percival Pott described the tubercular infection of the spine [3]. The first robust description of bacterial osteomyelitis, as we recognize today, dates to 1879 and was made by Lannelongue [4].

Despite the cumulative data on this disease and the improvement of knowledge on spine infection, cervical spine (C-spine) infections have a high mortality rate and account for 15% of all cases when complicated by abscess [5].

A. Barbanera (✉)
Chief of Neurosurgical Unit , Ospedale SS Antonio e Biagio e Cesare Arrigo, Alessandria, Italy

Neurosurgical Unit, Ospedale SS Antonio e Biagio e Cesare Arrigo-Alessandria, Alessandria, Italy

V. Grasso
Umberto Parini Hospital - USL Valle D'Aosta, Aosta, Italy

A. Cattalani · M. Vitali
Chief of Neurosurgical Unit , Ospedale SS Antonio e Biagio e Cesare Arrigo, Alessandria, Italy

E. Tessitore et al. (eds.), *Surgery of the Cranio-Vertebral Junction*,
https://doi.org/10.1007/978-3-030-18700-2_34

Infections at the C-spine [cranio-vertebral junction (CVJ) and subaxial cervical spine as a whole] are quite uncommon, accounting for less than 10% of all form of spine infections; nevertheless they are responsible of the majority of neurological impairment due to proximity to vital structure; they are the cause of 27% of all neurological deficits.

Infective process of the spine may be classified in various ways, considering the histologic response of the host to the specific organism, the primary anatomic location, the way of spreading, etc.

Infection can be classified according to:

- response to the host: *pyogenic* (due to bacterial infection), *granulomatous infection* (due to Mycobacteria, fungi, Brucella, and syphilis) or *parasitic infection* (Echinococcosis) [6, 7]
- primary anatomic localization: *discitis*, *spondylitis, spondylodiscitis* or *vertebral osteomyelitis* (*VO*), *spinal epidural abscess* (*SEA*) (primary or secondary), *pyogenic facet arthropathy* [6]
- spread: *hematogenous*, *contiguity*, *direct inoculation*
- duration: *acute* (<6 weeks); *subacute* (6 weeks–3 months); *chronic* (>3 months)
- age of host: adult or pediatric spine infection

Approximately 95% of pyogenic spinal infections involve the vertebral body, and only 5% the posterior elements of the spine. This discrepancy has been attributed to the blood supply to the vertebral body and its cellular marrow.

The key to understand the pathogenesis and the subsequent morphological aspect of spine infection is the lack of direct blood supply in adult intervertebral disk and, instead, the dense vascular network in vertebral body metaphyseal region. As bacteria follow vascular pathway, this explains why the vertebral body is usually infected within trabecular area by septic embolus and subsequently the infection settles down to the disk space.

In surgical procedure, the cause of iatrogenic infection is a direct inoculation of bacteria into the disk region and hence the resulting isolated discitis is the primary manifestation.

34.2 Cervical Spine Infection

The classification of c-spine infections is similar to that of thoracic and lumbar spine, so pyogenic and non-pyogenic forms are the main ones.

It could be also distinguished, as abovementioned, in discitis, spondylitis and spondylodiscitis, spinal epidural abscess, and pyogenic facet arthropathy depending on whether the causative germ is localized, i.e., to disk alone, vertebral body alone or both, epidural space, and facet joint, respectively. The pathogenesis and seeding, however, is quite different.

As a general rule, the most frequent way by which the pathogen can localize in spine is hematogenous spread, particularly arterial pathway; in C-spine, however, venous and lymphatic route, particularly in CVJ region, play a significant role; in this region contiguity and continuity spread are as important as hematogenous way.

The anatomy of CVJ, namely the anatomy of foramen magnum and occipital condyle, atlas, axis, and the complex of ligamentous structures makes this region of particular interest with regard to infections.

34.3 Anatomy of CVJ and Infections

An in-depth description of the anatomy of cranio-vertebral junction is beyond the scope of the present chapter, but is of paramount importance for understanding pathogenesis and subsequent clinical manifestation of spinal infections.

The CVJ is a complex of osteo-ligamentous components that joint the cranium to column [8].

The atlas, the first vertebra or C1, and axis, the second one or C2, are regarded atypical when compared with vertebrae of the subaxial cervical spine.

The two important anatomic features of the atlas are: (1) the anterior tubercle, located in the midline of the anterior arch: its importance lies on the close proximity to retropharyngeal space (RPS) and the dense venous plexuses inside it (see later); (2) the prominent tubercle of bone on each side of mesial lateral masses: it is the attachment of the transverse ligament that holds the dens confined to the anterior third of the atlantal ring; the ligament provides stability; hence its importance lies on onset of instability when destroyed from infection.

The second cervical vertebrae, axis or C2, has a characteristic upward projection, dens or odontoid process; it origins from the body and articulates with the posterior aspect of the anterior arch of the atlas. Between the lamina, posteriorly, and the lateral mass there is a not well-defined area known as pedicle/isthmus (this structure is important in posterior screw fixation). The laminae of the axis, the posterior elements, are thick and the spinous process is large and bifid; laterally, the transverse process projects and ends in a single tubercle: it contains a foramen transversarium.

The density of the trabecular bone of the axis varies: it is dense near the center of the tip of the dens and lateral masses beneath the superior articular surface, and hypodense at the center of the dens [9]. The importance of the density resides in the resistance to damage after seeding of bacteria.

The occipital condyles are the paired inferiorly and lateral prominences of the occipital bone that form the lateral part of foramen magnum together with the basi-occiput anteriorly and the squamosal segment posteriorly. They are commonly oval in shaped; they slope inferiorly from lateral to medial in the coronal plane. They have a canal, the hypoglossal or anterior condyloid canal, through which two structures travel: the hypoglossal nerve (cranial nerve XII) exits the skull, and a meningeal branch of the ascending pharyngeal artery enters it. The condyloid fossa, a recess behind the condyles, is frequently perforated by the posterior condylar foramen, through which an emissary vein runs from the sigmoid sinus. The dense anatomical structures that lie in these canals and travel from or to skull base and CVJ justify the frequent extension of infection upwards or downwards [10].

Two joints compose the CVJ: the atlanto-occipital and atlantoaxial joints.

The atlanto-occipital complex is composed of: (1) two membranes, the anterior and posterior atlanto-occipital ones that extended between the superior margin of anterior and posterior arch of C1 to foramen magnum; and (2) two synovial atlanto-occipital joints formed between the superior articular facet of the atlas and the occipital condyle.

The atlantoaxial complex is composed of three joints: the lateral joints are formed by the articulation between the superior articular facet of C2 and the inferior surface of the atlas; the median joint is formed between the odontoid posteriorly and the anterior complex composed by the anterior arch of the atlas and transverse ligament.

The important ligaments that connect C0 to C1-C2 complex are: the apical ligament (also known as "suspensory ligament") extends from the tip of odontoid to the anterior edge of the foramen magnum; the two paired alar ligaments extend from the tip of the dens to the medial aspects of each occipital condyle and on the lateral mass of the atlas [11]; the cruciate ligament composed of the transverse ligament of C1 and a ligamentous extensions, the superior and inferior ones, that connect it to the anterior edges of the foramen magnum and posterior surface of body of C2; the tectorial membranes extend from the upper surface of the basilar portion of the occipital bone and the anterior margin of the foramen magnum to the posterior body of the axis and the posterior longitudinal ligament. These structures are responsible for the majority of movement of the cervical spine being the bony structures determinant for mechanical properties of the atlanto-occipital joint, whereas ligamentous structures determine the properties of the atlantoaxial joint [12].

34.3.1 Blood Supply and Lymphatics

Blood supply to the CVJ region is provided by vertebral and occipital arteries. Two main arteries arise from vertebral arteries, anterior and posterior ascending vessels: they anastomose together to form an "apical arcade" around the alar ligament.

The anterior and posterior ascending vessels give off the small perforating branches to the body of the axis and the odontoid process; furthermore, in the apical arcade, small carotid arteries branches contribute to the vascularization by way of the base of the skull and apical ligament [13–15].

The primary lymphatic drainage of the CVJ region is into the retropharyngeal lymphatic nodes and then deep into the deeper cervical nodes. The nasopharynx, retropharyngeal area, and the paranasal sinuses also drain into the retropharyngeal nodes.

In an interesting paper, Parke et al. [16] described a complex of pharyngo-vertebral veins with a dense anastomosis between lymphatic and venous system; furthermore, the pharyngo-vertebral veins have a direct communication with the periodontal venous plexus that empty in the sinuses that lie in the suboccipital epidural space. As a primary consequence of this important anatomical relationship is that, in a retrograde fashion, an infection in the para- and prevertebral region, i.e., retropharyngeal space (RPS), can involve cranio-cervical joints resulting in osteomyelitis and subsequent instability with the impending development of neurological deficit. Thus, beyond the classical arterial pathway followed in thoracic and lumbar spine infection, there is a further route for septic involvement of the CVJ, the RPS [16, 17].

A straightforward example of the intimate relationship between RPS and CVJ is Grisel's syndrome. This condition is most common in patient less than 30 years old who suffered a recent or active upper respiratory infection or undergone recent ENT procedures [18, 19]. In this syndrome, the germ can spread through the pharyngovertebral venous plexus into the atlantoaxial articulation/facet joint. The odontoid inflammatory process leads to bone destruction, thinning of transverse ligament, and subsequent instability with the impending symptoms such as occipital and cervical pain, torticollis, and rotatory subluxation.

34.3.2 Retropharyngeal Space (RPS) Relevant Anatomy

RPS is the anatomical space that lies just behind oropharynx. It is bordered anteriorly by bucco-pharyngeal fascia and posteriorly by prevertebral fascia. The alar fascia, dependent from the deep cervical fascia, divides this space into anterior and posterior compartment. The former extends from the skull base to T4 vertebral body; the latter extends inferiorly to the diaphragm. RPS can be further classified as suprahyoid space or infrahyoid space relative to hyoid bone: the former contains retropharyngeal lymph nodes and fat, the latter only fat [20].

The relationship between RPS and CVJ is very close, especially with bony and ligamentous structure that forms anterior arch of C1 and odontoid process. As many others, Carlos R. Goulart et al. performed cadaveric endoscopic endonasal dissection that permitted to highlight the nearness among the oropharyngeal thin mucosa, anterior longus capitis and longus colli muscles, anterior longitudinal ligament, arteries (particularly vertebral arteries branches) and veins (the highest Batson plexus veins) and bony elements, particularly anterior tubercle and anterior arch of C1, odontoid process; apical and alar ligaments, tectorial membrane.

The oropharynx is colonized by normal flora and by potential virulent bacteria that in case of minor traumatic laceration of mucosa, can invade the RPS and give rise to infection [21].

For example a high-energy CVJ injury, in which anterior arch of C1 is the main cause of laceration of oropharynx epithelium, can lead to hematoma formation within deep muscles; oropharynx laceration is the cause of bacterial invasion of RPS and subsequent abscess formation due to the excellent pabulum represented by hematoma itself. Due to the dense anastomosis between vessel veins and lymphatic inside RPS, germ can multiply and spread with subsequent involvement of CVJ bones and epidural space [22, 23].

Also degenerative disease might be responsible of small tear of mucosal coating of oropharynx in minor hyperextension cervical injury [24].

In adult, another possible cause of apparently spontaneous retropharyngeal abscess formation is lacking of some kind of lymph node degeneration that involve this structure during adolescence: bacterial infection that originates from middle ear, sinuses or tonsils can therefore spread through nodes to RPS and give rise to abscess that can rarely complicate with vertebral osteomyelitis.

34.4 Pyogenic Spine Infection and C-Spine Involvement

The incidence of pyogenic vertebral osteomyelitis (V0) appears to have increased in recent years and is approximately 2.2/100,000 per year [25, 26] most likely due to improved diagnosis, the numbers of patients with immunosuppression and frequent use of intravascular catheters for therapies, the enlargement of people affected by chronic pathologies, such as diabetes, the rise of aging [27, 28], and a large amount of young people that abuse of intravenous drugs.

About the age, the incidence of infection increases with age; vertebral osteomyelitis is uncommon under the age of 20 years (0.3/100.000 persons), but over the age of 70 years, the incidence is 20-fold higher (6.5 per 100,000 persons).

Pyogenic cervical involvement by hematogenous source represents 6% of all cases of vertebral osteomyelitis [6, 29], whereas granulomatous infections are rare, and predominantly due to TB infection.

The importance of diagnosis of C-spine infection, particularly CVJ region, is due to the potential development of neurological deficits, reported between 24% and 64% of cases, due to extensively bony and ligament destruction and subsequent instability of C0-C1-C2 joints.

Pyogenic spine infection is believed to represent a spectrum of manifestation, but in 95% of cases in subaxial C-spine it manifests such as a spondylodiscitis and in CVJ localization such as spondylitis, epidural abscess, and pyogenic facet joint infection.

Any clinical condition that causes bacteremia may lead to hematogenous vertebral osteomyelitis and the major risk factors is a current active infection at any site of the body [30]; the most frequent one is recurrent urinary tract infection (28%), followed by soft tissue and respiratory tract infections [6]; older studies stated a frequency of infections in 1.5% of IV drug abusers, with increasing frequency [31, 32], but the percentage may be underestimated.

The most common isolated bacteria is *Staphylococcus* species (50% to 80% of cases), particularly *Staphylococcus aureus* methicillin-sensitive (MSSA), greater than 36% of species isolated in infected patients; methicillin-resistant *Staphylococcus aureus* (MRSA) is responsible of 6.8% of cases of infection. *Streptococcus* species were isolated in 19% of cases, whereas gram-negative bacteria in 14% of cases, with Pseudomonas (3.9%) and E. Coli (2.9%) the most commonly found. The cultures maybe negative in 24–40% of cases.

34.4.1 Pathogenesis

Spondylodiscitis, in adults, begins with seeding of bacteria into metaphyseal region of vertebra through hematogenous spread because of the lack of direct vascular supply of the disk. In children instead, due to the plentiful vascular supply of the disk that allow pathogen to directly seed into the nucleus pulposus, discitis alone is more frequently diagnosed than adult, with lumbar localization more commonly than cervical [33].

The acute phase of infection is characterized by vessels dilatation in vertebral body vascular network near the septic focus and subsequent edema formation (exudate) between the trabecula; this leads to an increased local pressure, reduction in blood flow, and the beginning of ischemic process. The exudate is mainly composed by neutrophil leukocytes that destroys the bone with lysosomal enzymes rapidly and necrosis develops within 48 hours; this process is responsible of infection's extension to the disk. In early regenerative phases, the neutrophil leukocytes are partially replaced by mononuclear cells (macrophages and lymphocytes) that enter in granulation tissue, composed by fine capillary vessels and a matrix of fibroblastic cells that proliferate: disk swelling is the main consequence. In late regenerative phase, the disk became sclerotic and fibrotic [34].

34.4.2 Clinical Presentation

The most important problem dealing with spinal infection, C-spine in particular, is the delayed diagnosis due to early vague symptoms.

In a literature review [35], the authors stated that 50% of patient suffered symptoms for >3 months prior to diagnosis and only 20% of individuals manifested symptom less than 3 weeks or between 3 weeks to 3 months. The clinical presentation is strictly related to the virulence of the organism, the immunocompetence of the host, and duration of the infection.

In general, neck and occipital pain are the most common presenting symptoms (92%) in patients with cervical and CVJ infection; fever is seen in only 50% of the patients: when it is the presenting symptom, the acute form should be suspected.

Signs of C-spine or CVJ infection, such as radiculopathy or myelopathy, are manifested in late phase of pathological complicated course and when present, an associated epidural abscess or spinal cord compression must be suspected. As a whole, the percentage of neurological deficit is about 17% in patients with spine infection and it is much more higher in C-spine infection [36]. A triad of neck pain, fever, and progressive radiculopathy should rise the suspicion of infection and should be used for early diagnosis [37]: unfortunately the triad is rarely seen. Cervical spine lymphadenopathy, spasm of neck musculature, and progressive torticollis have been described as early signs and symptoms [38], but are uncommon.

Atypical symptoms are present in about 15% of cases and they predominantly are meningeal irritation, headache, chest pain, or respiratory problems; less common findings may be muscle spasm, tenderness, weight loss, pain exacerbation with movement, limited motion, vague symptomatology such as, malaise, and decreased appetite.

Several more factors should contribute to the difficulty in diagnosis in this challenging region; the anatomy is the first one because it is quite different to that of other segments of spinal column. As described in the anatomical paragraph, the C0-C1-C2 joints consist only of synovial joint without disk between C1 and C2, and the infection often begins as a septic arthritis. The radiographic shrinkage of the disk space is evident in early subaxial cervical spine infection (spondylodiscitis and discitis); the widening of retropharyngeal soft tissue is easily missed until late.

34.4.3 Laboratory

Laboratory evaluation consists of blood count with erythrocyte sedimentation rate (ESR) and C-reactive protein (CRP); urine and blood cultures should be obtained.

The most sensitive and more specific inflammatory marker is CRP: the increase of its levels begins 6 h after onset of inflammatory process and reaches the peak 3–5 days after the infection; CRP drops rapidly with a half-life of 24 to 48 h after the resolution of the pathological process and normal values are reached in 10 days; conversely, ESR peaks at 5–7 days and for more than 3–4 weeks it remains at high values. Interestingly, Thelander and Larsson found that ESR and CRP values remain high for at least 10–14 days after routine spine procedures and thereafter an increase of their blood concentrations should rise the suspect of post-surgical infection [39].

34.4.4 Imaging

Radiographic changes are difficult to identify until advanced bone destruction is present; therefore the introduction and subsequent development of CT scan and MR images was of paramount importance and they have undoubtedly simplified the diagnosis [40].

In plain radiograph, early signs are focal osteopenia or osteolysis, paravertebral shadow, periosteal thickening. However, there is a delay of 3–4 weeks after onset of infection and that radiological signs clearly evident in subaxial spine, such as blurred endplates, disk space collapse, reactive bone formation should lack in CVJ spondylitis.

Lateral films are useful to visualize the prevertebral soft tissue swelling that usually is due to edema or retropharyngeal abscess, but they can be subtle and missed by an inexperienced radiologist.

CT scan with or without contrast agent injection is a useful tool that permits to clearly identify the degree of lytic vertebral body destruction, the extent of abscesses in soft tissue and also the boundary between abscesses and swollen paravertebral muscles; it is also more sensitive than MR image in localization of bone sequestration [41]. Furthermore, CT scan is able to differentiate pyogenic spondylitis from tuberculous or fungal ones; in the latter, the soft tissue extension is more prominent [42]; in the lumbar spine CT scan is able to identify the disk hypodensity that is specific for infection but is less useful in the thoracic and cervical region. Finally it is a useful and safe toll to guide biopsies of the spine for definitive identification of pathogen.

MRI is the imaging method of choice in spine infection. It, indeed, provides more anatomic information than CT scan or radionuclide studies and allows early signs of infection with identification of soft tissue swelling and abscess: MRI has 96% sensitivity, 93% specificity, and 94% accuracy in detecting vertebral osteomyelitis in general [43]. In addiction, MRI is particularly useful in atlas or odontoid osteomyelitis [44–46]. For example in early phase of dens osteomyelitis, T1- and T2-weighted MR images are able to identify findings consistent with uncomplicated osteomyelitis; however, the difference between normal and abnormal bone marrow is difficult to evaluate. Short tau inversion recovery (STIR) and chemical fat-saturated post-contrast sequences are able, indeed, to do that, i.e., to reveal intraosseous abnormal signal or enhancement [41, 47].

Spondylodiscitis has MRI characteristic findings: decreased signal intensity on T1-weighted images of vertebral endplate or compact bone (i.e., dens or anterior/posterior C1 arc), increased signal intensity on T2- weighted images and contrast enhancement of the disk and/or vertebral endplates; ring-enhancement on post-gadolinium T1-weighted images of abscesses.

Of interest, Chang et al. have conducted a study in whom they compare MR imaging features of granulomatous spondylitis, tuberculous mostly, with pyogenic spondylitis and identified five findings useful to differentiate these pathological entities [48]. The features were: degree of bone destruction, degree of disk preservation, paravertebral abscess appearance, and post-contrast agent injection abscess rim enhancement. Degree of vertebral body and disk destruction are the key findings that permit to distinguish the two entities: in almost all tuberculous patients (82%) there is a near complete vertebral body destruction, whereas this involves 30% of the patients with pyogenic spondylodiscitis.

Radionuclide studies are very useful because they could detect infection early in the course of pathology and seldom before plain films become positive. Gallium scan shows an increase of the uptake in a butterfly fashion around the area of infection. It has an 89% of sensitivity, 85% of specificity, and 86% of accuracy; it becomes positive before technetium scan [49, 50]. Gallium scanning exams return to normal during healing so this study could be used in follow-up to evaluate the response to therapy. Technetium scan shows an increase of the uptake in a diffuse fashion in the region of the infected vertebrae. It has a 90% of sensitivity, 78% of specificity, and 86% of accuracy. This exam remains positive for a long period after the end of the therapy, hence it could not be used in follow-up [50].

Both the technique may result negative in cases of occult infection due to low virulence of the organisms [51] and false-negative results are possible in case of regional ischemia, mainly in elderly people with technetium bone scan [51] or in leukopenic patients in gallium bone scan exams [52].

Single-photon emission computed tomography (SPECT) is used for early detection of spine infection and has the mainly advantage of contrast resolution and three-dimensional localization. In a recent study by Love et al. [53], gallium SPECT was compared to technetium SPECT and MRI with the results that gallium SPECT had comparable accuracy to MRI in detecting infection, hence the former should be used when MRI is contraindicated or in case where the diagnosis is inconclusive.

34.5 Tuberculosis of the Cervical Spine

Tuberculosis (TB) is still a world challenge despite antitubercular therapy with a prevalence of 14 million cases and 9.4 million new cases/every year [54].

Of patients with TB, 10–15% have involvement of musculoskeletal system and in nearly half of these patients, the spine is involved. Only 10% of all cases of spinal TB are localized in C-spine and among patients with tubercular spondylitis, CVJ involvement, C1-C2 complex particularly, is seen only 0.3–1% [55, 56]. However, in two published series [56, 57], until 5% of cases of spinal TB was at CVJ.

C-spine bone localization is usually secondary to direct extension from retropharyngeal lymph nodes, unlike thoracic or lumbar spine in whom the infection is secondary to hematogenous spread [58]. Extensive late destruction of bony elements of C1 and C2, such as in TB infection, can lead to instability and rotatory deformities of the CVJ. The lateral masses of atlas are involved in 72% of cases and the dens in 62% of the patients [59, 60].

34.5.1 Pathology

The Mycobacterium tuberculosis is responsible of the human infection. The bacterium is an obligate aerobe, i.e., with affinity for tissues rich in high oxygen tension.

Three types of tubercular lesions have been described:

- exudative lesions: these are the result of association of polymorphonuclear leukocytes, monocytes, and lymphocytes with an exudative reaction in the infected area (vasodilation and edema formation).
- proliferative lesion is the typical one, known as "tuberculous granuloma": it is formed by bacilli surrounded by two types of inflammatory cells: mononuclear cells that engulf the bacterium and then coalesce to form epithelioid cells; lymphocytes cells that encircled the epithelioid ones. The center of granuloma is then featured by caseating necrosis.
- composite lesions: as the inflammatory process progresses, the abscess, which is a collection of caseous material, bony sequestra, serum and inflammatory cells with scant tubercular bacilli, forms. The abscess may be confined, such as in the pre-odontoid space, or it can follow the tissue planes to flow distant to origin, for example the anterior or posterior neck triangles or in the axilla.

From a pathogenetic point of view, the incidence and type of neurologic deficit in cervical TB varies between the upper and lower cervical spine because of the close proximity of spinal cord; in fact, it occupies one-third of the spinal canal at the level of C1 and C2, hence the free space available makes neurologic deficit uncommon until extensive destruction and large abscesses form and mechanical compression or ischemia of the spinal cord secondary to vascular thrombosis result.

Clinical presentation and outcome are influenced by age of the patient: in children less than 10 years old and young people, fulcrum of movement is at C2-C3 disk, hence increased mechanical stress to this level makes it susceptible to infection; extensive destruction of growth plates and severe kyphosis in this age group are due to ligamentous laxity and horizontally oriented facets.

In patients more than 10 years old and in adult, the shape of articular joint is more vertical, and fulcrum of movement is shifted more inferiorly, hence lower C-spine is more susceptible to infection.

The understanding of the site of involvement of tuberculosis in the CVJ and the pattern of its spread and nature of its pathogenetic effects on the osteo-ligamentous assembly is crucial for defining the strategy of the management.

Tuberculosis involves the bone primarily and ligaments are affected only secondarily. Bones are involved by destruction while the ligaments are involved by displacement and disruption [61, 62].

The pattern of involvement of CVJ by TB can be divided into three stages, as described by Lifeso in 12 patients, on the basis of radiological features [63]:

Stage 1: in this stage, the ligaments are intact; there is minimal bony destruction and involvement of the cancellous part of the bone: usually unilateral involvement of the facet of atlas; less frequently, isolated and/or unilateral involvement of the facets of axis or the odontoid process.

There is no deformation and no evidence of C1-C2 dislocation. It may be seen inflammatory granulomatous reaction, usually around the involved facet joints, and caseous necrosis. The other parts of the atlas or axis bone and the contralateral facet are not involved. Clinically neck pain and reduction of neck movements are presenting symptoms of this stage.

Stage 2: the disease progresses with extension of the inflammatory reaction to atlantoaxial joint and to other parts of the atlas and/or axis bones and ligaments with the result of minimal, irreducible or, less frequently, reducible atlanto-axial dislocation (AAD), which is probably due to ineffectiveness of the alar and transverse ligaments. The contralateral joint is still unaffected and, hence, the dislocation is of "fixed" and rotatory variety. Prevertebral or extradural spinal caseous necrosis or pus formation is usually encountered. The joint space on the involved side is seen to be reduced or absent. Clinically the patient presents with neck pain, neck muscle spasm, and severe neck movements restriction. Torticollis is characteristic and appears to be the results to defense in an attempt to reduce stress to the affected joint and to protect the cord from compression. The patient may or may not have neurological symptoms or deficits.

Stage 3: there is an extensive involvement of the contralateral atlantoaxial joint and other bones with complete loss of odontoid and atlas arches; all ligaments of the region are destroyed. Instability of the CVJ is usually seen. Thus, the patient presents neurological deficit.

34.5.2 Clinical Features

Neurological deficits are delayed and initially less pronounced despite the aggressive destruction and deformation by the disease that is initially unilateral with spare of contralateral atlantoaxial joint. Due to the presence of relatively stable CVJ region and the effectiveness of the modern antituberculous drugs, symptomatology is initially subtle.

Severe pain and reduction of neck movements are presenting symptoms of C-spine TB; suboccipital headache is the early symptom in the course of CVJ localization; swelling in the neck, secondary to cold abscess, and torticollis can rarely be present at early stages and may reflect sternocleidomastoid spasm or lateral mass destruction of atlas with instability.

In subaxial c-spine TB patients, neurologic symptoms are seen in 25% of cases, while in only 15% to 20% of cases with CVJ TB localization, although reported incidence of spinal cord compression on imaging is quite high, i.e., 45% of cases [64].

Symptoms of spinal cord compression include a wide variety of weakness, spasticity, altered gait; paresthesias of extremities with loss of bowel and bladder control; and spinothalamic tract alterations; paresis of ninth and tenth cranial nerves manifests with a vary degree of dysphagia, nasal regurgitation, and hoarseness of voice; atlantoaxial instability and cervico-medullary compression may be responsible of sudden death, as reported by Fang et al. [65]. History of systemic signs of TB may be present and consist of weight loss, night sweat, and fever.

Vertebral and basilar artery thrombosis due to extensions of the exudative form of TB infection are also be described and manifest as brainstem symptomatology.

All the movements of the neck are severely restricted by pain and spasm; rarely, kyphotic deformity can be visualized.

Atypical clinical presentation is reported to vary from 0.2 to 10% [66], and it consists of: involvement of the posterior elements of the spinal column, skip lesions, extradural spinal cord compression without evidence of bony involvement, destructive lesions of the sacrum or acute hemiplegia or monoplegia due to one-side compression on cervico-medullary junction, or just above it [67].

34.5.3 Imaging

As a general rule, in TB the cancellous part of bone is most susceptible to destruction than the compact part that is affected late in the pathology with secondarily involved joint.

In TB, two types of radiological features are recognized: the granular type characterized by less destructive imaging of the affected bony elements; then the caseous exudative type that is characterized by more destructive features and more frequently associated to abscess.

Based on the radiologic location of the tuberculous focus, the lesions are classified as paradiskal, central, anterior, and appendicular.

Hence, in the early stages of C-spine and CVJ TB, the only first suspicion on lateral plain radiograph is an increased prevertebral soft tissue shadow (>7 mm at the lover border of the axis) without any extensive bony destruction that became visible first if the lesion involves at least 50% of the vertebral body and second if enough time has elapsed from beginning of host reaction (generally after 2–6 months) [68]. Other radiographic features are: reabsorption of dens margin and end plate of C2 body; obliteration or narrowing of C2-C3 disk space (as a general rule, in C-spine infection, changes of disk space and blurring of end plates are visible after a delay of 2–3 weeks); lytic destruction of anterior portion of the body; erosion of occipital condyles and, more importantly, extensive destruction of facet joints, that can quickly lead to an unstable spine with AAD and severe instability, are late visible.

Although not as effective as MRI, CT scans better delineate than plain radiographs the bony anatomy and show the bony destruction earlier; it can also identify the extent of paravertebral abscess and soft tissue shadows. CT scan can provide details of facet joints integrity, which are important in deciding the timing and nature of surgical intervention. An important additional benefit of CT scan is its use for CT-guided biopsy of the lesion to obtain the cultural specimen [69]. Contrast-enhanced CT scans better delineate the abscess walls and infected granulation tissue.

MRI is the imaging study of choice because it is able to show the earlier signal intensity changes in the bone marrow and spinal cord.

MRI changes include: early decreased signal intensity in T1-weighted images and increased signal changes in T2-weighted images as a result of bone marrow edema; subligamentous extension of infection to the adjacent vertebrae, mainly anteriorly, is commonly observed. MRI can also provide information on the cause of the neurologic deficits. It can help identify mechanical compression by the abscess, granulation tissue, bony fragments, instability, and basilar impression. Intrinsic signal changes within the spinal cord can be clearly visualized.

A multilocular, calcified abscess in the retropharyngeal and paraspinal region with a thick, irregular enhancing rim and associated bony fragmentation is characteristic of TB; intraosseous, paravertebral, and epidural abscesses are clearly visualized by fat-suppressed, gadolinium contrast-enhanced MRI, and contrast-enhanced MRI can also help in differentiating granulation tissue, which shows homogeneous enhancement, from abscess, which has only rim enhancement.

A conclusive diagnosis cannot be achieved from radiologic features alone, hence a biopsy is of paramount importance. Lesions located in the anterior aspect of C1 and C2 can be approached by the transoral route; in the presence of instability or neurologic deficit, the definitive procedure can also be performed at the same stage.

34.5.4 Management

The goals of management of C-spine TB include cure of the disease and prevention or reversal of any neurologic deficit. In early stages of the infection, effective medical therapy has made conservative treatment possible, whereas, in patients at risk for instability, deformity, or impending neurologic deficit, surgical intervention is favored.

Conservative choice remains the standard of care for most patients. Indeed, antibiotics and improving imaging modalities have made mortality and morbidity dropped from 25% to 56% in past years to <5% in modern era [70–72].

Factors that influence CVJ TB management are response to medical therapy, the extent of bone destruction with presence of AAD and invariably neurological patient status and degree of cord compression.

34.5.4.1 Surgical Management: Indications

Decision-making regarding surgery must take into account the modality of spread, degree of bone destruction, with occipital condyle and articular joints involvement being more important, nature and progression of neurological symptoms [62].

Although chemotherapy achieves disease clearance, it cannot arrest instability and development and progression of deformity; medical therapy, furthermore, may not be successful in some kind of patients with neurologic deficit caused by mechanical conditions such as retropulsed bony fragments and pathologic dislocation.

The present opinion regarding CVJ TB management switches from total conservative [73] to total surgery [74] and once surgical treatment is chosen, posterior vs anterior and posterior route or anterior transoral or endoscopic modality is the second step.

To date, there are sparse grading systems that help to guide treatment modalities. Lifeso's system, for example, is based only on radiological features (as early mentioned) [63] and supports, as Edward et al. sustained [74], a 2-stage surgical procedure with transoral decompression and posteriorly successive fixation. On the other hand, Gupta et al. [73] treated all patients with immobilization and external brace, regardless of clinical grade.

Recently Behari et al. [75] described a clinical grading system and grouped patients on the basis severity of clinical manifestation into two categories: those with minor deficit and those with major deficit. The former include patients with neck pain and minor disability that not interfere with daily life; the latter include patient with major disability and totally or partly dependent daily activity by other. On the basis of this system, both treatments, medical and surgical ones, are advocate: all patients with minor deficit were treated with antitubercular medical therapy alone, whereas all patients with major deficit were treated with surgery and medical therapy.

More recently, Teegala et al. [76] have developed a grading system in which radiological and clinical data were assessed and guided initial treatment. They grouped their patients (71 patients) into 3 grade: grade 1 (score 3–4); grade 2 (score 5–6); grade 3 (score 7–8) on the basis of three parameters: restriction of active neck movement (score 1–2); motor strength: minimal (Medical Research Council power > 4), severe (Medical Research Council power < 4), none (score 1–3); radiological score: retropharyngeal collection and/or evidence of bone destruction on C2 (score 1–3). The author treated all grade 3 patient [8] surgically (single-stage transoral decompression and posterior fusion) and grade 1 [27] and 2 [36] patients initially conservatively and only patient with reducible residual AAD [5] underwent surgical posterior fixation.

Therefore, in CVJ TB, surgery is less frequently indicated and may be required early in patients with severe disability and presence and progression of neurological deficits [77] with AAD or in patients that are responsive to medical therapy and residual AAD.

Qureshi et al. [56] recommended that all patients with CVJ TB and symptoms and signs of neurological deficits due to instability who fail to respond to 4–6 weeks of conservative treatment (medical therapy and external brace) should undergo posterior surgery (C0-C1/C2 fusion), with or without posterior decompression; anterior surgery is reserved in those few cases that do not improve neurologically after posterior fusion.

In either treatment, as short-term (6 months) chemotherapy has been associated with poor outcome, the authors suggested a prolonged (up to 18 months) medical regimen [73, 75, 78].

Hence in general, in CVJ TB, surgical treatment with the goals of debridement of the infected tissues, bony fragments, and disk to achieve spinal cord decompression and restore stability should be reserved in the following instances:

1. failure of clinical and radiologic improvement after medical therapy for at least 6–8 weeks.
2. acute and severe neurologic deficit following destruction of at least 50% of vertebral body with impending spinal cord compression.
3. instability in the form of AAD and subluxation.
4. retropharyngeal abscess associated to dyspnea, dysphagia, and dysphonia.
5. early mobilization in patients at risk for complications.

Surgical options depend on whether the site of TB involvement is atlantoaxial or axial-subaxial cervical spine and whether basilar invagination exists.

Posterior surgical procedures, in terms of occipito-axial or occipito-subaxial fusion, are performed as adjuncts to anterior surgical ones (either micro- or endoscopically). An isolated posterior surgical procedure for an anterior located lesion, irrespective of the cause, is contraindicated, as stated by Menezes AH [79] because it does not hit the anterior lesion and compromises the stability provided by the retained normal posterior structures.

As mentioned earlier, the antero-lateral routes should be the endonasal endoscopic or transoral/retropharyngeal technique.

Transoral technique has been the standard surgical corridor to decompress C1-C2 and is performed through transpharyngeal mucosa and provides exposure rostral from inferior tip of clivus to caudally the C2–3 space and laterally for 2 cm to either side of the midline.

The disadvantage of transoral approach is a long surgical corridor to traverse, limited visualization: laterally, the exposure is limited by the hypoglossal condylar canals, the Eustachian tubes, and the vertebral arteries; inferiorly by the degree of depression of the tongue, a lack in a sufficient working distance (2.5–3 cm) between the upper and lower incisor teeth; upward the exposure may be limited by soft palate (some authors advocate division of soft palate to achieve more rostral exposition:

transoral-transpalatopharyngeal approach); impairment of mucosal healing, CSF leakage; oropharyngeal swelling with necessity of tracheostomy.

Retropharyngeal approach is performed medial to sternocleidomastoid muscle through transverse submandibular incision via suprahyoid dissection. The latter has the disadvantage of wide anatomical dissection of cervical fasciae and a superior oblique trajectory that makes difficult a decompression of wide spread of infection.

Several authors have described the transnasal approach to CVJ [80–83] and have a comparison to standard transoral approach [84, 85]. The advantage of endoscopic endonasal approach (EEA) to CVJ is full visualization of deep seated structures, early nasal mucosal healing, and reduction of post-operative intubations; it appears to be superior to standard approach, when lesion extends upstairs over the inferior third of the clivus. The disadvantages are the anatomical limit of hard palate that prevents the use of endoscopy below C2; a long learning curve with instrumentation; and a multidisciplinary team.

Therefore, the appropriate choice is based on surgeon's experience, on extension and type of CVJ involvement, and on anatomical consideration as stated by a recent cadaveric study [82].

References

1. Capps E, Page TE, Rouse WHD. Hippocrates: on joints. In: Withington ET, editor. Hippocrates: the loeb classical library, vol. 3. London: W. Heinemann; 1927. p. 200–397.
2. Kuhn CG. Galen: De usupartium corporis humani. In: ClaudiiGaleni Opera Omnia, vol. 4. Hildesheim: Georg Olms; 1964. p. 42–119.
3. Pott P. Remarks on that kind of palsy of the lower limbs which is frequently found to accompany a curvature of the spine. London: Johnson; 1779.
4. Lannelongue OM. On acute osteomyelitis. Miscellaneous, pathological and practical medicine tracts. Paris; 1897
5. Reihsaus E, Waldbaur H, Seeling W. Spinal epidural abscess: a meta-analysis of 915 patients. Neurosurg Rev. 2000;232:175–204.
6. Hadjipavlou AG, Mader JT, Necessary JT, Muffoletto AJ. Hematogenous pyogenic spinal infections and their surgical management. Spine (Phila Pa 1976). 2000;25(13):1668–79.
7. Kaufman DM, Kaplan JG, Litman N. Infectious agents in spinal epidural abscesses. Neurology. 1980;30:844–50.
8. Yoo JU, Hart RA. Anatomy of the cervical spine. In: Emery SE, Boden SC, editors. Surgery of the cervical spine. Amsterdam: Elsevier; 2003. p. 1–10.
9. Heggeness M, Doherty B. The trabecular anatomy of the axis. Spine. 1993;18:1945–9.
10. Panjabi M, Duranceau J, Goel V, et al. Cervical human vertebrae. Quantitative three-dimensional anatomy for the middle and lower regions. Spine. 1991;16(8):861–9.
11. Dvorak J, Panjabi M. Functional anatomy of the alar ligaments. Spine. 1987;12:183–9.
12. Steinmetz MP, Mroz TE, Benzel EC. Craniovertebral junction: biomechanical considerations. Neurosurgery. 2010;66(3 Suppl):7–12.
13. Parke WW. The vascular relations of the upper cervical vertebrae. Orthop Clin North Am. 1978;9(4):879–89.
14. Schiff DCM, Parke WW. The arterial supply of the odontoid process (dens). Anat Rec. 1972;172:399–400.
15. Sherk HH, Parke WW. Normal adult anatomy. In: Bailey RW, Sherk HH, et al., editors. The cervical spine. Philadelphia: JB Lippincott; 1983. p. 8–22.

16. Parke WW, Rothman RH, Brown MD. The pharyngovertebral veins. An anatomical rationale for Grisel's syndrome. J Bone Jt Surg Am. 1984;66:568–74.
17. Menezes AH. Congenital and acquired abnormalities of the craniovertebral junction (children and adults). In: Youmans J, editor. Neurological surgery. 4th ed. Philadelphia: Saunders; 1995. p. 1035–89.
18. Patel A, Madigan L, Poelstra K, et al. Acute cervical osteomyelitis and prevertebral abscess after routine tonsillectomy. Spine J. 2008;8(5):827–30.
19. Samuel D, Thomas DM, Tierney PA, Patel KS. Atlanto-axial subluxation (Grisel's syndrome) following otolaryngological disease and procedures. J Laryngol Otol. 1995;109(10):1005–9.
20. Ueki Y, Watanabe J, Hashimoto S, Takahashi S. Cervical spine osteomyelitis and epidural abscess after chemoradiotherapy for hypopharyngeal carcinoma: a case report. Case Rep Otolaryngol. 2014;2014:141307.
21. Goulart CR, Mattei TA, Fiore ME, Thoman WJ, Mendel E. Retropharyngeal abscess with secondary osteomyelitis and epidural abscess: proposed pathophysiological mechanism of an underrecognized complication of unstable craniocervical injuries: case report. J Neurosurg Spine. 2016;24(1):197–205.
22. Nurata H, Yilmaz MB, Borcek AO, Oner AY, Baykaner MK. Retropharyngeal hematoma secondary to whiplash injury in childhood: a case report. Turk Neurosurg. 2012;22(4):521–3.
23. Lin JY, Wang CH, Huang TW. Traumatic retropharyngeal hematoma: case report. Auris Nasus Larynx. 2007;34(3):423–5. Epub 2006 Dec 11.
24. Robinson MH, Young JD, Burge PD. Retropharyngeal abscess, airway obstruction, and tetraplegia after hyperextension injury of the cervical spine: case report. J Trauma. 1992;32(1):107–9.
25. Kapeller P, Fazekas F, Krametter D, et al. Pyogenic infectious spondylitis: clinical, laboratory and MRI features. Eur Neurol. 1997;38(2):94–8.
26. Beronius M, Bergman B, Andersson R. Vertebral osteomyelitis in Göteborg, Sweden: a retrospective study of patients during 1990-95. Scand J Infect Dis. 2001;33(7):527–32.
27. Doutchi M, Seng P, Menard A, et al. Changing trends in the epidemiology of vertebral osteomyelitis in Marseille, France. New Microbes New Infect. 2015;7:1–7.
28. Akiyama T, Chikuda H, Yasunaga H, Horiguchi H, Fushimi K, Saita K. Incidence and risk factors for mortality of vertebral osteomyelitis: a retrospective analysis using the Japanese diagnosis procedure combination database. BMJ Open. 2013;3(3):e002412.
29. Malawski SK, Lukawski S. Pyogenic infection of the spin. Clin Orthop Relat Res. 1991;272:58–66.
30. Perrone C, Saba J, Behloul Z, et al. Pyogenic and tuberculous spondylodiskitis (vertebral oseteomyelitis) in 80 adult patients. Clin Infect Dis. 1994;19(4):746–50.
31. Sapico FL, Montgomerie JZ. Pyogenic vertebral osteomyelitis: report of nine cases and review of the literature. Rev Infect Dis. 1979;1(5):754–76.
32. Koppel BS, Tuchman AJ, Mangiardi JR, et al. Epidural spinal infection in intravenous drug abusers. Arch Neurol. 1988;45(12):1331–7.
33. Fernandez M, Carrol CL. Baker Cj: discitis and vertebral osteomyelitis in children: an 18-year review. Pediatrics. 2000;105(6):1299–304.
34. Rosenberg AE. Bones, joints, and soft-tissue tumors. In: Kumar V, Abbas AK, Fausto N, et al., editors. Robbins and Cotran pathologic basis of disease. 8th ed. Philadelphia: Saunders Elsevier; 2010. p. 1221–3.
35. Sapico FL, Montgomerie JZ. Vertebral osteomyelitis. Infect Dis Clin North Am. 1990;4(3):539–50.
36. Stone JL, Cybulski GR, Rodriguez J, Gryfinski ME, Kant R. Anterior cervical debridement and strut-grafting for osteomyelitis of the cervical spine. J Neurosurg. 1989;70(6):879–83.
37. Ross J, Brant-Zawadzki M, Chen M, Moore K, Salzman K. Diagnostic imaging: spine. 1st ed. Altona: Amirsys; 2004. p. 1–14.
38. Busche M, Bastian L, Riedemann NC, et al. Complete osteolysis of the dens with atlantoaxial luxation caused by infection with Staphylococcus aureus. Spine (Phila Pa 1976). 2005;30(13):E369–74.. Review

39. Thelander U, Larsson S. Quantitation of C-reactive protein levels and erythrocyte sedimentation rate after spinal surgery. Spine (Phila Pa 1976). 1992;17(4):400–4.
40. Halla JT, Bliznak JG, Finn S. Septic arthritis of the C1–C2 lateral facet joint and torticollis: pseudo- Grisel's syndrome. Arthritis Rheum. 1991;34(1):84–8.
41. Marin C, Sanchez-Alegre M, et al. Magnetic resonance imaging of osteoarticular infections in children. Curr Probl Diagn Radiol. 2004;33(2):43–59.
42. Brant-Zawadzki M, Burke VD, Jeffrey RB. CT in the evaluation of spine infection. Spine (Phila Pa 1976). 1983;8(4):358–64.
43. Modic MT, Feiglin DH, Piraino DW, et al. Vertebral osteomyelitis: assessment using MR. Radiology. 1985;157(1):157–66.
44. Noguchi S, Yanaka K, Yamada Y, et al. Diagnostic pitfalls in osteomyelitis of the odontoid process: case report. Surg Neurol. 2000;53(6):573–8; discussion 578–9. Review.
45. Haridas A, Walsh DC, Mowle DH. Polymicrobial osteomyelitis of the odontoid process with epidural abscess: case report and review of literature. Skull Base. 2003;13(2):107–11.
46. Shamim MS, Tahir MZ, Jooma R. Isolated tuberculosis of C2 spinous process. Spine J. 2009;9(4):e30–2.
47. Schmit P, Glorion C. Osteomyelitis in infants and children. Eur Radiol. 2004;14(Suppl 4):L44–54. Review.
48. Chang MC, Wu HT, Lee CH, Liu CL, Chen TH. Tuberculous spondylitis and pyogenic spondylitis: comparative magnetic resonance imaging features. Spine (Phila Pa 1976). 2006;31(7):782–8.
49. Bruschwein DA, Brown ML, McLeod R. Gallium scintigraphy in the evaluation of disk-space infections: concise communication. J Nucl Med. 1980;21(10):925–7.
50. Haase D, Martin R, Marrie T. Radionuclide imaging in pyogenic vertebral osteomyelitis. Clin Nucl Med. 1980;5(12):533–7.
51. Schofferman L, Schofferman J, Zucherman J, Gunthorpe H, Hsu K, Picetti G, Goldthwaite N, White A. Occult infections causing persistent low-back pain. Spine (Phila Pa 1976). 1989;14(4):417–9.
52. Staab EV, McCartney WH. Role of gallium 67 in inflammatory disease. Semin Nucl Med. 1978;8(3):219–34.
53. Love C, Patel M, Lonner BS, Tomas MB, Palestro CJ. Diagnosing spinal osteomyelitis: a comparison of bone and Ga-67 scintigraphy and magnetic resonance imaging. Clin Nucl Med. 2000;25(12):963–77.
54. World Health Organization. Global tuberculosis control, WHO report. Geneva: World Health Organization; 2010.
55. Akhaddar A, Gourinda H, Gazzaz M, Elmadhi T, Elalami Z, Miri A. Craniocervical junction tuberculosis in children. Rev Rhum Engl Ed. 1999;66(12):739–42.
56. Qureshi MA, Afzal W, Khalique AB, Pasha IF, Aebi M. Tuberculosis of the craniovertebral junction. Eur Spine J. 2013;22(Suppl 4):612–7. Epub 2012 Oct 5.
57. Allali F, Benomar A, El YM, Chkili T, Hajjaj-Hassouni N. Atlantoaxial tuberculosis: three cases. Joint Bone Spine. 2000;67(5):481–4.
58. Mohindra S, Gupta SK, Mohindra S, Gupta R. Unusual presentations of craniovertebral junction tuberculosis: a report of 2 cases and literature review. Surg Neurol. 2006;66(1):94–9; discussion 99.
59. Hsu LC, Leong JC. Tuberculosis of the lower cervical spine (C2 to C7). J Bone Joint Surg Br. 1984;66(1):1–5.
60. Kim NH, Lee HM, Suh JS. Magnetic resonance imaging for the diagnosis of tuberculous spondylitis. Spine (Phila Pa 1976). 1994;19(21):2451–5.
61. Goel A, Goel N, Shah A. Pathogenesis of tuberculosis of the craniovertebral junction: its implication in surgical management. In: Goel A, Cacciola F, editors. The craniovertebral junction: diagnosis, pathology, surgical techniques. Stuttgart: Georg Thieme Verlag; 2011. p. 415–22.
62. Goel A, Shah A. Lateral atlantoaxial facetal dislocation in craniovertebral region tuberculosis: report of a case and analysis of an alternative treatment. Acta Neurochir. 2010;152:709–12.
63. Lifeso R. Atlanto-axial tuberculosis in adults. J Bone Joint Surg Br. 1987;69(2):183–7.

64. Tuli SM. Tuberculosis of the craniovertebral region. Clin Orthop Relat Res. 1974;104:209–12.
65. Fang D, Leong JC, Fang HS. Tuberculosis of the upper cervical spine. J Bone Joint Surg Br. 1983;65(1):47–50.
66. Bhattacharya A, Banerjee S, Mukherjee SC, Gangopadhyay S. Atypical spinal tuberculosis. J Indian Med Assoc. 1996;94(9):353–4.
67. Dhammi IK, Singh S, Jain AK. Hemiplegic/monoplegic presentation of cervical spine (C1-C2) tuberculosis. Eur Spine J. 2001;10(6):540–4.
68. Sharif HS, Morgan JL, al Shahed MS, al Thagafi MY. Role of CT and MR imaging in the management of tuberculous spondylitis. Radiol Clin North Am. 1995;33(4):787–804. Review.
69. Stoker DJ, Kissin CM. Percutaneous vertebral biopsy: a review of 135 cases. Clin Radiol. 1985;36(6):569–77.
70. Mavrogenis AF, Igoumenou V, Tsiavos K, Megaloikonomos P, Panagopoulos GN, Vottis C, Giannitsioti E, Papadopoulos A, Soultanis KC. When and how to operate on spondylodiscitis: a report of 13 patients. Eur J Orthop Surg Traumatol. 2016;26(1):31–40.
71. Hoshino C, Narita M. Craniovertebral junction tuberculosis: a case report and review of the literature. J Infect Chemother. 2010;16(4):288–91.
72. Arora S, Sabat D, Maini L, Sural S, Kumar V, Gautam VK, Gupta A, Dhal A. The results of nonoperative treatment of craniovertebral junction tuberculosis: a review of twenty-six cases. J Bone Joint Surg Am. 2011;93(6):540–7.
73. Gupta SK, Mohindra S, Sharma BS, Gupta R, Chhabra R, Mukharjee KK, Tewari MK, Khandelwal N, Suresh NM, Khosla VK. Tuberculosis of the craniovertebral junction: is surgery necessary? Neurosurgery. 2006;58(6):1144–50; discussion 1144-50.
74. Edwards RJ, David KM, Crockard HA. Management of tuberculomas of the craniovertebral junction. Br J Neurosurg. 2000;14(1):19–22.
75. Behari S, Nayak SR, Bhargava V, Banerji D, Chhabra DK, Jain VK. Craniocervical tuberculosis: protocol of surgical management. Neurosurgery. 2003;52(1):72–80; discussion 80-1.
76. Teegala R, Kumar P, Kale SS, Sharma BS. Craniovertebral junction tuberculosis:a new comprehensive therapeutic strategy. Neurosurgery. 2008;63(5):946–55.
77. Goel A. Tuberculosis of craniovertebral junction: role of facets in pathogenesis and treatment. J Craniovertebr Junct Spine. 2016;7(3):129–30.
78. Chadha M, Argawal A, Singh AP. Craniovertebral tuberculosis: a retrospective review of 13 cases managed conservatively. Spine (Phila Pa 1976). 2007;32(15):1629–34.
79. Menezes AH, VanGilder JC, Graf CJ, McDonnell DE. Craniocervical abnormalities. A comprehensive surgical approach. J Neurosurg. 1980;53(4):444–55.
80. Kassam AB, Snyderman C, Gardner P, Carrau R, Spiro R. The expanded endonasal approach: a fully endoscopic transnasal approach and resection of the odontoid process: technical case report. Neurosurgery. 2005;57(1 Suppl):E213, discussion E213.
81. Burns TC, Mindea SA, Pendharkar AV, Lapustea NB, Irime I, Nayak JV. Endoscopic transnasal approach for urgent decompression of the craniocervical junction in acute skull base osteomyelitis. J Neurol Surg Rep. 2015;76(1):e37–42.
82. Seker A, Inoue K, Osawa S, Akakin A, Kilic T, Rhoton AL Jr. Comparison of endoscopic transnasal and transoral approaches to the craniovertebral junction. World Neurosurg. 2010;74(6):583–602.
83. Nayak JV, Gardner PA, Vescan AD, Carrau RL, Kassam ABSC, Snyderman CH. Experience with the expanded endonasal approach for resection of the odontoid process in rheumatoid disease. Am J Rhinol. 2007;21(5):601–6.
84. Visocchi M, Di Martino A, Maugeri R, González Valcárcel I, Grasso V, Paludetti G. Videoassisted anterior surgical approaches to the craniocervical junction: rationale and clinical results. Eur Spine J. 2015;24(12):2713–23.
85. Visocchi M, Germano A, Umana G, Richiello A, Raudino G, Eldella AM, Iacopino G, Barbagallo G. Direct and oblique approaches to the craniovertebral junction: nuances of microsurgical and endoscope-assisted techniques along with a review of the literature. Acta Neurochir Suppl. 2017;124:107–16.

Rheumatoid Cervical Myelopathy

35

Kuntal Kanti Das, Satyadeo Pandey, Shruti Gupta, and Sanjay Behari

35.1 Introduction

Rheumatoid arthritis (RA) is a chronic, systemic inflammatory disorder affecting primarily the synovial joints of the body [1–3]. Although the peripheral joints of the hands and feet bear the brunt of the disease, cervical spine remains the second most commonly affected site [4–6]. As a matter of fact, RA is the commonest inflammatory disorder of the cervical spine. The occipito-atlanto-axial complex is most severely affected by the rheumatoid process. Progression of the inflammatory process leads to a combination of atlanto-axial subluxation (AAS), cranial settling (CS) or basilar invagination (BI) and subaxial subluxation (SAS) [1, 2, 6, 7]. The resultant clinical manifestations are the major causes of morbidity and mortality in RA. Although the advent and widespread use of the disease-modifying antirheumatic drugs (DMARD) and the molecular targeted therapies (MTT) have improved the overall outcome in RA, these medications are largely unable to prevent the progression of symptomatic cervical rheumatoid disease [3, 6, 7].

Surgical fixation of the diseased spinal segment has remained the treatment of choice over the years [1, 2, 6–8]. Progressively, these patients are being operated earlier in their disease course, unlike in the past. The surgical fixation techniques as well as the instrumentations have significantly changed over the last few decades, paralleling the changes in the management of congenital cranio-vertebral junction (CVJ) anomalies. Segment sparing surgery (atlanto-axial fusion rather than occipito-cervical fusion) is rapidly becoming the initial treatment of choice unless the disease is rather advanced [8]. A number of recent studies have shown promising results of surgery even in the patients with worst preoperative

K. K. Das · S. Pandey · S. Gupta · S. Behari (✉)
Department of Neurosurgery, Sanjay Gandhi Postgraduate Institute of Medical Sciences, Lucknow, India

E. Tessitore et al. (eds.), *Surgery of the Cranio-Vertebral Junction*,
https://doi.org/10.1007/978-3-030-18700-2_35

neurological grades (Ranawat IIIb) [9–12]. Despite all these advancements, the role and timing of prophylactic surgery in the asymptomatic radiological disease still remains unclear [1, 13, 14].

35.2 Disease Burden and Natural History

35.2.1 Burden of Disease

The exact incidence of RA is not known. Approximately 41 new cases of RA over the age of 18 every year are diagnosed per 100,000 individuals worldwide [1, 14, 15]. It is estimated that 1–2% of the world's population is affected by RA at any given point of time [15]. Similarly, the exact figures of the cervical spine involvement in RA are not known, although it is believed to affect more than half of the RA patients. The figures vary from studies to studies and the incidence of radiological involvement of CVJ is thought to be higher than the symptomatic clinical disease. It is also possible that the advent and widespread use of newer drugs in RA have affected the incidence and the prevalence in the relatively newer publications. The prevalence of radiological cervical spine involvement is reported to be between 17 and 85% worldwide [1, 3, 6, 7, 14]. However, it is to be noted that only about 7–34% of these patients will present with neurological deficits secondary to these changes [1, 16]. A number of factors like severity of the peripheral joint disease, DMARD failure, prolonged corticosteroid usage, and the severity of RA itself (elevated levels of rheumatoid factor (RF) and erythrocyte sedimentation rate (ESR)) are known to be associated with the development as well as prognosis of the cervical spine disease [1, 7, 17, 18].

35.2.2 Natural History

The natural history of the rheumatoid cervical spine is variable although a large majority of the patients eventually progress to severe morbidity and death [14, 16, 19]. Earlier studies probably underestimated the natural history by labeling it rather benign. However, nowadays, we know that cervical spine involvement is seen in up to 85% of patients that is frequently progressive and potentially devastating [1, 5, 7, 13, 16–18, 20–23].

Most of the information on the natural history of the ailment has been derived from the experience of conservative management in rheumatoid cervical spine disease. In a relatively recent prospective study of 140 patients with definite RA followed over a period of 5 years, Yurube et al., [22] noted a 43.6% incidence of cervical instability, with a clinically severe disease prevalent in nearly 12.9%, of the patients. Administration of corticosteroids, established mutilating changes at baseline, and the development into mutilating changes during the follow-up period were identified as risk factors for "severe" instability in their study. Other authors have reported progression rates as high as 80 to 87% over 6 to 10 years [20, 21]. In the latest update of their patient cohort prospectively followed for more than 10 years, Yurube et al. [23] documented a highly significant conversion to spinal instability and severe clinical disease with increasing duration of follow-up. They noted an additional requirement of surgery for peripheral joint disease as another factor contributing to accelerated disease progression in the cervical spine.

It is believed that the evolution of medical therapy in RA has probably affected the natural history of the disease in recent times. Optimal treatment of RA using these agents can delay the involvement of the cervical spine. Of particular note, these drugs largely fail to prevent the progression of symptomatic cervical rheumatoid disease [3, 6, 7]. As far as the timing of cervical spine involvement is concerned, it can be as early as within 2 years of detection of RA or alternatively, it may be delayed for many years. This large variation in the lag period is probably related to the activity of the primary disease. AAS is the earliest pathological change observed in these patients. As the disease progresses, facet joint erosion results in progressive cranial settling (CS). Eventually, subaxial subluxations (SASs) begin to appear potentially leading to dire consequences including death. In one study, none of the patients survived after 7 years of developing clinical disease progression. Of particular note, nearly 50% of the mortalities take place within the first year of diagnosis of instability. Appearance of the CS is particularly associated with a dismal outcome [24].

A number of predictors have been proposed to signify the likelihood of disease progression. These include the disease duration, male gender, RF seropositivity, severe peripheral disease, prolonged steroid use, and increased C-reactive protein level [22–26]. Imagama and colleagues found that the presence of severe large joint disease (disease of shoulders, elbows, hips, and knees) called as the "large joint index" correlated significantly with AAS, CS, and an increased posterior atlanto-dental interval (PADI) [26].

35.3 Pathogenesis and Pathology

35.3.1 Pathogenesis

RA affects the synovial joints throughout the human body. This condition results from a complex interplay of genetic, environmental, and immune system related factors. The initiating factor is probably exposure to certain unknown antigens displayed by the synovial tissues of the genetically predisposed patients. Abnormal proliferation of the plasma cells occurs under the influence of the helper T cells (CD4+) to deal with this unknown event. These plasma cells lead to abnormal and excessive production of auto-antibodies like rheumatoid factor (RF) and anti-citric citrullinated peptides (anti-CCP) that target unknown antigens expressed by the synovial tissues of the target joints. Elaboration of cytokines like interleukin I and VI, and tumor necrosis factor alpha accentuate the inflammatory onslaught on the synovial membranes [4]. There is formation of an expanding mass of proliferating inflammatory cells and fibroblasts, known as the pannus. The inflammatory pannus elaborates certain enzymes/biproducts like tissue metalloproteinase and osteoclast-like factors leading to destruction of the joint capsules, the articular cartilage, and the subchondral bone [26]. There is loosening, tear, or even rupture of the surrounding ligaments giving rise to the classical joint dislocations and deformities. In addition, the poor nutritional status, prolonged immobilization, and long-term steroid/cytotoxic drug usage contribute to the osteopenia and fractures associated with this condition.

In the cervical spine, the zygapophyseal and uncovertebral joints are synovial in nature. Moreover, there are two synovial joints, one each on the anterior and the posterior aspects of the odontoid process of the axis. With such a dense aggregation of the synovial joints, it is not surprising that the cervical spine is so commonly and so severely affected in RA. The intervertebral disk spaces are not affected primarily as these are fibrous joints and are avascular. Therefore, the lack of an intervertebral disk, an inherently increased mobility, and the presence of multiple synovial joints make the occipito-atlantal-axis complex the most vulnerable segment for rheumatoid involvement. The intervertebral disks, however, eventually get affected from the extension of the surrounding inflammatory pannus. This explains the delayed appearance of subaxial cervical instability.

35.3.2 Pathology

The clinical manifestations and resultant morbidity in rheumatoid cervical myelopathy are the direct results of the underlying pathological changes in the bony spine. These pathologies lead to a combination of static and dynamic damage to the underlying neurovascular structures. The static compression is usually due to the retro-odontoid mass and less commonly due to fixed or locked bony dislocations [27, 28]. The different dynamic mechanisms of cord damage include the atlanto-axial subluxation (AAS), cranial settling (CS) or basilar invagination (BI) and subaxial subluxation (SAS) [1, 2, 6, 7]. In addition, there may be atraumatic fractures of the odontoid process and destruction of the lateral masses.

The vertebral arteries are not affected directly. Compression and kinking of VA may, however, add to the neurological decline in the advanced stages [4]. While all these local changes are happening in the cervical spine, other systems of the body like the pulmonary, cardiovascular, and the musculocutaneous systems develop various complications that may affect the final outcome after surgery in these patients [29].

35.3.2.1 Retro-Odontoid Soft Tissue (ROST)

The soft tissue mass that typically forms behind the odontoid process in RA has been a matter of much debate [27, 28]. It is commonly referred to as the "retro-odontoid pseudo tumor." ROST is generally believed to represent the inflammatory pannus, comprising inflammatory cells and necrotic fibrocartilage. Although the exact incidence is not known, it is believed that only some patients with rheumatoid cervical spine affliction go on to develop ROST. When present, ROST may cause persistent and static ventral compression on the cervico-medullary junction. These masses are thought to be derived from the inflammation of the para-odontoid synovial joints with thickening of the transverse atlantal ligament (TAL) and the tectorial membrane. Concurrent spinal instability is paramount for their maintenance and growth. The size of the ROST, and accordingly, their contribution to the patients' symptomatology may vary from patient to patient. Grob [30] proposed a radiological classification scheme for ROSTs comprising 4 grades: Grade 1 represents absent or minimal ROST, grade 2 indicates a moderate sized ROST, grade 3 indicates a large sized ROST but not causing cord compression, while grade 4 ROST is associated with spinal cord compression. Not all ROSTs are of the same character both histologically and on imaging. Yonezawa et al. [27] noted three different radiological types of ROST based on their intensity on T1- and T2-weighted magnetic resonance imaging (MRI). Type 1 ROST typically resembled the classic inflammatory pannus containing fluid inside the mass (T2 hyperintense); Type 2 ROST represented the "pseudo tumor" like pattern with T2-hypo- intensity suggesting the presence of fibrosis inside. Type 3 ROST displayed a mixed picture having features of both the previous types. ROSTs rarely require direct surgical approach and almost always regress or disappear following posterior fusion of the associated spinal instability. Yonezawa et al. [27] noted that type 1 ROST resolved the fastest after surgery while the type 2 ROST was much slower in regressing.

In a recent study, Dohzono et al. [28] noted that the thickness of ROST reduced with increasing severity of the atlanto-axial subluxation (AAS) and the peripheral joint disease. They postulated that the apparent decrease in the size of the ROST was probably because of the rupture and subsequent contracture of the TAL when atlanto-dental interval (ADI) exceeded 3–4 mm.

35.3.2.2 Atlanto-axial Subluxation (AAS)

AAS is the commonest (65%) and probably the earliest pathological change caused by rheumatoid involvement of the cervical spine. Rheumatoid AAS may be anterior, posterior, lateral, or a combination of these types. Anterior AAS accounts for nearly 75% of the dislocations seen clinically [1]. It usually results from incompetence of the transverse atlantal ligament (TAL). It should be remembered, however, that subluxations beyond 3–4 mm of the upper limit of the physiological range (also known as the anterior atlantodental interval [ADI, normal value: <3 mm]) require additional incompetence of the alar and the apical ligaments to manifest [22]. Asymmetric involvement of the C1/2 facet joints may give rise to lateral AAS. It accounts for 20% of all such cases and presents clinically with torticollis. Interestingly, a lateral radiograph may fail to diagnose the presence of lateral subluxation necessitating an open mouth odontoid view to appreciate the subtle joint asymmetry and neck tilt [16]. Posterior AAS is the rarest of all rheumatoid AASs (occurring in around 7% of the patients). It results from destruction/fracture of the odontoid process which enables posterior displacement of C1 arch over the C2 [31]. The lateral and the posterior types of AAS, although rare, result in significant cord compression and add to the difficulties in the surgical management [16, 19]. The AAS in RA is reducible in the initial stages. As the disease worsens further, the instability may become non-reducible. Non-reducibility is more likely when there is associated cranial settling or subaxial subluxation [29].

35.3.2.3 Cranial Settling (CS) or Basilar Invagination (BI)

Destruction of the C1/2 joint and C1 lateral mass leads to progressive invagination of the axis into the foramen magnum (incidence 4–35%) [32–34]. The odontoid and at times, the body of C2 vertebra end up compressing the cervico-medullary junction or the medulla oblongata itself. Associated local kyphosis may accentuate the compression further. The possibility of vertebral artery compression as well as sudden-onset death increases many folds with the development of this complication [32]. It is worthwhile to note that ADI spuriously normalizes when CS develops, thereby giving a false impression of improvement in the AAS [33, 34]. The obliquity of the anterior surface of the odontoid is responsible for this curious observation. Thus, as BI becomes more pronounced, the broader inferior aspect of the odontoid and C2 comes to lie at the level of the C1 arch with an apparent decrease in the ADI producing the erroneous impression of improvement in the AAS.

35.3.2.4 Subaxial Subluxation (SAS)

SAS is the last and the least commonly (7–29%) seen abnormality in rheumatoid involvement of the cervical spine [19, 23]. The destruction of the zygapophyseal/uncovertebral joints initially and intervertebral disks subsequently leads to sagittal displacement of the subaxial cervical spine. In addition, the cervical spines of these patients demonstrate disappearance of the normal interspinous bursae [35]. As mentioned previously, SAS may develop after the surgical fixation of the symptomatic CVJ disease [14, 29, 36, 37]. Chances of SAS are thought to be higher if the CVJ is fixed in a manner to leave an occipito-axial angle greater than 30 degrees [38].

35.4 Clinical Features

The manifestations of rheumatoid cervical spine may vary from no symptoms at all to the severest form of myelopathy where the patient is completely unable to ambulate. Although RA, as a whole, is more common in female patients, advanced cervical spine affection is probably commoner in male patients [14, 19]. Severe peripheral joint arthritis with muscle atrophy and contractures often mask the early myelopathic symptoms. Neck pain is usually an early manifestation and indicates instability at the level of the atlanto-axial complex. There may be associated restriction of the neck movements, particularly the rotational movement. Patients may additionally complain of clicking sounds with neck movements, a specific and often a characteristic symptom [1, 3]. Many patients complain of a feeling of their head falling forwards. Relief in neck pain on lying supine and the need to support the head while getting up from the bed are commonly reported. In addition, sub-occipital and occasional ear pain may be reported secondary to the irritation of the C2 nerve root.

Spasticity, limb weakness, and paresthesias herald the onset of myelopathy. As the disease progresses, the severity of myelopathy increases proportionately, eventually restricting the patient to the bed if the condition is not treated timely.

Table 35.1 Ranawat's classification of cervical myelopathy secondary to rheumatoid arthritis [50]

Class of myelopathy	Description of the disability
Class I	Neurologically intact
Class II	Subjective weakness with hyperreflexia and dysesthesia
Class IIIa	Objective weakness with long tract signs but ambulatory
Class IIIb	Objective weakness with long tract signs with disability to walk or feed oneself, quadriparesis

Of particular note, peripheral joint disease always precedes spinal manifestations. Therefore, signs of myelopathy are not as classical as observed in other causes of compressive myelopathy. Worsening of existing status of ambulation is unanimously agreed to be a harbinger of clinical myelopathy in RA [1, 3]. Pathological reflexes and Lhermitte's phenomenon are often demonstrable in the established cases.

Lower cranial nerve involvement in the form of difficulty in swallowing, nasal regurgitation of liquids, and change in voice with features of vertebro-basilar insufficiency (VBI) indicate CS [39]. VBI manifests as syncope, giddiness, tinnitus, and transient cerebellar signs, especially with attempted neck movements. Autonomic manifestations like bladder-bowel impairment and facial hypoesthesia appear rather late in the course of the disease.

35.5 Clinical Grading of the Functional Status in Rheumatoid Cervical Myelopathy

The conventional grading systems of compressive myelopathy like the modified Japanese Orthopedic Association Score (m-JOA), Nurick grading system, etc. do not apply in these patients due to severe pre-existing/accompanying musculoskeletal disability. The ability to walk forms an important parameter of judging the functional status of rheumatoid myelopathy. Therefore, certain specific grading systems have been proposed to qualify the functional status in rheumatoid cervical myelopathy. These include Ranawat's grading system and the American Rheumatologic Association (ARA) grading [1, 2, 40]. However, the most commonly utilized and widely validated scoring system across the world is the system proposed by Ranawat et al. Table 35.1 shows the details of Ranawat's grading system.

35.6 Role of Neuroimaging

Imaging plays an important role in assessing the extent of disease, establishing a baseline status for monitoring the disease progression over time, and most importantly, guiding the treatment. Plain radiographs, computed tomographic (CT) scan, and magnetic resonance imaging (MRI) of the CVJ including the entire cervical spine are necessary to properly characterize the disease.

35.6.1 Plain Radiographs

Plain radiographs of the cervical spine and the CVJ have played an important role in the evaluation of rheumatoid cervical myelopathy. These investigations remain relevant even in the current era of advanced imaging studies like CT scan and MRI. Different views utilized are the open mouth odontoid view, antero-posterior and trans-table lateral cervical radiographs including the dynamic lateral cervical spine flexion-extension views. The plain radiographs may reveal bony erosion and help in estimating the atlanto-dental interval (ADI), effective canal diameter (ECD), basilar invagination as well as subaxial cervical subluxation [1, 3, 6].

Certain specific points regarding the role of plain radiographs in rheumatoid cervical disease vis-à-vis congenital CVJ anomalies are worth mentioning here. An anterior atlanto-dental interval (ADI) more than 3 mm indicates pathological dislocation of the atlas over the axis in sagittal plane. This may not be a good indicator in rheumatoid CVJ disease for two reasons. First, the quality of bone and the resultant visualization on plain radiographs are not as good due to associated osteopenia, odontoid tip erosion, and pannus. Secondly, the ADI may appear within normal limits if there is associated CS, thus underestimating the grade of the disease [33, 34]. Therefore, the effective canal diameter (ECD), also known as the posterior atlanto-dental interval (PADI), is a more reliable indicator of anterior AAS in RA [1–3, 6, 24, 29]. The ECD or PADI of less than 14 mm indicates severe canal stenosis and correlates well with clinical status of the patient [1, 3, 6, 29]. Figure 35.1 depicts the typical findings on dynamic lateral radiographs in rheumatoid AAS.

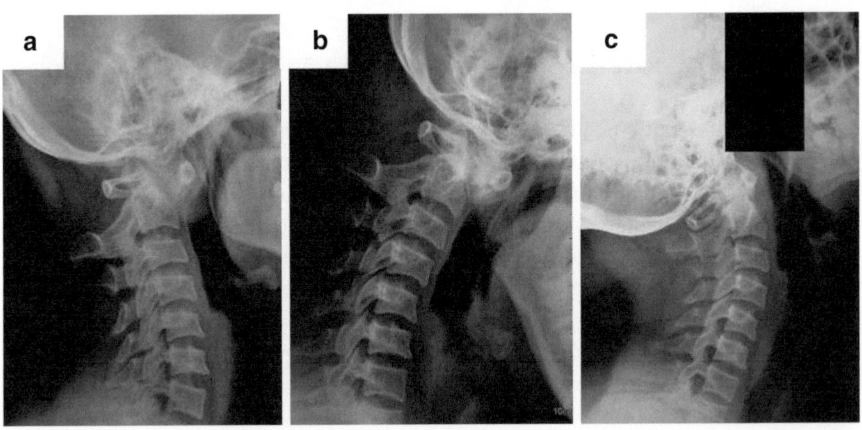

Fig. 35.1 Lateral cervical spine radiograph in neutral (**a**), flexion (**b**), and extension (**c**) views. The distance between anterior arch of atlas and the anterior surface of the odontoid, known as the anterior atlanto-dental interval (ADI), is increased in neutral film suggesting AAS. The distance between the posterior surface of the odontoid and the posterior arch of the atlas, known as the effective canal diameter (ECD) or the posterior atlanto-dental interval (PADI), is reduced. The ADI is increased in flexion (**b**) which becomes normal in extension (**c**) suggesting reducibility of the AAS. Also to be noted is the relative radiolucency of the odontoid compared to the axis body and the overlapping mastoid tip that hinder these assessments in the advanced stages of the disease

Similar to AAS, the conventional lines utilized for diagnosing BI or CS in congenital anomalies cannot be utilized in RA patients. Erosion/atraumatic fractures of the odontoid, presence of inflammatory pannus and osteopenia from a combination of causes affect clear visualization of the odontoid tip in these patients, thereby limiting the utility of the conventional lines [41]. Rather, lines that consider the odontoid height as a whole or the base of C2 body/pedicle, that are structures relatively well-preserved, are more useful. These lines/measurements include the Clark station, and the Redlund-Johnell and Ranawat's criteria [1, 2, 6, 8, 42, 43]. It has been proven that a combination of these 3 lines has better predictive value (nearly 90%) in diagnosing BI associated with RA than their use in isolation [42, 43]. These lines and criteria for diagnosing CS are detailed in Table 35.2.

Subaxial subluxations (SASs) are characterized by a step-like deformity of the vertebrae on lateral cervical radiograph. Typically, the posterior margin of the dislocated vertebra lies more than 3 mm ahead of the posterior margin of the inferior vertebra in flexion [1, 3, 6, 29, 43]. Similar to AAS, the space available for cord (SAC), a distance from the posterior margin of the vertebra to the spino-laminar line is a better predictor of the clinical disease. A diameter less than 10–12 mm at the level of dislocation indicates severe canal stenosis [1, 3, 6, 29, 43].

Despite their definite usefulness, the poor resolution, inability to assess the soft tissues, poor bone quality, and overlapping of structures like the mastoid tip are certain major limitations in the interpretation of plain radiographs in RA.

Table 35.2 Different craniometrics indices and their interpretations for making the diagnosis of cranial settling (CS) or basilar invagination (BI) in rheumatoid arthritis [42, 43]

Craniometric index	Description	Interpretation
Clark station	In the sagittal plane, the odontoid process is divided into three equal parts which are labeled as "stations." The stations are numbered I–III from odontoid tip to the base. The level at which the anterior arch of the atlas falls is determined	Normal: When anterior arch of atlas falls at the superior third, i.e., station I Mild CS: When anterior arch of atlas falls at the middle third, i.e., station II Severe CS: When anterior arch of atlas falls at the inferior third, i.e., station III
Redlund-Johnell criteria	In the sagittal plane, the distance between the inferior margin of C2 vertebral body and the McGregor line, i.e., the line drawn from the posterior end of the hard palate to the caudal cortical margin of the occiput is determined along the axis of C2	In CS or BI, the distance is less than 34 mm (males) or 29 mm (females)
Ranawat's criteria	In the sagittal plane, the distance between the center of the C2 pedicle and the transverse axis of atlas (Mc Rae's line) is measured along the axis of the odontoid process	In CS or BI, the value is typically less than 15 mm (males) or 13 mm (females)

35.6.2 Computed Tomographic (CT) Scan of the Cervical Spine Including CVJ

CT scan provides a better visualization of the bony anatomy compared to the plain radiographs. It is being increasingly used to study the pathologic bony anatomy before surgery [41, 43]. Moreover, volume rendering allows reconstruction of the complex anatomy in this area for proper surgical planning. Bony erosions or subluxation are better seen on CT scans. In the patients in whom an MRI cannot be performed, CT myelogram may be utilized to determine the level of spinal cord compression. Another advantage of the CT scan is the ability to image the vertebral arteries using CT angiography. The latter information is very useful during surgical exposure and instrumentation. CT scan allows exact measurement of the pedicles, laminae, and lateral masses to facilitate intraoperative decision-making pertaining to the choice and technique of instrumentation. Although dynamic study is possible in the CT scan as well, it probably underestimates the dynamic subluxation when compared to the plain films [41]. As Soderman et al. noted, this discrepancy between the plain radiographs and the CT scan is primarily due to different positioning employed for both these investigations [41]. They, however, found the CT scan to be better than the MRI in demonstrating dynamic changes inside the spinal subarachnoid space during spinal flexion. Figure 35.2 demonstrates the CT findings in a case of rheumatoid AAD. Note the ability to assess the lateral joints, their symmetry as well as the visualization of the pedicles on CT scan images.

35.6.3 MRI of the Cervical Spine Including the CVJ

MRI provides excellent soft tissue details of this region. The multiplanar images help in estimating the extent of the disease. The extent of inflammatory synovitis, pannus formation, and cord compression as well as the intramedullary changes secondary to the compression are clearly revealed on MR images [1, 7, 27, 28, 44]. The ROST, as previously mentioned, may have different signal intensities that may have different prognostic significance. In a recent study, Izuka et al. demonstrated that the intramedullary T2 hyperintensity correlated well with preoperative symptomatology. They noted disappearance of the T2 hyperintensity in 100% of their patients after surgery [44]. By taking into account the periodontoid soft tissue, MRI probably gives a better measurement of the effective canal diameter (ECD) than radiographs or CT scans. Additionally, cerebrospinal fluid pathway obstruction and associated hydrocephalus, if present, can be detected. Some authors have noted a relationship of the cervico-medullary angle measured on MRI and the patients' neurological status. This angle formed between ventral surface of the cervical spinal cord and the brainstem on midsagittal MRI normally measures

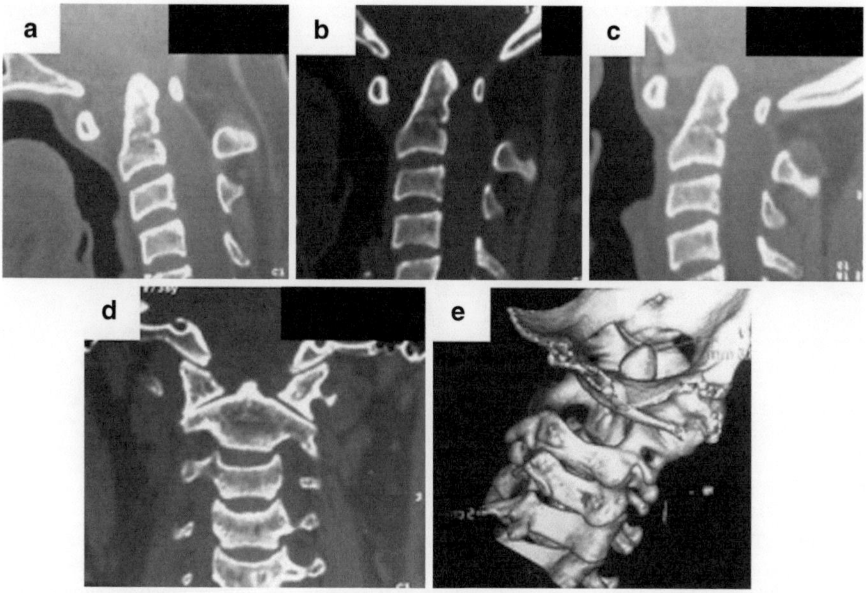

Fig. 35.2 CT scan of the cervical spine in a patient with rheumatoid cervical myelopathy shows excellent bony details with increased ADI with reduced ECD in neutral position (**b**). Note the subtle erosions/sclerosis on the posterior border of the odontoid. There is not much change in the ADI in flexion (**a**) and extension (**c**), a limitation of the CT scan over the plain radiographs. CT scan provides clear visualization of the lateral elements of occipito-atlantal-axial complex (**d**) for determining suitability of the newer instrumentation techniques and segment sparing atlanto-axial fusion. Reconstructed images help to estimate the sizes of the pars interarticularis/pedicle/lamina for choosing the size of the screws to be placed during fusion

between 135 and 175°. A value less than 135° usually implies significant CS and correlates well with clinical myelopathy [45]. Figure 35.3 demonstrates the MRI findings in a case of rheumatoid affection of the CV junction.

35.7 Management

Natural history studies have documented a progressive neurological decline and eventual death in the majority of these patients. The landmark study by Casey and Crockard highlighted the poor outcome of surgery in the advanced stages of the disease (Ranawat IIIb) [46]. Numerous studies have proven that timely surgical stabilization of the rheumatoid cervical spine can successfully prevent both radiological and clinical disease progression [8–12, 14, 43]. Therefore, it is unanimously agreed now that once a patient is diagnosed with rheumatoid cervical instability manifesting either as pain or as myelopathy, surgical fixation should not be delayed.

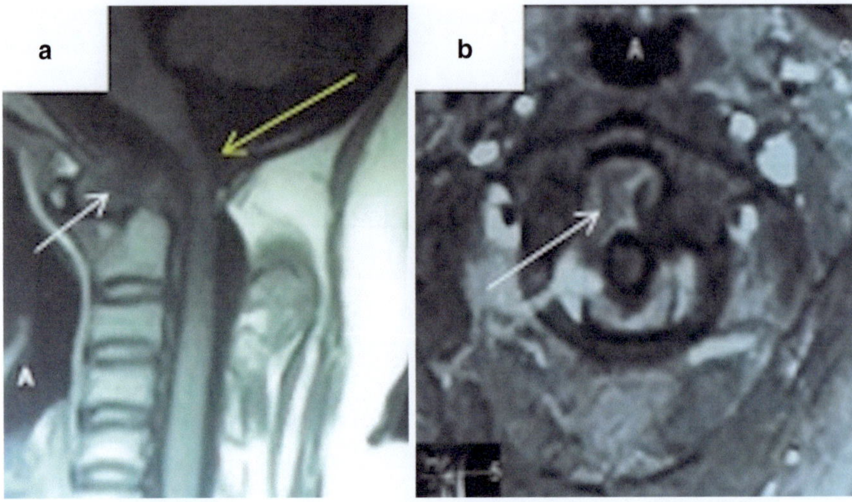

Fig. 35.3 T1-weighted MRI of the cervical spine shows destruction of the odontoid and a soft tissue mass consisting of the inflammatory pannus behind the anterior arch of the atlas shown with a white arrow (**a**). The compression and flattening of the cervico-medullary junction (shown with a yellow arrow) is well visualized (**a**). A T2 axial section shows the hyperintense pannus (marked with a white arrow) with compression and distortion of the spinal cord between the odontoid and the posterior arch of atlas. There is hyperintensity inside the cord suggesting myelomalacic changes secondary to the chronic compression

Prophylactic surgery in asymptomatic radiological disease, however, remains controversial at this point in time [13, 14, 43]. Continued radiological surveillance under cover of DMARDs/MTTs is probably the best thing to do until definitive evidences in favor of prophylactic surgery are published.

35.7.1 The Place of Conservative Treatment

Due to the lack of strong clinical evidence for recommending prophylactic cervical spine fusion at present, most rheumatologists prefer non-operative treatment in the early asymptomatic stages of the disease. Patients who do not have symptoms of the disease but show one or more of the radiological changes may be treated with a combination of medical therapy, neck immobilization using halo or cervical collars, supervised neck physiotherapy, and proper health education [14].

Medical therapy consists of DMARDS and MTTs as well as medications to treat osteopenia (calcium and vitamin D supplements, bisphosphonates) [14]. There are reports that active medical management of RA may delay the development of the symptomatic disease and may even lead to reduction in AAS. Immobilization of the spine is an important component of non-operative management. This can be achieved using a halo brace or a collar. Halo brace is very effective in reducing motion to enable healing to take place while the best medical treatment of RA is ongoing. Nannapaneni et al. [9] used halo brace preoperatively in their patients to relieve neurologic symptoms and to maintain realignment of the spine till the time of surgery. Miyomato et al. [29] maintained their patients on a preoperative halo for a period of 7 days that allowed them to achieve intraoperative alignment and fixation without much manipulation. The main problem with a halo is poor compliance on the part of the patients. Hard cervical collar, although often advised, hardly limits motion at the cervical spine. Supervised physiotherapy to strengthen the neck muscles may help in the initial part of the disease but its role is questionable and rather discouraged once neck pain starts.

Some people advocate non-operative treatment in Ranawat's stages I and II [14]. A recent systematic review has supported this understanding by documenting similar survival between operated and non-operated Ranawat's grade I and II patients. The same study, however, demonstrated higher chances of disease progression from Ranawat grade II onwards [14]. As the surgical results and postoperative care have improved drastically in recent times, the scope of non-operative treatment is getting limited day by day and an overwhelming majority of neurosurgeons over the world would advise surgery once symptomatic instability/myelopathy sets in.

35.7.2 Surgical Treatment

The surgical treatment aims to decompress the neural structures and at the same time to provide stability to the affected segment of the spine. The type and extent of surgery has changed a lot over time [9]. Earlier, ventral cord compression was almost always treated using transoral decompression (TOD) [47]. Recently, the endoscopic endonasal approach has been utilized for performing TOD [48]. The latter is reported to reduce complications of the traditional surgery while giving similar surgical outcomes. The technique and complications are similar to those seen in congenital CV junction malformations. TOD has, however, gradually diminished in popularity. This is mainly because of the realization that inflammatory pannus resolves after stabilization of the diseased spine and that the recent joint manipulation techniques render the so-called fixed AASs to reducible AASs on most occasions [49].

The posterior approach to the rheumatoid cervical spine/CVJ has become very popular as a standalone procedure in the recent times. In a recent review of the largest experience of such patients in the world, Bhatia et al. noted a gradual shift from the uniform occipito-cervical fusion to C1/2 fusion over the last 30-year period in their institute [9]. This could be attributable to the earlier referrals for surgery when the pathological changes are not fully developed so that a segment sparing C1/2 fusion may be all that is required. C1/2 fusion addresses the epicenter of the pathology and spares motion at the occipito-atlantal and subaxial joints that may be relatively normal in the initial stages of the disease. Reduction of motion at C1/2 level is known to halt the disease progression sufficiently to delay or at times obviate the need for an occipito-cervical fusion later [14, 29, 43].

There has been a change in the techniques of spinal fusion as well. Once popular, fusion procedures like Gallie's and Brooke's fusion or their modifications are seldom performed now-a-days. Rather, current techniques like Magerl's transarticular fusion and Goel-Harm's C1-C2 fusions focus on the lateral joints to ensure maximal reduction of motion and promote a solid bony fusion. Apart from treating AAS, these joint manipulations and joint jamming techniques using spacers/bone grafts help in the correction of BI as well as the rotational dislocation [49]. Nevertheless, poor bone quality and inflammatory erosion of the articular masses in the advanced stages of the disease coupled with inherent risks of VA injury remain major challenges with these recent techniques. Irrespective of the technique of fusion, adequate decompression of the spinal cord is the key. This may include a laminectomy, foramen magnum decompression, and rarely, removal of the inflammatory pannus. Intraoperative restoration of the C1/2 dislocation and distraction of the joints can also lead to indirect decompression of the cord akin to the ligamentotaxis for thoraco-lumbar fractures. Bony fusion is an important aspect of surgery and may be augmented by autologous grafts from ribs/iliac crest or bone substitutes.

Occipito-cervical fusion (OCF) in rheumatoid cervical spinal instability is usually indicated when the disease is relatively advanced radiologically and the patients have more than just a reducible AAS. In addition, posterior AASs are best treated using an OCF [29]. The techniques of OCF have also changed from the times of Ransford's loop to the current screw and rod fixation technique. The subaxial spinal disease determines the caudal limit of the fusion. Figure 35.4 shows the pre- and postoperative images in a patient with OCF for atlanto-axial instability secondary to RA.

SAS requires cervical fixation from a posterior approach as mentioned above. Very rarely, an acute kyphosis necessitates an anterior approach. Posterior approach

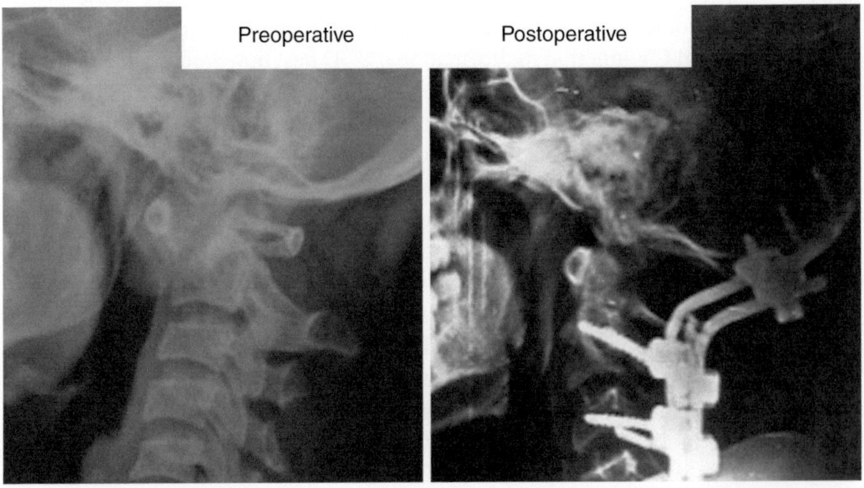

Fig. 35.4 Lateral cervical shows AAS with increased ADI preoperatively. The subluxation has been completely reduced with occipito-C2/3 fixation with normalization of the ADI postoperatively

usually involves a laminectomy and lateral mass fusion. The currently popular techniques are transarticular screw fixation or lateral mass fusion using screw and rod [14, 43]. However, SAS in the setting of RA is almost always preceded by AAS with or without CS. Therefore, OCF remains the treatment of choice in SAS [29].

35.7.3 Complications of Surgery

The current fixation techniques are very robust and do not need prolonged external immobilization anymore. The general complications of surgery are similar to those seen with congenital anomalies. Complication rates after surgery vary across different studies. The operative mortality ranges from 4 to 17%. Mortality rates increase with increasing duration of the systemic disease, severity of the RA, and preoperative clinico-radiological severity of the cervical myelopathy. As noted by Miyamoto et al., the incidence mortality rose from 26.5% in reducible AAS to 37.2% when there was additional SAS [29]. The main reasons for the underlying postoperative mortality are medical complications like pneumonia, massive gastrointestinal bleed, myocardial infarction, heart failure, etc. [29].

A higher incidence of surgical site infections, poor wound healing, and pseudoarthrosis are specific complications of surgical fixation in RA [29, 37]. Deep surgical site infections are particularly more common with OCF. More extensive dissection, increased operative times, more tissue handling, more blood loss, and an extensive hardware predispose to postoperative infections. Zygmunt et al. noted a 66% incidence of wound infection in their series of patients undergoing OCF [37]. More recently, Miyamato documented a relatively lesser incidence of 12.9% [29].

Progression of the subaxial disease remains another bane in the surgery of rheumatoid cervical spine [2, 14, 29, 43]. While the progression of the rheumatoid process in itself is the cause of this progression in some of the patients, failure to recognize and address any pre-existing SAS at the time of first surgery remains an important factor. Moreover, adjacent segment degeneration after a rigid spinal fusion may give rise to this not so uncommon complication. It has been reported following both C1/2 and OC fusion. The incidence of SAS after C1/2 fusion can be as high as 39% to 57% [43]. Krause et al. noted subaxial instability in 36% of their cases at a mean duration of 2.6 years after an initial short segment (O-C2) OCF [2]. Miyamato et al., while analyzing their experience over three decades with cervical spine fusions in RA, noted a 30% incidence of SAS after a short segment OCF (C2/3/4) [29]. They noted that patients undergoing a long segment (C0-C7 or T2) OCF often did not require revision surgery on account of SAS or pseudoarthrosis.

35.8 Surgical Outcome

The surgical outcome in rheumatoid cervical myelopathy is variable. A number of factors are involved in determining the outcome. Table 35.3 shows the different factors affecting outcome of rheumatoid cervical myelopathy following surgical

Table 35.3 Factors affecting outcome after surgery in rheumatoid cervical myelopathy

Clinical factors
Duration of RA
Severity of peripheral joint disease
Large joint disease
Peripheral joint surgery
Long standing use of steroids and other drugs
DMARD failure
Preoperative Ranawat's grade
Extent of visceral disease
Radiological factors
Number of pathologies
Posterior/lateral AAS
Presence of CS
Posterior atlanto-dental interval
Space available for cord in the midcervical spine
Laboratory values
RF levels
ESR level
CRP level
Postoperative factors
Progression of RA itself
Pseudoarthrosis
Infections
Progression of subaxial disease

treatment. A long duration of illness prior to surgery, severity of peripheral joint disease as well as the severity of the rheumatoid inflammatory process are important clinical determinants of the surgical outcome [1–3, 6, 22–26]. Peripheral joint disease severity has been reported by many to be predictive of not only the severity of the myelopathy but also the surgical outcome [26, 29]. Severe systemic inflammation, as indicated by high RF and C-reactive protein levels, indicating the presence of an uncontrolled systemic disease, is a poor prognostic factor. Poor response to DMARDs has also been recognized as a cause of suboptimal surgical outcome [43].

The most important determinant of surgical outcome is probably the preoperative functional grade. Numerous studies have found that the surgical outcome worsens with increasing preoperative Ranawat's grade. The utility of surgery in the neurologically "most devastated patients," i.e., in Ranawat grade IIIb, has been long debated. These patients constitute 24–36% of all rheumatoid cervical myelopathy patients [14, 43]. A number of recent studies have reported encouraging improvements in the functional grade (by at least 1 grade) in these patients after surgery [9–12]. van Asselt et al. reported neurological improvement in 73% and 67% of the myelopathic patients, 3 months and 2 years after surgery, respectively [11]. Likewise, Nannapaneni et al. [9] reported a 56% ambulatory rate after surgery in non-ambulatory patients. They also emphasized on the better outcomes obtained with long segment fusion of the cervical spine than with short segment ones. Tanouchi et al. [12] analyzed these patients and found that patients who could at least sit (IIIBa) fared better than those who were bedridden (IIIBb). The extent of improvement after surgery is variable and the majority of the patients improve to grades IIIa and II. Even a one grade improvement in these patients may enable them to ambulate, a point that is strongly propagated by the papers that have focused on the surgical outcome in Ranawat IIIb patients. While surgery may only provide marginal benefit in the advanced stages of the disease, it can still translate in to a substantially better quality of life. On the other hand, non-operative treatment uniformly leads to severe disability and death. Thus, the consensus at present is that all patients suffering from advanced rheumatoid cervical myelopathy must be considered for surgery.

Preoperative radiological extent of the disease remains an important factor affecting the outcome after surgery. A combination of pathologies like AAS, CS, and SAS responds poorly to surgery than AAS alone [3, 6, 12, 14, 29, 43]. Miyamoto et al. noted that reducible AAS had a significantly higher improvement in functional status than the other pathological manifestations and this improvement persisted beyond 10 years of surgery [29]. Reduced PADI is also reported to affect postoperative outcome adversely. In one study, PADI less than 10 mm was associated with a poor outcome compared to patients with values more than 10 mm [24, 29, 43]. Presence of subaxial subluxation, either alone or in combination, is an added reason for a poorer surgical outcome. Mid cervical spinal canal diameter less than 14 mm indicates a poor postoperative outcome. Unrecognized SAS remains a major cause of disease progression and pseudoarthrosis which impair the quality of the life of these patients [29, 43].

As noted above, postoperative complications may mar the results of an otherwise successful surgery [9, 29, 43]. Progression of RA after surgery has been noted by many authors to lead to a worsening of neurological status after an initial improvement following surgery [9, 29]. Nannapaneni et al. [9] brought attention to this particular aspect of the disease. Miyamoto et al. [29] also noted disease progression after surgery in their series. Deterioration of RA was seen in 36.8% and 25.6% of cases of irreducible AAS and SAS, respectively, in their series.

35.9 Conclusions

Involvement of the cervical spine in RA is relatively more common than previously assumed and increases the disease-related morbidity and mortality manifolds. Once involved, the inflammatory process leads to progressive joint damage and subluxation causing severe neurological manifestations. A combination of plain radiograph, CT scan, and MRI of the cervical spine is needed to comprehensively evaluate the extent of the disease and make surgical treatment decisions. Knowledge regarding the specific nuances involved in the interpretation of the radiological investigations is warranted. There is a large body of evidence today to suggest that surgical fusion of the spine not only halts the disease progression but also improves the quality of life of these patients. There has been a major change in the philosophy of the surgical management of rheumatoid cervical myelopathy over the last few decades. It is very important to address all the existing pathological instabilities during the first surgery itself to avoid disease progression. When performed timely, surgery can provide gratifying results. The extent of the systemic disease and the preoperative Ranawat's grade are probably the most important factors determining the surgical outcome. Currently, the role of prophylactic spinal fusion in asymptomatic rheumatoid cervical spine disease is not clear.

References

1. Nguyen HV, Ludwig SC, Silber J, Gelb DE, Anderson PA, Frank L. Rheumatoid arthritis of the cervical spine. Spine J. 2004;4:329–34.
2. Krauss WE, Bledsoe JM, Clarke MJ, Nottmeier EW, Pichelmann MA. Rheumatoid arthritis of the craniovertebral junction. Neurosurgery. 2010;66:83–95.
3. Wasserman BR, Moskovich R, Razi AE. Rheumatoid arthritis of the cervical spine—clinical considerations. Bull NYU Hosp Jt Dis. 2011;69:136–48.
4. Delamarter RB, Bohlman HH. Postmortem osseous and neuropathologic analysis of the rheumatoid cervical spine. Spine (Phila Pa 1976). 1994;19:2267–74.
5. Oda T, Fujiwara K, Yonenobu K, Azuma B, Ochi T. Natural course of cervical spine lesions in rheumatoid arthritis. Spine (Phila Pa 1976). 1995;20:1128–35.
6. Mallory GW, Halasz SR, Clarke MJ. Advances in the treatment of cervical rheumatoid: less surgery and less morbidity. World J Orthop. 2014;5:292–303.
7. Joaquim AF, Appenzeller S. Cervical spine involvement in rheumatoid arthritis—a systematic review. Autoimmun Rev. 2014;13:1195–202.
8. Bhatia R, Haliasos N, Vergara P, Anderson C, Casey A. The surgical management of the rheumatoid spine: has the evolution of surgical intervention changed outcomes? J Craniovertebr Junct Spine. 2014;5:38–43.
9. Nannapaneni R, Behari S, Todd NV. Surgical outcome in rheumatoid Ranawat class IIIb myelopathy. Neurosurgery. 2005;56:706–15.
10. Casey AT, Crockard HA, Bland JM, Stevens J, Moskovich R, Ransford A. Predictors of outcome in the quadriparetic nonambulatory myelopathic patient with rheumatoid arthritis: a prospective study of 55 surgically treated Ranawat class IIIb patients. J Neurosurg. 1996;85:574–81.
11. van Asselt KM, Lems WF, Bongartz EB, Hamburger HL, Drossaers-Bakker KW, Dijkmans BA. Outcome of cervical spine surgery in patients with rheumatoid arthritis. Ann Rheum Dis. 2001;60:448–52.
12. Tanouchi T, Shimizu T, Fueki K, Ino M, Toda N, Tatara Y, et al. Neurological improvement and prognosis after occipito-thoracic fusion in patients with mutilating-type rheumatoid arthritis. Eur Spine J. 2012;21:2506–11.
13. da Côrte FC, Neves N. Cervical spine instability in rheumatoid arthritis. Eur J Orthop Surg Traumatol. 2014;24:S83–91.
14. Wolfs JF, Kloppenburg M, Fehlings MG, et al. Neurologic outcome of surgical and conservative treatment of rheumatoid cervical spine subluxation: a systematic review. Arthritis Rheum. 2009;61:1743–52.
15. Linos A, Worthington JW, O'Fallon WM, Kurland LT. The epidemiology of rheumatoid arthritis in Rochester, Minnesota: a study of incidence, prevalence, and mortality. Am J Epidemiol. 1980;111:87–98.
16. Dreyer SJ, Boden SD. Natural history of rheumatoid arthritis of the cervical spine. Clin Orthop. 1999;366:98–106.
17. Neva MH, Isomäki P, Hannonen P, Kauppi M, Krishnan E, Sokka T. Early and extensive erosiveness in peripheral joints predicts atlantoaxial subluxations in patients with rheumatoid arthritis. Arthritis Rheum. 2003;48:1808–13.

18. Yurube T, Sumi M, Nishida K, Miyamoto H, Kohyama K, Matsubara T, et al. Incidence and aggravation of cervical spine instabilities in rheumatoid arthritis: a prospective minimum 5-year follow-up study of patients initially without cervical involvement. Spine (Phila Pa 1976). 2012;37:2136–44.
19. Shen FH, Samartzis D, Jenis LG, An HS. Rheumatoid arthritis: evaluation and surgical management of the cervical spine. Spine J. 2004;4:689–700.
20. Pellicci PM, Ranawat CS, Tsairis P, Bryan WJ. A prospective study of the progression of rheumatoid arthritis of the cervical spine. J Bone Joint Surg Am. 1981;63:342–50.
21. Fujiwara K, Owaki H, Fujimoto M, Yonenobu K, Ochi T. A long-term follow-up study of cervical lesions in rheumatoid arthritis. J Spinal Disord. 2000;13:519–26.
22. Yurube T, Sumi M, Nishida K, Takabatake M, Kohyama K, Matsubara T, et al. Progression of cervical spine instabilities in rheumatoid arthritis: a prospective cohort study of outpatients over 5 years. Spine (Phila Pa 1976). 2011;36:647–53.
23. Terashima Y, Yurube T, Hirata H, Sugiyama D, Sumi M. Predictive risk factors of cervical spine instabilities in rheumatoid arthritis: a prospective multicenter over 10-year cohort study. Spine (Phila Pa 1976). 2017;42(8):556–64.
24. Wollowick AL, Casden AM, Kuflik PL, Neuwirth MJ. Rheumatoid arthritis in the cervical spine: what you need to know. Am J Orthop (Belle Mead NJ). 2007;36:400–6.
25. Boden SD, Dodge LD, Bohlman HH, Rechtine GR. Rheumatoid arthritis of the cervical spine: a long-term analysis with predictors of paralysis and recovery. Bone Joint Surg Am. 1993;75:1282–97.
26. Imagama S, Oishi Y, Miura Y, Kanayama Y, Ito Z, Wakao N, et al. Predictors of aggravation of cervical spine instability in rheumatoid arthritis patients: the large joint index. J Orthop Sci. 2010;15:540–6.
27. Yonezawa I, Okuda T, Won J, Sakoda J, Nakahara D, Nojiri H, et al. Retrodental mass in rheumatoid arthritis. J Spinal Disord Tech. 2013;26:E65–9.
28. Dohzono S, Suzuki A, Koike T, Takahashi S, Yamada K, Yasuda H, et al. Factors associated with retro-odontoid soft-tissue thickness in rheumatoid arthritis. J Neurosurg Spine. 2016;25:580–5.
29. Miyamoto H, Sumi M, Uno K. Outcome of surgery for rheumatoid cervical spine at one institute over three decades. Spine J. 2013;13:1477–84.
30. Grob D, Würsch R, Grauer W, Sturzenegger J, Dvorak J. Atlantoaxial fusion and retrodental pannus in rheumatoid arthritis. Spine (Phila Pa 1976). 1997;22:1580–3.
31. Lipson SJ. Cervical myelopathy and posterior atlanto-axial subluxation in patients with rheumatoid arthritis. J Bone Joint Surg Am. 1985;67:593–7.
32. Neo M. Treatment of upper cervical spine involvement in rheumatoid arthritis patients. Mod Rheumatol. 2008;18:327–35.
33. Casey AT, Crockard HA, Geddes JF, Stevens J. Vertical translocation: the enigma of the disappearing atlantodens interval in patients with myelopathy andrheumatoid arthritis. Part I. clinical, radiological, and neuropathological features. J Neurosurg. 1997;87:856–62.
34. Casey AT, Crockard HA, Geddes JF, Stevens J. Vertical translocation: the enigma of the disappearing atlantodens interval in patients with myelopathy and rheumatoid arthritis. Part I. clinical, radiological, and neuropathological features. J Neurosurg. 1997;87:856–62.
35. Bywaters EG. Rheumatoid and other diseases of the cervical interspinous bursae, and changes in the spinous processes. Ann Rheum Dis. 1982;41:360–70.
36. Kraus DR, Peppelman WC, Agarwal AK, DeLeeuw HW, Donaldson WF 3rd. Incidence of subaxial subluxation in patients with generalized rheumatoid arthritis who have had previous occipital cervical fusions. Spine (Phila Pa 1976). 1991;16:S486–9.
37. Zygmunt SC, Ljunggren B, Alund M, Brattström H, Säveland HG, Holtås S, et al. Realignment and surgical fixation of atlanto-axial and subaxial dislocations in rheumatoid arthritis (RA) patients. Acta Neurochir Suppl (Wien). 1988;43:79–84.
38. Inada T, Furuya T, Kamiya K, Ota M, Maki S, Suzuki T, et al. Postoperative increase in occiput-C2 angle negatively impacts subaxial lordosis after Occipito-upper cervical posterior fusion surgery. Asian Spine J. 2016;10:744–7.

39. Oshima K, Sakaura H, Iwasaki M, Nakura A, Fujii R, Yoshikawa H. Repeated vertebrobasilar thromboembolism in a patient with severe upper cervical instability because of rheumatoid arthritis. Spine J. 2011;11:e1–5.
40. Ranawat CS, O'Leary P, Pellicci P, Tsairis P, Marchisello P, Dorr L. Cervical spine fusion in rheumatoid arthritis. J Bone Joint Surg Am. 1979;61:1003–10.
41. Söderman T, Olerud C, Shalabi A, Alavi K, Sundin A. Static and dynamic CT imaging of the cervical spine in patients with rheumatoid arthritis. Skeletal Radiol. 2015;44:241–8.
42. Riew KD, Hilibrand AS, Palumbo MA, Sethi N, Bohlman HH. Diagnosing basilar invagination in the rheumatoid patient. The reliability of radiographic criteria. J Bone Joint Surg Am. 2001;83:194–200.
43. Gillick JL, Wainwright J, Das K. Rheumatoid arthritis and the cervical spine: a review on the role of surgery. Int J Rheumatol. 2015;2015:252456.
44. Iizuka H, Iizuka Y, Kobayashi R, Nishinome M, Sorimachi Y, Takagishi K. The relationship between an intramedullary high signal intensity and the clinical outcome in atlanto-axial subluxation owing to rheumatoid arthritis. Spine J. 2014;14:938–43.
45. Bundschuh C, Modic MT, Kearney F, Morris R, Deal C. Rheumatoid arthritis of the cervical spine: surface-coil MR imaging. Am J Roentgenol. 1988;151:181–7.
46. Casey AT, Crockard HA, Bland JM, Stevens J, Moskovich R, Ransford AO. Surgery on the rheumatoid cervical spine for the non-ambulant myelopathic patient—too much, too late? Lancet. 1996;347:1004–7.
47. Crockard HA, Calder I, Ransford AO. One-stage transoral decompression and posterior fixation in rheumatoid atlanto-axial subluxation. J Bone Joint Surg Br. 1990;72:682–5.
48. Ponce-Gómez JA, Ortega-Porcayo LA, Soriano-Barón HE, Sotomayor-González A, Arriada-Mendicoa N, Gómez-Amador JL, et al. Evolution from microscopic transoral to endoscopic endonasal odontoidectomy. Neurosurg Focus. 2014;37:E15.
49. Goel A, Sharma P. Craniovertebral realignment for basilar invagination and atlantoaxial dislocation secondary to rheumatoid arthritis. Neurol India. 2004;52:338–41.

Index

E. Tessitore et al. (eds.), *Surgery of the Cranio-Vertebral Junction*,
https://doi.org/10.1007/978-3-030-18700-2

W

MIX
Papier aus verantwortungsvollen Quellen
Paper from responsible sources
FSC® C105338

If you have any concerns about our products,
you can contact us on
ProductSafety@springernature.com

In case Publisher is established outside the EU,
the EU authorized representative is:
Springer Nature Customer Service Center GmbH
Europaplatz 3, 69115 Heidelberg, Germany

Printed by Libri Plureos GmbH
in Hamburg, Germany